Triage Nursing SECRETS

Triage Nursing SECRETS

POLLY GERBER ZIMMERMANN, RN, MS, MBA, CEN
Assistant Professor
Department of Nursing
Harry S Truman College
Chicago, Illinois

ROBERT D. HERR, MD, MBA, FACEP
Medical Director
PacifiCare of Washington
Attending Emergency Physician
Northwest Emergency Physicians/Team Health
St. Joseph Hospital
Tacoma, Washington

SERIES EDITOR
LINDA SCHEETZ, EDD, APRN, BC, CEN
Assistant Professor
College of Nursing
Rutgers, The State University of New Jersey
Rutgers, New Jersey

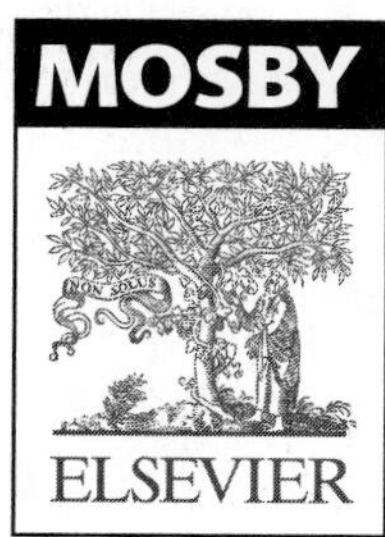

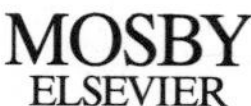

11830 Westline Industrial Drive
St. Louis, Missouri 63146

TRIAGE NURSING SECRETS

ISBN-13 978-0-323-03122-6
ISBN-10 0-323-03122-6

Notice

Knowledge and best practice in this field are constantly changing. As new research and experience broaden our knowledge, changes in practice, treatment, and drug therapy may become necessary or appropriate. Readers are advised to check the most current information provided (i) on procedures featured or (ii) by the manufacturer of each product to be administered, to verify the recommended dose or formula, the method and duration of administration, and contraindications. It is the responsibility of the practitioner, relying on their own experience and knowledge of the patient, to make diagnoses, to determine dosages and the best treatment for each individual patient, and to take all appropriate safety precautions. To the fullest extent of the law, neither the Publisher nor the Editors/Authors assumes any liability for any injury and/or damage to persons or property arising out of or related to any use of the material contained in this book.

ISBN-10 0-323-03122-6
ISBN-13 978-0-323-03122-6

Acquisitions Editor: Sandra Clark Brown
Developmental Editor: Cindi Anderson
Publishing Services Manager: Deborah L. Vogel
Senior Project Manager: Ann E. Rogers
Senior Design Project Manager: Bill Drone
Marketing Manager: Tricia Schroeder

Printed in United States of America

Last digit is the print number: 9 8 7 6 5 4 3 2

To my nephew and nieces
The children of my sister and brother-in-law Kelly and Mark Gerboth:
Benjamin Mark
Robin Renee
Deborah Kelly
You light up my life!

and

To my husband Rudi
Thanks for always being my beacon of support.

Polly Gerber Zimmermann

To my Belinda, the Woman of my Dreams
To Tyler, the Apple of my Eye
To Kathryn, the Light of my Life
To Benjamin, the Star of my Stage
Thanks for Choosing Me with my Cat Allergy
Over the Cat, Who is Cuter, Cuddlier, and Wiser.

Bob Herr

Contributors

Bernard "Bo" Ball, RN
Educator
TriageFirst, Incorporated
Fairview, North Carolina
69. Violence and Security Issues

Susan Bednar, RN, NP
Nurse Practitioner
Emergency Services
Evanston Northwestern Healthcare
Glenbrook Hospital
Evanston, Illinois
54. Toxicologic Emergencies

Lt. Kevin Richard Brooks
Anti-Terrorism/Hazardous Materials Training Lieutenant
Training Division
Broward Sheriff's Office
Department of Fire Rescue and Emergency Services
Fort Lauderdale, Florida
62. Weapons of Mass Destruction/Mass Casualty Incident

Patricia M. Campbell, RN, MSN, CCRN, ANP, CS
Emergency Nurse Practitioner
Emergency Professional Services, Incorporated
Banner Good Samaritan Medical Center
Phoenix, Arizona
28. Cough

Jill Cash, RN, NP
Nurse Practitioner
Southern Illinois OB-Gyn Associates
Carbondale, Illinois
56. Domestic Violence

SHARON SAUNDERSON COHEN, RN, MSN, CEN, CCRN
Clinical Nurse Specialist
Department of Emergency Preparedness/Weapons of Mass Destruction
North Broward Hospital District
Fort Lauderdale, Florida
15. Cultural Competencies in Triage
62. Weapons of Mass Destruction/Mass Casualty Incident
66. Prehospital/Emergency Medical Services Triage

SHELLEY COHEN, RN, BS, CEN
Educator/Consultant
Health Resources Unlimited
Hohenwald, Tennessee
58. Child Abuse
59. Elder Abuse

STEPHEN M. COHEN, MPAS, PA-C
Associate Professor
School of Graduate Medical Science
Barry University
Miami, Florida
15. Cultural Competencies in Triage

DARCY EGGING, MS, RN, CNP, CEN
Nurse Practitioner
Department of Emergency Services
Valley Emergency Care Incorporated at Delnor Community Hospital
Geneva, Illinois
32. Upper Abdominal Presentations

NINA M. FIELDEN, MSN, RN, CEN
Clinical Nurse Specialist, Forensic Nurse Specialist
Department of Emergency Services
The Cleveland Clinic Foundation
Cleveland, Ohio
53. Depression and Suicide
69. Violence and Security Issues

JAN FRUSTAGLIA, RN, BS, CCM, COHN-S
Program Coordinator
Health Professions Institute
Austin Community College
Independent Consultant
OccHealth Concerns
Austin, Texas
68. Occupational Health Considerations

MARY E. FECHT GRAMLEY, PHD, RN, CEN
Clinical Instructor
School of Nursing
Waubonsee Community College
Sugar Grove, Illinois;
Staff Nurse
Emergency Department
Delnor Community Hospital
Geneva, Illinois
44. Amputations
19. Headache
40. Lacerations and Puncture Wounds
67. Trauma Systems and Triage

VALERIE G. A. GROSSMAN, RN, BSN, CEN
Senior Nurse Counselor
Via Health Call Center
Via Health
Rochester, New York
65. Telephone Triage

JIN H. HAN, MD
Assistant Professor
Vanderbilt University Medical Center
Nashville, Tennessee
27. Chest Pain

BERNARD HEILICSER, DO, MS, FACEP
Medical Director, South Cook County EMS System
Director of Medical Ethics Program
Ingalls Memorial Hospital
Harvey, Illinois
72. Ethics in Triage: One Ethicist Speaks

ROBERT D. HERR, MD, MBA, FACEP
Medical Director
PacifiCare of Washington
Attending Emergency Physician
Northwest Emergency Physicians/Team Health
St. Joseph Hospital
Tacoma, Washington
14. Gender-Related Considerations
20. Closed Head Injury
21. Dental Pain/Tooth Avulsion
22. Ear Pain
23. Stiff or Sore Neck
24. Sore Throat
41. Foreign Bodies

45. Minor Motor Vehicle Crashes
46. Falls in the Older Adult Population
47. Dizziness, Vertigo, and Weakness
48. Syncope
49. Bites and Stings

SUSAN M. HOHENHAUS, RN, BS
Editor, PEMSoft Pty, Ltd;
Project Manager, Enhancing Pediatric Patient Safety
Patient Safety Center
Duke University Medical Center
Durham, North Carolina
12. Using a Color-Coded System to Estimate Weight at Triage
57. Bullying

DONA MARTIN LAING, RN, MSN, CEN, CNOR
Clinical Nurse Specialist
Department of Perioperative Services
MetroHealth Medical Center
Cleveland, Ohio
43. Burns

LINDA LEDRAY, PHD, RN, SANE-A, FAAN
Director
Sexual Assault Resource Service
Hennepin County Medical Center
Minneapolis, Minnesota
60. Sexual Assault

JERROLD BLAIR LEIKIN, MD
Professor of Medicine
Feinberg School of Medicine
Northwestern University
Pharmacology and Health Systems Management
Rush Medical College
Chicago, Illinois;
Director of Medical Toxicology
Evanston Northwestern Healthcare-OMEGA
Glenbrook Hospital
Evanston, Illinois
54. Toxicologic Emergencies

GAIL LENEHAN, RN, EDD, FAAN
Psychiatric Clinical Nurse Specialist
Emergency Department
Massachusetts General Hospital
Boston, Massachusetts
52. Triage of the Psychiatric Patient

Janet Marsden, MSc, BSc
Senior Lecturer
Postgraduate Programme Director
Department of Health Care Studies
Manchester Metropolitan University
Manchester, England
80. Manchester Triage Scale

Rebecca S. McNair, RN, CEN
President, Triage First, Inc.
Fairview, North Carolina
1. Triage Essence and Process
2. Triage Systems and Acuities
10. Documentation Issues
16. Heavy Users
69. Violence and Security Issues
78. ENA/ACEP Five-Level Triage Work Group
83. Process of Changing an Emergency Department from a Three-Level to a Five-Level System

Marylou S. Moeller, RN, BSN, CEN
Trauma Coordinator and Staff Nurse
New Hanover Regional Medical Center
Wilmington, North Carolina
29. Nausea and Vomiting

Toni G. McCallum Pardey, NP, RN, Gen Cert, A&E Cert, MNurs(NursPrac)
Clinical Nurse Specialist
Emergency Department
ED Wyong Hospital
Central Coast, New South Wales, Australia
81. Australian Triage Scale: A Five-Tier Triage Emergency Scale

Susanne A. Quallich, APRN, BC, NP-C, CUNP
Andrology Nurse Practitioner
Division of Andrology and Microsurgery
Michigan Urology Center
University of Michigan Health System
Ann Arbor, Michigan
35. Male Genital Pain
37. Dysuria

Karen L. Rice, MSN, APRN, BC
Adult Nurse Practitioner/Clinical Specialist, Acute Care Geriatrics
Department of Nursing
Ochsner Clinic Foundation
New Orleans, Louisiana
55. Differentiating Dementia from Delirium

Carol J. Schwartz, RN, SANE-A
Sexual Assault Resource Service
Hennepin County Medical Center
Minneapolis, Minnesota
60. Sexual Assault

Maureen S. Smith, MD
Emergency Department
Good Samaritan Hospital
Puyallup, Washington
26. Shortness of Breath

Audrey Snyder, RN, MSN, ACNP-BC, CEN
Advanced Practice Nurse-1
Clinical Nurse Specialist/Nurse Practitioner
Emergency Department
University of Virginia Health Sciences Center
Charlottesville, Virginia
77. PDA Use

Joan Somes, RN, MSN, PhD, NREMT-P, FAEN
Staff Nurse/Department Educator
Emergency Department
St. Joseph's Hospital
St. Paul, Minnesota
17. Rashes
33. Lower Abdominal Pain

Robert W. Stein, III, BSN, MSHA, RN, CEN, CHE
Director, Emergency Department
Health Central
Ocoee, Florida
39. Extremity Trauma

Rebecca A. Steinmann, RN, MS, CEN, CCRN, CCNS
Clinical Educator
Emergency Department
Children's Memorial Hospital
Chicago, Illinois
25. Vision Changes

Jared Strote, MD, MS
Clinical Instructor
Division of Emergency Medicine
University of Washington Medical Center
Seattle, Washington
42. Piercings (Voluntary)

Vicki Sweet, RN, MS, CEN, CCRN
Manager, Emergency Services
St. Jude Medical Center
Fullerton, California
18. Fever
51. Environmental Thermo-Emergencies

Barbara A. Weintraub, RN, MSN, MPH, PCCNP, CEN
Coordinator, Pediatric Emergency Services
Pediatric Emergency Department
Northwest Community Hospital
Arlington Heights, Illinois
50. Near-Drowning

Michael L. Wilkerson, EMT-P
Flight Paramedic/Firefighter
Department of Fire Rescue and Emergency Services
Broward Sheriff's Office
Fort Lauderdale, Florida
66. Prehospital/Emergency Medical Services Triage

Abigail R. Williams, RN, JD, MPH
President, Abigail Williams & Associates, PC
Worcester, Massachusetts
63. Health Insurance Portability and Accountability Act (HIPAA)

Darleen A. Williams, RN, MSN, CEN
Clinical Nurse Specialist for Emergency Services
Department of Education and Development
Orlando Regional Medical Center
Orlando, Florida
34. Gynecologic-Related Abdominal Pain
36. Pregnancy Considerations

Joseph E. Williams, MSN, ANP/ACNP-C
Acute Care Nurse Practitioner
Medicine Hospitalist Service
Ochsner Clinic Foundation
New Orleans, Louisiana
55. Differentiating Dementia from Delirium

Mary Ellen Wilson, RN, MS, CEN, FNP
Nurse Manager, Emergency Department
Cherry Point Naval Hospital
PhyAmerica Government Services
Havelock, North Carolina
29. Nausea and Vomiting

Jill Windle, RGN, MSc, BA
Lecturer Practitioner in Emergency Nursing
Department of Emergency Medicine
Salford Royal Hospitals (NHS) Trust/Salford University
Manchester, England
80. Manchester Triage Scale

Polly Gerber Zimmermann, RN, MS, MBA, CEN
Assistant Professor
Department of Nursing
Harry S Truman College
Chicago, Illinois
1. Triage Essence and Process
2. Triage Systems and Acuities
3. History Secrets
4. Physical Assessment
5. Vital Signs
6. Pain Assessment and Management
7. Triage Diagnostics
8. Protocol Samples
9. Decision-Making and Prioritization Principles
10. Documentation Issues
11. Pediatrics
13. Geriatric Considerations
17. Rashes
18. Fever
19. Headache
30. Diarrhea and Dehydration
31. Acute Abdomen and Peritonitis
33. Lower Abdominal Pain
34. Gynecologic-Related Abdominal Pain
38. Low Back Pain
40. Lacerations and Puncture Wounds
61. Alcohol Use and Abuse
64. Fast Track
65. Telephone Triage
70. Waiting Room Management
71. Language and Interpretation Issues
73. Customer Service/Patient Satisfaction
74. Personnel Qualifications
75. Education and Training for Triage Nurses
76. Taking Care of Yourself and Your Staff
79. The Emergency Severity Index Triage Scale
82. Canada Triage and Acuity Scale

Reviewers

KATHRYN C. ANDERSON, RN, BCEN, BA, ACLS
Nurse Manager
Vernon Urgent Care
Vernon, New Jersey

MELISA BAILEY, RN, LNC
Legal Nurse Consultant
Bailey Consultants
Houston, Texas

SANDRA K. BRANNON, MSN, RN
Assistant Professor
Department of Nursing
Lamar University
Beaumont, Texas

TERESA COCHRAN, RN, TNS, ENPC, ACLS
RN Emergency Department Coordinator
CGH Medical Center
Sterling, Illinois

NIKKI F. COOK, BSN, ACLS, PALS, TNCC
Staff Nurse
Medcenter One Health Systems
Bismarck, North Dakota

KAREN CROUSE, EdD, FNP(BC) CEN
Assistant Professor
Department of Nursing
Western Connecticut State University
Danbury, Connecticut

Eugenia E. Giguere, RN, BSN, CEN
Staff Nurse
O'Connor Hospital
San Jose, California

Patricia Gillett, MSN, C-FNP, C-ACNP
Faculty
College of Nursing
University of New Mexico
Albuquerque, New Mexico

Thomas H. Hodges, RN, BSN
Charge Nurse
Emergency Department
St. Claire Hospital
Clinical Instructor
Clover Park Technical College
Lakewood, Washington

Christopher D. Jenkins, RN, EMT-P
Independent Duty Medic
Cascade, Idaho

Michelle J. Klosterman, RN, CEN
Emergency Department Manager
Adams County Hospital
West Union, Ohio

Ronald Napier, LVN
EliteCare Staffing
Fresno, California

Jessica Ann Trivett, RN, BSN, PCCN
Travel Nurse
Medical Express
Westminster, Colorado

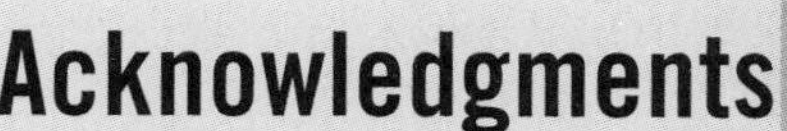

Acknowledgments

If it takes a village to raise a child, it must take an entire country to publish a secrets book. This book would not have been possible except for the many individuals who shared their hard-earned wisdom from the school of lived professional experience. Through their generosity, often in the context of the Managers Forum column in the *Journal of Emergency Nursing* and the Emergency Nursing Association's listservs, we all are enriched toward achieving the desired result of excellent patient care.

I am grateful to Bob Herr for being willing to do this "nursing" project. He is one of the best ED physicians I've ever been privileged to work with and has always regarded nurses as his colleagues.

I thank my husband, Rudi, for his endless support and belief in me and his willingness to put up with spousal neglect. I thank my sister, Kelly, for her consistent enthusiastic encouragement. I appreciate Rebecca McNair, President of TriageFirst, Inc., for being willing to share so much of her copyrighted material, expertise, and time to do unofficial reviews for many chapters. I am grateful to Gail Pisarcik Lenehan, the *Journal of Emergency Nursing's* editor-in-chief, for her efforts and willingness to mentor my writing and editing skills through the many years.

I acknowledge the following at the Harry S Truman College for their support: Retired President Phoebe Helm, President Margarite Boyd, Deans Michael Schoops and Rahman Pervez, Past Department of Nursing Chairperson Patricia DeWitt Corbett, and my ever-helpful teaching colleague, Tom Worms.

And finally I am grateful to Linda Scheetz for conceiving the Nursing Secrets series and allowing triage to be a part of it; to Elsevier, particularly editor Sandra Brown for embracing the series and triage, and senior project manager Ann Rogers, and especially to senior developmental editor Cindi Anderson for her tireless assistance, patience, and organization. She must have felt as many labor pains as we editors did.

POLLY GERBER ZIMMERMANN, RN, MS, MBA, CEN

I'd like to thank my many teachers in emergency triage, including the nurses at:

1976-1980:
St. Raphael's Hospital, New Haven, Connecticut
1980-1984:
Sudan Interior Mission/ELWA Hospital, Monrovia, Liberia
Washington University Medical Center, St. Louis, Missouri
1984-1988:
Northwestern Memorial Hospital, Chicago, Illinois
Columbus Hospital, Chicago, Illinois
Evanston Hospital, Evanston, Illinois
Glenbrook Hospital, Glenview, Illinois
Sherman Hospital, Elgin, Illinois
Crystal Lake Ambutal, Crystal Lake, Illinois
1988-1998:
University of Utah Hospital, Salt Lake City, Utah
FHP Utah Hospital, Salt Lake City, Utah
St. Mark's Hospital, Salt Lake City, Utah
Pioneer Valley Hospital, West Valley City, Utah
Lake Hospital, Yellowstone, Wyoming
Blackfeet Memorial Hospital, Browning, Montana
1998-1999:
University of Arkansas for Medical Sciences, Little Rock, Arkansas
1999-present:
Group Health Eastside Hospital, Redmond, Washington
Group Health Central Hospital, Seattle, Washington
Virginia Mason Hospital, Seattle, Washington
St. Joseph Medical Center, Tacoma, Washington
SS Universe Explorer Medical Clinic Nursing Staff, Nene Benavidez, and Medical Director Jack Putnam, MD

And most of all that 1972 volunteer coordinator at New Britain General Hospital (Connecticut) who redirected me from joining my friends in the Mercury Messenger Service to Central Sterile, where I got to wash bedpans and learn what hospital care is really about!

I have learned far more from you than I could ever teach,
—But in your honor I gave it a try!

BOB HERR, MD, MBA, FACEP

Contents

TOP SECRETS

1. The most common specific emergency department (ED) diagnoses for abdominal pain are gastroenteritis and appendicitis.
2. About a third of patients older than age 65 years who are admitted for abdominal pain will need surgery.
3. Clues that the cause of a patient's abdominal pain may be surgical are pain preceding vomiting and severe pain that persists for 6 or more hours.
4. Mittelschmerz should not be a consideration if there is vaginal bleeding (rule out ectopic pregnancy), a history of taking birth control pills (because they prevent ovulation), or a general sick appearance.
5. The rule for the older adult is that the atypical is typical.
6. Ask personal questions by facing the patient directly, in their "personal space," and speaking in a low voice.
7. Improve customer service/patient satisfaction by repeating (mimicking) the chief complaint back in the same words. It makes people feel that they have been "heard."
8. Deal with complaints about the wait by talking to the feelings, using a broken record technique, and providing a blameless apology.
9. Tongue furrows are unaffected by mouth breathing or age. With fluid volume deficit, additional longitudinal furrows are noted.
10. An early sign of dehydration (and dementia) is the decreased ability to focus. Ask the patient to name as many fruits as possible within 1 minute: the patient should be able to name at least 15.
11. The best indication of the elderly person's recent fluid intake is recent food intake.
12. Do not use Jell-O mixed with water or sports drinks to rehydrate infants.
13. Unilateral extremity findings are significant.
14. Key clues to the need for an extremity x-ray are the inability to bear weight and pinpoint tenderness. Use the Ottawa Ankle Rules and the Pittsburgh Decision Rules for knees.
15. Check the palmar side of the hand for injury when there is swelling on the dorsal side.
16. Any conditions that cause ischemia to the genitals are urologic emergencies.
17. Studies show that maternal estimate of the presence of a fever determined by touching the child's skin is accurate 50% to 80% of the time.
18. Ibuprofen is the better choice for treating fever in children (in single dosing, if older than 6 months).
19. 91% of parents still have fears about serious consequences from a fever.
20. Pediatric bradycardia should be assumed to be hypoxia until that is ruled out.
21. Children who are longer than the Broselow Tape will probably need adult equipment.
22. It is better, from a psychological standpoint, to overestimate the time of any wait. Communicate frequently during that wait.

23. The ACEP/ENA Five-Level Triage Task Force recommendation is to adapt a five-level triage acuity system. CTAS and ESI are good options.
24. The Emergency Severity Index (ESI) triage scale is based on an algorithm of acuity and anticipated resource consumption. The Emergency Nurses Association (ENA) publishes ESI but has not officially endorsed one particular five-level triage system.
25. It is estimated that 7.9% of all ED visits are alcohol related.
26. Use the SBIRT (screen, brief intervention, referral treatment) approach to screen for alcohol abuse.
27. Never assume a patient is "just a drunk."
28. Benzodiazepines are used for alcohol withdrawal. Agitation in an elderly person without alcohol abuse should not be treated with benzodiazepines because of the risk of a paradoxical reaction.
29. Muscular back pain (compared with pain from a disc) tends to be more gradual in onset, poorly localized, does not radiate below the knee, and does not exhibit spinal point tenderness.
30. Red flags for low back pain are evolving neurological deficits, direct trauma to the back, an inability to walk, cauda equina syndrome, or signs of infection, metastasis, or abdominal aortic aneurism.
31. Never automatically assume the caregiver of the older adult patient is acting in the patient's best interest. The most common perpetrator of elder abuse is a family member.
32. Prioritization considerations include acute before chronic, sudden onset before gradual onset, ruling out the worst-case scenario, life before limb, potential for worsening, and trends.
33. Patient-specific conditions to consider for increased prioritization are immunosuppression, very young or very old age, recent discharge from the hospital and/or medication change, and multiple comorbidities.
34. Obtain the 5T history pertinent for near-drowning.
35. The Canadian Triage and Acuity Scale (CTAS) is based on sentinel events and the usual presentation, providing objective data to help validate and assess the condition when establishing a triage level.
36. The ENA standard indicates that safe, effective, and efficient triage can be performed only by a registered professional nurse who is educated in the principles of triage.
37. Accomplish triage with impartiality, without being influenced by the patient's religion, level of attractiveness, wealth, or social habits.
38. Ask the patient with a respiratory complaint to rate the effort of breathing on a scale of 1 to 10 (Borg scale).
39. Perform a quick check for adequate oxygenation and perfusion with 30-2-CAN DO.
40. Orthostatics are not reliable as a sole indicator of dehydration and tend to be less accurate in the older adult.

41. The hop test/heel jar test is sensitive for peritoneal/lower abdominal pathology.
42. Have the patient cough, instead of using palpation, to test for rebound tenderness if the patient is in severe discomfort.
43. All heavy (repeat) ED users need a thorough and unbiased assessment every time.
44. Consider the patient's culture's differences in personal space, voice tone and volume, eye contact, gestures, primary caretaker, and perspective of time.
45. Rapidly assess for the possibility of a stroke by checking for palmar drift and by asking the patient to show you his or her teeth and say "Can't teach an old dog new tricks."
46. Call a rape victim advocate/sexual assault nurse examiner (SANE) automatically when a victim arrives.
47. Some victims do not initially label the sexual assault as a "rape." Ask, "Did anyone touch you sexually in a way that was against your will or that hurt you?"
48. Never write "alleged rape" as a chief complaint. Use "sexual assault" or "sexual assault examination."
49. A patient's identity is not protected health information (PHI) under Health Insurance Portability and Accountability Act (HIPAA). Sign-in sheets and flow boards can be used if the chief complaint/diagnosis is not identified with the patient's name.
50. Patients taking more than six different drugs per day are at a high risk for an adverse drug reaction. The average elderly person is taking four prescription drugs and two over-the-counter (OTC) medications.
51. It is estimated that 25% to 30% of women who seek care in the ED are victims of domestic violence. Use the mnemonic SAFE to screen for domestic violence and GUNS and FISTS to screen for the risk of violence in their life.
52. Acknowledge your observation that the patient's or family members' emotions are escalating. Do not quote authoritative rules, and attempt to make a verbal contract.
53. When a person is escalating to agitation or aggression, stand an arm's length away, at an angle with your arms at the side, and allow clear access to an exit.
54. Regardless of the triage system used, always err on the side of caution. Assume the patient is sick until proven otherwise.
55. Use a finger span scale (spreading the forefinger and thumb apart to indicate the degree of pain) with young, verbal children.
56. With a psychiatric patient triage, ask specific questions, such as "What did you hope that we could do for you here today?" rather than a vague "What's wrong?"
57. Be alert to the "Yes, but never this bad" syndrome from a family.
58. Rashes that are emergent are highly contagious, have coexisting systemic instability, new-onset petechia or purpura, or skin sloughing.
59. The ENA position is that no telephone advice is given unless a telephone triage program is in place or a life-threatening emergency is occurring.
60. Patients with visual changes should always have a visual acuity test done unless a chemical burn is suspected.

61. Use the acronym TRACEM for potential harm from or exposure to weapons of mass destruction.
62. For a burn patient, stop the burning process first. Remove all clothing and jewelry.
63. Flame events in closed spaces cause inhalation injury.
64. The palm of the patient's extended hand is equal to 1% of body surface area for that patient.
65. Chart the objective and subjective assessment of the patient's chief complaint. Do not be lulled into a premature conclusion or medical diagnosis.
66. Control bleeding and pain from a mouth laceration by having the patient suck on an ice cube.
67. Do not automatically obtain an initial routine urine specimen in triage from a man with urinary symptoms or urethral discharge (unless there has been recent instrumentation).
68. Rarely are positive home pregnancy tests falsely positive, but negative tests often are falsely negative.
69. Any suicidal act or threat must be taken seriously. Remove personal clothing and belongings and place the person in a safe environment.
70. Screening for depression can be accomplished by using the mnemonic SIG E CAPS or asking two questions. They are, "During the past month, have you often been bothered by feeling down, depressed, or hopeless?" and "During the past month, have you often been bothered by little interest or pleasure in doing things?"
71. Pediatric trauma patients are more prone than adults to have multiple injuries, hypothermia, airway obstruction, and internal injuries without overlying fractures.
72. The common saying is that 90% of what you need to know to make a diagnosis is in the history. Get a thorough one.
73. Ask about the use of botanical dietary supplements and herbs. Although 68% of middle-age women in one study used them, only 30% told their clinician.
74. Do not let the patient with abdominal pain eat or drink while waiting for care because all abdominal pain carries the potential for surgery.
75. Consider that pain in the upper abdomen in the older adult patient may be an atypical cardiac presentation.
76. Most mistriage occurs because of lack of education, inexperience, and empathy burnout.
77. One of the most frequent causes of acute mental status changes in the older adult is a urinary tract infection (UTI).
78. Approximately 30% of children in grades 6 through 10 are involved in bullying. Screen for it by asking "Has anyone at school made you sad or afraid?"
79. The headache that is the most concern is acute with a sudden, severe onset.
80. Use TACO to assess a patient with ruptured membranes.
81. Be concerned if a pregnant woman (more than 20 weeks' gestation) has urinary symptoms, low back pain, hypertension, vaginal bleeding, edema, or seizures.
82. Ask about fetal movement in any pregnancy after the 12th to 13th week.

Section I

Overview

Chapter 1

Triage Essence and Process

Polly Gerber Zimmermann and Rebecca S. McNair

1. What is triage?

The formal function of emergency department (ED) triage as the term is commonly used is the initial assessment and sorting by acuity for the immediate medical treatment needs in newly arriving patients. In disaster nursing, it is to maximize the number of survivors, or the greatest benefit for the largest number. A global sense of the concept involves the dynamic prioritization between multiple needs and continues throughout a patient's waiting and treatment. It is the constant who or what to do first.

2. What is the purpose of ED triage?

The purpose of ED triage is to get the right patient to the right place at the right time for the right reason. It is not diagnosing.

3. Describe the history of triage.

Triage comes from the French word *trier,* which means to sort or to choose. It started in the 1800s battlefield with the goal of determining who was salvageable. In the United States, it became more formalized in the late 1950s and 1960s as the ED volume increased beyond the resources for all incoming patients to have immediate care.

4. How have the goals of triage changed since the 1800s?

Today, beyond salvageability, triage seeks to decrease morbidity, disfigurement, and patient pain, while being a positive experience (and public relations) for the patients.

5. Is triage necessary?

Any time every presenting patient cannot receive immediate treatment; some level or form of triage must take place to prioritize between the various, competing needs. The process is working: while waiting times have increased overall, the wait for the *seriously* ill has decreased.

6. Are triage and assessment the same concept?

No. Assessment is a rapid, systematic collection of appropriate and necessary data about each patient. It is relevant to the patient's chief complaint, age, cognitive level, and social situation. Assessment is done in order to determine the appropriate care acuity level and immediate physical or psychosocial intervention. The conclusion of the nurse's interpretation of the assessment results in a triage decision.

7. Discuss EDs that advertise immediate placement of every patient into a treatment area.

The goal of this approach is avoid the triage process becoming a roadblock, such as the nurse obtaining a detailed history of a patient's chest pain while a treatment bed and staff are available. Regardless of where the person is placed, it is still essential to have a form of initial timely assessment to determine and prioritize needs. It is not effective or efficient to have someone sitting in a treatment area (even if the person is "happy") if no initial assessment of the current status is done for 30 minutes.

8. Who should do triage?

The Emergency Nurses Association (ENA) Standard (1999) indicates "safe, effective and efficient triage can be performed only by a registered professional nurse educated in the principles of triage with a minimum of 6 months' experience in emergency nursing." See the chapter on staff qualifications for further discussion.

9. Could a technician do triage alone if there are good triage protocols in place?

No. Protocols still require expertise in knowledge, interpretation, and application. For instance, is the pulse bounding or thready? The triage nurse is more than a scribe recording the verbal responses. The triage nurse hears what is not said or knows astute follow-up questions.

A trained paramedic or technician could initially greet the patient, obtain the data (name, date of birth, etc.) for a quick registration and be trained to elicit the chief complaint. However, a nurse must still do a visual rapid triage of all arriving patients and the formal triage interview and assessment (either in the triage area or at the bedside).

10. How long should triage take?

The goal for comprehensive triage is 2 to 5 minutes.

11. Is the 2- to 5-minute goal being met?

Travers (1999) found this goal is being met only 22% of the time. More time is needed for older adult patients, pediatric patients, and if a full set of vital signs is taken in the triage area. Keddington (1998) found that an average of 7 minutes was needed for pediatric patient if a full set of vital signs was included.

12. Is it essential to have a nurse in triage 24 hours a day?

A health care professional must initially assess the arriving patients 24 hours a day before registering the patient. Most hospitals make this a station-filled position. In a situation of routine low census periods, someone by the door (security, unit secretary) can immediately call for nurse or direct the patient into the treatment area upon their arrival. In the opposite situation of high census, a form of two-tier can occur.

13. What are the essential components of comprehensive triage?

- An across-the-room visual assessment (to determine stability of ABCD)
- A rapid triage (60 seconds or less) of an "appropriately elicited" chief complaint and/or a key question or visualization (such as feeling for a pulse in the extremity). This gives the information to determine the appropriate acuity and disposition or then a priority for the comprehensive triage assessment.
- Based on priority of patients in the triage area, the nurse completes a more thorough triage history and a focused physical assessment on those who were not emergent/immediate. This includes vital signs and documentation.
- A triage decision is made and the patient's acuity or level is assigned.

14. How does the triage nurse quickly assess stabilization of the ABCs in this quick glance for a pediatric patient?

The ENA national standardized Emergency Nursing Pediatric Course (ENPC) recommends the pediatric assessment triangle, which consists of appearance, circulation, and work of breathing.

15. How does the triage nurse quickly assess ABC stability in an adult?

This is often referred to as the "primary" survey. A "trick" from the EMS system is 30-2-CAN DO. If the patient's respirations are less than 30, the person knows their name and where they are (2), and the person follows your verbal commands (CAN DO), they probably have adequate initial oxygenation and perfusion.

16. What are other quick factors that could be considered for ABCD stability?

Quick assessments for this primary survey of airway, breathing, circulation, and disability could include:

A: Can the person verbalize? (There is an open airway.)
B: Are respirations quiet and effortless? (This is "normal.")
C: Is the person alert and oriented? (There is adequate perfusion to the brain.)

Capillary refill/blanching ≤2 seconds? (There is perfusion in the extremity.)
Does the person look pink?
Radial pulse present? (The blood pressure is at least 80 systolic.)

D: Mental disability, physical disability/neuro, and pain.
Responds appropriately to questions (alert and probably orientated × 4)
Moving all extremities (No physical disability)
Body language indicating a reasonable degree of comfort (e.g., no moaning)
No self-report of an intense discomfort (e.g., "my side is killing me")
No history of an ominous complaint and/or previous etiology

For further discussion, see the chapters on history and physical assessment.

17. Talk about obtaining the detailed history and physical assessment.

Obtaining the history and a focused physical assessment are part of the "secondary" assessment, after the ABCDs. See the chapters on these topics for further discussion.

18. Does every patient need a full set of vital signs taken?

Travers (1999) found, in ambulatory patients, the mean triage time was 4.0 minutes if complete vital signs were taken. If not taken, the mean time drops to 2.4 minutes. Pediatric patients were the majority of the patients (53%) that vital signs were deferred.

Some EDs only perform select vital signs (e.g., no blood pressure) for younger pediatric patients if the child has a localized complaint. However, other ways of determining the vital "status" should be noted, such as sucking on a bottle and capillary refill. These are often more indicative of the pediatric patient's oxygenation and circulation status than late vital sign changes. See the chapter on vital signs.

Others believe that a complete set of vital signs is always important as a screening tool. The American Society of Hypertension's 2004 federal guidelines call for health care providers to check children's blood pressures (starting at age 3 years) during routine office visits (http://hin.nblbi.nih.gov/nhbpep.htm).

19. Where should the waiting patient's chart be located?

Keep the chart with the waiting patient, whether that is the waiting room or the treatment area. This aids ongoing assessment and documentation.

20. Describe the triage acuity decision.

It is determining the patient's severity and assigning them an acuity that determines the urgency and order for the medical screening examination (MSE) and treatment. See the chapter on triage systems for further discussion.

21. What is the ENA standard of practice about assigning a triage acuity?

The ENA Comprehensive Specialty Standards (1999) indicates that triage determination is based on physical, developmental, and psychosocial needs as well as factors influencing access to health care and patient flow through the emergency care system.

22. What triage acuity level systems are United States EDs using most?

In the 2001 ENA Benchmark Guide, 69.4% were using a three-level, 11.6% were using a 4-level, and 3% were using a 5-level triage system. In addition, 11.7% of the reporting EDs were using no triage urgency scale at all: almost all of these were smaller facilities. The ENA benchmark study is being repeated in 2005.

23. Discuss ENA's work toward a 5-level system.

ENA passed a resolution in 2002 for a work group to review 5-level triage systems. In 2003, an American College of Emergency Physicians (ACEP)/ENA joint work group policy statement indicated support of the adoption of a reliable, valid 5-level triage scale. In 2004, the workgroup indicated the Canadian Triage and Acuity Scale (CTAS) or the Emergency Severity Index (ESI) are good options. See the chapters on 5-level triage systems and the ACEP/ENA work group for further discussion.

24. What are the most common medical reasons for an ED visit?

According to the 2002 Centers for Disease Control and Prevention (CDC) report, the most common medical reasons are:

- Abdominal pain (6.5%)
- Chest pain (5.1%)
- Fever (4.8%)

25. What about accidents?

Injury, poisoning, and adverse effects of medical treatment accounted for 35.5% of ED visits. Falls, striking or being struck, and motor vehicle incidents were the leading causes of injuries, accounting for about 40% of the visits related to injury. Head injuries among children under age 18 continue to decline, falling 75% since 1992.

26. What were the most frequently reported final primary diagnoses?

The CDC data indicated:

- Contusions (4.3%)
- Acute upper respiratory infections (4%)
- Open wounds except to the head (3.8%)
- Abdominal pain (3.7%)

27. What does EMTALA require?

EMTALA is the Emergency Medical Treatment and Active Labor Act. EMTALA is the extension of the original 1986 COBRA (Consolidated Omnibus Budget Reconciliation Act) or "anti-dumping" law, whose purpose was to prevent the unethical practice of refusing to treat some emergency patients or inappropriately transferring "charity" cases.

EDs are required to screen and stabilize life- or limb-threatening medical conditions. EMTALA is applicable to all patients (even if they have private insurance) and related to the patient's condition, not the type of facility (e.g., psychiatric patient who presents to a medical hospital is still screened.

28. What EMTALA requirements relate to triage?

EMTALA mandates a "decent" and "consistent" MSE for every patient who presents to the ED for care. A complete triage assessment should be done for each patient according to the hospital's protocol.

The term "complete MSE" refers to the care provided after triage, not the triage process itself. It is providing the necessary testing and on-call services within the capability of the hospital to reach a diagnosis that excluded the presence of legally defined emergency medical conditions. Insurance information cannot be collected if it delays the MSE.

29. Is there an EMTALA violation if the patient leaves from the triage waiting room without completing an MSE?

A competent adult may withdraw the initial request for evaluation at any time and EMTALA therefore no longer applies. However, no coercion can be used to dissuade patient from consenting to further examination or treatment, such as suggesting that continued care could be prohibitively expensive or triage process inequities that keep an "undesirable" patient waiting longer than other patients. Attempt to obtain a signature indicating an informed decision to leave; at a minimum document that the patient was left. Many hospitals consider these patients high risk and do a follow-up call.

30. What is an emergency medical condition?

An emergency medical condition could put the person at risk for loss of life or limb impairment. This can include undiagnosed acute pain sufficient to impair normal functioning, pregnancy with contractions, psychiatric disturbances, and substance abuse/intoxication.

31. Can managed care deny payment if there is not an emergency medical condition?

Would a "prudent lay person" be likely to seek ED care for these symptoms? If so, then the insurance should cover the visit. A common example is "chest pain" that is eventually diagnosed as costochondritis. Therefore it is helpful to put the patient's initial complaint in quotes, such as "I can't bear the pain in my arm."

32. Is it ever appropriate to tell a patient that an ED visit is not necessary, such as someone with a "cold"?

First, consider that any patient may not be forthcoming for the real reason for the visit at triage, such as being a victim of domestic violence or homeless. Similarly, the patient may sense something is wrong but not articulate it clearly. True scenarios that occurred:

- A teenager who came in without a parent for a "sore shoulder" after swimming had a septic joint.
- An elderly woman complaining of a headache was septic.
- An elderly patient with a "cold" (her chest was "tight") was having an acute MI.

Regardless, *all* patients must have an MSE. However a facility can have a "triage out" or "expedited MSE" procedure.

33. Describe the "triaging out" process.

Since 1995, the University of California-Davis triaged out nonemergent patients who could safely go to community resources. They found that, of the more than 30,000 patients in the last 10 years they have "triaged out", 73% were able to obtain follow-up care within 3 days and found it could be done safely with community support. Harbor-UCLA Medical Center's study gave next-day appointments at a clinic to nonemergent patients that could safely wait 24 hours. In 2002, the University of Colorado Hospital started referring nonemergent patients to community resources, without a scheduled follow-up appointment. All three programs claim no adverse outcomes. It is estimated that approximately 1000 hospital EDs now perform some form of this process.

34. Describe the process used by University of California-Davis.

The initial medical screening examiners are highly trained, mid-level providers. They evaluate all patients uniformly, according to a series of questions:

- Chief symptom: Chronic condition? At risk? Or a true emergency?
- Vital signs
- Mental state: Evidence of change?
- General appearance: Does the patient look sick?
- Degree of pain: Does the patient have moderate or severe pain?
- Skin: Evidence of dehydration, poor perfusion?
- Focused physical examination?
- Ability to walk?
- Pregnancy: Is the patient near term?

No questions are asked regarding payer information. The ED physician performs a formal examination if the screening reveals a need for physician intervention or a diagnostic test. If not, the patient is "stable" and referred to an off-site care center.

35. Explain how the University of Colorado's "Expedited Medical Screening" process works.

All patients still receive a traditional triage. Patients who are triaged at a Level 4 or Level 5 (in a 5-level system) then receive an expedited MSE to rule-out a medical conditioning needing immediate care. ED nurses receive a special 3-hour training to be qualified to perform the MSE on category 5 patients. Physicians or physician assistants perform MSEs on Category 4 patients.

If it is determined that patient does not need immediate care, the patients go to the financial desk after the MSE and a deposit is requested. If the patient chose not to give a payment, referrals to alternative community providers and resources are given.

36. Is it legal for EDs to ask for money during a patient's visit?

Yes, *if* it is after the MSE and the *same* process is done for *all* patients, regardless. Increasingly, EDs are asking for funds (and providing financial counseling) upon discharge. Vanderbilt University Medical Center requests deposits or co-payments and collected approximately $28,000/month in the first months.

37. Is the "triaging out" process the eventual goal for all EDs?

No. "Triaging out" depends heavily on triage nurses being expert, strict protocol, and sufficient community resources to meet the patient's needs in a timely and appropriate manner. EMTALA expert Mark Moy warns the risks for violations elsewhere are high. Some also question the ethics of this process. If the ED is a safety net, where will these patients go if that ED protection is removed?

38. Must a physician perform the MSE?

Appropriate medical people according to the hospital's bylaws must perform it, which are physicians for most hospitals. An essential criterion is that the MSE is performed by the same personnel for all similar patients in a similar acuity, regardless of their insurance status.

39. Can a patient be sent directly to a specialty clinic within the hospital?

A patient can be sent, with the patient's consent, to another in-house facility, especially if it is a higher or specialized level of care. However, a patient cannot be sent out of the facility, e.g., to their doctor's office or the public health sexually transmitted disease clinic, without an MSE.

40. Why is there overcrowding in EDs?

The CDC data indicates the number of visits to the nation's EDs climbed 23% the past decade (110.2M in 2002, up from 90 million in 1992), while the number of U.S. EDs fell 15%, because of closures and mergers. Some of the other reasons attributed to this increase include:

- *Aging population.* "Baby boomers" reaching their senior years now have more medical needs.
- *Shorter hospital stays.* This leads to complications that accounted for 1.4 million ED visits in 2001. (According to the CDC, the average length-of-stay in 2001 was 4.9 days compared to 1970, when it was 7.8 days. The most dramatic decrease was in the elderly, who went from 12.6 in 1970 to 5.8 in 2001.)
- *Public perception of need.* In another study, regardless of race or socioeconomic status, the majority believed that a healthcare provider should evaluate even their minor illnesses within 24 hours. In one study, 94% of the presenting ED patients thought they had a true need to be seen that day compared to the ED physicians' evaluation (based on presenting reason) that only 66% needed same-day care.
- *A convenient, ever-present option.* The ED has become the principle provider of primary medical care during off-duty hours. The CDC report classified 10% of the ED visits as "nonurgent". Pediatric admissions peak at night, probably because no pediatrician's office is open at 2:00 AM. The demand on "instant" care by insured patients is also on the rise.
- *Lack of inpatient beds.* While the average visit is 3 hours (from arrival to discharge), more than half spend 2 to 6 hours and more than 400,000 visits lasted 24 hours or longer (the "boarders").
- *Uninsured or underinsured patients.* Estimated to be at least 44 million (with 8.5 million children), these populations use the ED since they do not have routine medical care and the ED becomes their source of primary care.
- *The ED is a "safety net" but with uneven distribution.*

41. What is meant by ED "safety net" with uneven distribution?

The CDC reported that 36% of EDs serve a high volume of the "safety net" patients in the year 2000. This was defined as serving a patient population who were at least 30% Medicaid eligible, 30% uninsured, or 40% in either category. The complete report is available at http://www.cdc.gov/nchs/data.

42. Is low income the only factor that is causing overcrowding?

High population density is another consideration. The Government Accountability Office (GAO, formerly called the General Accounting Office) studied 3 indicators of crowding: ambulance diversion, the percentage of patients boarded in the ED for 2 hours or more, and the proportion of patients who leave without medical evaluation. It found hospitals in areas with populations of 2.5 million or more reported higher levels of all three indicators. Overall, while 60% of the EDs were located in metropolitan areas, they handled 81% of the U.S. ED visits.

43. Elaborate on the ED safety net being strained.

In 2004, Urgent Matters reports there are an increased number of patients relying on safety net resources and that EDs are struggling to absorb the impact of the unraveling safety net. In all ED visits that did not result in hospital admission, 42% were for patients with conditions that could have been safely treated by a primary care physician and 41% of ED visits occur during normal business hours when primary care is generally available (http://www.urgentmatters.org).

44. Has the American College of Emergency Physicians (ACEP) voiced an opinion about this issue?

An ED physician survey indicated that they believed 30% of the ED patients they treated had no medical insurance. Most (74%) believed that these patients were sicker, suffer from more critical medical problems, and had more difficulty with follow-up care (94%) than patients with insurance.

The ED physicians said their EDs were operating at or over capacity on weekdays (82%), worsening on weekends (91%). The number of uninsured patients treated in their EDs had increased in the past year (72%) and 79% of the physicians anticipate it will continue to increase in the next 1 to 2 years.

45. Discuss the increased use by insured patients.

There is an increased use by patients with insurance because it is convenient and insured patients want what is commonly described as "on demand" health care. The Center for Studying Health System Change found that hospital ED visits increased 16.3%, but, during the same time period, the visits by privately insured patients jumped 24.3% (Medicare patients 10%, uninsured patients 10.3%, Medicaid the same). According to the 2002 CDC report of all ED patients, 29% have private insurance, 20% have Medicaid, and 15% have Medicare.

46. Is the triage nurse responsible to go out and retrieve patients on the street?

The hospital is responsible for retrieving any individual who "comes to the ED." This includes hospital-owned property within 250 yards. However, the hospital should have a policy and process to retrieve appropriate patients that prevents abandonment of the triage role/patients in the waiting room and protects the safety of the staff. A policy can include activation of the EMS system.

47. What are some of the more common potential pitfalls with triage?

- *Falling into the first come, first serve mentality.* Patients should always be seen in order of need, not arrival.
- *Failing to monitor the waiting patient.* Just because a patient is waiting for a treatment room or a physician examination does not abdicate responsibility. See the chapter on waiting room management for further discussion of this topic.
- *Prioritizing the "who" rather than the "what."* Triage is based on the patient's condition or chief compliant, not who they are.

- *Focusing on a red herring.* Focusing on the most obvious symptom or patient-initiated presenting complaint rather than the real problem. One man came for his knee wound after falling, mentioning his leg wasn't working right. The knee had an abrasion, but the real problem was his one-sided weakness (e.g., new stroke).
- *Giving priority to the patient who complains the most.* Sometimes the patient who needs care the most is too sick to complain.
- *Known patient: "same ol', same ol'."* Old patients can get new complaints. Even a hypochondriac eventually dies of some physical ailment.
- *Failing to rule-out the "zebra."* As the adage goes, "When you hear hoof beats, think horses, not zebras." It is easy to be lulled into complacency by the commonness of some complaints, such as upper respiratory infection. But there are zebras out there, rule out the worse case scenario first. The tendency is to undertriage, rather than overtriage.
- *Basing the triage decision on other factors, such as the department environment, instead of the patient's condition.* A patient's acuity rating is based on the patient's need, regardless if there are no empty treatment beds and the waiting room is overflowing. Showing empathy to move ahead a young mother with five other children in tow can be done, but it is a management (not triage acuity) decision.
- *Using "cookbook" rules to make decisions.* Triage is continual critical thinking applied to *this* individual patient. All of those with the identical chief complaint or all children are not automatically assigned the same number.
- *Falling into (subconscious) age or gender bias.* Young, thin females can have a heart attack. Use population statistics to consider a possible etiology, not to rule it out.
- *Allowing the patient to lead you to your triage decision based on what they think the problem is.* Self-reports are helpful, especially comparing to their "normal." However, the patients' conclusions can be wrong.
- *Failing to document enough to validate the triage decision.* The criteria: will you be able to validate your triage conclusion 3 years from now based on what is written? Be sure to include specifics, such as "child wearing long sleeves despite 110° F heat" (consider abuse).

Key Points

- All arriving patients receive a "quick look" to determine ABCD stability and "sick" versus "not sick." Emergent patients go immediately into the treatment area; the rest are prioritized for the more thorough triage history and assessment.
- The ENA Comprehensive Specialty Standards (1999) indicates that triage determination is based on physical, developmental, and psychosocial needs as well as factors influencing access to health care and patient flow through the emergency care system.
- Avoid common pitfalls including first come, first served mentality, focusing only on the obvious or patient-initiated complaint, and giving priority to who (important, complaining) rather than the what between the waiting patients.

Internet Resources

CDC National Hospital Ambulatory Medicine Care Survey: 2002: 2002 ED Summary
http://www.cdc.gov/nchs/about/major/ahcd/ahcd1.htm

Center for Medicaid and State Operations/Survey and Certification Group: Revised Emergency Medical Treatment and Labor Act (EMTALA) Interpretive Guidelines
http://www.cms.hhs.gov/medicaid/survey-cert/sc0434.pdf

Bibliography

Brillman JC, Doezema D, Tandberg D, et al: Triage: Limitations in predicting need for emergent care and hospital admission, *Ann Emerg Med* 24:498-500, 1996.

Canadian Association of Emergency Physicians: Canadian Emergency Department Triage and Acuity Scale Implementation Guidelines, *J Can Assoc Emerg Physicians* Oct 1999.

Cohen S: *101 Triage Tips,* Hohenwald, Tenn, 2002, Health Resources Unlimited.

Derlet RW, Kinser D, Ray L, et al: Prospective identification and triage of nonemergency patients out of an emergency department: A 5-year study (comment), *Ann Emerg Med* 25:215-223, 1995.

Diesburg-Stanwood A, Scott J, Oman K, Whitehill C: Nonemergent ED patients referred to community resources after medical screening examination: Characteristics, medical conditions after 72 hours, and use of follow-up services, *J Emerg Nurs* 30(4):312-317, 2004.

Emergency Nurses Association: *ENPC provider manual,* ed 2, Des Plaines, Ill, 1998, Author.

Emergency Nurses Association: *Standards of emergency nursing practice,* ed 4, Des Plaines, Ill, 1999, Author.

Fackelmann K: Report: ER visits climb while emergency departments fall, *USA Today,* June 5, 2003:5A.

Gilboy N, Travers D, Wuerz R: Re-evaluating triage in the new millennium: A comprehensive look at the need for standardization and quality, *J Emerg Nurs* 25:468-473, 1999.

Gill JM, Reese CL, Diamond JL: Disagreement among healthcare professionals about the urgent needs of emergency department patients, *Ann Emerg Med* 28:474-478, 1996.

Keddington RK: A triage vital sign policy for a children's hospital emergency department, *J Emerg Nurs* 24:189-192, 1998.

Knaut AL, Sknau CS: EMTALA. In Markovchick VJ, Pons PT, editors: *Pons' emergency medicine secrets,* ed 3, Philadelphia, 2003, Hanley & Belfus.

Mason D: Collecting money at discharge (Managers Forum), *J Emerg Nurs* (in press).

McNair R (President): In the Nature of the Beast: Comprehensive Triage and Patient Flow Workshop, Fairview, NC, 2003, Triage First, Inc.

Moy MM: *The EMTALA answer book: 2002 edition,* New York, 2002, Aspen.

Paulson DL: A comparison of wait times and patients leaving without being seen when licensed nurses versus unlicensed assistive personnel perform triage, *J Emerg Nurs* 30(4):307-311, 2004.

Prutzman L, Oman K: Expedited medical screening exams (Managers Forum), *J Emerg Nurs* 30(6):560, 2004.

Slovis CM, Wrenn KD, Meador CK: *A little book of emergency medicine rules,* Philadelphia, 2000, Hanley & Belfus.

Travers D: Triage: How long does it take? How long should it take? *J Emerg Nurs* 25:238-240, 1999.

Washington DL, Stevens CD, Shekelle PG, Henneman PL, Brook RH: Next-day care for emergency department users with nonacute conditions: A randomized controlled trial, *Ann Intern Med* 137:707-714, 2002.

Zimmermann PG: Lessons learned: On watching for zebras, *J Emerg Nurs* 29(1):85-86, 2003.

Zimmermann PG: Triage. In Oman KS, Koziol-McLain J, Scheetz LJ, editors: *Scheetz's emergency nursing secrets,* Philadelphia, 2001, Hanley & Belfus.

Chapter 2

Triage Systems and Acuities

Polly Gerber Zimmermann and Rebecca S. McNair

1. What is a triage system?

A triage system is the basic framework in which patients are sorted, using one of the acuity rating scales, to determine priority of treatment.

2. What is a "traffic director" form of triage?

In the most simplistic form of triage, a "traffic director" greets and directs the patient to the correct treatment area. This is often performed by a nonlicensed staff member and is not recommended by the Emergency Nurses Association (ENA). It is illegal for a clerk to obtain any financial information (e.g., only identifying information, such as name and date of birth) if that process delays the medical screening exam (MSE).

3. Describe spot check.

Spot check is a more detailed "quick look" during which a patient, based on his or her presenting complaint is assigned a category within 2 minutes. A spot check system refers to when this is the only triage done and works best in a low-volume situation where treatment area space and staff are readily available for immediate involvement.

4. Describe bedside triage.

This is the term used for patients sent back immediately to the treatment bed and the information is now obtained at the bedside. Patients tend to perceive their care as faster since the waiting room was bypassed.

5. Discuss comprehensive triage.

In some sense, this involves a single person performing a form of two-tier triage.

There is an initial across-the-room look or visualizing the patient (general appearance, work of breathing, circulation) to ensure stability of the ABCDs (airway, breathing, circulation, and disability). Any unstable patient is immediately sent to the treatment area for interventions.

If multiple patients are waiting, there is then a rapid triage. This is a 60-seconds or less survey that elicits the chief complaint and a key assessment or focused history question to rule out the worse case scenario.

For patients who ABCDs are stable, the triage then continues with:
- Vital signs (weight)
- A focused history
- A focused triage physical assessment as appropriate (including appropriate "exposure" of the relevant area(s), pain rating, pulse oximetry, diagnostic point-of-care testings by protocol)
- Department-designated additional information (such as a screenings for domestic abuse, nutrition, etc., or inquiring about advanced directives)

As appropriate, some secondary survey is accomplished. Triage relies on eliciting a good history. See also the chapters on the waiting room management and history.

6. What is the standard of the ENA?

The ENA Practice Standard (1999) is comprehensive triage.

7. Discuss two-tier triage.

Two-tier is seen mainly in larger emergency departments. It usually refers to the use of two individuals and builds on a combination of spot-check and comprehensive systems. A registered nurse does an initial "quick look" to sort all incoming patients and identifies those who are emergent. This nurse also often handles any family and visitor concerns or needs. A second nurse performs the in-depth (and now less-interrupted) history and assessments for urgent and nonurgent patients.

Variation including temporarily sending out a second nurse to assist when triage is backing up or having the triage nurse initially sort out nonurgent patients and send them directly to a fast-track area for the history, assessments and vital signs. This is allowed under the Emergency Medical Treatment and Active Labor Act (EMTALA) regulations as long as all patients with the same type of complaints are treated in a similar manner.

8. When should an emergency department consider stationing two people in triage?

Triage consultant Rebecca McNair recommends that a second person (can be a non-RN) should be stationed in triage once the department's annual census reaches 30,000/year.

9. Provide guidelines for having a second person temporarily assist in triage.

One hospital has the rule of sending out a second nurse when there are five or more patients waiting. McNair recommends temporarily bringing out the second person for dual triage when there are five or more patients waiting for triage more than 15 to 30 minutes.

The primary triage nurse should do the rapid assessment of all patients and decide what aspects she wants the assisting person to do. That way the primary triage nurse will know something about everyone in the waiting room after the assisting person leaves.

10. Is it necessary for both of the individuals in triage to be registered nurses?

A nonmedical person may "greet" or collect basic patient identification information but should not be eliciting a chief complaint. A trained paramedic or EMT can obtain the chief complaint and/or perform some functions under the nurse's direction, such as obtaining vital signs, weight, or diagnostic tests per protocol. However, only a registered nurse should obtain the complete triage history and physical assessment.

11. What is "expanded" or "advanced" triage?

This term is usually by departments who have added protocols to initiate diagnostic work-up or treatment in the triage area. It can be "added on" to either comprehensive or two-tier triage.

Common items in protocols include first aid measures, visual acuity, extremity x-rays, screening lab work (urinalysis, urine pregnancy, urine dipstick, fingerstick blood glucose), analgesics/antipyretics administration, or tetanus immunizations. Examples are illustrated in the topic-specific chapters and the chapter on protocols.

12. Can financial information and registration be completed before all treatment is completed?

Yes, if the MSE is not delayed in order to obtain it. Hospitals often indicate the MSE is complete for patients in the treatment area by a check-off box. See the discussion of the expedited MSE in the Triage Essence chapter.

13. How does acuity rating fit into that?

The patient's acuity is determined and the patient is assigned a level of urgency and order in which to receive the MSE and treatment. In traditional 3-level triage or disaster triage, the terms for the levels of the triage acuity decision are emergency (red), urgent (yellow), and nonurgent (green).

14. What triage acuity level systems are U.S. EDs using most often?

In the 2001 ENA Benchmark Guide, 69.4% were using a 3-level, 11.6% were using a 4-level, and 3% were using a 5-level triage system. In addition, 11.7% of the reporting EDs were using no triage urgency scale at all: almost all of these were smaller facilities. The ENA benchmark study is being repeated in 2005. In 2003, the ENA Board of Directors approved to support the adoption of a reliable, valid 5-level triage scale. For further discussion, see the section of 5-level triage systems.

15. Why does ENA support adopting a 5-level triage system?

The current 3-level (and 4-level) acuity scales lack reliability and replicability in comparing determinations made by different persons (interrater agreement) and/or the same persons on different occasions (test-retest reliability). Gill et al (1996) found that, using a 3-level acuity scale, emergent determinations made by nurses of the same patient varied from 11% to 63%. Wuerz et al (1998) did a study with 87 nurses who used a 3-level triage scale to triage five standardized patient scenarios. There was poor agreement with poor test-retest agreement: only 24% of the nurses rated all five cases the same on both occasions, and 46% changed the rating by more than one severity level. There is currently no 3- or 4-level triage scale that is being researched, supported, required, or promoted by any professional or governmental organization. There are 5-level triage systems, in comparison, that have statistical reliability and validity.

16. Is it really important to have a statistically reliable and valid 5-level system as long as the triage nurse knows in his/her mind who will be seen next?

Yes. It is to everyone's advantage to have a triage acuity scale that is reliable, reproducible, and independent of which nurse is performing the role. The ACEP/ENA work group indicated it would improve the quality of care, patient safety, and ED operations while helping to support benchmarking, surveillance activities, and research.

Comparisons can be made within and between EDs if a standardized system is used. When these criteria are met, triage acuity categories can have a significant role in legal defense, federal funding, case mix data, staffing levels, predictable resource consumption, budgeting, managed care decision making, and outcome measures for admission rates, ED length of stay, and complexity of care. England, Australia, and Canada have accomplished some of these uses of triage data with their standardized 5-level triage system.

More importantly, a valid and reliable system maximizes triage accuracy and treatment of patients in the most expeditious manner, whereas one with poor reliability and validity undertriages and/or overtriages patients.

17. List some goals for the "ideal" 5-level triage system.

The ACEP/ENA work group identified that triage process and rules should be easily understood, rapidly applied, have high rates of inter-observer agreement, facilitate appropriate placement, correlate with ED resource use requirements, and predict clinical outcome.

18. List other characteristics of triage acuity scales that may be compared when evaluating different scales.

McNair indicates that some important features are:

- Nurse-Driven Process
- Rapidly identifies patients in need of immediate care
- Easily understood and rapidly applied
- Clear definitions of each acuity level
- Reflects the severity of illness or injury
- Incorporates discriminators to the chief complaint: Bleeding, Pain, Vital-Sign parameters, Age, Mental Status changes, Immunocompromised states, Trauma criteria
- Ability to use rapid and comprehensive triage
- Includes both subjective and objective observation
- Is applicable across all patient populations and age groups
- Ability to incorporate both pediatric vital signs and activity level
- Allows for nursing judgment to override any acuity rating proposed by system
- Allows for triage of psychological and social as well as physical presentations
- Able to accommodate nurse implementation of protocols and treatment plans
- Facilitates appropriate placement
- Incorporates "Time" Objectives for patient to be seen by caregivers (In order to benchmark)
- Incorporates Fractile Responses to Objectives
- Reflects the characteristics of reliability, validity, utility, and relevance
- Predicts clinical outcome (e.g., admit/discharge)
- Predicts ED resource use
- Ascending Scale or Descending Scale
- Is adaptable to computer documentation/systems integration
- Matches reimbursement

19. How else do the 5-level systems differ besides having additional, more precise categories?

The 5-level systems all recognize unstable patients for immediate treatment. Then:

- The Canadian Triage and Acuity Scale (CTAS) is built on the Australian method and works most similarly to the traditional 3-level system. Based on the chief complaint, the nurse obtains the focused history and physical assessment and makes an unofficial presumptive major symptom/disease categorization.
- The Manchester Triage Group works off of complaint-specific presentation flow charts, rather than a medical diagnosis. Under the presentation, it looks at six general key discriminators: life threat, pain, hemorrhage, conscious level, temperature, and acuteness. Discriminators specific to the complaint are applied within the flow chart.
- The Emergency Severity Index (ESI) is a triage algorithm that looks at high risk, mental status alteration, severe pain, or abnormal vital signs/pO_2 and then incorporates the number of anticipated different types of resource interventions. It expands the concept of triage from beyond what might be the patient's diagnosis to also what does the patient need done to determine what is wrong.

- Both the Canadian and ESI have statistical validity and reliability and are recognized by the ENA/ACEP 5-level triage workgroup as acceptable systems to adapt. See also the chapters on each specific triage system.

20. Do all of the standarized international 5-level systems identified above include the essential components that were discussed under triage essence and process?

Yes. All involve some type of quick look/rapid across the room assessment, a triage history, a triage physical assessment and then making a triage decision. The extent of which particular key information is assessed may vary.

21. What are the terms used for the different acuity levels in the 5-level systems?

Level	Canadian Triage and Acuity Scale (CTAS)	Manchester	Australian Triage Scale (ATS)	Emergency Severity Index (ESI)
1	Resuscitation (Immediate)	Immediate (Red) (0 minutes)	Immediately Life-Threatening (Immediate)	ESI-1 Immediately
2	Emergent (≤15 minutes)	Very Urgent (Orange) (10 minutes)	Imminently Life-Threatening (10 minutes)	ESI-2 Minutes
3	Urgent (≤ 30 minutes)	Urgent (Yellow) (60 minutes)	Potentially Life-Threatening (30 minutes)	ESI-3 Up to 1 hour
4	Less Urgent (≤60 minutes)	Standard (Green) (120 minutes)	Potentially Serious (60 minutes)	ESI-4 Could be delayed
5	Non Urgent (≤120 minutes)	Non-Urgent (Blue) (240 minutes)	Less Urgent (120 minutes)	ESI-5 Could be delayed

22. Are the patients given the time guidelines stated above?

Many tell the patients their triage rating, give a written explanation of the triage concept, and/or have a wall chart indicating the priority. Most indicate the times are meant to be a guide and a goal and do not tell the patients the specific times. CTAS uses the time objectives in light of fractile responses, i.e., it is a goal for a certain percentage of people to meet those times as benchmarked with other like facilities. Inability to meet those time objectives can provide leverage for change or obtaining needed resources.

23. Why doesn't the ESI system have more specific times stated?

The late Richard C. Wuerz, MD, co-developer of the ESI, believed not stating specific times is more appropriate for the litigious American society. Triage is really a prioritization of the needs in the department, not an absolute.

24. I am often pressured by patients to give them a time estimate. Patients get upset if the time is not met because of unexpected factors.

Be honest but vague. You can indicate how long current non–life-threatening patients are waiting, that the treatment area is full, and/or ambulances are expected or could come at any time. Psychologically, it is better to overestimate and take the person early than underestimate and have them wait additional time. Remember to talk to the inquirer's feelings ("I know it can be hard to wait") and keep them updated. Just because someone does not like the answer you initially give does not mean you need to change it.

25. How should I handle it if the patient is between two acuity categories?

Always give the patient the benefit of the doubt and assign the higher category. In McNair's consulting work, she consistently finds that nurses are more prone to mistakenly "undertriage" rather than "overtriage."

26. Are there any exceptions to the decision rules in traditional 3-level or 4-level triage?

Many facilities and/or practitioners will either officially, or unofficially as a management decision, use some factors to move a patient up in prioritization. They include:

- Presenting within 2 hours of a respiratory treatment
- Experiencing very severe pain (including a condition for which lying on a stretcher would help the patient's comfort)
- Arriving directly from a physician's office
- Returning to the emergency department within 24 hours after ED discharge
- Young children, especially late at night
- Behaving in a disruptive, violent, out-of-control, or incompetent manner
- Any abuse or neglect case
- "Mystery" patients, e.g., symptoms are not a recognizable common presentation

See also the chapter on prioritization and decision making for further discussion

27. Talk about the concept of ED treatment beds in the hallway.

The best departments have a systematic plan for when the ED patients "spill out" over into the hallway to insure timely and the same quality of care. These can include:

- Stored "fanny packs" with portable equipment
- Second "flow board" or method to track these patients in the "expanded" area
- Assigning staff (besides the triage nurse) for ongoing patient care

28. Discuss the concept of "saturation plans."

Hospitals have a policy, sometimes called an internal disaster plan, for when the emergency department is at "full capacity" and can no longer evaluate and treat patients in a timely fashion. Criteria to consider for activation:

- Triage flow and tone
- Impending known ambulance arrivals with high acuity levels
- Acuity levels of patients presently in the ED treatment area
- Inability to see waiting urgent patients in a timely manner
- Estimated time for discharge for current ED patients
- Numbers and expected bed availability time for "held" admitted ED patients

29. List measures that can be instituted.

All indicate it must be a hospital-wide solution. Possible actions (often in "tiered" responses) include:

- Calling in additional ancillary staff (x-ray, lab, housekeeping)
- Calling in ED staff, and/or floating inpatient staff, to the emergency department
- Moving admitted patients to the floor immediately without completing the usual admission orders, consultations, and so on in the ED
- Using other locations (such as recovery area after hours) for observation/holding
- Expediting discharges
- Holding admitted patients on the inpatient hallways
- Limiting elective surgeries
- Denying direct admissions
- Activating the disaster plan
- Transferring stable waiting admitted patients to other facilities

30. Tell me more about that concept of holding patients on the inpatient units.

Patients wait for an inpatient bed on a stretcher in the hallway of the floor unit (instead of the emergency department) where the eventual inpatient bed placement will be made. Stony Brook University Hospital in New York is probably the best-known pioneer of this concept. Their criteria exclude patients who are:

- ICU admissions
- Unstable (including those having an active myocardial infarction)
- Require frequent suctioning
- Have isolation requirements
- Using more than 4 liters of oxygen per minute

31. What are some of Stony Brook University Hospital's specific policies?

- No unit can receive more than 2 hallway patients.
- The "held" hallway patient receives the next available inpatient bed on the unit.
- All unoccupied acute floor beds must be utilized, taking into account that unit's staff nurses' routine competences.

32. What happened to Stony Brook's "hallway" patients?

Overall, 28% of patients assigned to a hallway bed actually go into a "found" bed by the time the patient arrives on the floor unit. Of the remaining patients, 26% are in the hallway bed less than an hour and 46% spend an average of 10.3 hours in the hallway.

Key Points

- The ENA Practice Standard (1999) is comprehensive triage.
- ACEP and ENA support the adoption of a reliable, valid 5-level triage scale. At this point, either the Emergency Severity Index (ESI) or Canadian Triage and Acuity Scale (CTAS) is acceptable.
- Regardless of the system used, error on the side of caution when unsure.

Internet Resources

Triage First: Triage Acuity Systems
www.triagefirst.com

Health Resources Unlimited
www.hru.net

Emergency Nurses Association
www.ena.org

Canadian Association of Emergency Physicians
http://www.caep.ca

Bibliography

Australasian College for Emergency Medicine (ACEM): Guidelines for implementation of the Australasian Triage Scale in emergency departments. ACEM (serial online), 2000; available at: http://www.acem.org/au.open/documents/triageguide; accessed March 4, 2004.

Australasian College for Emergency Medicine (ACEM): Policy document—The Australasian Triage Scale: ACEM (serial online), 2000; available at: http://www.acem.org.au/open/documents/triage; accessed March 4, 2004.

Barraco CA, Kelly-Sproul K, Santora C: Holding "Held" ED patients on inpatient units (Managers Forum), *J Emerg Nurs* 29(6):555-556, 2003.

Beveridge RC, Ducharme J, Janes L, Beauliu S, Walter S: Reliability of the Canadian ED triage and acuity scale: Inter-rater agreement, *Ann Emerg Med* 34:155-159, 1999.

Brillman JC, Doezema D, Tandberg D, et al: Triage: limitations in predicting need for emergent care and hospital admission, *Ann Emerg Med* 24:498-500, 1996.

Canadian Association of Emergency Physicians: Canadian Emergency Department Triage and Acuity Scale (CTAS), *J Can Assoc Emerg Physicians* 1:3, 1999.

Emergency Nurses Association: *Benchmark data,* Des Plaines, Ill, 2001, Author.

Emergency Nurses Association: *ENPC provider manual,* ed 2, Des Plaines, Ill, 1998, Author.

Emergency Nurses Association: *Standards of emergency nursing practice,* ed 4, Des Plaines, Ill, 1999, Author.

Emergency Nurses Association: *Triage: Meeting the Challenge,* Des Plaines, Ill, 1997, Author.

Fackelmann K. Report: ER visits climb while emergency departments fall, *USA Today,* June 5, 2003:5A.

Gilboy N, Travers D, Wuerz R: Re-evaluating triage in the new millennium: A comprehensive look at the need for standardization and quality, *J Emerg Nurs* 25:468-473, 1999.

Gilboy N et al: Emergency Severity Index (ESI), Des Plaines, Ill, 2003, Emergency Nurses Association.

Gill JM, Reese CL, Diamond JL: Disagreement among healthcare professionals about the urgent needs of emergency department patients, *Ann Emerg Med* 28:474-478, 1996.

Grossman VAG: *Quick reference to triage, ed 2,* Philadelphia, 2003, Lippincott.

Huff D: ED saturation internal disaster plan, *J Emerg Nurs* 27(6):583-584, 2001.

Mackway-Jones K: *Emergency triage: Manchester Triage Group,* London, 1997, BMJ.

McNair R (President): Triage and patient throughput. In the Nature of the Beast: Comprehensive Triage and Patient Flow Workshop, Fairview, NC, 2003, Triage First, Inc.

Prutzman O: Expedited medical screening exam (Managers Forum), *J Emerg Nurs* 30(1):22-29, 2004.

Simpson S: Verbal orders (Managers Forum), *J Emerg Nurs* (in press).

Tanabe P, Gimbel R, Yarnold PR, Adams JG: The Emergency Severity Index (version 3) 5-Level Triage System scores predict ED resource consumption, *J Emerg Nurs* 30(1):22-29, 2004.

Wuerz RC, Fernades CMB, Alarcon J: Inconsistency of emergency department triage, *Ann Emerg Med* 32:431-435, 1998.

Zimmermann PG: The case for a universal, valid, reliable 5-tier triage acuity scale for U.S. emergency departments, *J Emerg Nurs* 27(3):246-254, 2001.

Zimmermann PG: Triage. In Oman KS, Koziol-McLain J, Scheetz LJ, editors: *Scheetz's emergency nursing secrets,* Philadelphia, 2001, Hanley & Belfus.

Chapter 3

History Secrets

Polly Gerber Zimmermann

1. What should every triage history include?

Triage by its nature has a heavy focus on the patient's history. Generically, every triage history should include:

- Chief complaint (including onset, PQRST, mechanism of injury, treatment prior to arrival)
- Allergies
- Medications (prescriptions, over-the-counter, and environment). This could include sildenafil (Viagra) within the past 24 hours (ACC/AHA, 1999), illicit drug use, or risk of "date rape" drug ingestion.
- Past medical conditions
- Immunizations for patients less than 18 years old per protocol and last dT for all patients more than 18 years old
- Infectious? (Exposure to known illness, recent travel)
- Last menstrual period (in women of childbearing age). If the woman is pregnant, obtain the GPA (gravida, para, abortus). (See chapter on pregnancy complications.)
- Pain assessment
- Weight (and height) per protocol
- A Glasgow Coma Scale score (GCS) for all patients who have had a trauma, altered level-of-consciousness, or head injury

2. Give examples of phrases to help elicit the chief complaint.

Usually the patient's statement is documented (in quotes) to a question such as "What brings you to the emergency department today?" or "Tell me what's wrong today."

3. How should I handle a patient who complains of everything being wrong? It seems as if a total physical is desired.

Set limits. Indicate that it is not possible to take care of everything today, so what is most important. Ask "What is different or what made you come in *today?*"

4. What about a patient who is vague and nondescript about the chief complaint?

Indicate in a sincere tone of voice that you want to understand. Ask if there is anything else that is going on that the patient thinks might be contributing. I've never had any patient become offended by the question, and I've gotten some interesting answers. One woman complaining of "not feeling well" shared that her husband had died that very day 1 year ago. A man who said he "hurt all over" confided that it probably was stress because he recently lost his job and was going through a divorce.

5. What if the patient answers affirmatively to every single question you ask while obtaining the history?

Ask the patient if their toenails itch. It is not physiologically possible for nails to have that sensation. If the patient answers "yes" to that, then it is cause to question every other "yes" answer. However, if the patient thoughtfully answers "no," then the other positive answers would be regarded more seriously.

6. What should be included when the chief complaint involves a chronic condition?

- Their impression of how they are doing compared with their "normal"
- If there is anything that they know that they should be doing or that they should stop doing
- Is there anything that they know that they are not doing that they know they should be doing?

7. What could help improve the answers patients provide about allergies?

Patient populations who have English as a second language may not know the term "allergies." Try asking if there is any medication that makes them sick.

Always follow-up a "yes" answer to allergies by asking them what happens when they have their allergic reaction. One investigator found that 20% of responding individuals indicated an allergy to penicillin, but only 20% of those individuals had a true allergy. Patients will often attribute side effects, such as gastric upset or diarrhea, to an allergy.

8. Why should I include food allergies?

Prevalence of allergic disease is increasing worldwide (although some attribute it to increased awareness and reporting). Food allergies can be an alert to other potential reactions, such as seafood to dye with iodine or bananas to latex. For instance, although overall the current prevalence of allergy to peanuts and tree nuts is 1% to 2% in adults and children, in one study the percentage of allergic children doubled from 1997 to 2002.

9. How can I find a potential sensitivity to latex?

Ask them if their lips swell when they blow up a balloon or if they experience itching and burning after wearing rubber gloves.

10. Why is it so important to include nonprescription medications?

There can be drug interactions/poly-pharmacy concerns with nonprescription drugs use. Up to one-half of patients seeing a conventional physician are also seeing complementary and alternative medicine providers. Approximately 62% of the U.S. population uses alternative remedies, 19% of them indicated using natural products.

The most common uses for "complementary medication" is to treat back problems, colds, neck pain, joint pain or stiffness, or anxiety and depression. Mahady et al's (2003) survey of middle-aged women found 68% used botanical dietary supplements (BDS), most often soy products (42%), and green tea (35%). Interestingly, only 4% had obtained BDS information from a clinician and 70% did not tell their physicians.

11. Are there any herbs that are at higher risk?

The Consumers Union has warned Americans to avoid "the dirty dozen" supplements because they may cause cancer, kidney, or liver damage, or even death. They are aristolochic acid (birth wort), comfrey, germander, androstenedione, chaparral, kava, bitter orange, organ or gland extracts, lobelia, pennyroyal oil, skullcap, and yohimbe. In addition, there is more concern raised by the common use of St. John's Wort for depression. This herb alters cytochrome P450 enzymes, the hepatic system involved in the metabolism of more than 50% of all marketed drugs.

12. What if I suspect that the patient may be taking medication in an inappropriate manner, such as abusing laxatives? It is hard to get patients to be forthright.

What the patient is most comfortable discussing is often not the real source of trouble. Give the patient "permission" to discuss the atypical by bringing it into the realm of possibility. For instance, say, "Some people take only a tablespoon of milk of magnesia a day, some take two or three bottles a day. How much do you take?"

13. What can help obtain an accurate accounting of past medical conditions?

Review the medications and ask about any that may be for a chronic condition not listed, such as hypertension. As one explained, "I *used* to have high blood pressure but pills took it away." During the physical exam, look for distinct diagnostic scars. One man denied other medical conditions although he had a scar typical of post-open heart surgery. When asked, he replied, "I use to have heart problems but the surgery took care of that."

14. Why is immunization history so important?

- *Up to one third of U.S. toddlers are not up-to-date on immunizations.* Some parents are still choosing not to vaccinate their children although two large-scale studies have found no causative link between autism and the MMR shot and childhood vaccines and Type 1 diabetes.
- *Diphtheria-tetanus booster is required every 10 years.* Many adults are not current. Although 84% of young girls had immunity to both diseases in one study, only 41% of women aged 60 years and older did.
- *Flu and pneumonia screening for elderly patients.* Influenza and pneumonia together are the fifth leading cause of death among U.S. elderly persons. Yet only approximately 67% of the elderly people in the United States receive the flu vaccine and approximately 55% received the pneumonia vaccine.

15. Why are flu and pneumonia vaccinations important for seniors?

In one study, elderly patients who received a flu shot reduced their hospitalization for pneumonia (29%), flu (32%), heart disease (19%), and stroke (16% to 23%). Vaccinated patients' risk of death from any cause was also lowered by approximately half.

16. Why don't more seniors receive these vaccinations?

Recent shortages aside, self-reported reasons for not being vaccinated included their doctor did not recommend one (59%); did not know they needed it (50%), and/or believed that they were unlikely to get pneumonia (45%).

17. How can the ED make a difference in this vaccination rate? Most EDs don't offer routine vaccinations.

Norwalk et al's study (2004) found that physician offices that use three or more immunization promotion activities had twice as many of their patients receive pneumonia vaccinations. Practices that were able to provide information about a source of free vaccines (elsewhere) had four times more of their patients eventually receiving influenza vaccinations.

Overall, however, they found that the patients' attitudes and knowledge about vaccine were the most important factors. The ED visit is an opportunity to promote awareness and provide teaching. An interesting side note is that only 36% of health workers receive the influenza vaccination each year.

18. Any tips on how to readily obtain a reproduction history?

It is normal to record a woman's GPA, e.g., gravida, para, abortion (elective and spontaneous), and living children. Ask how many pregnancies and then "What happened?" because many women do not attribute a spontaneous miscarriage as an "abortion." If the woman hesitates, I initiate matter-of-factly, "Did you have an abortion?" The woman often seems relieved that I am accepting that option.

19. What about screening for alcohol abuse?

It is recommended to screen everyone. The Emergency Nurses Association (ENA) Board of Directors passed a position statement in support of alcohol screening and brief intervention. See the chapter on alcohol use.

20. What about screening regarding tobacco use?

Despite 70% of smokers saying they would like to quit, only half of those are encouraged to do this by health care providers. The average smoker requires multiple attempts over time to be successful (fewer than 5% of smokers are successful on their first attempt). Many departments have started to add this to their screening and health promotion.

21. Are there mnemonics to help obtain a thorough history?

Several are covered in other chapters, including PQRST (Chapter 6), OLD CART (Chapter 10), POSHPATE and TICOSMO (Chapter 7), CIAMPEDS (Chapter 10), and SAVE A CHILD (Chapter 11). Many standardized charts are designed to have spaces marked for these key areas. See related chapters for further discussion.

22. Why is a thorough history so important?

A medical adage is that 90% of what you need to know to make a "diagnosis" or determination is in the history. "The god is in the details." Consultant Shelley Cohen stresses, "If you don't ask, how will you know?" Specifically, never assume the following is not a consideration:

- The patient didn't fill or take the prescription he or she was given.
- The patient takes insulin but didn't list as medicine but you should know that because they are diabetic.
- The patient already saw a physician about the problem but didn't like the advice.
- The patient already tried their inhaler before coming in.
- Lists _____ as medications, but is not currently taking them.
- The patient lives alone and does not have adequate access to health care resources.

23. Any other tips for obtaining the history?

Slovis et al's (2000) suggestions include:

- Rare manifestations of common diseases are more common than common manifestations of rare diseases.
- Listen to any prehospital clinician's history and then thank them.
- If an ancillary person (secretary, aide, etc.) indicates someone looks sick, they probably are. They deserve to be checked immediately.
- People's faces reflect internal emotions. Watching people's faces will tell you when you or your question has caused/uncovered a painful area.
- Insist on a language of symptoms, feelings, and thoughts. Avoid "organ" talk, such as "How are your sinuses?"
- Be wary of an "accident" in the elderly. Ask how they felt prior to the fall (40% are a result of intrinsic factors, such as syncope or stroke).

- Alcoholics can be drunk and sick. (Alcoholics are never "just drunk" until they are sober.)
- HIV+ patients with respiratory complaints should have respiratory isolation and oxygen saturation.
- Most poisonings will manifest itself within 6 hours. (Two exceptions are acetaminophen and sustained-released pills.)
- If you suspect carbon monoxide poisoning, ask if the patient's pet is sick too.
- Acute loss of unilateral vision or true diplopia is never benign, even if it has totally resolved.
- Think "testicle" with abdominal pain in a young boy or old man.

24. I've heard I should ask if there is anything else the patient wants to say.

In one study, only 4 of 35 patients voiced *all* of the items they wanted to discuss. Items commonly *not* discussed included worries about diagnosis or prognosis, ideas about possible diagnosis, concern about symptoms of side effects, wanting or not wanting prescriptions, or information related to social context. Every problem the patients experienced afterward (such as nonadherence, etc.) was connected to an unvoiced item.

25. How can I handle the Joint Commission on Accreditation of Healthcare Organizations' (JCAHO) requirement for nutritional assessment?

The JCAHO standard PE1.2 states, "nutritional status is assessed when warranted by the patient's need or condition." Methods departments use to meet this need include asking:

- "What did you eat in the last 3 days?"
- "Has there been any recent unexpected weight loss of 10 pounds or more?"
- "Are you on a special diet for which you need additional information?"
- "When was the last time you ate or drank something?"

Others provide a one-page self-screening sheet with listed resources. (See the Internet Resource Box for a link.) Another ED meets the requirement by including and checking it in the discharge instructions if diet modifications were included (e.g., clear-liquid diet today, take ibuprofen with food).

26. What are common causes to consider for a patient with decreased level of consciousness?

Use the mnemonic **TIPS AEIOU:**

T Trauma, Temperature
I Infection
P Psychiatric
S Stroke, Shock, Seizure
A Alcohol
E Endocrine, Exocrine
I Insulin
O Opiate
U Uremia

Key Points

- Obtain a thorough history: "Ninety percent of what you need to know is in the history."
- Ask patients with vague or multiple complaints what made them come in *today.*
- Teach the importance of immunization to the elderly. Only 67% get flu vaccinations and 55% get pneumonia vaccinations.
- Ask about the use of botanical dietary supplements/herbs. Although 68% of middle-aged women used them, only 30% told their clinician.

Internet Resource Box

Emergency Nursing World: Frederick Memorial Hospital—Examine your Nutrition Health
http://www.enw.org/NutritionalScreening.doc

FDA's consumer advice on supplements
www.crsan.gov

National Clearinghouse for Alcohol and Drug Information
www.health.org/about/

National Council on Alcoholism and Drug Dependence, Inc.
www.ncadd.org

Tobacco Information and Prevention Source (TIPS) at National Center for Chronic Disease Prevention and Health Promotion
www.cdc.gov/tobacco

Bibliography

ACC/AHA Expert Consensus Document: Use of sildenafil (Viagra) in patients with cardiovascular disease, *Circulation* 199:168-177, 1999.

Barry CA: Patients' unvoiced agendas in general practice consultations, *BMJ* 320:1246-1250, 2000.

Cohen S: *101 triage tips,* Hohenwald, Tenn, 2002, Health Resources Unlimited.

Fielden NM: ED flu/pneumonia vaccine screening for elderly patients (Managers Forum), *J Emerg Nurs* 30(5):493-494, 2004.

Grossman VGA: *Quick reference to triage,* ed 2, Philadelphia, 2003, Lippincott.

Kruszon-Moran DM, et al: Tetanus and diphtheria immunity among females in the United States: Are recommendations being followed? *Am J Obstet Gynecol* 190:1070-1076, 2004.

Mahady GB, et al: Botanical dietary supplement use in peri- and postmenopausal women, *Menopause* 10:65-72, 2003.

Markowitz JS, Donovan JL, et al: Effect on St. John's wort on drug metabolism by induction of cytochrome P450 3A4 enzyme, *JAMA* 290(11):1500, 2003.

McNair R (President): In the Nature of the Beast: Comprehensive Triage and Patient Flow Workshop, Fairview, NC, 2003, Triage First, Inc.

McNair R (President): *TRIAGE First EDucation: A comprehensive emergency department triage course,* Fairview, NC, 2004, Triage First, Inc.

Nichol KL, Nordin J, Mullooly J, Lask R, Fillbrandt K: Influenza vaccination and reduction in hospitalizations for cardiac disease and stroke among the elderly. *N Engl J Med* 348:1322, 2003.

Noone J: Nutritional Assessment (Managers Forum), *J Emerg Nurs* 28(3):244-245, 2002.

Norwalk MP, Bardella IJ, Zimmerman RK, Shen S: The physician's office: Can it influence adult immunization rates? *Am J Manag Care* 10(1):13-19, 2004.

Rockett IR, Putnam SL, et al: Assessing substance abuse treatment need: A statewide hospital emergency department study, *Ann Emerg Med* 41(6):802, 2003.

Rolniak S, Browning L, MacLeod BA, Cockley P: Complementary and alternative medicine use among urban ED patients: Prevalence and patterns, *J Emerg Nurs* 30(4):318-324, 2004.

Sicherer SH, et al: Prevalence of peanut and tree nut allergy in the United States determined by means of a random digit dial telephone survey: A 5-year follow-up study, *J Allergy Clin Immunol* 112:1203-1207, 2003.

Siks JE, et al: Cost-effectiveness of vaccination against invasive pneumococcal disease among people 50 through 64 years of age: Role of comorbid conditions and race, *Ann Intern Med* 17(138):960-968, 2003.

Slovis CM, Wrenn KD, Meador CK: *A little book of emergency medicine rules,* Philadelphia, 2000, Hanley & Belfus.

U.S. Department of Health and Human Services: Clinical practice guideline: Treating tobacco use and dependence, Washington, DC, 2000, U.S. Public Health Service.

Zimmerman RK, Santibanez TA, Fine MJ, et al: Barrier and facilitators of pneumonococcal vaccination among the elderly, *Vaccine* 21:1491-1512, 2003.

Zimmerman RK, Santibanez TA, Janosky JE: What affects influenza vaccination rates among older patients? *Am J Med* 114:31-38, 2003.

Zimmermann PG: Guiding principles at triage: Advice for new triage nurses, *J Emerg Nurs* 28(1): 24-33, 2002.

Chapter 4

Physical Assessment

Polly Gerber Zimmermann

1. Describe what looking at a patient's general appearance means.

Considering multiple aspects of the patient's physiological status and draw a conclusion about the patient being "well" versus "not well." It starts with ABCDs, but progresses beyond that. See also "across the room assessment" (see Chapter 1) and toxic appearance (see Chapter 11). Other things the nurse would note include:

- Personal Hygiene and Dress—appropriate for temperature, clean
- Overall size—emaciated, obese
- Affect—depressed, energetic
- Posturing/Gait—Limp, steady
- Body Language—grimacing, favoring something
- Pattern of Speech—Clear, Logical

2. What is meant by a focused assessment?

The history and assessment is narrowed to the areas related to the complaint and its possible causes.

3. Suggest a quick determination for whether a patient's ABCs are adequate.

- Use 30-2-CAN DO. There is adequate oxygen and perfusion/circulation if the adult:
  - Has respirations less than 30 per minute (30)
  - Is oriented to person and situation (2)
  - Obeys verbal commands (CAN DO)
- In addition, watch the patient walk. Someone who cannot tolerate the mild stress of walking without a serious effect is working hard to maintain oxygenation.

4. What is a quick way to know if someone's airway is open?

Anyone talking has an open airway. Stridor or drooling is an ominous sign.

5. Describe breathing assessment.

Normal respirations are effortless and quiet. Beyond the respiratory rate, depth, and rhythm, respiratory assessment can include the:

- Ability to speak/breathlessness (sentences, phrases, words)
- Peak Expiratory Flow Rate (PEFR) or Pulse Oximetry (adequacy for oxygenation). The Canadian Emergency Department Triage and Acuity Scale (CTAS) places a higher importance on the patient's PEFR.
- Mental status (oxygen perfusion through the brain)
- Lung sounds
- Work of breathing
- Color: cyanosis is a late sign.

6. Discuss evaluation of the work of breathing.

Increased work is indicated by retractions, grunting, flaring, or the patient's self-rating on the valid, reliable Modified Borg Scale. Have the patient rate how hard they are working to breathe on a 0 to 10 scale. It provides an objective way to monitor the subjective degree of effort to maintain the oxygenation status. A level 8 or above on the Modified Borg Scale is likened to breathing for 5 minutes through a coffee stirrer. This is a person who is likely to suddenly "tire out" despite an adequate current pulse oximeter reading.

7. Provide some guidelines for determining the severity of respiratory distress.

Be concerned about patients with known asthma who come in because there has been an increase in their respiratory symptoms. At the very least, place them in an area where they can be watched and tell them to report any worsening to the emergency staff. Ask, "Is this attack the same or different from your usual attacks?" The CTAS and Manchester Triage Group provide these distinguishers:

SEVERE

CTAS (Level 2, ≤15 minutes)

- PEFR <40% predicted or previous best
- PO_2 <92%

Manchester Triage Group (Level 2, 10 minutes)

- Unable to talk in sentences
- Marked tachycardia (in adult, HR >120), bradycardia (<60 minutes), irregular rhythm
- PEFR ≤33% of best
- PO_2 <95% on O_2 or <90% on air
- Altered conscious level
- Exhaustion

MODERATE

CTAS (Level 3, ≤30 minutes)

- PEFR 40% to 60% predicted/previous best

- Po_2 ≥92% to 94%
- Mild/moderate shortness of breath with exertion
- Frequent cough or night awakening (unable to lie down flat without symptoms)

Manchester (Level 3, 60 minutes)
- PEFR ≤50% of best or predicted best
- Po_2 <95% on room air
- Significant history of asthma (brittle)
- No improvement with inhalation treatment (by self or doctor's office)

MILD
CTAS (Level 4, ≤60 minutes)
- PEFR >60% predicted/previous best
- Po_2 >95%

Manchester (Level 4, 120 minutes)
- Wheeze (audible, auscultated, or "feels" it)
- History of chest infection or chest injury
- Recent problem (within the last 7 days)

8. Should a blood pressure be taken on all adults?

Most do as a screening tool. It is now estimated that 65 million adult Americans (or approximately one-third) have hypertension. One study found that one-third of the ED patients with high blood pressure did not know that they had it.

9. What is now considered a "normal" blood pressure for an adult?

The Seventh Report of the Joint National Committee on Prevention, Detection, Evaluation, and Treatment of High Blood Pressure (JNC 7) for adults (in mm Hg):
- Normal: systolic blood pressure (SBP) ≤120 and diastolic blood pressure (DBP) ≤80
- Prehypertension: SBP 120 to 139 or DBP 80 to 89
- Stage 1 hypertension: SBP 140 to 159 or DBP 90 to 99
- Stage 2 hypertension: SBP ≥160 or DBP ≥100

See Chapter 5 for further discussion.

10. Do emergency nurses play a role in making patients aware of hypertension?

Tanabe et al (2004) found that 73% of the low acuity patients who presented with elevated blood pressures had no documentation of the blood pressure being rechecked and no documentation of the patient being referred for follow-up care. Similarly, don't assume the patient with hypertension is taking the medications on a regular basis.

11. Is it important to adapt these new guidelines in our recommendations?

The National Committee for Quality Assurance estimates that approximately 57,500 patients die each year because they did not receive "best practice" care as recommended by evidence-based medicine. Hypertension is one of the chief identified diagnoses.

12. Is it an Emergency Medical Treatment and Active Labor Act (EMTALA) violation to take the blood pressure for a requesting visitor without providing a medical screening exam (MSE)?

Not if the individual does not request ED evaluation and care. Many departments offer this as a community service and public relations. However, keep interventions to generic teaching and recommendations.

13. Discuss evaluation of "D" or disability.

Disability includes mental status (see also Chapter 55), neuromuscular dysfunction, and pain rating (see Chapter 6).

14. What should be evaluated first when a patient is restless or has a mental status change?

Hypoxia and hypoglycemia.

15. What is traditionally included in assessing a patient's orientation?

Person, place, and time are traditionally noted, with time being the first to show an alteration. We have 4 years to practice who is the president, but only 24 hours for the day of the week. Patients must have all of the items correct to have credit, e.g., city, state, county, hospital name, and floor/room or year, season, date, day, and month. We all know them: if they don't, they are "impaired" in some way.

The social persona can be the last thing to be lost. Do not be fooled by a person's sociability or humor as an answer, such as "Around here, it doesn't matter what day it is because one day is the same as the next."

16. Discuss assessing for recent events.

A more thorough assessment also includes the fourth evaluation for recent events (last 5 days). This is useful in assessing frontal lobe function and is commonly done with stroke evaluations. For instance, "How did you get to the hospital today?" An alternative is to indicate this is a memory quiz and state three things, indicating you will ask about them later. Use unrelated items, such as apple, ball, dog and have the patient repeat them. Do not ask obvious things, such as January, February, or March. At the end of the interview, ask the person to repeat them back to you.

Early dementia will have only some of the information and/or will "hunt" for clues (the day on the newspaper, etc.). In addition, an early sign of dementia or dehydration is a decreased ability to focus (unable to say the days of the week backwards).

17. Discuss assessment of the movement and strength of the extremities.

Many elderly patients have the effects of arthritis (or even deconditioning) in their hands and forearms that can contribute to subtle weakness in an assessment. Instead of the traditional hand grasp, try:

- The examiner's second and third middle index finger grasped by the patient: you should have to work hard to remove it when they are tightly holding it.
- Have the patient hold both arms straight up, palm forward for 20 seconds. Try to force an arm down (there should be significant resistance). Watch for any drifting. Another version is to have the patient hold their arms straight out, laterally from the body, and try to force the arm down.
- Palmar drift. The patient holds both arms straight out, palm side up for 10 seconds, with their eyes closed. There should be no drifting; a positive palmar drift is the weaker side's arm moving down and turning the palm medially.

18. What is a good way to distinguish the various levels of best motor?

Lower suggests asking the person to hold up two fingers for "obeys commands." Then you know there was no reflex involved. For withdrawing, apply peripheral pain and continue to hold the painful stimulation as the patient withdraws. If the patient continues to pull away after an initial movement, then it is withdrawing and not a reflex.

19. What is essential to do in a nursing neurologic exam?

A typical nursing neurologic check includes a Glasgow Coma Scale (GCS) score, a pupillary examination, and a brief motor assessment. In essence, can the patient walk, talk, and move their eyes? The "C" in ABCD should also include stabilization of the C-spine in appropriate patients.

20. What should guide a good neurologic assessment?

- Maximum stimulation for maximum response. Nurses are often reluctant to inflict pain on a comatose patient, but it is necessary to have an accurate trending of the important subtle changes.
- Pain stimulation should be applied for at least 15 seconds.
- On a sternal rub, use a knuckle like a pestle and mortar, not like rubbing a washboard.
- Vary the site. Bruising may result, so also use a trapezius squeeze or pressure on the supraorbital rim. Twisting the nipples or squeezing the scrotum is no longer considered ethical.

21. Any other recommendations in doing a good neurologic assessment and documentation?

- Avoid vague terms (lethargic, stuporous, or obtunded) that mean different things to different observers. The best practice is to describe the state of arousal (alert?) and the mental functions the patient can perform (e.g., knows city and president but unable to state month).
- Approach the patient silently. Nurses often talk while approaching the patient, but then you do not know if the patient is spontaneously opening their eyes to sensing the nurse's presence or to the voice.
- Use the best response in the GCS. If one side has flexion and one side has extension, the patient gets credit for the extension. However, also test for a peripheral nerve response/paralysis by pressing a pencil into the patient's nail bed.
- Inadequate or inaccurate baseline assessments, can lead to failure to pick up subtle clues.

Lower explains that nurses often fail to:

- Obtain adequate details. In future assessments, the lack of previous details is an early warning.
- Ask the questions of all patients. Lower's study found that ED nurses would not ask basic orientation questions of patients who looked affluent or well-educated because they would feel silly. Simply preface the assessment with an explanation such as "I have to ask you some questions that might sound a little silly, but they really will help me to have a good idea of your brain function so I can take the best care of you."

22. What if we suspect the unresponsiveness may be purposeful (i.e., faking), such as someone who "faints" right as the check is brought in the restaurant?

As a Navajo proverb says, "You can't wake up a man pretending to be asleep." Telltale signs can include peeking or nonrhythmic seizure activity (check the tongue for a laceration as a clue that a real seizure has occurred). Other "tricks of the trade" include:

- Looking for a response to calculated statements, such as "We'll need to insert a large urinary catheter if he doesn't wake up."
- Instilling natural tear eyedrops (and watching for resistance)
- Introducing noxious stimuli (such as ammonia). It is ethical to do some neurological testing (pain stimuli, Babinski reflex), which are not only noxious, but provide helpful clinical data also.
- Placing the patient's hand directly above his or her face and allowing the hand to drop (protecting the patient's face with your hand). If there is a physiologic reason for the patient's condition, the hand will smack the patient's face/your hand (because of gravity). If the reason is psychogenic, the patient lets the hand drift to the side.
- Opening the eyelids. If the eyes deviate upward and only the sclera show (Bell's phenomenon) you should suspect psychogenic causes. The eyelids close slowly and incompletely (a movement difficult to fake) when opened in a patient with a true coma.

- If all else fails, cold caloric testing can be done, looking for nystagmus.

23. Is the blink test reliable?

A patient with a suspected psychogenic cause may blink when you rapidly flick your hand at a comatose patient who has open eyes. However, the flow of air may also have been the stimulation for a corneal reflex in a patient who is truly comatose.

24. What can cause a coma or altered mental status?

Use the mnemonic TIPS AEIOU

Trauma, Temperature
Infection (central nervous system and systemic)
Psychiatric
Space-occupying lesion, Stroke, Subarachnoid hemorrhage, Shock
Alcohol and other drugs
Endocrine, Exocrine, Electrolytes
Insulin (diabetes)
Oxygen (lack of), Opiates
Uremia

Another mnemonic for Altered Mental Status is VITAMINS

Vascular
Infections
Trauma
A lot of toxins
Metabolic
Intussusception
Neoplasms
Seizure

25. What is recommended for screening a patient who is possibly having an acute stroke?

The Los Angeles Prehospital Stroke Screen (LAPSS) (which uses patient history, blood glucose level, and brief examination) and the Cincinnati Prehospital Stroke Scale (CPSS) (which uses three assessment parameters: facial droop, palmar arm drift, and speech). Assess facial droop by asking the patient to smile or show their teeth. Assess speech impairment/slurring by asking the patient to say, "You can't teach an old dog new tricks." Developed and validated for prehospital use, they are beneficial for triage.

26. What is recommended for ongoing assessment in a patient who is possibly having an acute stroke?

The past level of nursing neuro assessment is not adequate for evaluation of the acute stroke population. The GCS was developed for traumatic brain injury populations, but is not sensitive to subtle changes.

What is now recommended is the National Institutes of Health Stroke Scale (NIHSS). It is capable of identifying stroke severity, documenting subtle serial changes in status, and assigning a numeric value to findings. The 2001 American Heart Association's Advanced Cardiac Life Support Provider Manual indicates that this valid and reliable tool has become the standard for neurologic function and should be used by those who care for ED acute stroke patients.

27. Discuss the role ED nurses can have in stroke/brain attack, cerebral vascular accident (CVA) awareness.

One study found that 43% of the public knew no signs or symptoms of a brain attack, compared to 80% to 90% of the public knowing the signs and symptoms of a heart attack. Provide information about the symptoms, and also the need to call 911 if the patient notes facial droop, arm drift, or speech alteration. In the same study, only 43% indicated they would call 911. The time for arrival to the emergency department is 2 to 3 times longer if arranging one's own transportation and 3 to 4 times longer if calling one's physician first.

28. What percentage of patients with a vertebral column fracture or dislocation present with neurologic impairment?

That would be 14%-15%. Injury to the cervical spine has a higher rate of neurologic compromise than do lower spine injuries.

29. How should I approach the potential risk in patients?

Consider mechanism of injury (MOI). The most common causes of spinal injury of vehicular crashes (39%); violence, primarily gunshot wounds (26%); and falls (22%). Consider the patient's mental status. If alcohol, drugs, head injury, shock, or any other cause alters pain perception, the injury should be assumed to be present.

McNamara and Klevens (2003) suggest that a helpful reminder for a potential spine injury is that "a proper history is A MUST":

- Altered mental state. Check for drugs or alcohol.
- Mechanism. Does the potential for injury exist?
- Underlying conditions. Are high-risk factors for fractures present?
- Symptoms. Is pain or paresthesia part of the picture?
- Timing. When did the symptoms begin in relation to the event?

30. What is physically examined in the spine for spinal cord trauma?

Parameters to assess on physical examination are a neurologic examination and palpating the spine for tenderness, deformity, and muscle spasm. However, the examiner feels only the posterior elements and a fracture may be present despite a lack of tenderness.

31. Can nurses routinely assess the need to apply or remove a cervical collar?

Yes. Many emergency medical systems (EMS) have a standard operating procedure for an initial assessment of spine injuries. A positive finding in any of the criteria results in immediate immobilization. The four components of the examination include:

- Determination of an uncertain or questionable MOI
- Patient ability to participate in the examination (e.g., altered mental status, distracting injuries, communication problems, patient younger than 8 years of age, intoxication)
- Spinal pain or tenderness (by questioning and palpitation)
- Motor/sensory examination

Based on the EMS success, some emergency departments (EDs) use a similar nursing assessment to determine if an ambulatory patient needs immobilization and/or if an immobilized patient can be removed from the backboard.

32. Is it dangerous for patient with a severe brain injury to wear a cervical collar?

It could be. Some recent studies have shown that the hard cervical collar can cause increases in intracranial pressure (ICP) because it can contribute to jugular venous compression and obstruction of venous outflow from the brain.

33. Discuss how to remember the cranial nerves.

The cranial nerves are:

I	Olfactory nerve
II	Optic nerve
III	Oculomotor nerve
IV	Trochlear nerve
V	Trigeminal nerve
VI	Abducens nerve
VII	Facial nerve
VIII	Vestibulocochlear nerve
IX	Glossopharyngeal nerve
X	Vagus nerve
XI	Accessory nerve
XII	Hypoglossal nerve

Many use the timeless saying, "On Old Olympus' Towering Top, A Finn and German Viewed Some Hops" to remember the cranial nerves. However, you still need to remember the functions with the names, such as oculomotor, trochlear, and abducens effect eye movement. Rayfield's saying, "3,4,6, make my eyes do tricks" helps the nurse recall that these cranial nerves affect pupil constriction, eyelid movement, and eyeball movement (six points of gaze).

The seventh cranial nerve, facial, effects expression, tearing, and saliva. The most common dysfunction is a one-sided droop, Bell's palsy. Picture a bell with a VII on it to help recall which cranial nerve is involved. Note that the clapper is an eyeball to remember the eyelid involvement and need for eye care.

The eighth cranial nerve, acoustic, controls balance and hearing. Picture a cheerleader with the accompanying saying, "3,4,6,8: how do we accommodate?" A cheerleader obviously needs balance to accommodate and picture her cupping her ear to "hear" the cheer. Her circling eyes remind you of the 3,4,6 for eye tricks.

34. How can I distinguish petechiae and purpura from other rashes?

These rashes do not blanch.

35. What causes paired or butterfly-shaped bruises on the skin?

Pinching. They are usually self-inflicted or signs of abuse.

36. How do most departments handle weights on children and adults?

Most obtain actual weights on children and stated weights on adults. Regardless of the method, it is good to indicate if the weight noted on the chart is actual or stated.

37. What should I consider in a patient who is reporting hearing loss or vertigo?

Excessive earwax. If you can't see the tympanic membrane, the wax needs to be removed.

38. Any tips about performing a physical assessment?

- Always put your hand on and examine the body area that the patient reports is hurting.
- Remove the patient's clothing when examining the patient in the treatment area.
- Don't assume anything is as bad as it looks: most things are not. This is helpful to remember when approaching very bloody or critically ill appearing patients.
- Ask about the amount of blood loss at the scene for lacerations to vascular areas, such as the scalp or thigh.
- Nonexertional sweating and new fecal incontinence are serious findings.

39. What is Sudden in Custody Death Syndrome?

This syndrome refers to young, "healthy" adults who have an unexpected cardiac arrest after being in police custody. It occurs when there was a physical struggle of some type and its cause is hypothesized to be a result of the sudden release of excessive adrenaline.

Key Points

- Use 30-2-CAN DO for an across-the-room assessment of stability of the ABCs.
- Ask a patient with shortness of breath/breathlessness to rate the work or effort of their breathing on a scale of 0 to 10 (Modified Borg Scale).
- Rapidly assess for the possibility of a stroke by facial droop (show your teeth), speech impairment (say "Can't teach an old dog new tricks") and palmar drift. Perform initial and on-going neurologic assessments on a potential stroke patient with the NIH stroke scale.
- Assess for a faking "coma" by the hand drop and lifting the eyelids.

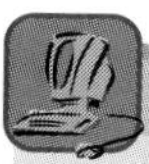

Internet Resource Box

Women: Stay Healthy at Any Age: Checklist for Your Next Checkup
http://www.ahrq.gov/ppip/healthywom.htm

Men: Stay Healthy at Any Age: Checklist for Your Next Checkup
http://www.ahrq.gov/ppip/healthymen.htm

NCQA: Measuring the Quality of America's Health Care
http://www.ncqa.org/Communications/News/sohc2003.htm

Bibliography

American Heart Association: Acute ischemic stroke. In Cummins R, editor: *ACLS provider manual,* Dallas, 2001, American Heart Association.

Baren JM, Alpern ER: *Emergency medicine pearls,* Philadelphia, 2004, Hanley & Belfus.

Bickley LS, Szilagyi PG: *Bates' guide to physical examination and history taking,* ed 8, Philadelphia, 2003, Lippincott.

Chobanian AV, et al: The seventh report of the Joint National Committee on Prevention, Detection, Evaluation, and Treatment of High Blood Pressure: The JNC 7 report, *JAMA* 189:2560-2572, 2003.

Criddle LM, Bonnono C, Fisher SK: Standardizing stroke assessment using the National Institutes of Health Stroke Scale, *J Emerg Nurs* 29(6):541-546, 2003.

Hammerschmidt R, Meador CK: *A little book of nurses' rules.* Philadelphia, 1993, Hanley & Belfus.

Jackimczyk KC: Altered mental status and coma. In Markovchick VJ, Pons PT, editors: *Pons' emergency medicine secrets,* ed 3, Philadelphia, 2003, Hanley & Belfus.

Kendrick KR: Can a self-rating 0-10 scale for dyspnea yield a common language that is understood by ED nurses, patients, and their families? *J Emerg Nurs* 26(3):233-234, 2000.

Kendrick KR, Baxi SC, Smith RM: Usefulness of the modified 0-10 Borg scale in assessing the degree of dyspnea in patients with COPD and asthma, *J Emerg Nurs* 26(3):216-222, 2000.

Kothari R, Pancioli A, Lui T, Brott T, Broderick J: Cincinnati prehospital stroke scale: Reproducibility and validity, *Ann Emerg Med* 33:373-378, 1999.

Lester O: Weight measurements (Managers Forum), *J Emerg Nurs* (in press).

Loving G: EMS field spine clearance (Managers Forum), *J Emerg Nurs* 27:286-288, 2001.

Lower JK: Facing neuro assessment fearlessly, *Nursing* 32(2):58-64, 2002.

McNamara RM, Klevens MJ: Spine and spinal cord trauma. In Markovchick VJ, Pons PT, editors: *Pons' emergency medicine secrets,* ed 3, Philadelphia, 2003, Hanley & Belfus.

Metheny NM: *Fluid & electrolyte balance nursing consideration,* ed 4, Philadelphia, 2000, Lippincott.

Rayfield S, Manning L: *Nursing made insanely easy!* ed 3, Gulf Shores, Al, 2002, ICAN, Inc. Publishing.

Slovis CM, Wrenn KD, Meador CK: *A little book of emergency medicine rules,* Philadelphia, 2000, Hanley & Belfus.

Tanabe P, Steinmann R, Kippenhan M, Stehman C, Beach C: Undiagnosed hypertension in the ED setting: An unrecognized opportunity by emergency nurses, *J Emerg Nurs* 30(3):225-229, 2004.

Zimmermann PG: Guiding principles at triage: Advice for new triage nurses, *J Emerg Nurs* 28(1): 24-33, 2002.

Zimmermann PG: Tricks for the ED trade, *J Emerg Nurs* 29(5):453-458, 2003.

Chapter 5

Vital Signs

Polly Gerber Zimmermann

1. Is a complete set of vital signs needed on patients with localized complaints?

Some do not require routine universal vital signs for a clearly localized problem (e.g., sprained ankle) or children less than 3 years of age. Additional considerations include:

- *Nursing time.* Travers (1999) found triage lasted 1.6 minutes longer if a complete set of vital signs were taken.
- *Screening role.* Nearly one third of those with hypertension are unaware of it. Routine vital signs can provide a teaching opportunity.
- *Public Relations.* Patients equate vital signs with "good care." Emergency department (ED) staff nurse Tom Trimble, RN, uses the experience with children to demystify the process (an "officer friendly" program for nursing) and to encourage nursing as a career.

2. Give some examples of EDs' policies regarding children's vital signs.

Schneck Medical Center (Seymour, IN)
Source: Melissa Anderson, RN; ED Staff Nurse
Blood pressures taken:

- ≥3 years
- Having an IV
- Being admitted
- Any child of any age who, in the nurses' judgment, has symptoms or a history that could affect the blood pressure (vomiting, diarrhea, trauma, etc.)

MetroHealth Medical Center (Cleveland, OH)
Source: Barbara Wolfe, RN, ED Staff/Charge Nurse
Blood pressures for:

- Children ≥4 years
- Any systemic condition that would warrant it
- Temperatures (only rectal) on all pediatric patients regardless

Iroquois Memorial Hospital (Watseka, IL)
Source: Abby Purvis, RN CEN; ED Director

- No blood pressure for minor illness or extremity injury on a patient <18 years
- Temperature on all patients
  - Tympanic or rectal for <6 years of age
  - No tympanic thermometer for <3 months or a suspected abnormal body temperature

Children's Memorial Hospital (Chicago, IL)
Rebecca Steinman, RN MS CEN CCRN CCNS, ED Clinical Educator

- Blood pressures are taken on all children as part of the initial assessment and p.r.n. (as needed)

3. Is there a simple way to remember the "normal" pediatric ranges?

Use Rayfield and Manning's chart (2002). Recall that neonates have a heart rate of 140. Pull out the 40 for the respiration rate. Then the heart rate goes down approximately 20 and the respiration rate decreases by approximately 10 for each age group.

Neonate	
Respiratory	40
Heart rate	140
Toddler (age 2 to 4)	
Respiratory	30
Heart rate	120
Child (age 6 to 10)	
Respiratory	20
Heart rate	100
Adult	
Respiratory	12 to 18
Heart rate	60 to 100

4. Give some guidelines for evaluating the respiratory parameters and triage acuity for severe respiratory distress.

The Canadian Triage and Acuity Scale (CTAS) indicates Level 2 (Emergent, ≤15 minutes)

- Peak Expiratory Flow Rate (PEFR) <40% predicted or previous best
- Po_2 <92%

The PEFR is preferred, but for patients unable to do that, particularly for children under age 6, use oxygen saturation and clinical features.

The Manchester Triage Group Level 2 (Very Urgent, 10 minutes)

- Unable to talk in sentences
- Marked tachycardia (in adult, HR >120)
- Increased work of breathing (increased respiratory rate, use of accessory muscles, grunting) in children
- Exhaustion (e.g., appears to have reduced respiratory effort despite the same continuing respiratory insufficiency)
- Acute onset immediately or shortly after a recent physically traumatic event
- PEFR ≤33% of best
- Po_2 <95% on O_2 or <90% on room air

5. How about moderate respiratory distress?

CTAS Level 3 (≤30 minutes)

Moderate shortness of breath

- PEFR 40% to 60% predicted/previous best
- PO_2 ≥92% to 94%

Mild shortness of breath

- PEFR >60%
- PO_2 ≥95%
- Considerable shortness of breath with exertion, frequent cough, or night awakening (e.g., unable to lie down flat without symptoms)
- Considerable past medications (e.g., inhaler overuse) and/or previous attack patterns (history of intubation, ICU admission, frequent hospitalizations)
- Indicates tightness in the throat or that the respiratory symptoms are worsening

Avoid low triage ratings in an asthmatic that has come in because of increased respiratory symptoms. Always keep under observation in the waiting room.

Manchester Level 30 (Urgent, 60 minutes)

- PEFR ≤50% of best/predicted best
- PO_2 <95% on room air
- Significant history of asthma (brittle or previous life-threatening episodes)
- No improvement with inhalation therapy (either self- or doctor-administered prior to arrival)

6. How about examples of mild dyspnea triage?

CTAS (Less Urgent, ≤1 hour)

- PO_2 = 95% or better

Flulike symptoms

Manchester Triage Group (Standard, 120 minutes)

Any sense of "wheeze" (audible wheeze or even a subjective feeling of wheeze)

Presence of chest infection or injury

Recent (less than 1 week) problem

7. Describe use of the Borg scale.

On a scale of 0 to 10 (sometimes with a visual scale), have the patient rate the *effort* that is being expended for breathing. Although pulse oximetry indicates current oxygenation, the effort indicates the *work* to maintain that level of oxygenation. A rating of level 8 or higher is likened to breathing through a coffee stirrer.

8. How is bradycardia in a child approached?

Bradycardia in a child equals hypoxia until proven otherwise and is considered emergent. Fluid volume deficit, acidosis, and drug ingestion could be other causes.

9. Where should a pulse be taken on a child?

Apical is recommended if the child is less than 3 years of age. Use the brachial, popliteal, or femoral pulses to feel for the presence of a pulse.

10. What is a quick way to tell if someone has adequate oxygen and perfusion to the brain?

30-2-CAN DO. The patient is considered to have adequate oxygen and perfusion to the brain if:
- Respirations are <30 per minute (30).
- The person knows who he or she is and the current situation (2).
- The person obeys a verbal command (CAN DO).

11. What is a quick assessment to be sure a patient has an adequate blood pressure?

Studies have found variation, but as a general rule-of-thumb
- A palpable radial pulse, the systolic blood pressure (SBP) is at least 80.
- A palpable femoral pulse, the SBP is at least 70.
- A palpable carotid pulse, the SBP is at least 60.

12. List alternative sites for a blood pressure measurement if the upper arms can't be used as a result of injury.

- The forearm with the radial artery: systolic pressure is 10 mm Hg lower than the brachial artery
- The thigh with the popliteal artery: systolic pressure is 10 mm Hg higher than the brachial artery
- Just above the malleoli with the dorsal pedis or posterior tibial artery: systolic and diastolic values are the same as the brachial artery

13. What are the current recommendations for a "normal" adult blood pressure?

The Joint National Committee on Prevention, Detection, Evaluation, and Treatment of High Blood Pressure (JNC) classified the new target blood pressure as below 120/80 mm Hg (2003). "Prehypertensive" is classified as 120 to 139/80 to 89.

14. Why is it important to talk to patients about hypertension?

Approximately 50 million Americans have hypertension. For every 20-mm increase in the systolic pressure, the risk of heart disease doubles. Tanabe et al found that opportunities for education were not routinely taken in the ED.

15. Describe orthostatic vital signs.

The blood pressure and pulse are taken lying, sitting, and standing, with at least 1 minute between each position change. A range of 10 to 20 beats increase in the pulse and a 10 to 20 beats decrease in the systolic blood pressure with standing is considered "positive" for dehydration. Pulse is the more sensitive indicator.

16. Are orthostatic vital signs an absolute accurate indicator of dehydration?

They are not reliable as a sole indicator and with the older adult. In normal hydrated patients who are 65 years or older, there will be a false positive more than 25% of the time. Normal physiologic response variability is also wider than previously thought. One study found that a blood pressure drop of 20 mm Hg has only 25% sensitivity and 81% specificity for ≥5% fluid deficit. Another study found routine heart rate increases from 5 to 39 beats per minute, probably from baroreceptor stimulation.

17. Give some formulas to help estimate normal pediatric blood pressure.

- Systolic over 2 years = 90 + (2 × age)
- Diastolic is two thirds of the systolic
- Lower systolic limit over 2 years = 70 + (2 × age)

18. Discuss pulse pressure.

Pulse pressure is the difference between systolic and diastolic blood pressures. Normally systolic pressure exceed diastolic by approximately 40 mm Hg. Narrow pulse pressure occurs with increased peripheral vascular resistance, decreased cardiac output, and fluid volume deficit. A widening pulse pressure can be a normal response to conditions (fever, exercise, etc.) but can also be evident with increased intracranial pressure.

19. Do rectal, oral, and axillary temperatures correlate?

Rectal is the most accurate method for a core temperature. There is no absolute reliable correlation for the different methods. Oral temperatures vary by up to 2.9°F (1.6°C) depending on where the probe is positioned in the mouth. Oral temperatures are usually 1.3°F (0.7°C) lower than rectal temperatures, and are significantly influenced by respiratory rate, heart rate, recent smoking, and recent ingestion of hot or cold liquids. Axillary temperature is reportedly 1.3°F (0.7°C) lower than oral temperatures. The normal diurnal variation for temperature in children is up to 1.1°C (~1.9°F) and 2°C (3.6°F) in adults. This circadian variation remains in febrile individuals.

20. Does the degree of fever always directly correlate with the severity of illness?

No. Fever magnitude is not helpful in predicting the presence of bacteremia in adult patients. However, Barkin and Rosen (2003) indicates each degree elevation from approximately 39°C (102.2°F) increases the risk of occult bacteremia.

21. What is the effect of fever on the other vital signs?

Each 1°F (0.55°C) of fever increases the basal metabolic rate by 7%. The pulse typically increases approximately 10 beats per minute for each 0.6°C (1°F) increase in temperature. Tachycardia inappropriate for the degree of fever can occur in early septic shock, hypoglycemia, hypovolemia, or an overdose. Tachypnea out of proportion to the fever can occur in pneumonia, gram-negative bacteremia, CNS lesion, or a systemic acidoses (DKA) (see Chapter 18).

22. Should every patient with a fever have an absolute white blood cell count (WBC) done?

There is no laboratory or historical factor that can definitely exclude a serious underlying bacterial disease. Any absolute WBC and band count should be interpreted in light of the patient's clinical picture. Some believe that a normal WBC count and differential have a high negative predictive value for serious bacterial illness (i.e., normal values imply that serious disease does not exist).

23. How can I obtain an optimal pulse oximeter reading?

Oxygen saturation measured by pulse oximetry closely correlates with arterial blood gas levels if the patient does not have peripheral vascular disease and the oxygen saturation is >70%. The source must be warm, with good circulation (test the capillary refill), and without impeding artifact (dark nail polish). Although the finger tends to give the best reading, alternative sites include the toe, ear lobe (which tends to run slightly higher), bridge of the nose, or side of the hand (especially in children). Readings can be affected by localized edema, use of noninvasive automatic blood pressure cuff on the extremity, intravascular dye, severe anemia, carbon monoxide inhalation, or nitrate therapy.

24. What else is called the fifth vital sign?

A pain rating on all patients. The Joint Commission for Accreditation of Healthcare Organizations (JCAHO) requires that facilities must have specific procedures for pain assessment and management. Most EDs apply this standard as minimally assessing the pain on arrival in triage and on discharge (if present). For further discussion, see Chapter 6.

25. Is rechecking vital signs required prior to discharge?

It is a standard of care to *reassess* a patient after the initial assessment/triage before discharge (which often includes vital signs). However, it would be more informative to evaluate pain relief and an ability to take oral fluids in a patient with a migraine.

26. Give an example of a reassessment policy.

Rex Healthcare (Raleigh, NC)
Source: Elizabeth Murphy, RN CEN BSBA, Quality Assurance Representative
Department standards are:

- Nurses' notes after the patient has been in the department for 2 hours (or sooner as warranted)

- Reassessment of the chief complaint (or new ones) every 2 hours.
- Vital signs retaken every 4 hours (or more often as clinically indicated)
- Reassessment of all patients at time of discharge for changes in vital signs, pain scale, and current clinical status at the time of discharge.
- Nurse documents the vital signs and notifies the provider of abnormal results prior to the patient's discharge when the patient's vital signs fall within the parameters in the following table:

	ADULT	CHILD 1 to 8 years	INFANT 0 to 12 months
Blood Pressure	>150/90	<80/60	
Pulse	<50	<80	<100
	>100	>120	>140
Respirations	>28	>28	>32
Temperature	>100.5°F (38°C)	>100.5°F (38°C)	>100.5°F (38°C)

Key Points

- Ask the patient with a respiratory complaint to rate the effort of breathing on a scale of 1 to 10 (Borg scale). It indicates the work for oxygenation and who might arrest.
- Quick check for adequate oxygenation and perfusion is 30-2-CAN DO.
- Orthostatics are not reliable as a sole indicator of dehydration, and tend to be less accurate in the older adult.
- The new recommended target blood pressure is 120/80 (prehypertensive is 120 to 139/80 to 89).
- Degree of fever is not helpful in predicting bacteremia in adult patients.
- Each 1°F (0.55°C) of fever increases the metabolic rate by 7% (increases pulse by 10 bpm)

Internet Resources

Emergency Nurses Association
www.ena.org

Emergency Nursing World
www.enw.org

Canadian Association of Emergency Physicians
www.caep.ca

Emergency Nursing Journal Online
http://emj.bmjjournals.com/

Sylvia Rayfield & Associates, Inc.
www.sylviarayfield.com

Bibliography

Anderson M: Pediatric routine vital signs (Managers Forum), *J Emerg Nurs* (in press).

Barkin RM, Rosen P: *Emergency pediatrics: A guide to ambulatory care,* ed 6, St Louis, 2003, Mosby.

Canadian Association of Emergency Physicians: Canadian Emergency Department Triage and Acuity Scale implementation guidelines, *J Can Assoc Emerg Physicians* 1:3, 1999.

Chobanian AV, et al: The seventh report of the Joint National Committee on Prevention, Detection, Evaluation, and Treatment of High Blood Pressure: The JNC 7 report, *JAMA* 289:2560-2572, 2003.

Danzl DF: Hypothermia and frostbite. In Markovchick VJ, Pons PT, editors. *Pons' emergency medicine secrets,* ed 3, Philadelphia, 2003, Hanley & Belfus.

De Jong M, Moser D, An K, Chung M: Anxiety is not manifested by elevated heart rate and blood pressure in acutely ill cardiac patients, Abstract at the NTI & Critical Care Exposition, AACN, May 2004, Orlando, Fla.

Eibert W: Febrile adults. In Hamilton GC, Sanders AB, Strange GR, Trott AT, editors: *Emergency medicine: An approach to clinical problem-solving,* ed 2, Philadelphia, 2003, WB Saunders.

Graneto JW, Soglin DF: Maternal screening of childhood fever by palpation, *Pediatr Emerg Care* 12: 183-184, 1996.

Grossman VGA: *Quick reference to triage,* ed 2, Philadelphia, 2003, Lippincott.

Hurley ML: The latest hypertension guidelines, *RN* 66(8):43-45, 2003.

Kentrick KR, Baxi SC, Smith RM: Usefulness of the modified 0-10 Borg scale in assessing the degree of dyspnea in patients with COPD and asthma, *J Emerg Nurs* 16:216-222, 2000.

Lamb RP, Birnbaumer DM: Fever. In Markovchick VJ, Pons PT, editors: *Pons' emergency medicine secrets,* ed 3, Philadelphia, 2003, Hanley & Belfus.

Mackway-Jones K: Emergency triage: Manchester Triage Group, London, 1997, BMJ Publishing Group.

McConnell EA: Performing pulse oximetry, *Nursing* 11:17, 1999.

Murphy E: Reassessment times (Managers Forum), *J Emerg Nurs* 31(2):189, 2005.

Murphy KA: *Pediatric triage guidelines,* St Louis, 1997, Mosby.

Nelson DS: Emergency treatment of fever phobia, *J Emerg Nurs* 24(1):83-84, 1998.

Purvis A: Pediatric routine vital signs (Managers Forum), *J Emerg Nurs* (in press).

Rayfield S, Manning L: *Nursing made insanely easy!* ed 3, Gulf Shores, Al, 2002, ICAN, Inc. Publishing.

Steinman R: Pediatric routine vital signs (Managers Forum), *J Emerg Nurs* (in press).

Tanabe P, Steinmann R, Kippenhan M, Stehman C, Beach C: Undiagnosed hypertension in the ED setting—An unrecognized opportunity by emergency nurses, *J Emerg Nurs* 29(3):225-229, 2004.

Travers D: Triage: How long does it take? How long should it take? *J Emerg Nurs* 25(3):238-240, 1999.

Trimble T: Routine pediatric vital signs (Managers Forum), *J Emerg Nurs* (in press).

Wolfe B: Routine pediatric vital signs (Managers Forum), *J Emerg Nurs* (in press).

Zimmermann PG: Guiding principles at triage: Advice for new triage nurses, *J Emerg Nurs* 28(1): 24-33, 2002

Zimmermann PG: Tricks for the ED trade, *J Emerg Nurs* 29(5):453-458, 2003.

Chapter 6

Pain Assessment and Management

Polly Gerber Zimmermann

1. Why is pain assessment important for the triage nurse?

Pain relief provides physiologic and psychologic benefits and is a patient's right. The American Pain Society (APS) identifies pain assessment as the fifth vital sign.

2. Is the pain experience the same for every patient?

The classic definition is that pain is "whatever the experiencing person says it is and it exists whenever he says it does" (McCaffery, 1989). Research showed that patients perceived the same stimuli anywhere from a "1" to "9" sensation. In addition, circumstantial factors could temporally alter any individual's pain threshold or tolerance.

3. Why should the triage nurse ask rather than wait to see if the patient initiates the complaint about pain?

Patients do not always initiate reporting their pain because of fear, mistaken beliefs (e.g., analgesics are addictive, relief is unavailable), or altered mental status.

4. Are vital signs a dependable indicator of severe pain?

Research shows that elevated vital signs related to pain may occur for only a short time. The body seeks equilibrium: in an hour or less the vital signs usually return to what they were previously regardless of the patient's relief.

5. When should pain be assessed?

It is considered a part of an initial nursing assessment, usually performed in triage. Pain reassessment should be done in a timely manner, at least after any intervention to relieve pain, and many practitioners routinely include it as part of the emergency department (ED) discharge assessment.

6. What patient descriptions could help determine when a patient's pain is serious?

- Comparison to a previous experience, such as "my typical migraine"

- History of significant events causing similar pain, such as a history of kidney stones or a myocardial infarction (MI)
- Identification of a new distinction, such as "the worse headache I've ever had"

7. What should initiate concern that the patient's pain is serious?

Pain that is the most concern is pain that:

- Begins abruptly, e.g., the patient can recall the exact time or activity when the pain began
- Has maximum severity at the onset, e.g., reaches the greatest intensity in less than 1 minute
- Awakened the patient from sleep
- Described as a constant ache, pressure, burning, or squeezing
- Has associated vital sign changes

8. Should pain medications routinely be withheld until the etiology is known?

That is no longer considered necessary. Studies found there were no differences in the physical findings or diagnostic accuracy between patients who received morphine and those who received a placebo.

- The APS (1999) guideline states that pain should be treated while investigation proceeds and withholding analgesia is rarely justified.
- The American College of Emergency Physicians' clinical policy statement (1994) encourages early pain relief in stable patients with nontraumatic acute abdomen.
- The Canadian Association of Emergency Physicians' (1994) consensus statement indicates that there is no "justification to not relieve the (abdominal) pain immediately. Judicious IV opioid titration to relieve most of the pain...allows a better abdominal examination.

9. What is a common way to assess the intensity of pain in an adult?

A numeric rating scale (NRS). The patient provides a self-rating on a scale of 0 to 10. Pain relief is ordinarily provided for a self-rating of 4 or higher.

10. Some patients can't seem to numerically rate their pain. Talk about other ways.

Overall, scales are less helpful (or reliable) at the extremes of age. Other options include:

- A descriptive word. Concern is raised if a foreboding word is used, such as "unbearable," "excruciating," or "disabling."
- Visual Analog Scale (VAS). A pencil and paper 100-mm line divided into 10-mm segments, labeled from 0 to 10. The patient indicates along the measurement bar.
- The FACES pain scale, developed for use with children, can be used with adults when a language barrier is present or the patient is cognitively impaired.

- Turning the horizontal scale vertically can be helpful for individuals who speak a language that reads vertically or from right to left. The scale should be positioned so that "10" is at the top because sequences that progress upward are more universally recognizable than those that progress downward.
- The Manchester Triage Group suggests comparing the disruption to the usual activities.
- If nothing works, treat the patient if it is believed they have severe pain.

11. Provide the PQRST mnemonic.

Provokes	What provokes the symptoms?
Quality	What makes it better/worse? What does it feel like?
Radiation	Where is it? Where does it radiate?
Severity	Rate on a scale of 1 to 10?
Time	How long?
Treatment	What has been done already?

12. What if the patient's self-rating is questionable, like 10 for a "cold"?

The first time any individual experiences a new type of pain, it actually is the "worst ever" or a 10 for that individual. Ask about the worst pain ever experienced before this. If the current pain is compared to an incident such as childbirth, renal colic, or a fracture, then the nurse knows the pain is probably severe. Slovis et al (2000) suggests before automatically accepting the "worst headache of your life," always ask, "Have you had many other worst headaches of your life before today?"

13. Why should the triage nurse ask about the type of pain?

The type of pain holds clues about the etiology. A superficial or local nerve tissue ending is pain that is more well-localized, sharp, constant, throbbing, or tingling. Generally, pain is less serious if it is crampy, intermittent, or sharp without vital sign abnormalities.

14. How do I handle patients who are "drug seekers"?

Do not automatically and/or independently make that conclusion about an individual. The Emergency Medical Treatment and Active Labor Act (EMTALA) considers "undiagnosed acute pain" as an emergency medical condition. Even if there was questionable behavior in the past, the patient could have developed a new condition. Pain consultant Margo McCaffery also emphasizes that a patient's behaviors could actually represent inadequate pain relief.

Avoid confrontation. Do not tell anyone that they will not receive pain medications or narcotics prior to the medical screening examination (MSE).

15. How do you handle questionable behaviors, such as one patient's actual request for "a pound of morfin" (morphine)?

Set limits. Pain can be treated while in the ED (including avoiding narcotics) without giving a prescription to take home. If a prescription is given for a controlled substance, encourage the number be written in three ways (script, numeric, and Roman) to avoid potential alterations. Consider involving a case manager.

16. Do we have an obligation to turn in these "drug seekers" in to law enforcement?

No. According to a U.S. Supreme Court ruling, doing that would be a violation of informed consent and the patient's right to privacy. These restrictions are true even if the patient sought medical care under a fictitious name for the alleged purpose of getting drugs. The only exception is if the patient commits a direct crime, such as stealing a prescription pad.

17. Describe how case management can work for a patient with frequent ED visits for pain.

The patient's primary medical doctor (PMD) is contacted for the recommended treatment plan. The patient is made aware of the existence and content of this plan (which often includes a "no narcotics" provision) and the coordination of the ED with the PMD. When the patient comes in, the agreed-on plan is provided to the attending ED physician to use after appropriate screening (to make sure there is nothing different occurring).

18. Is it acceptable to give a placebo to patients with questionable presentations?

The placebo phenomenon was believed to account for approximately 35% of patients' improvement. New analysis now questions the whole concept. The APS contends that placebos are appropriate only in approved, double-blind analgesic studies in which patients give informed consent. The deceptive use of placebos for analgesia is now considered unethical.

19. What about older adult patients with dementia? Do they have less pain?

Research demonstrated that cognitively impaired patients' reports about their pain were as valid as those in patients without cognitive impairment.

20. How can I obtain an accurate description of pain from a patient with dementia?

Ask simple questions, be specific, and stay in the here and now. Avoid general, broad questions, such as "Describe your pain." Instead ask, "Do you feel any burning sensations? Any aches? Soreness? Instead of saying, "Tell me where your pain is and where does it radiate?" specifically ask about each region, one at a time. Lightly press on the upper right hand quadrant and say, "Does it hurt here?"

21. Give some examples of pain scales for children.

Scale	Intended Age-Group	Description
PIPP Premature Infant Pain Profile	Neonates	Physical, behavioral, and contextual (circumstantial) indicators Gestational age and six other indicators rated on a four-point scale
CRIES Crying Requires O_2 for >95% oxygenation, Increased vital signs Expression, and Sleeplessness	Neonates	These five areas are scored for a total
FLACC Faces Legs Activity Cry Consolability	Postoperative children ages 2 months to 7 years	Child is observed for 1 to 5 minutes, and numbers most closely matching the observed behaviors are selected
Wong-Baker FACES Pain Scale	Young Children	Child points to the face that resembles their pain
Finger Span	Younger, verbal children (younger than age 7 years) who may have difficulty with ranking	Child ranks pain by altering the distance between their thumb and index finger

22. Give more information about the use of the finger span for rating pain.

Children are asked to rank their pain using their thumb and index finger. "No hurt" (often a preferred term over "pain") is the two digits together, "medium hurt" is fingers stretched halfway (inches) apart, and "most possible hurt" is the two fingers as wide apart as possible. The nurse should first demonstrate, using his or her own hand. It is documented by converting to a related number or the words the child uses.

23. Why wouldn't the FACES scale always be used on verbal children?

A child must be able to understand the concept of ranking to correctly use many of the scales, including the Wong-Baker FACES. One study found that only 26% of 5-year-olds could correctly rank when asked the question, "Which is larger, 9 or 5?"

24. Talk about physician standing orders for oral analgesia in triage.

Many departments have a protocol allowing medication to be administered (pending no contraindication). Campbell et al (2004) describes their use of a protocol led to a significant improvement in early pain management and patient satisfaction.

25. Give some examples of protocols.

MetroHealth Medical Center, Cleveland OH
Source: Barbara Wolf, RN, ED Charge Nurse
Adults: 650-1000 mg acetaminophen (Tylenol) or ibuprofen (Motrin); 600mg (if have taken the drug before, have no allergies or gastric disease, and are not taking warfarin).

Children (under age 13 years) are given a weight-based dose: 15-20 mg/kg for acetaminophen or 10-12 mg/kg for ibuprofen.

Protocol is not initiated if there is abdominal pain (traumatic or nontraumatic) or if the child has a painful extremity and fever (e.g., hip pain with a fever, rule out [r/o] septic joint).

Cleveland Clinical Foundation, Cleveland, OH
Source: Nina M. Fielden, MSN RN CEN, ED Clinical Nurse Specialist

- Assess pain using VAS, Wong-Baker, or FLACC with each vital sign measurement and within 1 hour of any intervention.
- Patient must be hemodynamically stable, without complaints of chest pain, abdominal pain, or traumatic pain.
- Patient is first asked if they have taken anything for pain in the last 4 hours, if they have allergies, history of liver, peptic ulcer, or renal disease, or are taking warfarin.
- Patient is offered acetaminophen (10-15 mg/kg PO for children or 650-1000 mg PO for adults) or ibuprofen (10 mg/kg PO children or 600-800 mg PO adults).
- Consider additional nonpharmacologic pain relief measure such as immobilization, elevation, cold application, cleansing/dressings, or distraction.

St. Joseph Hospital, Bellingham, WA
Source: Diana Meyer, RN MSN CCRN CEN, Emergency Services CNS
For complete listing of all six protocols, see Chapter 8.

- Acute pain protocol for pain ≥6/10, activated by the physician, allows hydromorphone (Dilaudid) 0.5 mg IVP to patients <65 years of age (0.2 mg if ≥65) every 5 minutes (assessing after each dose) to the maximum amount of 2.0 mg.
- Nurse-initiated protocols for extremity injury, back pain, dental pain (allowing acetaminophen and hydrocodone [Lortab], and eye pain (allowing Proparacaine [Alcaine])
- Nurse-initiated protocol for nitrous oxide (nitronox) for fracture and burn pain, prior to painful procedures, and to relieve anxiety associated with painful conditions and procedures

26. Our protocols allow either acetaminophen (Tylenol) or a nonsteroidal anti-inflammatory drug (NSAID). How do I decide which one to give?

- *Type of pain/cause of pain.* NSAIDs are particularly effective for muscle/joint pain.
- *Patient history.* NSAIDs should not be used if there is a history of bleeding disorders, taking anticoagulants, or gastric issues. Acetaminophen should not be used with a history of hepatic dysfunction or heavy alcohol intake.
- *What has been used before? Is it working?* Sometimes a drug "failure" is related to the dosing. Anecdotally, some viral syndromes respond better to one drug.
- *Patient Preference.*

27. List nonpharmacologic means of pain relief.

- Application of cold, elevation, immobilization
- Imagery, relaxation, deep breathing, music, massage
- Distraction. Children can blow bubbles to "blow the pain away." The deep and steady breathing helps relax muscles and assists the child in gaining self-control.
- Pressure at the P6 acupuncture point near the wrist (also known to control nausea and seasickness).

28. Discuss topical anesthetics.

Topical anesthetics have become one important tool. EMLA and ELA-Max are used for intact skin and topical anesthesia (TAC and LET) for broken skin (wound repair). In addition Ethyl chloride can be used as a topical skin refrigerant.

29. Is there anything else I can do to lessen the pain of an intramuscular injection?

Apply manual pressure to a site for 10 seconds prior to giving the injection. The research-validated technique works because it stimulates multiple nerve endings.

30. Tell me more about using oral glucose as an analgesic for infants.

Gradin, Eriksson et al (2002) found the use of 1 mL of 30% oral glucose solution during venipuncture was 20% more effective than EMLA. The glucose solution also has the advantage of taking effect almost immediately.

31. Why is meperidine (Demerol) used less now?

Meperidine has an accumulating active metabolite (normeperidine). It is a risk for neurotoxicity, especially in the older adult or for on-going needs. To detect early signs of central nervous system toxicity, look for a fine hand tremor.

32. If this is true, why weren't there more seizures from Demerol administration?

More toxicity has not been noted in the past because it was traditionally prescribed in subtherapeutic doses. For true adequate treatment of severe pain, most adults would require at least 75 to 100 mg every 2 to 3 hours and some would take up to 150 to 200 mg every 2 to 3 hours.

33. Should promethazine HCl (Phenergan) be used as a potentiator?

Promethazine neither relieves pain nor potentiates opioid analgesia. One study showed that promethazine increases sensitivity to pain and increased the amount of opioid needed. In 1999, the APS warned against its use.

34. Is respiratory depression a common complication for patients receiving a narcotic?

The actual likelihood of clinically significant, opioid-induced respiratory depression is less than 1%. Sedation will precede respiratory depression.

35. How about the risk of addiction with narcotic use?

In one survey, 46% of the responding nurses overestimated the risk of addiction from narcotics used for medical purposes. Research indicates that the medical use of opioids for pain relief is rarely associated with development of addiction.

36. Is there bias in analgesic administration?

Freeman and Payne (2000) concluded that there is a "subtle form of racial bias on the part of medical care providers." In one study, 55% of Hispanic ED patients received inadequate pain medication for bone fractures compared to 26% of white patients. In another study, blacks and Hispanics were 28% less likely than whites (reporting similar severity of pain) to receive an opioid analgesic.

37. What is necessary to meet the Joint Commission on Accreditation of Healthcare Organization's (JCAHO) standards regarding pain management?

Hospital procedures must include assessment measures of pain intensity and quality (pain characteristics, frequency, location, and duration), documentation that facilitates regular assessment, and staff eduction on pain assessment and management.

38. Talk about the use of prehospital analgesia.

Studies found accurate assessments can be done in the field but analgesia is often not provided, even for obvious causes such as a fracture. When prehospital analgesia was administered, the patients received significant pain relief earlier (up to 2 hours sooner) and had no serious side effects. One example is a system that allows up to 0.1 mg/kg morphine sulfate (with the standard contraindications, such as a closed head injury).

Key Points

- Try turning a horizontal pain scale vertically (with the "10") on the top if a patient has difficulty using it.
- The finger span scale, spreading the forefinger and thumb apart to indicate the degree of pain, works well with young, verbal children.
- It is not necessary to routinely hold analgesia until a final diagnosis is made.
- Prior to an intramuscular injection, apply manual pressure for 10 seconds to decrease the patient's discomfort.

Internet Resources

JCAHO: Pain: Current Understanding of Assessment, Management, and Treatments
http://www.jcaho.org/news+room/health+care+issues/pain+mono_npc.pdf

American Pain Society: Pain—the Fifth Vital Sign
www.ampainsoc.org/advocacy/fifth.htm

Pain Management in the ED Setting—What Works
http://www.aacpi.wisc.edu/images/15_pdf/GErvin.pdf

Academic Emergency Medicine: Pain Assessment in the ED—Nurse Underestimation of Patient Pain Intensity
http://www.aemj.org/cgi/content/abstract/6/5/514-a

State Of California—State and Consumer Services Agency—Pain Assessment: The Fifth Vital Sign
http://www.rn.ca.gov/practice/pdf/npr-b-27.pdf

Avoiding Misconceptions in Pain Management
http://www.medscape.com/viewarticle/418521

Narcotic Analgesic Dosage Conversion Chart
http://www.globalrph.com/narcotic.htm

Bibliography

Agency for Health Care Policy and Research: Acute pain management: Operative or medical procedures and trauma, Rockville, Md, 1992, AHCPR Pub No 92-0032, Department of Health and Human Services.

American College of Emergency Physicians: Clinical policy for the initial approach to patients presenting with a chief complaint of nontraumatic acute abdominal pain, *Ann Emerg Med* 23(4):906-922, 1994.

American Pain Society (APS): *Principles of analgesic use in the treatment of acute pain and cancer pain,* ed 4, Glenview, Ill, 1999, Author.

Campbell P, Dennie M, Dougherty K, Iwaskiw O, Rollo K: Implementation of an ED protocol for pain management at triage at a busy level I trauma center, *J Emerg Nurs* 30(5):431-438, 2004.

Canadian Association of Emergency Physicians: Canadian emergency department triage and acuity scale (CTAS) implementation guidelines, *J Can Assoc Emerg Physicians* 1(3):1-24, 1999.

Chung JWY, Ng WMY, Wong TKS: An experimental study on the use of manual pressure to reduce pain in intramuscular injections, *J Clin Nurs* 11:457-461, 2002.

Ducharme J: Emergency pain management: A Canadian Association of Emergency Physicians (CAEP) consensus document, *J Emerg Med* 12(6):855-866, 1994.

Fanurik D, Koh JL, Harrison RD, Conrad TM, Tomberlin C: Pain assessment in children with cognitive impairment: An exploration of self-report skills, *Clinical Nurse Res* 7(2):103-119, 1998.

Fielden NM: Nurse-initiated pain relief triage protocols (Managers Forum), *J Emerg Nurs* 30(6):561, 2004.

Frew JD: Pain control for "drug seekers" (Managers Forum), *J Emerg Nurs* 28(4):343-344, 2002.

Gradin M, Eriksson M, Holmquist G, Holstein SAS, Schollin J: Pain reduction at venipuncture in newborns: Oral glucose compared with local anesthetic cream, *Pediatrics* 110(6):1053, 2002.

Joint Commission on Accreditation of Healthcare Organizations: Joint Commission on Accreditation of Healthcare Organizations pain standards for 2001, Oak Brook Terrace, Ill, Feb 2001, Author.

Krechel SW, Bildner J: CRIES: A new neonatal postoperative pain measurement score: Initial testing of validity and reliability, *Paediatr Anaesthesia* 5(1):53-61, 1995.

Mackway-Jones K: *Emergency triage: Manchester Triage Group,* London, 1997, BMJ Publishing Group.

McCaffery M: *Pain: Clinical manual for nursing practice,* ed 2, St Louis, 1998, Mosby.

McCaffery M: Stigmatizing patients as addicts, *Am J Nurs* 101(5):77-79, 2001.

McCaffery M: Using the 0-to-10 pain rating scale, *Am J Nurs* 101(10):81-82, 2001.

McCaffery M, Robinson ES: Your patient is in pain: Here's how you respond, *J Emerg Nurs* 32(10): 36-47, 2002.

Merkel S: Pain assessment in infants and young children: The finger span scale, *Am J Nurs* 102(11): 55-56, 2002.

Merkel S, Malviya S: Pediatric pain, tools, and assessment, *J Perianesth Nurs* 15(6):408-414, 2000.

Merkel SL, Voepel-Lewis T, Shayevitz JR, Malviya S: The FLACC: A behavioral scale for scoring postoperative pain in young children, *Pediatr Nurse* 23(3):293-297, 1997.

Pasero C: Pain assessment in infants and young children: Neonates, *Am J Nurs* 102(8):61-63, 2002.

Pasero C: Pain assessment in infants and young children: Premature infant pain profile, *Am J Nurs* 102(9):105-106, 2002.

Pasero C, Reed BA, McCaffery M: Pain in the elderly. In McCaffery M, Pasero C, editors: *Pain: Clinical manual for nursing practice,* ed 2, St Louis, 1999, Mosby.

Slovis CM, Wrenn KD, Meador CK: *A little book of emergency medicine rules,* Philadelphia, 2000, Hanley & Belfus.

Stein RW: Drug seeking (Managers Forum), *J Emerg Nurs* 31(1):98, 2005.

Stevens B: Pain in infants. In McCaffery M, Pasero C, editors. *Pain: Clinical manual,* St Louis, 1999, Mosby.

Stevens B, Johnson C, Petryshen P, Taddio A: Premature infant pain profile: Development and initial validation, *Clin J Pain* 12:13-22, 1996.

Tamayo-Sarver JH, Hinze SW, Cydulka RK, Baker DW: Racial and ethnic disparities in emergency department analgesic prescription, *Am J Public Health* 93(12):2067-2073, 2003.

Victor K: Properly assessing pain in the elderly, *RN* 64(5):45-49, 2001.

Wolf B: Nurse-initiated pain relief triage protocols (Managers Forum), *J Emerg Nurs* 30(6):560-561, 2004.

Wong D: Topical local anesthetics, *Am J Nurs* 103(6):41-45, 2003.

Wong DL, Hockenberry-Eaton M, et al: *Wong's essentials of pediatric nursing,* ed 6, St Louis, 2001, Mosby.

Young D, Mentes JC, Titler MG: Acute pain management protocol, *J Gerontol Nurs* 26:10, 1999.

Chapter 7

Triage Diagnostics

Polly Gerber Zimmermann

1. Describe standing orders for diagnostic tests in triage.

Diagnostic tests, as part of the assessment, help to focus the options and determine acuity (see Chapter 9 for further discussion). The emergency department (ED) Medical Director signs off on the standing order protocol to allow the triage (or treatment) nurse to initiate this order if the patient meets the designated criteria. Common examples include antipyretic or analgesic medication, laboratory tests or radiographs, or initiation of an intravenous site. The order can be documented on the order sheet as "standing order" or "per protocol."

2. Will the hospital be reimbursed for these standing orders?

Yes, they are physician orders and the physician, by eventually signing the chart, is affirming these orders should be completed. The timing and location of the order being done does not effect reimbursement, even if the patient changes his or her mind and leaves without completing the medical screening exam (MSE). Having them entered on the order sheet usually resolves any reimbursement issues.

3. What point of care (POC) diagnostic testing are EDs doing?

The Voluntary Hospital Association (VHA) found that POC is widely used for glucose (95%), urine dip (54%), urine pregnancy (33%), ISTA (23%), rapid strep (21%), troponin (19%), and blood gas (18%). Hemoccult of stool is also frequently done. Overall, the VHA found the trend has been for performing less POC tests, except for capillary glucose.

4. What is needed to have successful POC testing besides protocols/standing orders?

- Education and competency verification of staff performing the test
- Quality control measurements performed consistently (with documentation)
- A process for obtaining reimbursement

5. Any other concerns regarding POC testing?

The Joint Commission of Accreditation of Healthcare Organizations (JCAHO) Standard: PC.16.30: is "Staff performing tests have adequate, specific training and orientation to perform the tests and demonstrates satisfactory levels of compliance." One hospital had a statement in the lab policies that board certified physicians were competent to do this type of bedside testing by virtue of their medical training. During this hospital's 2004 JCAHO survey, physicians were viewed as "staff" and not regarded as exempt from meeting these training and documentation requirements.

6. Give examples of when a triage nurse would consider performing fingerstick glucose.

Most ED nurses automatically do capillary fingerstick blood glucose on all diabetics, any patients with altered level of consciousness or neurologic deficits, or complaints of dizziness, weakness, or syncope.

7. Give some examples of an appropriate use of a urine dipstick or a urinalysis.

Most EDs have a protocol for a urine dipstick or urinalysis if there are urinary symptoms and hold a specimen. Urine dipstick or urinalysis of an ordinary voided specimen can be useful looking for:

- Blood, such as in possible renal calculi, abdominal trauma, back injuries
- Ketones, in a Type I diabetic or a patient who is dehydrated
- Nitrate, for urinary symptoms of infection
- Protein if pregnancy past the first trimester (with signs/symptoms of edema, headache, or elevated blood pressure)
- WBC, nitrate, blood for low back pain
- Amylase for upper abdominal pain or upper back pain
- Bilirubin for right-upper-quadrant abdominal pain, jaundice, IV history, or any signs or symptoms of hepatitis

8. Should all females reporting dysuria, frequency or urgency have a urine dipstick or urinalysis done?

That approach is under discussion. The sensitivities, specificities, and likelihood ratios vary widely in literature, and evidence suggests that the testing done in practice is not as reliable as when it is done under research protocol conditions. For women with these symptoms, the predictive value of a positive test ranges from 75% to 99% and the predictive value of a negative test ranges from 40% to 99%. Therefore, some EDs chose to treat uncomplicated urinary track infections (UTIs) without the screening tests and use the tests only on patients with low or moderate probability.

9. In what situations would EDs require a clean catch midstream or catheter urine specimen?

Situations requiring the more pristine collection process might include patients who:

- Have recurrent, previously treated UTIs
- Are pediatric patients
- Are geriatric patients
- Have potential septic signs and symptoms

10. Is there ever a situation when it is not recommended to obtain an initial urine specimen?

Men with uretheral discharge, complaints of penile discharge, or pain in the penile shaft or meatus. Some practitioners would prefer first obtaining a urethral swab for GC/chlamydia when a sexually active male has symptoms of urethritis. These results are more accurate when the man has not voided for several hours.

Another clinician's approach is to obtain the immediate urinalysis (when considering UTI, prostatitis, and urethritis). The location of the symptoms usually can be established on clinical grounds through an examination of the genitals, prostate, and urethra.

11. What are guidelines of obtaining a urine pregnancy test?

Most perform a urine pregnancy test if the female is of child bearing age (age 14 to 54) and:

- Will need a radiograph OR
- Has abdominal pain (possible ectopic pregnancy or spontaneous abortion)

Usually the only exception is if the woman's history reveals pregnancy is impossible (e.g., hysterectomy). Contraception, including birth control pills and tubal ligations, can fail.

12. Should I assume reliability when a woman indicates she is pregnant, or not pregnant, based on her home pregnancy test?

Although manufacturers of home pregnancy tests claim that their products are 99% accurate on the first day after a missed menstrual period (or earlier), the validity of these claims do not hold up in Cole et al's study. Overall, rarely are positive tests falsely positive, but negative tests often are falsely negative.

13. Any quick way to help discern if a pregnant woman is leaking urine or amniotic fluid?

Amniotic fluid has a pH of 7 to 7.5 and will turn Nitrazine paper black. Urine's average pH is 6.

14. Can nurses effectively order radiographs?

Fry studied trained triage nurses who ordered radiographs for patients with isolated distal limb injuries, excluding those with severe pain or evidence of acute neurovascular compromise. The nurse-ordered radiographs had a 43%

abnormal finding rate; the physician-ordered radiographs had a 33% abnormal finding rate. Lindley-Jones and Finlayson's study found that triage nurses (by protocol) ordered 8% fewer radiographs than the physician or emergency nurse practitioners and had a 6% higher "hit" rate. Both studies found that patient wait time decreased and the patient satisfaction increased.

15. Give examples of specific protocol/standing order for diagnostic testing.

Memorial Regional Hospital (Hollywood, FL)
Source: Melinda (Mel) Stibal, RN BSHC, Emergency/Trauma Administrative Director
Immuno-compromised with fever greater than 100.5°F (38°C)

- CBC, SMA7, urinalysis, urine C&S, blood cultures × 2
- Portable chest radiograph
- Saline lock
- Pulse oximetry
- New-onset seizures
- CBC, SMA7, Urine toxicology, ETOH level
- CT brain
- Accu-Chek
- Saline lock
- Pulse oximetry
- Ativan 2 mg IV for active seizures
- Drug levels (when appropriate) for digoxin, theophylline, Dilantin, Tegretol, Lithium, Depakote

Medical clearance for admission to psychiatric facility

- CBC, SMA7, urine toxicology, ETOH
- EKG (30 years and older)
- Pregnancy test (for all premenopausal women)

(See Chapter 8.)

16. How do EDs use electrocardiogram (EKG) rooms for triage of chest pain patients?

A trained technician or nurse practitioner performs the EKG within 5 to 10 minutes of the patient's arrival, using a small private area close to triage, and it is then interpreted by the attending ED physician or the nurse practitioner. The process also allows for a timely lab specimens and intravenous access. Depending on if there are significant findings, the patient returns to the waiting room or is immediately moved into the treatment area.

17. What are routine requirements regarding obtaining and measuring an EKG rhythm strip?

Most EDs require an initial rhythm strip when cardiac monitoring is initiated, and when there are changes, and documenting the patient's name, time, date, and lead. Often the heart rate, rhythm, heart sounds, and pulse characteristics are included as part of the systemic nursing history and physical.

Many do not require the nurse to measure the PR, QRS, and/or QT intervals because they are included on the concurrent 12-lead EKG. Others do because a visual interpretation without measurements (e.g., Mobitz II from a third degree A-V block) can be inaccurate or miss subtle aspects, such as lengthening of the QT interval.

18. Do you have any tips on remembering the different types of heart blocks on a rhythm strip?

American Medical Resource Foundation (AMRF) suggests the following chart:

Type of AV Block	QRS Rhythm	P-R Interval	P Waves	Cause
1st degree	Regular	>0.20 seconds, constant	Regular rhythm, 1 for each QRS	Drugs, ischemia, congenital
2nd degree Type I	Usually irregular	Change	Regular rhythm, more P's than QRS's	Drugs, ischemia, increased vagal tone
2nd degree Type II	Regular or irregular	Constant	Regular rhythm, more P's than QRS's	Organic damage to conduction pathways
3rd degree	Regular, either a junctional escape rhythm or ventricular escape rhythm	There is no actual P-R intervals, because there is no relationship between the P waves & WRS complexes	Regular rhythm, usually more P's than QRS's	AV node: drugs, ischemia, increase vagal tone Infranodal: damage to conduction pathways

19. Can you suggest a trick for helping new graduates interpret arterial blood gases (ABGs)?

My generic nursing students tend to do well with ABG number interpretation when using the figure "H" as suggested by Kirksey and Goodroad. Place Pa_{CO_2} values on the left axis of the "H", from 20 to 80 mm Hg (represents the respiratory component). Place bicarbonate (HCO_3^-) values from 12 to 48, on the right axis of the "H" (represents the metabolic component).

The normal ranges for these parameters are 35 to 45 mm Hg for the $PaCO_2$ and 22 to 26 mmol/L for the HCO_3^- level. The mean values, 40 mm Hg $PaCO_2$ and 24 mmol/L HCO_3^- are connected to form the centerline of the "H" or the "baseline." Write the pH on that line: normal pH values are 7.35 to 7.45.

First, analyze the pH. A pH less than 7.35 is acidic ("acid" and "low" are the two shorter words) and a pH higher than 7.45 is alkaline ("alkaline" and "high" are the two longer words).

Then plot the $PaCO_2$ and HCO_3^- values on the model and draw a line intersecting them. The side on which there is a deviation from the baseline indicates if this disturbance is respiratory or metabolic. Use of this visual aid makes it apparent, for example that a result with a pH of 7.2 $PaCO_2$ of 65 mm Hg and HCO_3^- of 24 mmol/L represents respiratory acidosis.

When a patient's acid-base imbalance is partially compensated, all three values are abnormal. The system with the greatest deviation from the baseline is the one primarily affected. The system with the lesser change is the one that is compensating.

20. Any precautions to observe in drawing blood for laboratory tests?

Do not reuse the blood tube holder. In one analysis of 9 years of data from 90 facilities, disassembling the blood tube holder device caused 11% of the contaminated needle sticks. Dispose of the holder and needle as a whole. Do not reuse tourniquet. Reuse of the holder and tourniquet have been implicated in the transmission of bloodborne disease, such as hepatitis B.

21. Why is glucose reading important on critical patients?

There is growing evidence that hyperglycemia in a critically ill patient has a negative impact on the clinical outcomes.

22. What is a quick way to understand blood urea nitrogen (BUN) and creatinine (Cr^-) results?

When the BUN and Cr^- are both elevated, think kidney. If just the BUN is elevated, think liver, dehydration, or some other cause.

23. Which electrolyte imbalance is the most crucial to intervene on?

Hyperkalemia, because of the cardiac effects.

24. Discuss anion gaps.

The anion gap (AG) measures the amount of negatively charged ions in the serum (unmeasured anions) that are not bicarbonate (HCO_3^-) or chloride (Cl^-). The anion gap is calculated by subtracting the sum of HCO_3^- and Cl^-

values from the sodium (Na^+) value, the major positive charge in the serum. Potassium (K^+) values are not generally used in the calculation because the huge amount of intracellular potassium (155 mEq) and the relatively low amount of potassium in the serum (only approximately 4 mEq). Normal AG is 8 to 12 (some use the value 10 to 14).

25. Is a wide or elevated anion gap important?

Yes. Metabolic acidosis is present and is probably as a result of cause represented by MUDPILES

M Methanol
U Uremia
D DKA and AKA
P Paraldehyde
I INH (isoniazid) and Iron
L Lactic acidosis
E Ethylene glycol
S Salicylates

26. What about a narrow AG acidosis?

This is often from diarrhea or renal tubular acidosis. Think HARDUPS for causes

H Hyperventilation (chronic)
A Acetazolamide: Acids (e.g., hydrochloric); Addison's disease
R Renal tubular acidosis
D Diarrhea
U Uterosigmoidostomy
P Pancreatic fistulas and drainage
S Saline

27. What should I think about if the patient is taking digoxin (Lanoxin) or theophylline or aminophylline and is sick, particularly "flu" symptoms?

The need for drug levels to rule-out drug toxicity. The well-known digoxin toxic signs of bradycardia and halos appear late.

28. Discuss the use of rapid influenza testing in a pediatric ED.

Rapid tests for influenza are becoming more accurate. In one study, knowing the results of a rapid influenza test reduced other testing of young, febrile children showed the possibility of reducing costs and unneeded antibiotic prescriptions.

Key Points

- Consider the need for a more pristine, clean-catch or catheterized urine specimen collection if the patient has reoccurring, previously treated UTIs, is geriatric, is pediatric, or has signs/symptoms of possible sepsis.
- Home pregnancy tests often do not match up to their advertised claims. Rarely are positive tests falsely positive, but negative tests often are falsely negative.
- Do not reuse blood tube holders or tourniquets.
- When considering etiology, use MUDPILES for an elevated AG and HARDUPS for a narrow AG.

Internet Resources

College of American Pathologists: Moving the Sicker Quicker with ER Point-of-Care
http://www.cap.org/apps/docs/cap_today/feature_stories/0304ERpointofcare.html

Bibliography

Bonner AB et al: Impact of the rapid diagnosis of influenza on physician decision-making and patient management in the pediatric emergency department: Results of a randomized, prospective, controlled trial, *Pediatrics* 112:363-367, 2003.

Capes S, Hunt D, Malmberg K, et al: Stress hyperglycemia and increased risk of death after myocardial infarction in patients with and without diabetes: A systematic overview, *Lancet* 355:773-778, 2000.

Cohn EG, Gilroy-Doohan M: *Flip and see ECG,* ed 2, Philadelphia, 2002, WB Saunders.

Cole LA et al: Accuracy of home pregnancy tests at the time of missed menses, *Am J Obstet Gynecol* 190:100-105, 2004.

Fry M: Triage nurses order x-rays for patients with isolated distal limb injuries: A 12-month ED study, *J Emerg Nurs* 2791:17-22, 2001

Johnson S: Measuring/documenting indicators on mounted EKG strips (Managers Forum), *J Emerg Nurs* 31(2):190, 2005.

Kirksey KM, Holt-Ashley M, Goodroad BK: An easy method for interpreting the results of arterial blood gas analysis, *Crit Care Nurse* 21(5):49-54, 2001.

Lindley-Jones M, Finlayson BJ: Triage nurse requested x-rays, *J Accident Emerg Med* 17:103-107, 2000.

Malmber K, Norhammer A, Wedel H et al: Glycometabolic state at admission: Important risk marker of mortality in conventionally treated patients with diabetes mellitus and acute myocardial infarction: Long term results from the DIGAMI study, *Circulation* 99:2626-2632, 1999.

McGrayne J: Hemoccult and POC testing (Managers Forum), *J Emerg Nurs* 31(2):193, 2005.

Murphy KA: *Pediatric triage guidelines,* St Louis, 1997, Mosby.

Pierce B: Triaging chest pain with an EKG (Managers Forum), *J Emerg Nurs* 30(2):162-163, 2004.

Ray C: POC and Hemoccult testing competencies and documentation (Managers Forum), *J Emerg Nurs* 31(2):192-193, 2005.

Schiebel NEE: Urinary tract infection: Cystitis, pyelonephritis, and prostatitis. In Markovchick VJ, Pons PT, editors. *Pons' emergency medicine secrets,* ed 3, Philadelphia, 2003, Hanley & Belfus.

Slovis CM: Fluids and electrolytes. In Markovchick VJ, Pons PT, editors. *Pons' emergency medicine secrets,* ed 3, Philadelphia, 2003, Hanley & Belfus.

Slovis CM, Wrenn KD, Meador CK: *A little book of emergency medicine rules,* Philadelphia, 2000, Hanley & Belfus.

Zimmermann PG: Tricks for the ED trade, *J Emerg Nurs* 29(5):453-458, 2003.

Chapter 8

Protocol Samples

Polly Gerber Zimmermann

1. What are the advantages of having protocols?

These "standing orders," agreed on by the attending physician staff results in:

- Administrating the same quality of care regardless of the staff member in triage by setting a minimum expectation for a given situation
- Serving as a reference for experienced nurses facing an infrequently seen situation
- Aiding the inexperienced nurse who needs more frequent guidance
- Using them as a teaching tool during orientation

As a result of instituting protocols, many departments report higher staff and patient satisfaction, with few patients leaving without being seen (LWBS).

2. How can we find triage protocols to use?

- Survey other hospitals in the community to see what they are using
- Ask a listserv (such as Emergency Nurses Association's [ENA] members or managers) about current policies/procedures they are using
- Search the Internet or literature
- Write your own, using current standards and census of the practicing physicians

3. What processes should we insure regarding our protocols?

Cohen (2002) recommends:

- That what triage nurses are doing in practice (e.g., ordering labs or radiographs) is in writing
- Protocols are reviewed and signed as standing orders/protocols by a physician
- That staff are in compliance and using the protocols appropriately (use retrospective chart audits)

4. Discuss continuous quality improvement in terms of protocols.

On a regular, ongoing basis, the department's protocols should be evaluated for such aspects as:

- Are they accomplishing what they were intended to?
- Are they safe?
- Are they in line with expert standard professional practice and recommendations?

Box 8-1. Mary Hitchcock Memorial Hospital Emergency Department

EMERGENCY DEPARTMENT POLICY/PROCEDURE	
SUBJECT: RN X-Ray Ordering Guidelines	APPROVAL:
RELATED POLICIES: ED Nursing Standard of Care	EFFECTIVE DATE: 04/2003 REVISION DATE: 01/2005

Policy

The following films may be ordered independently by ED-RNs for patients with recent extremity trauma.

General Guidelines for Extremity X-Rays

- If any of the following are present, an x-ray is indicated:
  - Deformity
  - Bony instability
  - Crepitus
  - Point tenderness
  - Ecchymosis or severe swelling
  - Moderate to severe pain with weight bearing (hip, thigh, foot)
  - Any penetrating injury in a joint area
  - Foreign body present or suspected

Guidelines for Specific Areas

Toes/Fingers:

- Order only the involved digit if all signs/symptoms are distal to web space
- Order foot/hand for any involvement proximal to web space

Foot:

- Signs/symptoms from the web space of the toes to the bend of the ankle
- Use Ottawa Ankle Rules
- Calcaneous films may be ordered for isolated heel pain after a fall from a height where the patient landed on the heels

Ankle:

- Use Ottawa Ankle Rules

Tibia/Fibula:

- Signs/symptoms not proximate to ankle or knee

Knee:

- Use Ottawa Knee Rule

Box 8-1. Mary Hitchcock Memorial Hospital Emergency Department—*cont'd*

Hand:

- Signs/symptoms proximal to the web spaces of the fingers and distal to the base of the thumb

Wrist:

- Signs/symptoms between the web space of the thumb and just proximal to the head of the radius/ulna
- Note the presence of snuffbox tenderness on x-ray request and in nurse's notes

Forearm:

- Localized tenderness or limitation/loss of supination/pronation

Elbow:

- Pain associated with limitation/loss of supination/pronation/extension
- Children <5 years old with suspected radial head subluxation (nursemaid's elbow) do not require x-rays

Humerus:

- Signs/symptoms in upper arm

Clavicle:

- Tenderness specific to clavicle

Shoulder:

- Decreased range of motion or tenderness and recent history of dislocation

Hip/Pelvis:

- Fall with hip pain, externally rotated and/or shortened extremity, unable to bear weight

Portable Chest:

- Unstable patients in significant respiratory distress or status post-extubation

X-Ray Requisition

- According to federal regulations regarding reimbursement for diagnostic testing, the x-ray requisition must include the following information:
  - Body part to be examined with laterality identified if appropriate
  - Clinical indication for the examination
  - History, Signs, Symptoms
  - What is the question we are trying to answer?
  - Attending MDs name (if two are on duty, list both)
  - Date

Box 8-2. St. Joseph Hospital ED acute pain management protocol

MEDICATION AND TREATMENT

Inclusion:

- ≥16 years
- Pain ≥6/10
- No known allergies to the medications on this protocol

Pain must be assessed and documented after each dose of medication.

Patients <65 years of age:

- Hydromorphone (Dilaudid) 0.5 mg IVP.
- If pain is ≥6, may continue with 0.5 mg hydromorphone (Dilaudid) q 5 minutes.
- Maximum amount of hydromorphone (Dilaudid) is 2 mg. Notify physician if pain remains ≥6.
- Discontinue administration of hydromorphone (Dilaudid) if sedation score is ≤1. Notify physician.
- Administer naloxone (Narcan) for sedation score of 0 and/or respiratory depression (RR ≤10/min and SaO_2 <92% on 3 L/min). Notify physician.

Patients ≥65 years of age:

- Hydromorphone (Dilaudid) 0.2 mg IVP.
- If pain is ≥6, may continue with 0.2 mg hydromorphone (Dilaudid) q 5 minutes.
- Maximum amount of hydromorphone (Dilaudid) is 2 mg. Notify physician if pain remains ≥6.
- Discontinue administration of hydromorphone (Dilaudid) if sedation score is ≤1. Notify physician.
- Administer naloxone (Narcan) for sedation score of 0 and/or respiratory depression (RR ≤10 and SaO_2 <92% on 3 L/min). Notify physician.

Nausea management:

Promethazine (Phenergan), 12.5 mg IV.
May repeat 12.5 mg in 15 minutes if no relief.
If patient remains nauseated 1 hour after the second dose of promethazine (Phenergan), notify physician.

Oversedation/Respiratory Depression Management:

Narcan for oversedation/respiratory depression (RR ≤10/min and SaO_2 <92% on 3 L/min)
Naloxone (Narcan) 0.4 mg vial prn

Procedure for titrating naloxone (Narcan) dose to reverse oversedation or respiratory depression:

1. Draw up 0.4 mg (1 cc) of naloxone in 10 cc syringe.
2. In the same syringe, draw up 9 cc of 0.9% sterile normal saline for a diluted concentration of 0.04 mg/cc.
3. Give 1 cc IVP naloxone solution into vein; repeat every minute until respiratory rate is satisfactory.

Do not exceed minimum dose required to provide acceptable respiratory rate of ≥10/min and SaO_2 >92% and sedation score >1.

Respiratory rate and quality are paramount. Reversal of analgesia may result.

Sedation Score

Score	Description	Definition
0	Unresponsive	Does not move with noxious stimuli
1	Responds to noxious stimuli	Opens eyes, raises eyebrows, or turns head toward stimulus, moves limbs with noxious stimulus (fingernail pressure, sternal rub)
2	Responsive to touch or name	Opens eyes, raises eyebrows, or turns head toward stimulus, moves limbs when touched or when name is spoken (shake and shout)
3	Calm and cooperative	No external stimulus is required to elicit movement, and patient appears calm and follows commands

Box 8-3. St. Joseph Hospital ED dental pain management nurse-initiated protocol

The registered nurse initiates this protocol at the time of initial assessment of patients (age ≥16) with dental pain.

Inclusion

- Age ≥16
- Chief complaint of dental pain presenting without any of the exclusion criteria
- No known allergies to protocol medications

Exclusion

- Age <16
- Do not administer ibuprofen to patients who have bleeding disorders or are taking anticoagulants
- Patients with the following symptoms are triaged as Level II and brought immediately to treatment area for physician evaluation:
  - Appear systemically ill with abnormal vital signs
  - Severe unilateral sore throat
  - Voice changes (muffled, hot potato voice)
  - Stridor
  - Unable to swallow, drooling
  - Pain radiating to ear
  - Elevation and edema of the tongue

Procedure

- Complete and document initial assessment, including pain severity score
- Identify allergies/potential drug reactions
- Provide pain management as indicated below. The RN may choose to use a lower level of pain management (as outlined by this protocol) based on the patient's condition or request
- Provide patient education: When patient has received narcotic, caution him/her not to drive
- Document intervention on ED order sheet and flowsheet

Mild Pain (1-3)

Ibuprofen
 600 mg PO
For patients unable to take ibuprofen, use
Acetaminophen
 975 mg PO

Moderate to Severe Pain (4-10)

Acetaminophen/hydrocodone (Lortab)
 1 tablet hydrocodone (7.5 mg)/acetaminophen (500 mg) + ibuprofen 600 mg PO

Consult with physician for additional medications when contraindications exist or pain relief has not been achieved.

Box 8-4. St. Joseph Hospital ED nitronox administration nurse-initiated protocol

Utilizing the clinical guidelines from nurse initiated interventions, the ED RN may initiate patient-administered nitronox:

- To treat pain associated with fractures and burns
- Before painful procedures such as IV insertion and wound care
- To relieve anxiety associated with painful conditions and procedures

General Information

- Nitronox provides rapid onset (2-6 minutes), quickly reversible (2-5 minutes) analgesia
- Children and older adults may use nitrous oxide as long as they can cooperate and self-administer the nitrous oxide. The nitronox delivery device (mask/mouthpiece) should never be held on the patient's face
- Nitronox causes drowsiness and is not used in patients with an altered LOC, head injuries, or those who are heavily sedated or intoxicated
- Nitronox collects in the dead air spaces and can expand the preexisting pockets of air associated with pneumothorax, otitis media, perforated viscus, bowel obstruction, air embolus, and decompression sickness

Contraindications

- Patient is unable to self-administer and/or understand instructions
- Altered LOC (risk of aspiration)
- Chest injuries (potential for pneumothorax) or COPD
- Pregnancy: actual or suspected (associated with fetal defects and SAB)
- Abdominal pain (potential of SBO or perforated viscus)
- Facial injuries that impair ability to create a seal
- Suspected air embolism or decompression sickness

Side Effects

- Vomiting
- Shortness of breath
- Excitement
- Drowsiness
- Confusion
- Light-headedness

Complications

- Propping or holding the mask against the patient's face may result in excessive sedation. The patient must hold the mask to prevent overdosage
- Aspiration may occur if the patient vomits with the mask in place

Patient Preparation

- Assess and document vital signs
- Instruct the patient to do the following:
    - Form a tight seal with the mask or mouthpiece and take slow, deep breaths
    - Exhale into the mask or mouthpiece so that exhaled gas is collected into scavenger and not dispersed into ambient air
    - Avoid unnecessary conversation to limit exhalation of nitrous oxide into the room
    - Discontinue if nausea, light-headedness, or other side effects occur

Procedure

- Allow the patient to inhale gas for 3 to 4 minutes before beginning any procedures. Some patients may require up to 6 minutes
- As the patient becomes relaxed, he or she will be unable to create an adequate amount of negative pressure to trip the demand valve
- Allow the patient to resume gas inhalation when he or she is able to hold the mask or mouthpiece
- Limit nitronox administration to 30 minutes
- Document vital signs, length of gas inhalation, and response to medication

Important

- Patient must be able to self-administer the nitronox
- Administration of nitronox is discontinued when the acute need for pain and/or anxiety relief has been met
- Consult with a physician for additional medications when contraindications exist or pain relief has not been achieved

Box 8-5. St. Joseph Hospital ED back pain management nurse-initiated protocol

The registered nurse initiates this protocol at the time of initial assessment of patients (age ≥16) with mechanical back pain.

Inclusion

- Age ≥16
- Chief complaint of back pain presenting without any of the exclusion criteria
- Assess:
  - Mechanism of injury
  - Exacerbation of chronic pain
  - Worse with movement or prolonged sitting or standing
  - Onset sudden or gradual over days
- No known allergies to protocol medications

Exclusion

- Age <16
- Do not administer ibuprofen to patients who have bleeding disorders or are taking anticoagulants
- Patients with the following symptoms are triaged as Level II and brought immediately to treatment area for physician evaluation:
  - Appear systemically ill with abnormal vital signs
  - Fever
  - New-onset back pain with age ≥60 or IVDA
  - Pain that is different than usual back pain
  - Unilateral or bilateral lower extremity motor and/or sensory abnormality
  - Dysuria
  - Cough
  - Bowel or bladder problems

Procedure

- Complete and document initial assessment, including pain severity score
- Identify allergies/potential drug reactions
- Provide pain management as indicated below. The RN may choose to use a lower level of pain management (as outlined by this protocol) based on the patient's condition or request
- Provide patient education: When patient has received narcotic, caution him/her not to drive
- Document intervention on ED order sheet and flowsheet

Mild Pain (1-3)

Ibuprofen
600 mg PO
For patients unable to take ibuprofen, use
Acetaminophen
975 mg PO

Moderate to Severe Pain (4-10)

Acetaminophen/hydrocodone (Lortab)
1 tablet hydrocodone (7.5 mg)/acetaminophen (500 mg) + ibuprofen 600 mg PO

Consult with physician for additional medications when contraindications exist or pain relief has not been achieved.

Box 8-6. St. Joseph Hospital ED eye pain management nurse-initiated protocol

The registered nurse initiates this protocol at the time of initial assessment of patients (age ≥12) with eye pain associated with trauma.

Inclusion
- Age ≥12
- Chief complaint of eye pain (e.g., foreign body sensation) presenting without any of the exclusion criteria
- Assess:
  - Mechanism of injury
  - Condition of eye
  - Pain level
- No known allergies to protocol medications

Exclusion
- Age <12
- Patients with
  - Allergies to the "caines"
  - Penetrating eye injuries

Procedure
- Complete and document initial assessment, including pain severity score
- Identify allergies/potential drug reactions
- Provide pain management as indicated below
- Provide patient education: Instruct patient not to rub the eye(s) after instillation of proparacaine (Alcaine). If a foreign body is under the upper lid, further damage may occur
- Document intervention on ED order sheet and flowsheet

Intervention
- Instill 2 drops of proparacaine (Alcaine) into the conjunctival sac of the affected eye(s)
- Assess and document relief of pain
- If not substantially relieved, may repeat dose × 1

Consult with physician for additional medications when contraindications exist or pain relief has not been achieved.

Box 8-7. St. Joseph Hospital ED extremity injury pain management nurse-initiated protocol

The registered nurse initiates this protocol at the time of initial assessment of patients with isolated extremity injuries.

For All Patients

- Complete and document circulation, sensation, and movement examination
- Ice
- Splint/immobilization
- Elevation
- Identify allergies/potential drug reactions
- Do not administer ibuprofen to patients who have bleeding disorders or are taking anticoagulants
- Provide pain management as indicated below. The RN may choose to use a lower level of pain management (as outlined by this protocol) based on the patient's condition or request
- Provide patient education: When patient has received narcotic, caution him/her not to drive
- Document intervention on ED order sheet and flowsheet

Intervention

Mild Pain (1-3)

Ibuprofen
- 10 mg/kg PO for pediatrics
- 600 mg PO for adults

For patients unable to take ibuprofen, use

Acetaminophen
- 15 mg/kg PO for pediatrics
- 975 mg PO for adults

Moderate Pain (4-6)

For Adults

Acetaminophen/hydrocodone (Lortab)
- 1 tablet hydrocodone (7.5 mg)/acetaminophen (500 mg) + ibuprofen 600 mg PO

For Pediatrics

<2 years old: Consult Md

≥2 and ≤12 years old:

Lortab elixir 2.5 mg + ibuprofen 10 mg/kg PO

>12 years old: Vicodin 5 mg + ibuprofen 400 mg PO

Severe Pain (7-10)

For Adults

Morphine 2 mg slow IVP q 5 min up to 10 mg

Notify physician if pain not managed after 10 mg

For Pediatrics

Notify MD immediately

Keep Patient NPO

Consult with physician for additional medications when contraindications exist or pain relief has not been achieved.

Box 8-8. Minor Care/Quick Care/FastER Care

Policy

In an effort to expedite patients in the ED, a Minor Care/Quick Care/FastER Care System has been implemented during peak hours. The patients are seen by the physician/ARNP on duty in the ED Minor Care/Quick Care/FastER Care area.

Procedure

1. Patient presents to ED and is triaged per the Triage policy.
2. Once patient is triaged to Minor Care/Quick Care/FastER Care, patient will be directed to the appropriate area.
3. See attached guidelines for Minor Care/Quick Care/FastER Care.

Minor Care/Quick Care/FastER Care Guidelines

ABRASIONS	With or without minimal localized infection
ABSCESS	Small abscesses with or without a fever
ALLERGIC REACTION	Without systemic symptoms
ASTHMA	<50 years of age in no apparent respiratory distress and no need for immediate treatment
BACK PAIN	Mild/moderate; ambulatory without leg numbness or weakness; may be chronic in nature; no serious trauma
BITES	Animal, human, aquatic animal (e.g., fish, man-o-war) or insect without systemic symptoms
BURNS	Non-circumferential and/or no greater than 5% of total BSA; sunburn
COLD SYMPTOMS	Temperature of <104°F; without respiratory distress and/or chest pain
COUGH	Non-cardiac; no hemoptysis; without chest pain and/or respiratory symptoms
DENTAL PROBLEMS	Without major facial trauma
DYSURIA/UTI SYMPTOMS	Without symptoms of pyelonephritis (e.g., flank pain, vomiting, temperature >101°F, or severe abdominal pain)
EARACHES	Without significant bleeding or CSF drainage
EMPLOYEE HEALTH	Minor illnesses; return to work; blood or body fluid exposure
EYE PROBLEMS	Red eye; corneal abrasions; foreign bodies; no penetrating trauma or chemical injury
FINGER/TOE NAIL PROBLEMS	Infection/injury
FOREIGN BODIES	Superficial; soft tissue, nasal, ear, or eye
HAND INFECTIONS	Paronychia, soft-tissue infections with or without trauma
HEADACHE	Mild to moderate; chronic history, no new onset, no trauma
HEMORRHOIDS	Bleeding controlled
IMMUNIZATIONS	Tetanus prophylaxis
JOINT PAIN	Without fever
LACERATIONS	Intact neurovascular status; no LOC with head or facial lacerations
MEDICATION ADMINISTRATION	Private physician orders

Box 8-8. Minor Care/Quick Care/FastER Care—*cont'd*

NOSEBLEED	Minor; bleeding subsided; without hypertension
ORAL INFECTIONS	Temperature >103°F; without trauma
ORTHOPEDIC INJURIES	Sprains; minor fractures; finger/toe dislocations; no injury that requires conscious sedation for treatment
PRIVATE PHYSICIAN ORDERS	For minor, non-urgent illness/injury
PUNCTURE WOUNDS	No major vessel, bone, or nerve involvement
RASHES	Simple history; no systemic allergic reaction
SEXUALLY TRANSMITTED DISEASES	Exposure; urethral discharge; males only
SOFT TISSUE INFLAMMATION/ INFECTION	Without temperature >103°F
SORE THROAT	Without temperature >104°F; no respiratory distress
VOMITING	Associated with flu symptoms; no significant abdominal pain; no hematemesis, without clinical signs of dehydration
VIRAL SYNDROME	Without temperature >104°F; nonspecific muscle aches and/or fatigue, URI symptoms, may include mild abdominal cramping
WOUND CHECKS	No dressing changes on burns that may need debridement
X-RAY RECALLS	

Bibliography

Cohen S: *101 triage tips,* Hohenwald, Tenn, 2002, Health Resources Unlimited.

Meyer D: ED pain relief protocols (Managers Forum), *J Emerg Nurs* 30(6):561, 2004.

Proehl J: X-ray protocols (Managers Forum), *J Emerg Nurs* 31(1):93-94, 2005.

Purvis A: Nurse-initiated pain relief triage protocols, *J Emerg Nurs* 30(6):560-561, 2004.

Stibal M: Fast track protocols (Managers Forum), *J Emerg Nurs* (in press).

Chapter 9

Decision-Making and Prioritization Principles

Polly Gerber Zimmermann

1. What factors go into the decisions nurses make in triage?

Multiple studies have found that experience and expertise are significant contributing factors in decision making, along with task complexity, presence of conflict, nursing experience, education, and expertise. The beginner nurse needs specific rules to make the decision, but expert nurses have a varied wholistic approach in seeing the "big picture."

2. Do nurses agree that these factors relate to triage decision making?

Cone and Murray (2002) interviews with emergency department (ED) expert nurses identifies the component of decision making for triage nursing as established criteria, assessment, appearance, communication, experience, intuition, and critical thinking.

3. What exactly is critical thinking?

Alfaro-LeFevre (1999) defines it as careful, deliberate, outcome-focused (results-oriented) thinking that is mastered for a context. It is based on scientific method, the nursing process, a high level of knowledge, skills, experience, professional standards, a positive attitude toward learning, and ethic codes. It includes an element of constant re-evaluation, self-correction, and striving to improve.

4. What are some characteristics of critical thinking?

- Open-mindedness. This includes awareness of one's own values and beliefs that might hamper decision making (e.g., subconscious prejudices).
- The ability to see things from more than one perspective
- Awareness of one's own strengths and weaknesses
- Ongoing striving for improvement

5. What can help develop critical thinking?

Alfaro-LeFevre recommends asking a negative question when setting priorities, such as, "What could happen if I don't do . . .?"

6. What are key aspects of critical thinking in a clinical setting?

Dorothy delBueno indicates the following key aspects:

- Can the nurse recognize the patient's problem?
- Can the nurse safely and effectively manage the problem within his or her scope of practice?
- Does the nurse have a relative sense of urgency?
- Does the nurse know why he or she is doing the actions? In other words, doing the right thing for the right reason.

7. How does the Manchester Triage Group describe the strategies used in triage decision making?

- *Reasoning.* Inductive (specific to general) reasoning considers all possibilities. It is used by the less experienced nurse and is time consuming. Deductive (general to specific) reasoning allows rapid sorting as it simultaneously weeds out the inappropriate information. It is the often (unrecognized) practice of experts.
- *Pattern recognition.* Information is pieced together in an analytical way, comparing the pattern in relation to previous cases. It is developed with experience, becomes intuitive, and is the most commonly used for rapid triage.
- *Repetitive hypothesizing.* Gathering (accumulative) data to confirm or eliminate a possibility. This is the process that continues with the diagnostic work-up.
- *Mental representation.* It is a simplification, often used in a confusing case, to try to focus on the most relevant ("What one thing made you come today...?").
- Intuition

8. Describe instinct or intuition.

It is often called a sixth sense that something is not quite right with the "conventional" decision for a particular patient. It is sometimes described as a nagging feeling in one's gut that a particular patient is more serious that he or she appears on the surface, that something else is wrong, or that this "minor" symptom needs more attention.

9. How does instinct or intuition develop?

Work-related "sixth sense" instincts develop from a subconscious processing of memory, physical clues, or subtle facial microexpressions (e.g., the woman says everything is fine but has a fleeting change in facial expression to make the nurse question that). Although nurses initially follow the "plan" that worked in earlier or similar situations, the unconscious mind is vigilant for anything odd or unexpected. The sense that "something is wrong" can cue the prefrontal cortex that a threat of danger is present (e.g., the patient is "sick") and a need to react. People who trust their trained instinct will often sense the need to act and intervene even if they cannot always articulate the complete rationale behind that knowledge. Fischer et al (2004) showed pediatric physicians had good discriminative ability in predicting which children were infectious prior to the lab results.

10. How do I develop my own instinct?

Obtain on-going knowledge, experience, learn from others' examples (including literature, such as Triage Decisions column in the *Journal of Emergency Nursing*), and continuous quality improvement. Review your patients' charts at the end of the shift. Did the treatment professionals pick up something you missed? One study found reflective learning (written narratives, critical incident reports, and mentored, post-experiential small group discussions) helped dental students improve their learning.

11. What processes does Edwards (2000) say nurses use to make triage decisions?

- Rationalist perspective-nursing process
- Intuitive reasoning
- Hypothetico-deductive

12. Describe the rationalist perspective nursing process.

This well-known problem-solving cycle is logical, but hinges on gathering adequate information. This sometimes takes the form of a systematic review of the body's systems. In triage, this approach is limited because it is inappropriate for situations that require rapid interventions or with high levels of uncertainty. Then action takes priority.

13. How does Edwards elaborate on the concept of intuition that was already discussed?

Calling it a "common-sense" understanding, it is a form of rapid reasoning performed unconsciously. The difficulty is passing it on to inexperienced nurses and/or if nurses are unable to see their weaknesses and consistently make intuitive "wrong" decisions.

14. Discuss the hypothetico-deductive approach.

The nurse immediately formulates a "range of possibilities" and then gathers more data to narrow down the tentative list. It can start with the prehospital report. For instance, the patient is an 80-year-old woman who was found on the floor by a throw rug versus a 40-year-old disheveled man found on the street outside a bar. Cues are gathered into clusters of interrelated information that looks at probability, seriousness, amenability to health care intervention, and novelty. Based on the nurse's knowledge, information is used to determine the presence or absence of (or differentiate) an abnormal state(s).

15. Provide the basic overarching principles for prioritization in ED triage.

- *Maslow Hierarchy of Needs.* His framework provides for the most basic needs to be met before the higher-level needs. They are physiologic, safety needs, love and belonging, esteem, and self-actualization (self-realization).
- *ABCD* (Airway, then Breathing, then Circulation, then Disability)

16. List more specific priority principles or guidelines for triage.

- *A before B before C before D, but consider the level of severity.* A severe C is before a mild B. A patient hemorrhaging is before someone with a mild asthma attack who can speak in sentences.
- *What is the worst-case scenario this patient could have with this complaint?* Do not miss the novelty, infrequent or high-risk complication. So the post–motor vehicle accident (MVA) patient complains of rib pain (probably from the lap belt) but rule out hitting the head/loss of consciousness (LOC) and punctured lung (clear and equal breath sounds).
- *Systemic over local and life before limb.* A possible overdose with potential systemic consequences takes priority over someone with a deformed arm (localized problem).
- *Acute over chronic.* Acute or sudden onset generally means the problem is more serious. This is defined if the individual knows the exact time or activity of the onset or the maximum intensity if reached immediately (in less than 1 minute).
- *Short-term over long-term.* Always go for the "lesser of the two evils"; something may have complications (e.g., start an intraosseous needle with a resulting osteomyelitis) but is done regardless for stabilization.
- *Actual over potential.* Treat the actual problem now before trying to prevent a future problem.
- *Trending.* More concern is warranted when associated with other definitive changes. A trend of minor symptoms that tend to reoccur repeatedly, to increase in severity, or indicate a steady progressive decline is of more concern.
- *Potential for worsening.* This is an overdose or allergic response, in which the true amount and final effect is not known. Complaints of a throat "tightening" is serious.
- *Stop any harm immediately.*
- *Patient before paperwork.*
- *First things first.* Do the most urgent first. Medications tend to be a priority.
- *Presence of other risk factors or co-morbidities.* The patient's physiologic coping status is already stressed before this new injury or illness insult.

17. List some risk factors or co-morbidities that would be more likely to make a patient a higher priority.

- *Very young or very old.* (Decreased immunity.) Those less than 7 days of age are considered very high risk.
- *Altered immunity from drugs (steroids, chemotherapy) or conditions (HIV+, leukemia, splenectomy).* This includes avoiding the exposure of susceptible individuals to nosocomial infection. The immunosuppressed patient may be stable, but should not be in a waiting room full of acutely ill people.

- *Recipient of a transplanted organ.* (Taking steroids, risk of electrolyte imbalance.)
- *Multiple other medical conditions.* The person has less physiologic reserve to fight. Diabetes is of particular concern because it decreases the immunity.
- *Does the patient have a history of an ominous outcome/etiology for this complaint before?* Did the patient with chest pain previously have a heart attack (because they probably still have most of the same risk factors they had the first time)?
- *Compare the patient's current condition with their normal states.* Consider the patient's response: do they think this is "different" or the "worst"?
- *Pregnancy.* Consider the risk of injury to the fetus if maternal condition is not resolved. Presenting complaints that are of specific concern in a pregnant patient include trauma (including ruling out abuse), hypertension (≥140/90), history of a seizure (rule out preeclampsia/eclampsia), dribbling "urine" (rule out leaking amnionic membranes), heavy blood loss after 24 weeks (rule out placenta previa), or back pain (rule out labor).
- *Decreased level of consciousness from any cause* (head injury, intoxication, etc.)
- *Trauma.* We cannot often externally see the extent of the injury. This includes a new onset neurologic deficit.
- *Significant pain* (usually considered ≥ 7 in a 0 to 10 scale)
- *Recent discharge from the hospital and/or medication changes.* There is an increased risk of drug reactions or inappropriate administration.
- *The patient received treatment prior to arrival without improvement and/or was seen by a physician prior to arrival.*
- *Recent foreign travel (within the past 3 months).*
- *Abuse/neglect, especially in an incident occurring within 4 hours before ED presentation.*
- *Psychiatric presentation.* Consider the patient's current state of agitation, self-control, willingness to stay, significant psychiatric history, and/or the presence of a responsible person with the patient.

18. Some staff criticize my triage decision making when it results in getting a new patient.

Unfortunately, staff are not always altruistic in their interactions with colleagues and some are just unhappy to have "more work." Ways to help deal with that can include:

- *Making them accountable for their opinion.* Consultant Shelley Cohen offers a "script": "If you have new patient information, please feel free to document the new assessment and change in triage acuity that you are going to make with your signature."
- *Cite a higher authority.* The higher authority can be a standardized course, such as Pediatric Advanced Life Support (PALS) or Emergency Nurse Pediatric Course (ENPC). Cohen offers this script:
  - "The department policy calls for the patient to be a ____ category. If you feel we need to change these triage policies, you should talk with the Nurse Manager and have it brought up at the next staff meeting."
  - *Consider their motive or communication style.*

19. Elaborate on what is meant by their motive or communication style.

Many departments have a few individuals on the sidelines who freely dispense cynical criticism, sometimes referred to as the "queen or king syndrome." Many of these individuals expect preferential treatment; at times it can degrade into a "bullying."

Try dealing directly with the individual about the behavior, but not in the middle of a tirade. Defensive arguing at that time only fuels the problem. Seek them out at the end of the shift and ask what literature or standard they were basing their protest on. One nurse indicates he will "apologize" for "overburdening" the protesting nurse because he values their collegiate relationship. Usually the person now has better insight into the inappropriateness of the previous reaction, and it can be an impetus for change. Allowing the behavior to go unchecked, however, lowers morale and has a negative impact on the department. If no change occurs, seek the manager's assistance.

20. What kind of things lead to errors in decision making?

- *Lack of knowledge.* You can't perceive what you can't know.
- *Confirmation bias.* Focusing on information that supports the initial or favored hypotheses.
- *Personal bias.* A high risk on a "known" patient. Assume the patient is sick this time (regardless of the past) until proven otherwise. Triage nurses were reluctant in one study to identify the symptoms as cardiac in middle-aged women because "… that could be me."
- *Considering too few possibilities or failing to assess completely.* This can be a result of the inexperienced nurse not knowing what he or she does not know or a failure to assess completely (e.g., the Bell's palsy triaged as a stroke). Avoid being the "court reporter" that only notes what the patient says.
- *Exposure frequency.* Nurses tend to draw on their most recent, frequent, or dramatic experiences for comparison with the current situation. They are less likely to consider something not commonly seen in their department.
- *Bias from other clinicians.* Information from prehospital health care providers or other nurses is essential, but can be unintentionally incomplete or biased.
- *"Oh my god!" distracters.* This is usually a visually repulsive initial finding that tends to pull everyone's attention, such as the hand of a child blown apart. The basic priorities still remain: life before limb.
- *Accepting the "patient's self-diagnosis."* A classic example can be the failure to have the patient who had an MVA undress for an appropriate assessment because "I only hurt my hand" (and they are in a hurry to leave).
- *Lack of a safety culture and processes*
- *Interpersonal interactions*
- *Cognitive errors*

See also Chapter 1.

21. Discuss cognitive errors.

Approximately half of all malpractice suits brought against emergency physicians arise from delayed or missed diagnoses. Croskerry (2003) looked at failures in perceptions and biases (so-called cognitive dispositions to respond). They found 32 types of cognitive errors, such as looking onto salient features of the initial presentation too early.

22. How can the triage nurse avoid cognitive errors?

Croskerry (2003) suggested:

- Always consider alternatives.
- Decrease reliance on memory and use cognitive aids, such as reference books.
- Use cognitive forcing strategies, such as protocols that minimize personal bias.
- Provide adequate time for thinking by having a reasonable workload.
- Establish clear accountability and follow-up. Provide rapid and reliable feedback so errors are immediately identified, understood, and corrected.

23. Discuss health care safety/error issues in the light of decision making.

Past solutions had been to find the people to blame and/or get better or different people. There is growing awareness that we need to look at the working conditions, including the shifts/fatigue (Rogers, 2004), and the involved process. The new focus is on creating more error-proofed systems with automatic checks, such as prompts. These standard operations helped create a culture and climate of safety in other fields, such as aviation.

24. Provide an example to support the concept of stressing safety climate.

In one study, safety climate surveys were given to employees from various hospitals and naval aviators. Overall, the problematic response (suggesting an absence of a safety climate) rate 5.6% for naval aviators versus 17.5% for hospital personnel. A problematic response rate was 20.9% in high-hazard hospital domains, such as EDs and operating rooms. Problematic responses among health care workers were up to 12 times greater than those of aviators on certain questions.

25. Discuss interpersonal relationships as a factor.

Up to 70% to 80% of medical errors include interpersonal interaction issues. Yet in one study of teamwork and patient safety attitudes for hospital nurses working in the ED and intensive care (ICU), 23% to 33% rated their experiences with the primary physician or consulting physician as low or very low. Feeling free to approach health care colleagues will promote essential communication in decision making.

Key Points

- Prioritization considerations include acute before chronic, sudden onset before gradual, consider the worst-case scenario, life before limb, potential for worsening, and trends.
- Patient-specific conditions to consider for increased prioritization is immunosuppression, comparison to their "normal," very young/very old, previous history of an ominous etiology, recent discharge from the hospital and/or medication change, and multiple co-morbidities.
- Help avoid triage errors by keeping current in knowledge, assuming the patient is sick until proven otherwise, avoiding premature conclusions, and incorporating protocols.

Internet Resources

National Association for Associate Degree Nursing: Critical Thinking in Nursing Practice—The Vignette Project
http://www.noadn.org/conf2003/critical_thinking.pdf

Healthgulf.com: Triage In The Emergency Department
http://news.healthgulf.com/ems/tn.pdf

AllNurses.com: Critical Thinking—How to Inspire It?
http://allnurses.com/forums/showthread.php?s=&threadid=38137

Emergency Nurses Association: Decision Making, Clinical Judgment, and Critical Thinking—Walking Around the Elephant
http://www.ena.org/conferences/annual/2004/handouts/239-o.pdf

Bibliography

Alfaro-LeFevre R: *Critical thinking in nursing: A practical approach*, Philadelphia, 1999, WB Saunders.

Arslanian-Engoren C: Gender and age bias in triage decisions, *J Emerg Nurs* 26(2):117-124, 2000.

Battles JB, Shea CE: A system of analyzing medical errors to improve GMEE curricula and programs, *Acad Med* 76(2):125-133, 2001.

Brennan M: "Queens" (and "Kings") (Managers Forum), *J Emerg Nurs* 39(2):164, 2004.

Canadian Association of Emergency Physicians: Canadian emergency department triage and acuity scale implementation guidelines, *J Can Assoc Emerg Physicians* 1:1-24, 1999.

Cohen S: 101 triage tips, Hohenwald, Tenn, 2002, Health Resources Unlimited.

Cone KJ, Murray R: Characteristics, insights, decision making, and preparation of ED triage nurses, *J Emerg Nurs* 28(5):401-406, 2002.

Croskerry P: The importance of cognitive errors in diagnosis and strategies to minimize them, *Acad Med* 78(8):775-780, 2003.

delBueno D: Assessing new hire competencies, *J Emerg Nurs* 29(3):271-272, 2003.

Edwards B: Clinical reasoning. In Dolan B, Holt L, editors. *Accident & emergency theory into practice*, London, 2000, Harcourt.

Fischer JE, et al: Quantifying uncertainty: Physicians' estimates of infection in critically ill neonates and children, *Clin Infect Dis* 38:1383-1390, 2004.

Gaba DM, Singer SJ, Sinaiko A, et al: Differences in safety climate between hospital personnel and naval aviators, *Hum Factors* 45(2):173-185, 2003.

Kaissi A, Johnson T, Kirschbaum MS: Measuring teamwork and patient safety attitudes of high-risk areas, *Nurs Economics* 21(5):211-218, 2003.

Mackway-Jones K: *Emergency triage: Manchester Triage Group*, London, 1997, BMJ Publishing Group.

McKay JI: "Queens" (and "Kings") (Managers Forum), *J Emerg Nurs* 39(2):163-164, 2004.

Strauss R, Mofidi M, Sandler ES, et al: Reflective learning in community-based dental education, *J Dent Educ* 67(11):1234-1242, 2003.

Zimmermann PG: Guiding principles at triage: Advice for new triage nurses, *J Emerg Nurs* 28(1):24-33, 2002.

Chapter 10

Documentation Issues

Rebecca S. McNair and Polly Gerber Zimmermann

1. What are the hallmarks of good documentation of the triage assessment?

Brevity *and* clarity. Both must be evident to ensure an efficient and thorough, safe patient course through the triage and transition of care process.

2. What are the minimum documentation requirements for the triage nurse?

Emergency Nurses Association's (ENA) "Making the Right Decision" outlines the essentials of documentation. I have found these requirements to be consistent and valid throughout our consulting work. They are as follows:

- Arrival time
- Time seen by triage nurse
- Chief complaint
- Meds and allergies
- Vital signs
- Subjective and objective assessment based on chief complaint
- Acuity category (including a generalized statement of the patient status, such as no acute distress [NAD])
- Diagnostic tests and care rendered
- Disposition
- Reevaluation and changes in condition

3. Any other suggestions for inclusions?

- Method of arrival (ambulance name, ambulatory, etc.). Patients who can't walk are at high risk for having a true emergent condition.
- Observations of abnormality (odor resembling alcohol, etc.)
- Teaching done
- Family awareness of the situation

4. How should the chief complaint be charted?

It should be a symptom, not a nurse- or patient-given conclusion or diagnosis. The patient has urinary burning and frequency, not a "urinary tract infection." The patient's previous history of urinary tract infections (UTIs) can be documented in the history. Accepting a premature conclusion can subconsciously influence the triage assessment and acuity.

5. Does subjective objective assessment plan (SOAP) charting have a role in the documentation of the triage assessment?

Yes. Even though we may not actually print the acronym on our documentation tools, include:

Subjective information (what the patient tells us voluntarily or in response to questions in a directed interview)
Objective information
Nursing **A**ssessment of the situation and patient status (may be a general statement, but also should include Acuity)
Nursing **P**lan (Placed in observation chairs, room placement, etc.)

SOAPIER can be an added help, meaning
Interventions,
Evaluation,
and **R**eassessment.

Although these are obvious components of a comprehensive assessment, a rapid triage should also have the same components unless the patient is taken immediately back for treatment as a result of a high acuity presentation.

6. Give an example of using SOAP.

An example of documentation of a Rapid triage using the SOAP acronym would be
S complaining mid sternal chest pain, shortness of breath × 2 hours
O alert/oriented × 4, pale, dry, respirations slightly labored
A Level 1–Emergent (Unstable)
P Acute treatment room immediately
Rapid Triage Nurse Signature ______________________________

7. What are some tools that are used to help with a rapid documentation of the triage assessment?

The mnemonic PQRST (see Chapter 6). Another is OLD CART (Tipsord-Klinkhammer and Andreoni, 1998):
Onset of symptoms
Location of symptoms
Duration of symptoms
Characteristics of symptoms described by patient
Aggravating factors
Relieving factors
Treatment administered before arrival and outcome

8. It seems that documenting the pain assessment has a more recent awareness and emphasis.

Pain, whether physical, emotional or psychological, is usually what brings a patient to the emergency department (ED). Patients have a right to assessment and management of their pain, regardless of the type. The ENA Course for Advanced Trauma nursing states (regarding physical pain), "There is no direct relationship between the strength of a stimulus and the perception of pain.

Therefore the correlation between the degree of pain and the type of injury is unreliable. Unfortunately it is often used as the basis for analgesia dosage."

9. Give some pointers on improving pain assessment.

- *The manner in which the complaint is properly elicited and documented.* When asking a patient about his pain, I consistently advise the use of the word "discomfort" in place of the word pain, "Are you having any discomfort?" Pain is often perceived as something sharp or stabbing.
- *Pain can be assessed using self-report, behavioral observation, or physiologic measures.* Often triage nurses ONLY use self-report. Although we don't want to do the opposite of only using behavioral observations or physiologic measures, good assessment and documentation rely on both subjective and objective components to support the acuity decision.

For example: A patient with a chief complaint of abdominal pain × 4 days, states his pain is 9/10. However, the patient has normal vital signs, smoking with his friends outside. The patient's perception of his pain may be a 9, but the nurse may support a lower acuity designation and the ability of the patient to wait.

10. List some common pain assessment tools.

See the chapter on pain assessment. PQRST is commonly used. Other pain severity tools used in the ED are:

- Visual Analog Scale (VAS)
- Spanish Pain Scale
- Faces Legs Activity Cry and Consolability (FLACC) Postoperative Pain Tool
- CRIES: A neonatal postoperative pain measurement score

A recent study found that the verbally administered numerical rating scales (NRS) from 0 to 10 could be substituted for the VAS in acute pain management.

11. What is the Pain Severity Scale?

0	None	Customer not reporting pain.
1	Mild	Customer says pain is mild, or does not appear distressed.
2	Moderate	Customer says pain is moderate or appears distressed from the pain, less able or willing to participate in care.
3	Severe	Customer says pain is severe or appears very distressed; function, mobility, or behavior is affected.
4	Very Severe	Customer says pain is very severe, significantly interferes with ADLs, independence, and quality of life.

ADL, Activities of daily living.

12. Is it okay to just document a brief focused objective assessment instead of addressing all the major body systems at triage?

Only if the nurse is performing a rapid triage, is confident of the acuity and appropriate disposition, and the patient will be placed in an open bed, with an available care provider immediately. Otherwise the triage nurse MUST show that the patient was stable at triage and therefore able to wait safely. This does NOT mean, however, that an in-depth secondary assessment is performed.

For example a brief statement is acceptable: *Amb w/o diff, A/O × 4, skin w/d, resp reg and unlab, NAD* (Ambulatory without difficulty, alert and oriented to person, place, time and purpose, skin warm and dry, respirations regular and unlabored. No acute distress.) A check box template allows efficiency and speed. This records the fact that the patient was stable on the triage assessment, and was able to wait or go to radiology. If the patient's status changes, and you have not documented a baseline, then the burden of proof resides with the caregiver in charge of that person at the time, which is the triage nurse.

Always move from general to the specific. Next comes the brief focused objective statement regarding the presenting chief complaint, i.e., *CMS intact, + pedal pulses, + edema left lat malleolus* (color, motor, sensation intact, pedal pulses palpable, edema noted to left lateral malleolus).

13. Are there any tips or tools for documentation of pediatric assessment?

Pediatric Mnemonic for triage assessment (emergency nurse pediatric course [ENPC]) is CIAMPEDS
Chief Complaint
Immunizations
Allergies
Medications
Past medical history, **P**arents' impression
Events surrounding
Diet, **D**iapers
Symptoms associated with illness/injury

The Pediatric Assessment Triangle for your quick-look assessment of the pediatric patient as recommended by ENPC (2004).

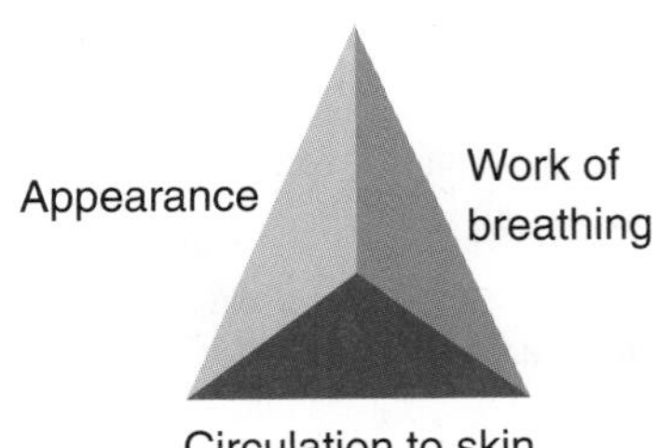

14. Discuss the terms to use in charting alertness for a child.

Care should be given when documenting the terms "lethargic" and "irritable."

Lethargic denotes significant neurologic sequelae, whereas *drowsy* means the child CAN be aroused easily. See the word "lethargic" when in fact the child just needs a nap, or has been crying from injury or not feeling well, and is just worn out.

Irritable denotes a serious neurologic event, whereas a fussy child can be consoled by caregiver or parent. My experience in consulting work reveals the word "irritable" frequently documented, when the child is just fussy because of illness, missing his or her nap, being with strangers, etc.

15. What is different in documentation of trauma?

Physiologic criteria, anatomic criteria, and mechanism of injury must be addressed. We may overlook critical information if we say a patient was involved in a motor vehicle collision (MVC), but omit that they were unrestrained and were struck in the driver's side by a vehicle traveling 40 mph. This info can be gathered and documented in the treatment area if the patient is seen by a primary nurse rather quickly. In our consulting work we often see the patient in the waiting area, with a lower acuity, and the only documentation is "Involved in MVC, NAD." This is not sufficient information to establish that a patient can safely wait.

16. Can documenting by exception be used successfully at triage?

There are many occasions in which certain aspects of assessment were not addressed, and therefore not documented. So often it is difficult to be sure that all the necessary components of an assessment were actually even considered when the triage nurse charts by exception. It is possible to chart by exception if the department has an excellent tool with all the normal parameters spelled out on the chart and a policy to support this practice.

It may be possible, and even expedient, to document by exception for the objective aspects of the exam (vital signs, body systems, pulses, etc.) and a few subjective aspects (Allergies, Meds). However, the objective components, which are amenable to documentation by exception, actually take little time to record with appropriate abbreviations, and the assessment must occur anyway to know if normal parameters are met.

It is necessary to record the chief complaint and subjective assessment regarding the presentation (e.g., onset of illness or injury). Then the factors that influence the triage decision are documented.

17. Regarding paper documentation forms, what is the best form to use at triage?

The best form to use is one that:

- Complements and blends with your actual triage process and patient flow
- Doesn't jump around from subjective to objective information
- Includes the essential components of documentation described by ENA
- Allows recording of the entire triage process and systematic decision making, such as interventions and plan
- Levels the playing field.

18. Explain what "levels the playing field" means.

Tools, as possible, must help pass on our knowledge to incoming nurses. With check box and template documentation tools, more inexperienced nurses are able to see a presentation and the proper associated assessment and documentation performed, thereby increasing their own armamentarium.

Many nurses may initially be overwhelmed by the sheer amount of type on a check boxed form, but once they are acquainted with and get used to the form, most admit that they are quick, comprehensive, and easy to use. See the Internet Resource Box for an example of this form.

19. What are the advantages of electronic documentation?

One study found that nursing documentation time went from 35.1% to 24.2%, with an increase in direct care from 31% to 40% of the nurses' time. Time spent on assessment doubled.

20. What are some of the things to look for in electronic triage tools?

In addition to all of the above points, the electronic triage template or tool must allow for the nurse to use a systematic decision-making process, and not be confined to simple or obvious clinical presentations. The human is a complex being, and a myriad of presentations (some atypical) are possible. The system should allow the nurse to override any acuity designations appointed by a computer, and to make general subjective and objective observations, which clarify and/or support your triage decisions.

21. What is key to remember with documentation?

Include enough documentation that it will be clear why you did what you did and who knew what, when, and why. Build your case. A common question asked in a deposition is, "What were you thinking at that time?"

22. I worry about the liability from patients who chose to leave after checking in with the triage nurse.

It is estimated that 29.6 million ED visits were not triaged (and records of triage were not made). Of these, 1.8 million patients left without being seen (LWBS), e.g., before a medical screening exam (MSE) was performed. If the triage nurse becomes aware of the patient leaving, attempt to give risks and obtain a signature or document the impossibility to obtain it. Documentation should illustrate that the patient is making an independent, informed decision and include the "why," competency, and understanding of risks. Sample statements could include:

- Patient states wants to see primary medical doctor (PMD) in the morning.
- Aware of risks including death.
- Judgment not clinically impaired.
- May return at any time.

23. Give an example that can be used if a patient decides to LWBS.

An Emergency Medical Treatment and Active Labor Act (EMTALA) expert recommends telling patients that the ED is still ready to see them if they change their minds, but then obtaining a signature on a related form. The wording he suggests is:

"I recognize that under federal and state law, I have the right to a medical screening examination and stabilizing treatment for any emergency condition found. I hereby withdraw any request for such an examination and/or treatment for myself or for ____________________ (relation) and hereby release the hospital from any obligations it has under the law to provide such examination and/or treatment."

24. What about handwriting legibility?

This area is receiving an increased focus during Joint Commission of Accreditation for Healthcare Organizations (JCAHO) surveys. When one surveyor finds handwriting that the surveyor cannot read; two different nurses will be asked to read it. If the nurses cannot read it, it can be a citation.

25. What about the use of nursing home transfer sheets?

A common problem is that nursing homes will send material more related to the client's chronic conditions than this visit. Paradise Valley Hospital (National City, CA) developed a "Hot Shot" transfer form on bright pink paper. The sheet includes why the patient is being sent today to the ED, the patient's attending physician, and if there are advance directives.

Key Points

- Brevity and clarity are the hallmarks of good documentation.
- Chart the objective and subjective assessments of the chief complaint. Do not be lulled into writing a premature conclusion or medical diagnosis.
- Document competency, why, understanding of risks, and explanation of high-risk symptoms for any patient who is LWBS.

Internet Resources

ED Documentation Form
http://www.triagefirst.com/ED%20Chart.pdf

EMTALA Online. Health Law Resource Center
www.medlaw.com

Bibliography

American Academy of Pediatrics: *The assessment and management of acute pain in infants, children, and adolescents,* Elk Grove Village, Ill, 2001, Author.

American Pain Society: *Task Force on Pain in Infants, Children and Adolescents,* Glenview, Ill, 2000, Author.

Baker S: Nursing home transfer sheet information (Managers Forum), *J Emerg Nurs* 30(4):351-352, 2004.

Emergency Nurses Association: *Emergency nurse pediatric course,* Des Plaines, Ill, 2004, Author.

Lawrence JD: Documenting left without being seen cases (Managers' Forum), *J Emerg Nurs* 29(6):564, 2003.

Lawrence JD: EMTALA Q & A, *ED Manag* 15:56-57, 2003.

McNair R (President): Documentation lecture and lab. In *The nature of the beast: Comprehensive triage and patient flow workshop,* Fairview, NC, 2003, Triage First, Inc.

McNair R (President): Systematic triage assessment. In *Triage First EDucation: A comprehensive emergency department triage course,* Fairview, NC, 2004, Triage First, Inc.

Sloan EP: *ED documentation: A systematic approach to the care of critically ill patients,* ICEP Resident Academic Forum, Northwestern Memorial Hospital, Chicago, Ill, April 29, 2004.

Tipsord-Klinkhammer B, Andreoni CP: *Quick reference for emergency nursing,* Philadelphia, 1998, WB Saunders.

Wong DH, Gallegos Y, Weinger MB, et al: Changes in intensive care unit nurse task activity after installation of a third-generation intensive care unit information system, *Crit Care Med* 31(10): 2488-2494, 2003.

Section II

Special Considerations

Chapter 11

Pediatrics

Polly Gerber Zimmermann

1. Define pediatric besides the definition of age ranges.

There is no one universal standard. The American Heart Association (AHA) guidelines indicate that infant is up to 1 year of age and a child is 1 year to 8 years of age. Various other organizations use different arbitrary "cut-off" ages of 12, 14, or 16 years.

The Emergency Medical System of North Caroline defines "pediatric," for the purpose of use of protocols and equipment, as a patient who fits on the Broselow tape. Although this guideline does not address developmental issues, any child that is "off the tape" will basically use adult-sized equipment and medication dosing. It is particularly helpful in a situation in which there is no confirmed weight or age, such as a disaster scenario.

2. What percent of the emergency department population is pediatric?

Pediatric patients constitute approximately 21% to 23% of all general emergency department (ED) visits. Critically ill children present with symptoms that are rapid in onset, involve the respiratory or central nervous systems, and require immediate intervention.

3. What is a key concept of pediatric care?

Children are not little adults.

4. List some basic different physiologic characteristics of children.

- The pediatric airway is smaller in diameter and more easily occluded.
- Infants are obligatory nose breathers; children are diaphragmatic breathers.
- The work of breathing is more obvious because they have a compliant chest wall.
- Early respiratory distress is characterized by increased work of breathing and tachypnea; bradypnea is a late sign.
- Children have a smaller circulating blood volume (80 mL/kg). Use capillary refill as an early indicator rather than pulse and blood pressure.
- Children are more susceptible for dehydration. Use weight, urine output, dry mucus membranes/dry cracked lips, and absence of tears as indicators of dehydration. (See also Chapter 30.)

5. What is considered a key pediatric problem?

Obesity. About 16% of children are now considered overweight, which is about three times higher than in 1960. This predisposes to future health risks, including hypertension, type 2 diabetes, liver disorders, dyslipidemia, hyperinsulinemia, and obstructive sleep apnea.

6. Describe how to do a quick look triage of a child.

Emergency Nursing Pediatric Course (ENPC) recommends the "across the room" triage of general appearance, work of breathing, and circulation. Circulation can be evidenced by color and capillary refill.

7. What is meant when it is said to evaluate if a child looks sick?

Consider the patient's level of alertness and activity, respiratory effort, muscle tone, eye contact, ability to feed, and interactiveness. Toxic-appearing children may show irritable behavior, poor feeding, lethargy, cyanosis, and unwillingness to interact.

8. Do I proceed if the child looks well and someone other than the parent or guardian brought the child?

The law implies parental consent for a child's treatment in an emergency. Obviously this is required to preserve life, limb, or alleviate pain or suffering. Ethicist and ED physician Bernard Heiliscer recommends a liberal interpretation of this standard. Ask this question: "Would I consider a parent negligent if they did not treat their child for this condition?" If so, treat and attempt to contact the parent or guardian.

9. Provide some mnemonics to help with obtaining the history of children.

ENPC uses CIAMPEDS (see Chapter 10). Another is **SAVE A CHILD:**
Save: observations made prior to touching the patient
A Child: history from caretaker, brief examination
Skin (mottled, petechiae, pallor)
Activity (responsive)
Ventilation (retractions, rate, stridor)
Eye contact (glassy stare, fails to engage)
Abuse (unexplained bruising, inappropriate parent)
Cry (high-pitched)
Heat (fever)
Immune system (sickle cell, corticosteroids)
Level of consciousness (irritable, lethargic)
Dehydration (capillary refill, severe diarrhea/vomiting)

10. How should level of consciousness be assessed in a child?

Besides the pediatric Glasgow Coma Scale, ENPC recommends AVPU (**A**lert, **V**erbal, **P**ain, **U**nresponsive).

11. List some tips when obtaining vital signs in children.

- All pediatric patients should have a weight. (Children have a large body surface area-to-weight ratio. The weight is needed for medication dosing.)
- Count respirations before handling the child. If crying, indicate it, e.g., "40/cry."
- Bradycardia should be considered hypoxia until it is ruled out.
- Blood pressure changes are a late indicator because of the compensatory vasoconstriction. Changes in blood pressure often do not occur until just before total circulatory collapse. Formulas for use, outside of charts, include systolic over 2 years = 90 + (2 × age); diastolic is two thirds of systolic; and lower systolic limit over 2 years of age is 70 + (2 × age). See also Chapter 5.

12. How can I get the weight of a young child who won't stand on the scale, but is too large for the infant scale?

Weigh the parent/caregiver alone and then holding the infant. Subtract the difference. Most obtain some form of obtained actual weight, rather than stated weight, on children.

13. Is a head circumference measurement required for all infants?

Head circumference on all infants is not an absolute requirement of the Joint Commission for Accreditation of Healthcare Organizations (JCAHO) for EDs as long as they follow their hospital's policy. While some do this assessment as a screening measure, others question the value because there are no past measurements for comparison and practitioner variation can be a factor. The ED needs a policy indicating its difference from the hospital's pediatric department. Some use a generic policy that assessments are individualized to the patient's need. Others obtain it if:

- Indicated by presenting condition in a child less than 12 months old
- Suspected head injury, abuse, or septic/meningitis is present
- Ordered by the attending ED physician

14. What can I suggest when a child is behind in routine immunizations?

The Trust for American Health indicates that although 80% of white children are current with immunizations, the percentage of children who are black, illegal immigrants, in a home with a single parent, or not covered by insurance who are current is much lower. Children can receive immunizations at a public health clinic without revealing their immigration status.

15. I worry that I might be wrong when suspecting abuse in a pediatric patient.

Any injury in pediatrics might be a result of abuse. It is acceptable to suspect child abuse and be wrong. It is not acceptable to fail to suspect when it has occurred.

16. Discuss the role of the caregiver with a pediatric patient.

The parent or primary caregiver knows the child better than anyone else. While the triage nurse can discern the difference between sound nursing judgment of how the child looks and parent's perception, listening to the parent will usually provide useful information.

17. Can you offer a tip for dealing with parents?

Compliment their child. It can sometimes disarm a "difficult" parent.

18. Don't parents often just want an antibiotic for their child, even if it isn't warranted?

One study found that 50% of parents expected an antibiotic for their child's upper respiratory infection, but only 1% directly asked the prescriber. (The prescribing physician perceived the parents' expectation 34% of the time.) Parents were the most satisfied, even if they did *not* receive antibiotics, if the physician initiated a discussion about antibiotics and offered a contingency plan if the child did not improve. Overall, nationwide, the use of antibiotics in children under age 5 has declined 23% from 1994-1995 to 1998-2000. The decline was greatest in physician offices (versus EDs and hospital-based clinics). Currently, only 27% of health care visits result in antibiotics being prescribed. The majority of prescriptions were for otitis media (about 50%) and upper respiratory infections or pharyngitis (about 20%).

19. Do ED prescribers feel pressure to give antibiotics to improve "customer satisfaction"?

Physicians are more likely to prescribe an antibiotic if they believe the parents expect it. However, Stivers et al (2003) found that caregivers may misperceive pressure for antibiotics, especially if the parent suggests a diagnosis rather than report symptoms (e.g., "He might have strep throat." versus "He has a sore throat."). The researchers found that the parents often simply want reassurance that the child is not seriously ill or it was correct to seek care. Try increasing your communication of those reassurances in triage.

20. Should all children be automatically given a higher triage category?

No, triage is the current condition, not age. At times a management decision may be made to prioritize within a triage category for a young child late at night.

21. Is it best to set up a separate pediatric area, with its own triage and staff?

Unless a pediatric hospital, most recommend keeping one triage area in a general hospital to maximize awareness and control of the entire department. While the children may be treated in their own area, with appropriate décor and activities, it is usually recommended that all staff have a comfort level with all types of patients to maintain flexibility.

22. What additional education should ED nurses have to care for pediatric patients?

The Emergency Nurses Association Position Statement indicates "ENA recommends the Emergency Nursing Pediatric Course (ENPC) be the minimum educational standard for nurses providing emergency care to children." It also indicates, "emergency nurses must be knowledgeable of injury and disease prevention strategies, pediatric triage assessment and prioritization, nursing assessment, diagnosis, intervention, and on-going evaluation of children and adolescents."

Key Points

- Children longer than the Broselow tape will probably need adult equipment.
- Consider the child's alertness, activity, respiratory effort, muscle tone, eye contact, ability to feed, and interactiveness to determine "sick" or "toxic."
- Bradycardia should be considered hypoxia until it is ruled out.
- Routine ED head circumference measurement on all infants is not required.
- Give credibility to a parent's report that his/her child is sick.

Internet Resources

Emergency Nurses Association: Position Statement: Care of the Pediatric Patient During Interfacility Transfer
http://www.ena.org/about/position/carepediatric-inter.asp

Iroquois Memorial Hospital—Emergency Department: Age-Specific Guidelines
http://www.ena.org/document_share/documents/age_specific.pdf

Hot Topics in Healthcare: New Guidelines Warn—You may not be able to take care of sick children
http://www.ahcpub.com/ahc_root_html/hot/archive/edn062001.html

Emergency Nursing Through the Eyes of a Child
http://southflorida.sun-sentinel.com/careers/vitalsigns/pfold2003/xiii21emergency.htm

Bibliography

Andreoni CP, Klinkhammer B: *Quick reference for pediatric emergency nursing,* Philadelphia, 2000, WB Saunders.

Bernardo LM, Lees WE: Infants and children. In Oman KS, Koziol-McLain J, Scheetz LJ, editors: *Scheetz's emergency nursing secrets,* Philadelphia, 2001, Hanley & Belfus.

Bruns C: Measuring head circumference (Managers Forum), *J Emerg Nurs* 28(1):61, 2002.

Emergency Nurses Association: *Emergency nurse pediatric course,* Des Plaines, Ill, 2000, Author.

Emergency Nurses Association: *Position statement: Educational recommendation for nurses providing pediatric emergency care,* Des Plaines, Ill, 2001, Author.

Finkelstein JA, Stille C, Nordin J, et al: Reduction in antibiotic use among US children, 1996-2000, *Pediatrics* 112(3):620-627, 2003.

Grossman VGA: *Quick reference to triage,* ed 2, Philadelphia, 2003, Lippincott.

Halasa NB et al: Differences in antibiotic prescribing patterns for children younger than five years in the three major outpatient settings, *J Pediatr* 144:200-205, 2004.

Hohehaus S: Defining "Pediatric" (Managers Forum), *J Emerg Nurs* (in press).

Hohenhaus SM: Is this a drill? Improving pediatric emergency preparedness in North Carolina's emergency departments, *J Emerg Nurs* 27(6):568-570, 2001.

Mangione-Smith R: Parent expectations for antibiotics, physician-parent communication, and satisfaction, *Arch Pediatr Adolesc Med* 155:800-806, 2001.

Shread P: Pediatric-only area in the ED (Managers Forum), *J Emerg Nurs* 28(5):460-461, 2002.

Slovis CM, Wrenn KD, Meador CK: A little book of emergency medicine rules, Philadelphia, 2000, Hanley & Belfus.

Stivers T, Mangione-Smith R, Elliott MN, et al: "Why do physicians think parents expect antibiotics? What parents report versus what physicians believe," *J Fam Pract* 52(2):140-148, 2003.

Chapter 12

Using a Color-Coded System to Estimate Weight at Triage

Susan M. Hohenhaus

1. Sometimes a child is very ill when arriving at the emergency department, yet we still need a weight to determine medication doses and emergency equipment sizes. Is there a way other than placing a child on a scale that I can get an accurate weight?

Yes. Many emergency departments (EDs) have utilized the Broselow Tape as a tool to estimate weight in children under the age of approximately 13. It represents an objective, validated way to estimate accurate weight when it is not possible to obtain that information in the traditional way.

2. What is the Broselow-Luten Resuscitation Tape and where did it come from?

The Broselow Tape was developed in the late 1980s by an emergency physician, James Broselow, who felt that there had to be a better way to conduct a pediatric resuscitation. Rather than guessing weights and using cumbersome formulas to calculate medication dosages and determine equipment sizes for pediatric patients, he found that length had a direct correlation to weight in the pediatric population and the Broselow Tape was a result of that research. Since then, the tool can be found in many EDs as a standard for estimating pediatric weight and selecting medication and equipment.

3. I see children in the ED all the time. Why can't I just "guesstimate" the child's weight?

Studies have shown that as clinicians we are not very adept at guessing the weight of our patients. In one study in which the health care providers claimed to be "fairly accurate" in their guesses, only about 50% were close enough for accurate dosing. Serious medication dosage errors may occur when relying on guessing.

4. Why can't I just get the weight from the parent or caregiver?

Parents are usually quite stressed when their child is critically ill or injured. Asking them to identify an accurate weight for the child may cause confusion and be reported inaccurately. Also, parents will usually report the child's weight in pounds rather than in kilograms, causing the risk for confusion and error.

5. How do I know which children will "fit" on the Broselow Tape?

In general, children less than 13 years old have heights/lengths that correspond to weights on the tape. Small infants (<3 kg) will require different methods of weight estimation, medication dosing, and equipment selection.

6. Is this concept only for emergency resuscitation?

No. Broselow recommends that every child under the age of 13 be measured at triage and assigned a color zone as a vital sign. Already some prehospital ambulances have resuscitation bags in each color on the Broselow Tape. Broselow envisions that this color concept can eventually follow the child through the health care visit, regardless of point of entry or destination, to establish a common resuscitation language for the child and as a guide in future product labeling.

7. How do I use the Broselow Tape?

With the child lying supine and the Broselow Tape with the side listing the weight visible, place the "red" arrow on the tape at the patient's head ("red to head"); using your hand in a sliding motion flatten the tape out next to the child; stop at the child's heel. The color zone found at the child's heel should be noted and assigned to this child. In general for resuscitation, a child who is too long for the tape should have adult protocols implemented.

Anecdotally, some emergency departments are reporting their Joint Commission for Healthcare Organizations (JCAHO) surveyor is asking ED nurses to demonstrate how they use the tape.

8. What information is on the Broselow Tape?

The Broselow Tape contains nine color zones that list recommendations for resuscitation, including medication dosage, fluid therapy, and rapid sequence intubation. Also included are equipment sizes for the most common items used during initial stabilization of a critically ill or injured child, including endotracheal tube, vascular access catheter, and blood pressure cuff sizes. Other items such as the Pediatric Trauma Score and suggested pediatric ventilator settings are also included.

9. Are there other tools like the Broselow Tape?

The Broselow Tape is currently the only method available that utilizes length to accurately predict weight. There are other methods of calculating medication dosages or selecting equipment; however, they each require an accurate weight as a starting point.

10. Are there other tools that can be used with the Broselow Tape?

Caution should be used when utilizing any other system in conjunction with the Broselow Tape. The color sequence of the Broselow Tape is copyrighted.

Many manufacturers use color to identify various items related to patient care. Some of these colors are similar to the Broselow color scheme, but others are not.

Unless there is identification on the device that it is directly linked to the Broselow Tape, the clinician should be cautious. The "Color Coded Kids" logo should be visible on any item that is designed specifically to be used with the Broselow Tape.

11. Are there references for the use of the Broselow Tape?

There is an educational website, developed with federal funding, that is designed to help clinicians learn more about how to use the Broselow Tape. Additionally there is a Pediatric Education for Prehospital Professionals course available from the American Academy of Pediatrics. It contains a video that outlines how to use the Broselow-Luten Tape. See Internet Resources for the URLs for these sites.

12. Why do you need education on how to use the Tape? Isn't it rather obvious?

During our mock resuscitation exercises, I observed critical safety issues in the use of the Broselow-Luten Resuscitation Tape. These included:

- Improper positioning of the tape during patient measurement
- Difficulty using the tape to determine the correct medication and equipment size to use
- Confusion regarding the items inside the complementing organizers, whether purchased commercially or created by individual institutions

13. What can help eliminate these types of errors?

I recommended:

- The red measuring arrow is always upright if the aid is placed in plastic or laminated.
- Replacing the 1998 version of the aid with the 2002 version, which "corrected" the confusing smallest zone
- Ensuring regular training that includes awareness of the "crash cart" contents and demonstrated competency on the use of the tape
- Marking individual items within the "crash cart" drawers according to the color zone they are included in

Key Points

- Weights must be obtained on all children. It is recommended that every child under the age of 13 be measured at triage and assigned a color zone as a vital sign.
- The Broselow-Luten Resuscitation Tape is an aid for emergent situations that uses the child's height/length, which statistically corresponds to weights.
- Verify staff competency with correct use of the tape and awareness of crash cart contents. Store the tape with the red measurement arrow upright.

Internet Resources

Duke Enhancing Pediatric Safety (DEPS)
www.DEPS.dukehealth.org

Pediatric Education for Prehospital Professionals (PEPP)
www.PEPPsite.com

Bibliography

Black K, Barnett P, Wolfe R, Young S: Are methods used to estimate weight in children accurate? *Emerg Med (Fremantle)* 14(2):160-165, 2002.

Hohenhaus SM: Assessing competency: The Broselow-Luten Resuscitation Tape, *J Emerg Nurs* 28(1):70-72, 2002.

Hohenhaus SM: Is this a drill? Improving pediatric emergency preparedness in North Carolina's emergency departments, *J Emerg Nurs* 27(6):568-570, 2001.

Hohenhaus SM, Frush KS: Pediatric patient safety: Common problems in the use of resuscitative AIDS for simplifying pediatric emergency care, *J Emerg Nurs* 30(1):49-51, 2004.

Lubitz DS, Seidel JS, Chameides L, Luten RC, Zaritsky AL, Campbell FW: A rapid method for estimating weight and resuscitation drug dosages from length in the pediatric age group, *Ann Emerg Med* 17(6):576-581, 1998.

Luten R, Wears RL, Broselow J, et al: Managing the unique size-related issues of pediatric resuscitation: reducing cognitive load with resuscitation aids, *Acad Emerg Med* 9(8):840-847, 2002.

Vilke GM, Marino A, Fisher R, Chan TC: Estimation of pediatric patient weight by EMT-PS, *J Emerg Med* 21(2):125-128, 2001.

Chapter 13

Geriatric Considerations

Polly Gerber Zimmermann

1. Describe the elderly population in the United States and their use of the emergency department.

- Currently people aged 65 or older in the United States makes up 13% of the population, but 18% of the emergency department (ED) patients.
- Out of every 100 ambulatory care annual visits (made to physician offices, hospital outpatient departments, or EDs), 47 were to EDs in people aged 65 and older, compared to 30/100 by people aged 45 to 64.
- Persons aged 75 and older have the highest rate of ED visits (61.1 per 100 persons). The next highest rate was for persons aged 15 to 24. Visits by nursing home residents accounted for 2% of all visits.
- In a benchmark study conducted by the Emergency Nurses Association (ENA), 60% of the ED managers reported an increase in the number of elderly and nursing home patient visits in 2000.

2. How are elderly patients different in their use of ED resources than younger patients?

Elderly patients are more likely to:

- Present to the ED with illnesses of higher acuity levels
- Arrive by ambulance
- Require longer triage interviews
- Have an ED visit last longer/require more staff time and resources
- Be admitted to the hospital (46%) or to be admitted to an intensive care unit
- Have repeat ED visits
- Experience higher rates of adverse health outcomes after discharge

3. Talk about the issues that contribute to the complexity of older adult patients.

- *Physiologic changes.* These include decreased elasticity in blood vessels, brittle bones, decreased glomerular filtration rate/creatinine clearance (up to 50% less by age 90), decreased gastrointestinal absorption (by 50%), decreased cardiac output (50%), decreased pulmonary function (30%), lower albumin levels, and slower thought processes.
- *Decreased immunity resulting in an atypical presentation.* The thalamus shrinks 90% and there is a loss of T-cell function. For example, a "classic" urinary

tract infection causes dysuria, frequency, and urgency, but the older adult patient is more likely to just exhibit incontinence, confusion, and anorexia. While "classic" pneumonia causes a purulent cough, fever, and leukocytosis, the elderly are more likely to be afebrile (25% to 30% of the time) with a normal white blood cell count (WBC) (more than 20% of the time). Tachycardia, tachypnea, and a sudden onset of confusion may be the only manifestations of the pneumonia.

- *Different physiologic response to medications.* They often require a smaller dose (up to one-third to one-half less) and have a higher risk of toxicity (as a result of the decreased glomerular filtration rate resulting in accumulation and toxicity).
- *More likely to be on medications (such as beta blockers) that mask hypovolemia.*
- *Co-morbidities.* The independent living senior has an average of three chronic medical problems; those living in care facilities have ten. This includes being more likely to have depression, dementia, incontinence, and immobility.
- *Blunted presentations, including less pain with a serious injury or lack of chest pain with a myocardial infarction.*
- *Decrease in social support.* There are more needs regarding risk for abuse, end-of-life decisions, palliative care, and family stressors.

4. What are the other top medical reasons for elderly patients' ED visits?

Chest pain, trauma, pneumonia, congestive heart failure, abdominal pain, electrolyte imbalance or dehydration, stroke, diabetes, change in mental status, and sepsis.

5. How seriously should I regard abdominal pain in the older adult?

Acute abdominal pain in the older adult is a serious complaint because the elderly tend to have a delay in the presentation and perforation is more likely. Cholecystitis is the most common surgical cause; two other common causes are diverticulitis and appendicitis. A general guideline for the older adult patient is the atypical is typical as the presentation.

6. How should I regard confusion in the older adult?

Acute onset of confusion in an older person is a "change in mental status." It can often be a sign of infection, dehydration, constipation, or withdrawal for sedative-hypnotic abuse.

7. What is the most common reason for injury-related ED visits in Americans?

According to the Centers for Disease Control and Prevention, 62% of the approximately 2.7 million older adults (65 years and older) treated for nonfatal injuries in hospital emergency departments were related to falls.

8. Discuss the related issue of backboard immobilization.

One study found that the total backboard time was 53.9 minutes if x-rays weren't taken and 181.3 minutes for patients who had x-rays. Yet immobilization of healthy subjects on a rigid spine board for 80 minutes may introduce tissue pressure high enough to result in the development of pressure ulcers.

9. What lab values may vary in the "normal" for patients older than age 65?

Elderly patients' "normal" lab values are similar to other adults' values, but a few exceptions include:

- Elevated serum alkaline phosphatase (may be 2.5 times higher than normal)
- Elevated fasting blood glucose (135 to 150 mg)
- Elevated erythrocyte sedimentation (40 mm per hour)
- Decreased hemoglobin (11 mg/dL in women or 11.5 g/dL in men)
- Elevated blood urea nitrogen (BUN) (28 to 35 mg/dL)

10. Describe polypharmacy in relationship with the older adult.

Polypharmacy refers to the use of multiple drugs on a routine basis. The elderly consume 33% of all prescribed medications and more than 70% of over-the-counter medications. The average elderly person uses more than four prescription medications and more than two over-the-counter medications daily: this "six" is viewed as the magic tolerable number.

The risk of polypharmacy-induced drug interactions directly increases as the number of drugs increase.

While the risk of an adverse drug reaction is only 6% with two drugs, it is 100% with eight drugs. One third of the geriatric population regularly takes eight or more drugs. Adverse drug reactions (ADR) account for 10% to 31% of hospital admissions and the severity of ADRs increases with age.

Additionally, Curtis et al (2004) found that 21% of elderly individuals filled a prescription for a drug that (in general) should be avoided in patients aged 65 and older. Of these, 44% were for drugs that carry a "substantial risk" of adverse effects in the older adult.

11. Describe a paradoxical reaction for elderly patients.

The typical side effects for benzodiazepines (such as diazepam [Valium] and lorazepam [Ativan]) include sedation or psychomotor impairment. The opposite effect occurs in as many as 29% of people, primarily children and the older adult. They have a "paradoxical" reaction characterized by emotional lability, agitation, and (sometimes) rage.

12. How can the triage nurse obtain an accurate list of current medications the patient is taking?

Some EDs actively encourage patients to bring a written list. When asking for a verbal list, always ask "anything else?" until the patient can't recall any more. Specifically ask about over-the-counter drugs and natural herbs.

The Pennsylvania State University Gerontology Center reported that when adults ages 65 to 91 in a primary care study were asked to bring in all of their prescription medications in a brown paper bag, the resulting list was more complete than their official pharmacy records.

13. Why is it important for the triage nurse to ask about a patient's adherence to a prescribed medication regimen?

One study found (understandably) that the more complex the medicine regimen, the more patient confusion and likelihood to have some non-adherence. Two out of three times, although, the prescriber did not realize that there was nonadherence occurring. The tendency, instead, is to attribute the patient's current status to drug failure and therefore prescribe stronger or more drugs.

All patients are noncompliant/nonadherent to some degree in up to 50% of chronic conditions. The complex reasons include misunderstanding, decreased cognition and comprehension, being unaware of the individual's non-compliance, poor communication, or physical limitations. After obtaining a list of drugs, consider asking if the patient has been able to take them regularly in the past week.

14. List some considerations regarding the older adult for an analgesic medication.

- Meperidine (Demerol) is not recommended because of possible toxicity, particularly if the patient has heart failure or renal impairment.
- Intramuscular injections are not recommended in older adults because they are likely to have diminished muscle and fatty tissue, which compromises the drugs' bioavailability.
- Remember the pain needs of patient with dementia. In several studies, this category of patients received less analgesic medications than those without dementia.

15. Why should the triage nurse be particularly alert for potential error when administering medications to the elderly?

The U.S. Pharmacopoeia 2004 report indicated that patients age 60 and older accounted for more than one third of all medication errors and 55% of fatal errors.

16. **What is being done to educate ED nurses about the special needs of the geriatric patient?**

The Emergency Nurses Association (ENA) has developed a standardized 8-hour course, GENE (Geriatric Emergency Nursing Education) with funding from a grant received from Nurse Competence in Aging. For more information, contact the ENA (www.ena.org).

17. **How should I deal with an accompanying caregiver?**

An older adult has the right to confidentiality. Verify the patient wants the caregiver present during the triage interview and question the patient alone when screening for abuse. Similar to parents with a young child, consider a caregiver's impression of a dependent elder. If they say the patient with Alzheimer's is acting different today, they are probably right.

18. **Should an older adult be triaged at a higher acuity level than someone younger with the same chief complaints?**

Triage criteria are based on the patient's condition. Avoid age discrimination: age alone is not a criterion, either young or old. However, the older adult is more likely to have other factors (such as co-morbidities, decreased immunity, etc.) to justify a higher priority.

Key Points

- The older adult patient is the proportionately highest user of ED visits and resources. Their atypical presentations, co-morbidities, and lack of social support can make them a more difficult category of patients to triage.
- Patients taking more than six drugs per day are at high risk for adverse drug reactions. The average elderly person is taking four prescription drugs and two over-the-counter medications.
- A more complete list of drugs was obtained (than the official pharmacy records) when older adults brought in all of their prescription medications in a brown paper bag.
- A general guideline with the older adult is that the atypical is typical. Their presentations often appear different or less acute than it actually is.

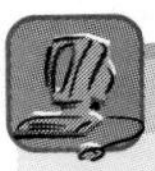

Internet Resources

National Center for Chronic Disease Prevention and Health Promotion: Healthy Aging
www.cdc.gov/aging

Emergency Nurses Association Position Statements: Care of Older Adults in the Emergency Setting
http://www.ena.org/about/position/CareofOlderAdults.asp

US Census Bureau: Elderly (65+) Population
http://www.census.gov/population/www/socdemo/age.html#elderly

Bibliography

Aminzadeh F, Dalziel WB: Older adults in the emergency department: A systematic review of patterns of use, adverse outcomes, and effectiveness of interventions, *Ann Emerg Med* 39(3):238-247, 2002.

Burt CW, McCaig LF: Trends in hospital department utilization: United States, 1992-1999, National Center for Health Statistics, *Vital Health Stat* 13:150, 2001.

Cohen S: *101 Triage Tips,* Hohenwald, Tenn, 2002, Health Resources Unlimited.

Cordell W, Hollingsworth J, Olinger M, Stroman S, Nelson D: Pain and tissue-interface pressures during spine-board immobilization, *Ann Emerg Med* 26:31-36, 1995.

Curtis LH, Ostbye T, Sendersky V, et al: Inappropriate prescribing for elderly Americans in a large outpatient population, *Arch Intern Med* 154:1621-1625, 2004.

Gutierrez MA, Roper JM, Han P: Paradoxical reactions to benzodiazepines, *Am J Nurs* 101(7): 334-340, 2001.

Hayes KS: Seniors. In Oman KS, Koziol-McLain J, Scheetz LJ, editors. *Scheetz's emergency nursing secrets,* Philadelphia, 2001, Hanley & Belfus.

Hayes KS: Research with elderly ED patients: Do we have any answers? *J Emerg Nurs* 26(3):268-271, 2000.

Jackimczyk KC, Tripp W: *Geriatric emergency medicine.* In Markovchick VJ, Pons PT, editors. *Pons' emergency medicine secrets,* ed 3, Philadelphia, 2003, Hanley & Belfus.

Lerner EB, Moscati R: Duration of patient immobilization in the ED, *Am J Emerg Med* 18:28-30, 2000.

MacLean SL: *2001 ENA benchmark guide: Emergency departments,* Des Plaines, Ill, 2001, Emergency Nurses Association.

The Pennsylvania State University Gerontology Center: Congruence of self-reported medications with pharmacy prescription records in low-income older adults, *Gerontologist* 44:176-185, 2004.

Richardson B: Overview of geriatric emergencies, *Mt Sinai J Med* 70(2):75-84, 2003.

Titler MG, Herr K, Schilling ML, et al: Acute pain treatment for older adults hospitalized with hip fracture: Current nursing practices and perceived barriers, *Appl Nurs Res* 16(4):211-227, 2003.

Travers D: Triage: How long does it take? How long should it take? *J Emerg Nurs* 25(3):238-240, 1999.

Chapter 14

Gender-Related Considerations

Robert D. Herr

1. Aren't gender-related differences at triage obvious?

Certainly the obvious difference in anatomy influences the potential causes of abdominal pain. Additionally, predilection of women for autoimmune-mediated disease indirectly influences potential causes of many conditions.

Other conditions not related to gender-specific organs nor autoimmune disease have been traditionally considered the same regardless of gender. It is no longer taken for granted that studies enrolling chiefly men or women can be generalized to both sexes. The past 10 years has exposed a systematic underenrollment of women to study certain chronic diseases such as heart and lung disease.

Only recently has research shown key differences in disease presentation. This is important to know at emergency department (ED) triage because rapid diagnosis and therapy can reduce morbidity and improve outcome. Chest pain/acute myocardial infarction (AMI) and stroke (cerebral vascular accident [CVA], brain attack) are two classic examples. Yet one study found that 25% of ED nurses thought there was no difference in the gender presentation of chest pain despite the fact numerous studies show that females have "typical" chest pain only around a fourth of the time when experiencing an AMI.

2. What key diseases do we currently know present significantly differently in the two sexes?

AMI, stroke, and consideration of domestic violence.

3. Talk about the difference in the AMI presentation.

Up to 75% of women present with "atypical" symptoms with an AMI. One study found that a woman is more likely to have:

- Vague pain located in the intrascapular, back (twice as common in women as men), epigastric, or right arm area
- Nausea and other gastrointestinal symptoms
- Shortness of breath
- Severe fatigue

In one study of 515 women diagnosed with AMI, the women frequently reported experiencing "prodromal symptoms" more than 1 month before the AMI. They were unusual, extreme fatigue (70.7%); sleep disturbances (47.8%); and shortness of breath (42.1%). Only 29.7% reported ever having any chest discomfort.

Acute chest pain was absent in 43% of them at the time of their AMI. The most frequent acute symptoms they experienced were shortness of breath (57.9%), weakness (54.8%), and extreme fatigue (42.9%).

4. These sound like the common symptoms for perimenopausal, overworked middle-aged women. What can help discriminate something serious is going on, especially when I work in an environment that doesn't have an electrocardiogram (EKG) immediately available?

A helpful discriminating question can be "Is this fatigue unusual for you?" The women described the feeling as "extreme" fatigue, not the usual tiredness one feels at the end of a busy day.

Additionally, consider other screening questions that indicate acute coronary syndrome. These include risk factors of smoking, hyperlipidemia, hypertension, family history, diabetes mellitus, or recent cocaine use. Consider also if there is a history of:

- Cardiac surgery/bypass, or angioplasty
- History of coronary artery disease, angina, or AMI
- Use of nitroglycerin for chest pain

5. Even though the presentations are different, are the outcomes the same for the two genders?

Women are more likely to have poorer morbidity and mortality results, partly because their heart problems occur later in life and are more severe. For women:

- 50% die in the first heart event, versus a 30% chance for death with a man
- 38% die within a year of surviving their first heart attack, versus 25% of men.
- 46% of women are disabled by heart failure after a heart attack, versus 22% of men.

Additionally, there appears to be a race factor: African American women have a 35% higher death rate.

6. What can help change this?

Awareness was the beginning; the majority of women think they are going to die from breast cancer, not heart disease. The reason for these differences in outcomes is still not well understood. Women wait longer to seek care (11 hours versus 5 hours for men), often because their symptoms did not match their expectation (74%), denial, or other (frequently care-taking) responsibilities. They are also less likely to be hospitalized and less likely to undergo thrombolytic therapy. Hopefully future advances in health care will help provide the answers for improvement in these outcome disparities.

7. Discuss differences in acute stroke presentation between the two genders.

Acute stroke studies show women have worse outcomes including higher mortality. Studies have shown men were triaged more rapidly than women with stroke symptoms and women tended to wait longer for head computed tomography.

A possible explanation for this is that women with stroke, similar to AMI, don't always have the obvious, expected symptoms. A study of acute stroke at ten community hospitals showed that women presented more with atypical stroke symptoms. Men had significantly more classic stroke symptoms such as gait abnormality, imbalance, aphasia, and hemiparesis. Women with an acute stroke more frequently complained of pain (headache, face pain, single limb pain), changed level of consciousness, and nonspecific symptoms including chest pain, shortness of breath, and palpitations.

8. Elaborate on the traumatic injury and domestic violence connection.

It is estimated that 20% to 30% of all U.S. women have been abused by one of their intimate partners; six out of ten assaults on women are caused by partners or former partners (not strangers).

Acute traumatic injury in women may be more likely to derive from domestic violence than the similar injury in men. Certain indicators that should raise the suspicion of an assault-related injury include contusions, internal injuries, and fractures of the skull, spine, or trunk. Pregnancy is a risk factor: 4% to 8% of all pregnant women are abused.

While studies have shown women assault men as commonly, women sustain more injuries as a result of these assaults. This is attributed to the difference in physical strength and the difference in the nature of the assault (women are more likely to throw things).

9. How will I be sure to identify a victim of domestic abuse?

Unfortunately domestic violence cannot be accurately identified by type of injury, nature of complaint, or demographic of patient. Somatic complaints of headache or abdominal pain may derive from stress of interpersonal violence.

It is estimated that the ED identifies that abuse is an element only about one third of the time. Currently, 92% of women who are abused indicated they did not discuss it with their health care provider. Advocacy for universal screening for each ED visit grows to help establish that the ED is a "safe place" to talk about these things. We also need to insure adequate plan for resources exists should the abuse be revealed to us.

It seems that at the least as ED providers, we could strive to do a better job of asking injured persons, especially women, about what happened in an atmosphere that encourages the most complete and honest response. In one study, identified abuse victims indicated that they felt embarrassed, afraid, and that they were "seen but not heard (understood)" by the staff. See Chapter 56 for further discussion.

Key Points

- Women have atypical presentations for AMI, stroke, and domestic violence.
- Women have worse outcomes for AMI and stroke than comparable men.
- AMI in women should be suspected by shortness of breath, weakness, and extreme fatigue.

Internet Resources

IWDA Recommendations for Integrating Gender Considerations into Emergency Operations: Addressing the Psychosocial Effects of Gender-Based Violence
http://www.iwda.org.au/features/darfur/psychosocial%20effects.pdf

Emergency Nurses Association: The Female Heart
http://www.ena.org/conferences/annual/2004/handouts/344-c.pdf

Emergency Nurses Association Position Statements: Diversity in Emergency Care
http://www.ena.org/about/position/DiversityEmergencyCare.asp

Nurses, Women, and Heart Disease: Making the Connection
http://nsweb.nursingspectrum.com/ce/ce143.htm

Heart Disease Studies find Gender-Specific Symptoms
http://www.npwh.org/newslettermar-01.htm

Second International Conference on Women, Heart Disease, and Stroke
http://www.americanheart.org/downloadable/heart/1093877882586PrePro.pdf

Knowledge of Heart Disease among Women in an Urban Emergency Setting
http://www.nmanet.org/OC1027jnma0804.pdf

Presentation, Delay, and Contraindication to Thrombolytic Treatment in Females and Males With Myocardial Infarction
http://www.nmanet.org/OC1027jnma0804.pdf

Bibliography

Abbott J: Assault-related injury: What do we know, and what should we do about it? *Ann Emerg Med* 32:363-366, 1998.

Fanslow JL, Norton RN, Spinola CG: Indicators of assault-related injuries among women presenting in the emergency department, *Ann Emerg Med* 32:363-366, 1998.

Gorman C: The no. 1 killer of women, *Time* April 28, 60-66, 2003.

Labiche LA, Chan W, Saldin KR, Morgenstern LB: Sex and acute stroke prevention, *Ann Emerg Med* 40:453-460, 2002.

Leneski L, Morton P: Delay in seeking treatment for acute myocardial infarction: Why? *J Emerg Nurs* 26(2):125-129, 2000.

McSweeney JC, Cody M, O'Sullivan P, et al: Women's early warning symptoms of acute myocardial infarction, *Circulation* 108:2619, 2003.

Washington DL, Bird CE: Sex differences in disease presentation in the emergency department. *Ann Emerg Med* 40: 461-463, 2000.

Chapter 15

Cultural Competencies in Triage

Stephen M. Cohen and Sharon Saunderson Cohen

1. Why do you have a chapter on this topic?

This needed focus arose after the 2002 Institute of Medicine's report: *Unequal Treatment: Confronting Racial and Ethnic Disparities in Health Care.* For instance, there was poorer pain management among racial and ethnic minorities compared with whites seen for the same complaint in the emergency department (ED). African American urban children receive less treatment (according to national guidelines) for asthma in the ED than white children. The ED milieu has unique features, such as time pressure, incomplete information, and high demands. These increase the likelihood that stereotypes and bias will (even subconsciously) affect decisions.

2. What is transcultural nursing?

Transcultural nursing is the formal study of nursing practice involving identifying the differences and similarities among patients of different cultures. The purpose is to provide a framework for culturally specific and sensitive health care.

3. What makes up an individual's culture or cultural identity?

An individual's culture is composed of the activities, beliefs, values, and practices that they learn from the identification with any particular group. Cultural identity guides thinking, decision making, and actions or reactions and response to health care.

4. What is the difference between ethnicity and race?

Ethnicity refers to commonality of traits and customs as in being a member of an ethnic group. Race is about biology and physical characteristics such as skin color, body morphology, and similar characteristics. Members of a single ethnic group can be of different races.

5. What is the goal in becoming "culturally competent"?

Cultural competence in health care is an individual's or organization's ability to display awareness of, and act consistent with, the health related cultural values or beliefs.

6. What are the standards of a culturally sensitive institution?

The fourteen Culturally and Linguistically Appropriate Services (CLAS) standards from the Office of Minority Health of the Public Health Service (see Appendix A).

7. We are a small, homogenous community and don't have diversity needs.

The idea behind diversity-sensitive measures is to simply treat everyone equally. In any community, there is variety if you simply look at people for who they are. Consider differences in religions, socioeconomic levels, or lifestyle. One area is which bias often exits without recognition is assuming heterosexuality.

8. List some examples of removing bias in triage questions related to sexuality.

- Instead of asking about sexual activity that assumes an opposite sex partner, ask "Do you have sex with men, women, or both?"
- Instead of asking about reaching a spouse, ask "Who would you like me to contact?"
- Instead of inquiring whether a woman is sexually active and/or using birth control, phrase it as "Do you have a need for birth control?" Then follow-up affirmative answers by asking what is used.

9. What about foreign languages?

Interviews conducted in one's native language are most effective. It is said there are two times an individual needs to speak in their native tongue: when they talk to their God and when they talk to their doctor. Fagan et al (2003) found that visits last longer with translation, but certainly contribute to better care. The family or ad hoc nonclinical staff are used in emergent situations, but should not be a primary resource as a result of privacy and accuracy concerns. See also Chapter 71.

10. What are the important cultural components of triage and assessment?

Aspects that could be a consideration in every ED visit:

- Current family organization and roles of members
- Beliefs and practices related to this presentation
- Impact of ethnically related social issues such as poverty
- Beliefs related to health care
- Implications of spirituality on the illness or injury
- Immigration status and history

A Framework for Culturally Competent Triage

Explanation: Explain to the patient why you are asking triage questions.
Treatments: Have the patient tell you at triage what treatments they have tried, what worked, what didn't, and are they willing to try allopathic treatment options?
Healers: Does the patient seek advice from alternative or folk healers? If so, describe.
Negotiate: Try to find options that are mutually acceptable to the health care team and patient and that incorporate the patient's beliefs.
Intervention: Determine any intervention that is mutually agreed on by health care team and patient.
Collaboration: Collaborate with the patient, family members, and health care team.

11. How should I handle it when patients indicate a traditional medical practice from their culture that I don't agree with?

Do not give a judgment but do not ignore it. (Practices can be linked with spiritual implications.) Document what help was sought and the results of that treatment.

12. When triaging a patient, what areas should the triage nurse consider in trying to be culturally sensitive?

Seven key areas include respect for personal space, voice volume, eye contact, gestures, primary caretaker, the patient's perspective of time, and encouraging feedback.

13. Talk more about respecting a person's personal space.

Stay at arm's length initially and observe the patient's reaction and interaction with other family members, if present. Some cultures prefer physical closeness (Spanish or Italian), in other cultures personal space and privacy are highly valued.

14. Discuss voice, eye contact, and gestures.

Speak clearly but in a soft tone. (We sometimes act like the patient will understand English if we only shout it.) In some cultures, such as the Vietnamese, direct eye contact or pointing may be viewed as being disrespectful.

15. Explain what is meant by determining the primary caretaker or historian.

Ask the patient and/or family member who will be responsible for providing the care. In the Asian culture, for example, the eldest son is traditionally responsible for making decisions and carrying out instructions. In the Indian (Native or India) culture, the husband (if the wife is the patient) will be the historian including questions about menses.

16. What is the ultimate goal?

The American Hospital Association (AHA) aims for hospitals to become culturally proficient, not just competent. Cultural proficiency involves holding different cultures in high esteem (as opposed to just accepting them), and goes beyond speaking the language. It also includes seeking to increase diversity in the health care workforce.

Culturally and Linguistically Appropriate Standards

Ensure that patients receive effective, understandable care that is provided in a manner compatible with their health beliefs and practices and preferred language.

Implement strategies to recruit, retain, and promote at all levels of the organization a diverse staff and leadership that are representative of the demographic characteristics of the service area.

Ensure that staff at all levels and across all disciplines receive ongoing education and training in culturally and linguistically appropriate service delivery.

Offer and provide language assistance services, including bilingual staff and interpreter services, at no cost to each patient with limited English proficiency at all points of contact, in a timely manner during all hours of operation.

Make available easily understood related materials and post signage in the languages of the encountered groups and/or groups represented in the area.

Develop, implement, and promote a strategic plan that outlines clear goals, policies, operational plans, and management accountability/oversight mechanisms to provide culturally and linguistically appropriate services.

Conduct initial and ongoing organizational self-assessments of class-related activities and integrate cultural and linguistic competence-related measures into internal audits, performance improvement programs, patient satisfaction assessments, and outcomes-based evaluations.

Ensure that data on the individual race, ethnicity, and spoken and written language are collected in health records, integrated into the organization's management information systems, and periodically updated.

Maintain a current demographic, cultural, and epidemiologic profile of the community and a needs assessment to accurately plan for and implement services that respond to the cultural and linguistic characteristics of the service area.

Provide to patients in their language both verbal offers and written notices informing them of their right to receive language assistance services.

Assure the competence of language provided to limited English proficient patients by interpreters and bilingual staff. Family and friends should not be used to provide interpretation services (except on request by the patient).

Develop participatory, collaborative partnerships with communities and utilize a variety of formal and informal mechanisms to facilitate community and patient/consumer involvement in designing and implementing CLAS-related activities.

Ensure that conflict and grievance resolution processes are culturally and linguistically sensitive and capable of identifying, preventing, and resolving cross-cultural conflicts or complaints by patients/consumers.

Culturally and Linguistically Appropriate Standards—*cont'd*

Regularly make available to the public information about their progress and successful innovations in implementing the CLAS standards and to provide public notice in their communities about the availability of this information.

From Assuring Cultural Competence in HealthCare: Recommendations for National Standards and an Outcomes-Focused Research Agenda—Recommendations for National Standards; Office of Minority Health, Public Health Service; U.S. Department of Health and Human Services; available at http://www.omhrc.gov/clas/culturalla.htm.

17. List suggestions to help health care professionals with cultural competence.

- Require cultural competency training in nursing and physician educational programs.
- Incorporate cultural competency within accreditation, certification, or credentialing.
- Use evidence-based guidelines in practice to decrease uncertainty and minimize individual discretion in decision making.
- Maintain continuous quality improvement programs to monitor adherence to clinical protocols to help identify clinical disparities at the individual or institutional level.
- Allow zero tolerance for stereotypical remarks in the workplace.
- Enhance linguistic services.
- Include cultural care disparity elements in other research projects.

18. How can I become more culturally competent?

- Continue to learn about the practices in the communities you serve.
- Take the time to listen and respond individually.
- Use family members and significant others to gain awareness and insight.

Most patients will respond favorably if sincerely asked, "Help me to understand. Tell me more about this practice."

19. What should be done if an employee is using inappropriate sexually-oriented comments, such as calling a homosexual patient by an offensive name?

Any human being, regardless of lifestyle, should feel comfortable in receiving care. Employee counseling should focus on the behaviors and potential negative impact (not the employee's personal values). That language essentially dehumanizes the person.

Key Points

- The celebration of difference is the next step beyond mere tolerance or acceptance.
- Consider cultural differences in personal space, voice tone and volume, eye contact, gestures, primary caretaker, and perspective of time.
- Avoid phrasing questions that assumes heterosexuality.

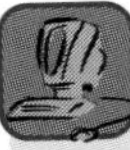

Internet Resources

Assuring Cultural Competence in Health Care: "The CLAS Standards"
http://www.omhrc.gov/clas/indexfinal.htm

Office of Minority Health
http://www.omhrc.gov/

Cultural Diversity in Nursing
http://www.culturediversity.org/

Cultural Diversity Rx
http://www.diversityrx.org/

Culture Med at the SUNY Institute of Technology
http://www.sunyit.edu/library/html/culturedmed/index.html

Bibliography

Emergency Nurses Association: *Position paper: Diversity in emergency care,* Des Plaines, Ill, 2003, Author.

Fagan MJ, Diaz JA, Reinert SE, et al: Impact of interpretation method on clinic visit length, *J Gen Intern Med* 18(8):677-678, 2003.

Rea R: Implementing diversity-sensitive measures (Managers Forum), *J Emerg Nurs* 29(5): 468, 2003.

Richardson LD, Ivin CB, Tamayo-Sarver JH: Racial and ethnic disparities in the clinical practice of emergency medicine, *Acad Emerg Med* 10(11):1184-1188, 2004.

Smith LS: Leading and managing a diverse workforce. In Zimmermann PG, editor: *Nursing management secrets,* Philadelphia, 2002, Hanley & Belfus, pp 156-161.

Chapter 16

Heavy Users

Rebecca S. McNair

1. Why are heavy users an issue for emergency nurses and physicians?

Triage by nature is constantly deciding between who is sick and who is not sick. Heavy users (also known as "frequent flyers") of the emergency department (ED) are familiar patients and can tempt health care providers to automatically assume they are not sick.

2. Are heavy users at any higher risk than other patients?

The Emergency Nurses Association (ENA) indicates that heavy users and patients who return within 72 hours are to be considered high risk. Heavy users often die earlier than the average person as a result of the nature of their noncompliance, abusive and/or social, and psychologic problems.

3. What are the usual presentations and demographics of the heavy user?

The demographics of heavy users are varied, as are their presentations. They include:

- Chronic medical condition
- Complex medical condition
- Drug-seeking behavior (see also Chapter 6)
- Violent behavior
- Abusive behavior
- Patients with serious medical problems, whose noncompliance put them in jeopardy
- Patients with social and/or psychologic problems who find the ED as their safety net

4. Why is the ED the safety net for heavy users?

EDs became that as a result of the Emergency Medical Treatment and Active Labor Act (EMTALA). It mandates that an "appropriate" medical screening examination be done for every individual who presents to the emergency department and requests care. EMTALA is a civil right for U.S. residents.

5. **Sounds wonderful. What is the problem?**

The problem is often that EMTALA is an unfunded mandate that falls unevenly on providers. Rural and inner-city areas, in which the uninsured are found in disproportionate numbers, are particularly hard hit.

6. **Does this relate at all to overcrowding in EDs?**

Surveyed ED physicians said their EDs were operating at or over capacity on weekdays (82%) and weekends (91%). They identified that the number of uninsured patients treated in their ED had increased in the past year (72%), and 79% anticipate it continuing to increase in the next year.

7. **Has anything been done to manage improper use of the ED?**

Managed Care Organizations created certain strategies to attempt to deal with the inherent problems of patients presenting to EDs with issues that were NOT considered to be life- or limb-threatening. This was an attempt to "rein in" the heavy users regarding "appropriate ED use" and help with ED overcrowding.

8. **List those strategies.**

- *Physician gate keeping*—The private HMO physician would approve or not approve the ED visit based on a conversation. Initially, even registration clerks held these conversations that were the basis for decisions.
- *Capitation*—The medical group is paid a certain amount per member per month that pays for emergency care, among other expenses. This was an incentive for physicians to reduce costs, including emergency visits, through expanded office hours and taking phone calls evenings/weekends from their patients.
- *Patient re-education*—Patients were sent a card that listed phone numbers to call when having a medical emergency so they could be told the right place to go. The difficulty is that when a person has what they perceive as an emergency; they may not be reading the cards. Also patients who are noncompliant with treatment regimens may also be the people who do not comply with these instructions regarding care options.
- *Primary medical care link for all patients*—Everyone does not have a relationship established with a physician. Some blame frequent turnover in providers or insurance coverage as interfering with establishing this connection.

9. **So why do we still have heavy users or "frequent flyers"?**

Ruth Malone's work (1996) found that all of the above strategies to control improper use were based on three implicitly linked, but *false,* assumptions

- The primary reason for most ED visits is to seek medical care.
- The problems for which the care is sought are, in most cases, bona fide emergencies.
- Patients are rational consumers who will make "better" (and predictable) choices if proper incentives (or disincentives) are provided.

10. Why is the first assumption about the reason for the visit wrong?

Malone found some of the heaviest utilizers of ED services do *not* visit the ED primarily to seek acute medical care or even primary medical care. Instead, they are really seeking safety, rest, shelter, comfort, showers, food, clothing, inclusion, and recognition, or in other words, "almshouse needs." Although there are "shelters," they are not always available when these individuals need them.

11. I don't understand. I've never heard a heavy user ask for help with these types of needs.

Malone says that patients have learned that it is unacceptable to state outright that they in fact have a social or psychologic problem. So they "medicalize" their problem for us.

12. Explain why the second assumption about seeking care for nonemergencies is wrong.

Although the needs may be "social" rather than "medical," they really are "emergencies" in one sense. Lack of rest, food, and shelter certainly constitute emergencies in the most basic sense.

13. Discuss the error in assumption number three about helping rational consumers to make choices based on incentives.

Economic factors don't make a difference for the indigent and homeless patients. They are unable to pay for medical care in any setting, under any circumstances (Malone, 1996).

14. What approach is needed for EDs to deal with heavy users?

Care plans/case management that addresses their social and psychologic concerns, and medical issues.

15. How can I personally begin to build a working relationship to deal with heavy users?

Malone (1996) encourages:

- Accept the person as he/she is, and tolerate the verbal ramblings.
- Recognizing the possibilities and encourage the person.
- Avoid a power struggle with the patient.
- Realize change can occur in different ways at different periods of time, and may not always be what or when we envision it.

16. What is most important to remember when caring for a heavy user?

Heavy users actually do *not* represent a large percentage of the volume in EDs, and yet they can be so frustrating to the staff. The triage nurse must remember that heavy users can have serious medical problems, and therefore not be biased in their assessment and treatment of these patients. As caregivers, we must strive to maintain a therapeutic, professional, and compassionate response to these patients as we would to any other patients. Meanwhile, as a profession, we must continue to move toward institutional and legislative ways of dealing with our ED issues, such as underfunding and overcrowding.

Key Point

- All heavy users ("frequent flyers") need a thorough and unbiased assessment every time.

Internet Resources

Triage First, Inc.
www.triagefirst.com

Emergency Nurses Association
www.ena.org

Centers for Medicare and Medicaid Services
www.cms.hhs.gov

Bibliography

Kne T, Young R, Spillane L: Frequent ED users: patterns of use over time, *Am J Emerg Med* 16:648-652, 1998.

Little GF, Watson DP: The homeless in the emergency department: A patient profile, *J Accid Emerg Med* 13:415-417, 1996.

Lucas RH, Sanford SM: An analysis of frequent users of emergency care at an urban university hospital, *Ann Emerg Med* 32:563-568, 1998.

Malone RE: Almost like "family": emergency nurses and "frequent flyers," *J Emerg Nurs* 22:176-183, 1996.

Malone R: Whither the almshouse? Over utilization and the role of the emergency department, *J Health Polit Policy Law* 23(5):795-832, 1998.

McNair R (President): *Taming the beast. In The nature of the beast: Comprehensive triage and patient flow workshop,* Fairview, NC, 2003, Triage First, Inc.

McNair R (President): Triage is a tiger. In TRIAGE First EDucation: A comprehensive emergency department triage course (caregiver and patient satisfaction), Fairview, NC, 2004, Triage First, Inc.

Pope D, Fernandez CMB, Bouthillette F, Etherington J: Frequent users of the emergency department: A program to improve care and reduce visits, *Can Med Assoc J* 162(7):1017-1020, 2000.

Spillane LL, Lumb EW, Cobaugh DJ, et al: Frequent users of the emergency department: Can we intervene? *Acad Emerg Med* 4:574-580, 1996.

Section III

Symptoms

Chapter 17

Rashes

Joan Somes and Polly Gerber Zimmermann

1. Why are rashes so troubling to deal with in the emergency department?

It has been said, "Everything can cause a rash and nothing can cause a rash!" A "rash" can cover a lot of ground, not to mention skin. Although bothersome, rashes are rarely serious, especially for pediatric patients.

2. What do people with a rash expect?

They want to know:

- What caused it?
- Is it contagious?
- What to do about it?

These include those who are asking for a "second opinion," such as the woman with an 8-month-old rash that had been already seen by three different dermatologists!

3. How do I approach assessing a rash?

- Determine stability of ABC (e.g., no anaphylactic reaction)
- Presence of associated (systemic) symptoms ("sick versus not sick")
- Appearance (color, shape, size, progression, distribution, and location)
- With gloves on, run your fingers across the rash to determine if it:
  - Is flat or raised
  - Blanches or remains same color

4. What should I note about location?

- Where did the rash begin?
- How did it progress? (from face toward trunk, trunk to extremities, warm creases, etc.)
- Where is the rash located now? (only by the wristwatch, all over the body, around the eyes or mouth [wet areas], etc.)

5. Provide a rule-of thumb for physically assessing a rash.

"Feel" the rash, but never without wearing gloves.

6. Tell me the terms to use to describe the lesions.

- *Macule:* Flat, nonpalpable lesion that is a different color from the surrounding skin (freckles, nevi, Mongolian spots, measles).
- *Papules:* Slightly raised and discolored lesions smaller than 1 cm in diameter (acne, insect bites, contact dermatitis).
- *Pustule:* Raised lesion containing an exudate giving it a yellowish appearance (folliculitis, impetigo, and candidiasis [yeast]).
- *Vesicle*: Blisters containing transparent fluid. Vesicles are less than 0.5 cm and the term "bulla" is used for greater than 0.5 cm (burns, chickenpox).
- *Nodule:* "Bumps" deep in the skin. The lesion will not move, even though the skin above the lesion can be moved around. This lesion may be seen and/or only felt (cysts, rheumatoid nodules, lymphadenitis).
- *Plaque:* Solid elevated lesions larger than 5 mm in size.
- *Wheal:* Swollen, circumscribed elevated lesions with a flat top. The irregularly shaped edges are somewhat circular and typically outlined in a red color with the center ranging in color from white to bright red.

7. What should I ask in the history of someone with a rash that is not life-threatening?

- When did the rash start?
- Has the rash changed and how? (bigger, redder, more oozing, painful, spreading)
- Constant or intermittent (pattern of reoccurrence)?
- Itching? (look for scratch marks)
- Painful?
- Known recent exposures to known infectious disease? (Are the patient's immunizations up to date?)
- Known bites?
- Recent changes in lifestyle/habits or exposures to common allergens (e.g., new laundry detergent, drugs, soaps)?
- Recent activities (traveling, swimming in the ocean, woods with poison ivy)?
- Any change in medications (including over-the-counter herbs)?
- What has the patient done to treat it?
- Have they already seen anyone before about this rash?

8. Give an example of triage acuities for a rash.

Manchester Triage Group

Level 1	Immediate	ABC compromise including stridor
Level 2	Very urgent (10 minutes)	Severe pain/itch Significant history of allergy (e.g., known sensitivity with severe reaction) Facial or tongue edema Acute, sudden-onset shortness of breath Purpura

Level 3	Urgent (60 minutes)	Moderate pain/itch Inappropriate history Widespread (>10% body surface area) of new unknown rash Blisters or discharge
Level 4	Standard (120 minutes)	Minor pain/itch Recent (within 1 week) problem

9. Which rashes should lead the nurse to take rapid action?

- Highly contagious (for example, varicella). The severe acute respiratory syndrome (SARS) outbreak illustrated the importance of a readily activated isolation procedure to protect other vulnerable patients. A unit secretary contracted chickenpox just by having the unmasked child in the registration area.
- Coexisting signs/symptoms of systemic instability (septic) or edema (stridor, wheezing, angioedema, periorbital edema, large systemic wheals)
- New onset-petechia or purpura (thrombocytopenia, sepsis, meningococcemia)
- Skin sloughing (Stevens-Johnson syndrome, necrotizing fascitis)

10. Give classic symptoms that would help me spot SARS and varicella.

SARS is suspect if there are respiratory symptoms, high fever, and recent travel to Eastern countries. Varicella (chickenpox, herpes zoster) starts on the trunk as a macule that turns into a vesicle, which eventually crusts over. New eruptions occur daily for several days as the rash spreads upward and outward so lesions will be in different stages. Both are infectious by respiratory route: immediately mask (airborne precautions) the patient. For further discussion, see Chapter 1.

11. How is smallpox presentation different than chickenpox?

Smallpox starts on the face and spreads to the trunk and the entire smallpox rash erupt at the same time, rather than in stages.

12. What are the most frequent allergic systemic (anaphylactic) causes of rash?

Nuts, berries, bee stings, medications, dairy, eggs, certain spices and preservatives, latex, seafood/shellfish, chocolate, perfumes, chemicals (like bleach), and pets

13. What is important to remember with a patient who is experiencing any degree of systemic allergic reaction (urticaria, wheals, pruritus, mild wheezing)?

These patients have a high potential for continuing or sudden deterioration to anaphylaxis and should be given a top priority. Clues regarding the severity include the:

- *Presence of constitutional symptoms* (tachycardia, hypotension, respiratory complaints, significant history, petechiae/purpura). True anaphylaxis involves multiple body systems. Does the patient look sick?
- *Speed of the reaction's onset* (e.g., slower is usually less severe)
- *Location of pruritus* (if itching is confined to one area of the skin, there is less likely a systemic problem) correlates with the acuteness of the reaction.
- *Amount of itching* correlates with severity of the reaction.

14. Can I feel reassured that there will be no reaction from a drug this time if the patient has safely taken a drug before?

No. Anyone can develop an allergic reaction to anything at any time. Many commonly used drugs have a reaction rate of 1%. A rash from drug hypersensitivity usually has red, flat lesion with symmetric distribution that are almost always on the trunk and extremities.

Some primary offenders include ampicillin, sulfa, penicillins, and cephalosporins. If there is angioedema of the lips, tongue, pharynx, and larynx, consider angiotensin-converting enzyme (ACE) inhibitors. Other offending "drugs" are hidden in foods such as tartrazine (FD&C yellow dye #5) and aspartame (NutraSweet).

This is also a good point to remember while administering drugs to patients *in* the ED. Many departments have a policy that a patient cannot be discharged until 20 to 30 minutes after an intramuscular (IM), intravenous (IV), antibiotic, or narcotic administration.

15. Sometimes we administer narcotics and then eventually discharge from the triage area when the census is high and it is a known situation, such as a reoccurring migraine. Give an example of a policy regarding a drug administration wait time.

Good Hope Hospital (Erwin, NC)
Source: Dennis M McCool Bed JD RN, Director of Critical Care Services

- Patients wait 30 minutes if given an antibiotic or other type of injection.
- If IM or IV medication would impair driving ability, patient has someone sign a "designated driver" form. The form indicates the patient has received a medication that makes it risky to operate a motor vehicle and this person is responsible to see the patient gets home safely. (If the patient does not have anyone, only prescriptions are given.)

16. What is angioneurotic edema?

It is a variant of urticaria with painless subcutaneous swelling of the face (eyelids, lips, tongue), and can occur in the hands, feet, and genitalia. It can be hereditary or idiosyncratic. A classic "diagnostic" assessment is to recreate it by drawing one's nails across the skin and watching the wheals develop.

17. I understand the rationale for emergent treatment using epinephrine, H_1 blockers (diphenhydramine [Benadryl]), and steroids for an allergic reaction. Why is cimetidine (Tagamet) or ranitidine (Zantac) sometimes ordered immediately too?

They are H_2 blockers that help block the histamine release. Although commonly used for gastric problems, they can lessen the histamine response in an allergy.

18. Describe petechia and purpura.

Petechia (pinpoint) and purpura (blotches) are flat, nonpalpable dark-red to purple lesions that do not blanch. Petechia is less than 1 cm in diameter; purpura is larger and can cover an entire extremity. These can indicate a systemic blood dyscrasia from life-threatening conditions, such as disseminated intravascular coagulation (DIC) or idiopathic thrombocytopenic purpura (ITP).

A new onset of these rashes is a harbinger of a worse condition and need to be triaged a higher priority. (Canadian Triage and Acuity Scale [CTAS] is Level 2, which is ≤15 minutes; Manchester Triage Group is Level 2, which is 10 minutes.)

19. I know *Neisseria meningitidis* meningococcemia causes new onset purpura and petechiae. List its classic symptoms.

- Toxic looking patient
- Purpura and petechial rash
- Fever
- Decreased level of consciousness (possibly signs of meningitis)

Even without knowing the etiology, the triage nurse would readily pick up that a patient with these symptoms is a "sick" patient and a priority.

20. Why do you make the distinction of a new onset purpura?

There are chronic skin conditions with purpura, such as pigmented purpuric dermatoses, that are not serious. They can be distinguished from acute conditions by its insidious and slow onset (months to years).

21. What are other important considerations with petechiae?

Petechiae following a blunt trauma (after vehicular trauma) are indicative of the severity of the force, although a patient with a major fracture exhibiting petechiae several days later could be having a fat embolus. Another is a "rash" that is actually from abuse, such as petechial hemorrhages from squeezing or strangling the neck).

The Manchester Triage Group indicates that any time the alleged mechanism does not explain the apparent injury or illness, it is considered inappropriate (possible abuse) and given at least a Level 3 Urgent (60 minutes). Therefore, if the patient presents with a petechial rash that is inexplicable from the stated mechanism, the patient should be assigned at least a Level 3 Urgent triage status. The CTAS places physically stable but abuse/potential abuse victim at Level 2 (Emergent [≤15 minutes]).

22. Discuss a rash in which the skin sloughs off.

Entire sheets of skin will peel off in Stevens-Johnson syndrome. Similarly, entire large areas of skin will peel off with bullous impetigo, scarlet fever, or staphylococcal scaled skin syndrome. These obviously sick patients are a high priority.

This is in comparison to any vesicular rash that forms a crust when they rupture and eventually flake (or slough) off (for example, chickenpox). Usually the crust and superficial skin flakes off the trunk and extremities (the fingers/toes remain intact). These are not emergent.

23. Tell me more about the rash from Stevens-Johnson syndrome.

- Involves up to 15% of the total body surface area (TBA)
- Symmetric, severe vesicobullous eruptions with high fever (10% to 30%) and pneumonitis (23%)
- 50% of the cases are from drug reactions

24. What is key in determining potential contact dermatitis in adults?

Look for a clear line of demarcation. Ask the patient what they have recently touched. Common sources are clothing, jewelry, soaps, perfumes, metals, and lotions.

For example, some believe today's widespread body piercing is leading to an increase nickel allergy. Is the rash where they had their watch? In one case, the man had a rash only in his axillae and groin (the only areas he washed with the hotel soap).

25. What are the four traditional childhood viral illnesses that cause rashes?

Incidence has decreased as a result of routine immunization, but they are:
- Rubeola (German measles)
- Rubella (3-day measles)
- Varicella (chickenpox)
- Erythema Infectiosum (Fifth's disease)

26. Tell me classic signs of Rubeola.

Classically 14 days after exposure to the virus, the patient develops:
- Erythematous maculopapular rash in the hairline and behind the ears that spread into one big red lesion (that blanches)
- An accompanying upper respiratory syndrome with the following symptoms (photophobia, runny nose, conjunctivitis, high fever, and cough)
- Koplik spots (1- to 3-mm bluish white spots) in the buccal mucosa within the first 48 hours

27. Discuss rubella classic signs and symptoms.

After 12 to 25 days incubation:

- Prodrome (1 to 5 days) of fever, malaise, headache, and sore throat
- "Blush" rash (or macules/papules) on the skin, starting on the face, and spreading downward into eventual total body redness that disappears in 3 days
- Swollen lymph nodes behind the ears and at the back of the neck

28. Describe *erythema infectiosum* (Fifth disease)

- High fever initially, that abruptly abates, before the rash develops.
- Fiery red rash on the cheeks ("slapped face" appearance).
- One to two days after the facial rash, a nonitchy macular erythema or erythematous, maculopapular rash occurs on the trunk and limbs.
- No rash on the palms or soles.
- Fever, malaise, headache, sore throat, cough, runny nose, nausea, vomiting, diarrhea, and muscle aches.

29. You mention a "slapped face" appearance. Aren't there other conditions that can cause that too?

Probably the best known are:

- Systemic lupus erythematous (SLE). It is a multisystem disease involving the connective tissue and blood vessels but the macular facial rash is distinguished because it is in the shape of a butterfly.
- Rosacea. It is an acneform inflammation combined with increased reactivity of the capillary system leading to flushing and burning of the face, but it is located on the chin, cheeks, nose, and forehead.

30. Provide a superficial overview of other diseases that cause a rash.

- *Scarlet fever (strep throat):* Fine, red papular rash (sandpaper) and a strawberry red tongue.
- *Psoriasis:* Chronic itchy scaling papules and plaques that tend to be located on areas of repeated pressure or trauma (e.g., palms, soles, knees, elbows, shins).
- *Herpes zoster (shingles):* A band of pain along a dermatome (does not cross the midline) followed by a maculopapular rash progressing to a vesicular rash.
- *Lyme disease:* "Bulls-eye" rash (up to 50% of the cases): circular red rash with white center with a history of exposure 7 to 10 days earlier in wooded areas with "deer ticks." Accompanying flulike syndrome is present.
- *Toxic shock syndrome (TSS):* Diffuse macular erythroderma (looks like a sunburn) that blanches when pressure is applied. Although the commonly perceived etiology is always a tampon left in too long, one-third of TSS patients are male infected with *S. aureus.* The patient is acutely ill, often with high fever, hypotension, vomiting/diarrhea, or sore throat.
- *Rocky Mountain spotted fever (RMSF).* It is caused by the *Rickettsia rickettsii,* which is transmitted by ticks. The rash starts out as small, red macular rash on the wrist and ankles (that blanch under pressure) and then spread to the extremities and trunk.

31. What other rashes do insects cause?

Any flying or crawling "bug" can and will bite, producing a localized papule/wheal. Scabies, lice, and fleas present similarly so it is often difficult to determine which is causing the itching and rash. Some patterns include:

- *Fleabites:* Tiny little punctures with redness in a zigzag line on the legs and waist area
- *Lice:* Small red dots with eggs on the hair follicles around the waist area, shoulders, axillae, neck, and hair
- *Scabies:* Zigzag skin course from the female mite burrows, located in web spaces of hands and feet, face, and scalp
- *Chiggers:* Red papules that itch fiercely (and then turn into a nodule that lasts up to 14 days) from a mite under the skin often after outdoor activity

32. What are sea bather's eruptions?

It is red macular or papular dermatitis, caused by stings from the stinging cells (also called nematocysts) of the larval forms of certain sea anemones. Patients may indicate they look like mosquito bites. They appear in areas covered by swimwear within a few hours of being in the Caribbean or off the coasts of Mexico, Florida, or Long Island. Prevention is removing swimwear immediately and then showering.

33. Can lightning cause a rash?

A classic keraunographic skin marking that is fern-like redness (which is actually a superficial burn). It appears within several hours of the burn and starts to fade in about 12 hours. The rash requires no special treatment, but it may suggest the etiology for the unconscious golfer's presentation.

34. What is a "huffer rash"?

The patient develops a contact dermatitis around their mouth from inhaling paint fumes from a plastic bag that has had spray paint sprayed into, so he could get "high."

35. I work alone in a clinic. Should I be worried if I cannot determine the cause of a rash?

Approximately 20% of the population will have urticaria sometime in their lifetime, but the cause can only be identified about 25% to 60% of the time. Regardless, the vast majority responds to an antihistamine, such as diphenhydramine hydrochloride (Benadryl), topical steroids, and time. The key determinant, as with any triage, is current patient stability and risk of deterioration.

36. Name resources that might be helpful to use.

- Dermatology or physical assessment textbooks that shows color pictures and provides descriptions of the most common skin disorders. See resources list for suggestions.
- Centers for Disease Control and Prevention (CDC) reports of rash-related diseases (e.g., smallpox) that are routinely sent to many health care facilities.

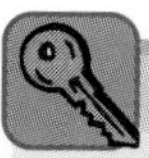

Key Points

- Emergent rashes are highly contagious, have co-existing systemic instability, new onset petechia or purpura, or skin sloughing.
- Symptoms indicating a systemic response include constitutional symptoms (multiple body systems), rapid onset, and generalized, severe pruritus (itching).
- Contact dermatitis usually has a clear line of demarcation.
- Approximately 20% of the population develops urticaria sometime in their life, cause is identified only 25% to 60% of the time, but most respond to standard treatment and time.

Internet Resources

Rash Diagnosis
http://www.nurseweek.com/news/features/02-08/lyme_web.asp

The Necessary Elements of a Dermatologic History and Physical Evaluation
http://www.ajj.com/services/pblshng/dnj/ceonline/14377383/default.htm

Nursing Assessment of the Patient With Primary HIV Infection: Key to Improving Clinical Recognition
http://www.centerforaids.org/rita/0202/nursing.pdf

Emergency Medicine On the Web: Rash Diagnosis Algorithm
http://www.ncemi.org/cgi-ncemi/edecision.pl?TheCommand=Load&NewFile=rash_algorithm&BlankTop=1

Bibliography

Ball AP, Gray JA: *Infectious disease,* London, 1993, Churchill Livingstone.

Buttaravoli P, Stair T: *Minor emergencies: Splinters to fractures,* St Louis, 2000, Mosby.

Canadian Association of Emergency Physicians: Canadian emergency department triage and acuity scale implementation guidelines, *J Can Assoc Emerg Physicians* 1:3, 1999.

Emergency Nurses Association: *Emergency nursing core curriculum,* ed 5, Philadelphia, 2000, WB Saunders.

Emergency Nurses Association: *ENPC provider manual,* ed 3, Des Plaines, Ill, 2004, Author.

Fitzpatrick TB, Johnson RA, Wolff K, Suumond R: *Color atlas and synopsis of clinical dermatology,* ed 4, New York, 2002, McGraw Hill.

Habif TP, Campbell JL, Quitadamo MJ, Zug KA: Skin disease diagnosis and treatment, St Louis, 2001, Mosby.

Hamilton GC, Sanders AB, Strange GR, Trott AT: Emergency medicine: An approach to clinical problem-solving, ed 2, Philadelphia, 2003, Saunders.

Jenkins JL, Braen GR: *Manual of emergency medicine,* ed 4, Philadelphia, 2000, Lippincott Williams & Wilkins.

Leung D: *Pediatric allergy principles and practice,* St Louis, 2003, Mosby.

Mackway-Jones K: Emergency triage, Manchester Triage Group, London, 1997, BMJ Publishing.

McCool D: Injection wait times (Managers Forum), *J Emerg Nurs* 30(6):563, 2004.

Rosen P: The five-minute emergency medicine consult, Philadelphia, 1999, Lippincott Williams & Wilkins.

Tinitinalli J, Kelen G, Stapczynski JS: *Emergency medicine: A comprehensive study guide,* ed 6, New York, 2004, McGraw-Hill.

Zimmermann PG: Triage and differential diagnosis of patients with headaches, dizziness, low back pain, and rashes: A basic primer, *J Emerg Nurs* 28(3):209-215, 2002.

Chapter 18

Fever

Vicki Sweet and Polly Gerber Zimmermann

1. Talk about temperature.

A fever is considered ≥100.4°F (38°C) in children (some consider 100.9°F/38.3°C in adults) and is a symptom, not a disease. This defense mechanism is blunted in the very young (under 3 months), very old, or those who are immunosuppressed from comorbidity (HIV+, splenectomy) or drugs (steroids, chemotherapy). Fever accounts for 6% of all adult and 20% to 40% of all pediatric visits to the emergency department (ED). Never disregard the patient who complains "only" of a fever without further evaluation. The etiology, and any coexisting fluid/electrolyte imbalances, must be determined.

2. What is the formula for converting Fahrenheit to Celsius (Centigrade)?

°C = (°F – 32) × 5/9 or (°F – 32) × 0.55

3. Give me an example of "normal" temperature ranges.

- Oral temperatures range from 96.0°F to 99.3°F (35.6°C to 37.4°C)
- Axillary temperatures, which are inaccurate, range from 98.6°F to 99.3°F (37°C to 37.4°C)
- Rectal temperatures (most accurate, "core") range from 97°F to 100.3°F (36.1°C to 38°C)

4. What is one of the most important initial assessments when looking at a patient with a complaint of fever?

"Sick versus not-sick" eyeball evaluation. One of the most important assessments for this determination is the patient's cerebral perfusion, e.g., level of consciousness.

5. Which temperature value is considered "emergent"?

Fever is one assessment in the triage determination, not an absolute. It does not necessarily reflect the seriousness of the patient's condition. Give a higher priority to:

- Infants under 12 weeks of age with a fever 100.4°F (38°C) rectally.
- A fever ≥104°F (40°C) that does not respond to previous antipyretic measures.
- A fever >102°F (39°C) that has not improved >72 hours.

6. Why should I be more concerned about an infant's fever?

Neonates (<28 days old) and young infants (<6 months old) have immature immune systems and are less capable of localizing infections and/or can harbor serious bacterial infections although appearing benign. Infants <3 months with rectal temperatures of ≥101.3°F (38.5°C) have 20 times more risk of serious infection than do older children. A "septic workup" must be done.

7. Are there times when I don't need to take a temperature in triage?

Some EDs' policy is to not take a temperature if the patient has a clear, localized problem (e.g., broken ankle) versus a systemic complaint (cough).

8. Is rectally the acceptable method to take children's temperatures in triage?

Children deserve dignity and respect. It may not necessarily be appropriate to take a rectal temperature in a triage environment that is visible to others.

9. Why are tympanic thermometers not always used? Patients prefer them.

Tympanic is more reliable than axillary, but studies found there was still a variation of 0.3°C to 1.12°C (the ear tug did not make a difference). Additionally, tympanic is invalid with otitis media, excessive earwax, or newborns. Most departments do not allow it in children <5 years or if there is a suspicion of febrile illness.

10. Talk about the "hand method" for measuring the temperature.

The Manchester Triage Group actually uses the "hand method" (e.g., tactile assessment) of touching the skin for a clinical impression, versus a thermometer reading, to determine the temperature for initial triage sorting. It is followed up with an accurate measurement as soon as possible.

Very hot adult	>41°C	>105.8°F	Level 2 (Very Urgent, 10 minutes)
Hot child	>38.5°C	>101.3°F	
Hot Adult	>38.5°C	>101.3°F	Level 3 (Urgent, 60 minutes)
Warmth	>37.5°C	> 99.5°F	Level 4 (Standard, 120 minutes)

11. These assessments sound like the mothers who know their child has a fever by touch.

Although a thermometer-measured temperature is best, studies confirm that mothers are accurate in assessing the presence or absence of a fever by touch for their children 50% to 80% of the time.

12. Why is it said that temperature is the "forgotten vital sign" in critical ED patients?

In the chaos of caring for a critical patient, temperature can be accidentally omitted. In the secondary survey, F = Full set of vital signs.

13. What are the most common causes of elevated temperatures in children as a whole?

Viral illness, gastroenteritis, and upper respiratory infection.

14. Must all fevers be treated with antipyretics?

Fever is a defense mechanism that inhibits microbes so the need for routine treatment is a controversy. In one study, 61% of pediatric residents agreed it is a defense and should not be treated, but said they do so anyway. They indicate they do it to make the child comfortable, to prevent febrile seizures, and to satisfy the parents (44%). Fevers are usually treated in pregnant women and patients with preexisting cardiac compromise (cannot tolerate the increased metabolic demands).

15. When do we give acetaminophen and when do we give ibuprofen?

The two drugs work through different mechanisms. Acetaminophen (Tylenol) works by blocking the release of prostaglandins. It is usually used first. Ibuprofen (Motrin) works by inhibiting prostaglandin synthesis. It is superior on temperatures greater than 102.5°F.

The meta-analysis of 17 trials published (Perrott et al., 2004) indicated that, in single dose administration, ibuprofen was the better choice for treating fever in children, especially at higher therapeutic doses. For pain relief, ibuprofen and acetaminophen were comparable.

Safety and efficacy of ibuprofen in children younger than 6 months of age has not been established. It is also not appropriate if there is an aspirin allergy or a viral infection (chickenpox). There is no link between ibuprofen and Reye's syndrome.

16. Should I teach about the possibility of alternating acetaminophen and ibuprofen for treating fever?

Teaching patients/parents to alternate these medications is somewhat controversial. Concern revolves around confusion in dosing with a potential for overdose. It addition, physiologically, ibuprofen inhibits glutathione production, which is required to prevent the accumulation of acetaminophen in the renal medulla. By administering these medications together, especially if incorrect doses, there is risk for renal damage.

17. Give examples of standing orders for antipyretics.

Source: Kathleen Murphy's Pediatric Triage Guidelines
Acetaminophen (Tylenol)
- Temperature is 101°F (38.3°C) or higher
- An additional dose may be given if acetaminophen was administered more than 2 hours prior to arrival.
- Contraindication with known hypersensitivity or a history of liver disease
- Administer 10 to 15 mg/kg based on the patient's *measured* weight

Ibuprofen (Motrin)
- Must receive an initial dose of acetaminophen
- May give if temperature is higher than 103°F (39.5°C) 1 hour after receiving an appropriate dose of acetaminophen.
- Patient is at least 6 months old.
- Contraindicated in patients with a history of chickenpox, asthma, ibuprofen or aspirin hypersensitivity, coagulopathy, emesis, moderate dehydration, renal or liver disease, or less than 2 weeks postoperative
- Administer 10 mg/kg based on the patient's measured weight

18. I want a triage protocol for antipyretics but my facility resists it.

Many hospitals have fever protocols for weight-based dosing for pediatrics and a standard dose for adults. However, some fear that the patient will begin to feel better and leave without receiving a medical screening exam if antipyretics are given in triage. To help justify a need for a policy like this, track the department's wait time for febrile patients from triage until receiving an antipyretic.

19. Why is it significant to ask about a previous febrile seizure?

Approximately 2% to 5% of all children aged 3 months to 5 years have a febrile seizure, usually in response to a *rapid* rise in temperature. Those with one simple febrile seizure have about a 30% chance of having a second one. Most children do outgrow them by age 5 and there is usually no lasting sequela (or lifelong epilepsy).

20. Can febrile seizures be prevented?

Some experts believe that rapid administration of an antipyretic may not necessarily prevent a febrile seizure, yet they agree that it has other positive benefits, such as making the child feel better.

21. Should every patient with a fever have a white blood cell count (WBC) done?

The absolute WBC and band count are neither sensitive nor specific and, if measured at all, should be interpreted in light of the patient's clinical picture. Some believe that a normal WBC count and differential have a high negative predictive value for serious bacterial illness (i.e., normal values imply that serious disease does not exist).

22. It seems that some parents panic and believe their child's fever is a serious illness, rather than a treatable symptom.

In 1980, nearly 94% of parents believed that fever could cause serious side effects. In 2001, despite our "better informed public," 91% of parents are still worried about the harmful effects of fever. One study found that parents who saw a video on fever management in the waiting room had decreased (30% to 35%) visits to an ED for fever in the following 6 months compared to a control group.

23. What should I do if parents of a school-age child gave him aspirin?

Determine whether it was really aspirin. People often use the generic term "aspirin" to mean any over-the-counter antipyretic. If it truly was aspirin, and the child has a viral illness, then the concern would be a risk for Reye's syndrome. Document and communicate this to the health care provider managing the care of the patient. Liver enzymes testing might be done.

24. Should I be concerned when parents insist on keeping the febrile infant bundled up in several blankets despite my education?

There are some cultures that have beliefs about heat and cold in the balance of health. Some experts believe that in many cases this will not increase the core temperature.

Key Points

- Besides the objective temperature measurement, use the eyeball "sick" versus "not sick" technique to help prioritize febrile patients
- Children less than 3 months with a fever (≥100.4°F/38°C) are a priority.
- Studies show that maternal estimate of the presence of a fever by touching the child's skin is accurate 50% to 80% of the time.
- A meta-analysis of 17 trials published in June 2004 identified that (in single dosing) ibuprofen is the better choice for treating fever in children, especially at higher therapeutic doses.
- Parents still have fears of serious consequences (91%) from a fever.

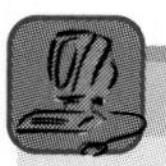

Internet Resources

Fever in the Toddler
http://www.emedicine.com/ped/topic3009.htm

Pediatrics, Febrile Seizures
http://www.emedicine.com/emerg/topic376.htm

Febrile Seizures
http://www.emedicine.com/neuro/topic134.htm

Fever, Children
http://www.emedicinehealth.com/articles/10035-1.asp

Pediatrics, Fever
http://www.emedicine.com/emerg/topic377.htm

Bibliography

Crocetti M, Moghbeli N, Serwint J: Fever phobia revisited: Have parental misconceptions about fever changed in 20 years? *Pediatrics* 107:1241-1246, 2001.

Graneto JW, Soglin DF: Maternal screening of childhood fever by palpation, *Pediatr Emerg Care* 12:183-184, 1996.

Grossman VGA: *Quick reference to triage,* ed 2, Philadelphia, 2003, Lippincott.

Lamb RP, Birnbaumer DM: Fever. In Markovchick VJ, Pons PT, editors: *Pons' emergency medicine secrets,* ed 3, Philadelphia, 2003, Hanley & Belfus.

Mackway-Jones K: *Emergency triage,* Manchester Triage Group, London, 1997, BMJ Publishing Group.

Murphy KA: *Pediatric triage guidelines,* St Louis, 1997, Mosby.

Nelson DS: Emergency treatment of fever phobia, *J Emerg Nurs* 24(1):83-84, 1998.

Perrott DA, Piira T, Goodenough B, Champion DG: Efficacy and safety of acetaminophen vs ibuprofen for treating children's pain or fever: A meta-analysis, *Arch Pediatr Adolesc Med* 158:521-526, 2004.

Zimmermann PG: Guiding principles at triage: Advice for new triage nurses, *J Emerg Nurs* 28(1): 24-33, 2002.

Chapter 19

Headache

Mary E. Fecht Gramley and Polly Gerber Zimmermann

1. How common are headaches?

It is estimated that 75% to 80% of the population in the United States suffers from a headache annually. Approximately half of these are migraine headaches.

2. How often do individuals seek medical attention for headaches?

Traumatic events result in 1% to 2% of headaches and the individual seeks medical attention. Only 4% to 5% of nontrauma related headaches become severe enough to seek medical attention.

3. When should I be the most concerned about a headache? When the pain is the worst?

No. The degree of pain does not necessarily correlate with the seriousness of the symptom. A headache is more concerning if it occurs along the following "red flags":

- Patient >55 years of age. Up to 15% of the older adult with a new onset headache will have a serious condition.
- Children. Headaches are less common in children. Only 35% have infrequent headaches by age 7; a little over 50% by age 15.
- Headache is different than ever before. This includes the worse ever or increasing in frequency or severity. "Ordinary" headaches tend to be similar.
- Sudden onset
- Awakens a patient from sleep
- First-ever headache. Someone who never gets headaches now suddenly gets one.
- Significant correlating symptoms. This includes fever, stiff neck, seizure, confusion/forgetfulness, change in level of consciousness (could be as a result of an infection or bacterial meningitis)
- History of head trauma. This is especially of concern in patients who are older adult, taking anticoagulants, or an alcoholic (could be as a result of a subdural or epidural hematoma).
- History of a loss of consciousness
- Current change in neurologic status, including new onset of unilateral weakness
- Fever

4. List some questions I could ask in assessing the headache.

- On a scale of 0 to 10, what is the level of the pain?
- Exactly where is the pain?
- Describe the quality (pounding, stabbing, etc.) and intensity (severe, etc.).
- Did the headache come on over a period of time and get progressively worse?
- When did the headache start? (length of time it is present).
- What were you doing when the pain started? (could be as a result of injury, carbon monoxide poisoning from an enclosed space)
- Can you associate any food intake with the onset of the pain? (could be as a result of exposure to toxins)
- What other symptoms are you experiencing with the headache? (could be as a result of seizure, visual changes, signs/symptoms of migraine)
- What have you done to treat the headache?
- What makes the pain worse?
- What makes the pain better?
- Have you had a headache like this previously? How often?
- What made you come in today for your headache?

5. Why would you ask the last question? Isn't it obvious the patient wants relief?

Headaches are an ordinary, occasional complaint for most people, but few patients go to an emergency department. Something, even if it is the intensity or the inability to get relief, made this patient decide more advanced medical help was needed. You want to know what that is.

I was working independently in an occupational health clinic when a man presented extremely worried about his relatively sudden, severe right temporal headache that didn't improve despite taking his usual acetaminophen (Tylenol). I sent him to a hospital for what turned out to be temporal arteritis. The aspect that influenced me the most to make that decision was how distraught the man was about *this* headache.

6. List some questions to ask about the history of someone with a headache.

- When was the last time you ate? (Ask to rule out hypoglycemia.)
- Have you had any recent infections?
- Do you have any other medical conditions? (e.g., hypertension, glaucoma, personal or family history of migraines, liver disease, kidney disease, insomnia, bipolar disorder, cancer)
- What medications are you currently taking? (e.g., beta blockers, anticoagulants, eye drops, natural herbs, over-the-counter [OTC] medications)
- Have you had any recent exposure to chemotherapy? (Some chemotherapy agents may precipitate long-term headaches, even after the therapy concludes.)
- Have you recently stopped drinking coffee, eating chocolate, or smoking?
- What usually works for your headache pain?

7. Why would you care about herbal intake?

It is estimated that about a third of the population uses herbs and often do not volunteer that information because they are "natural." However, they can affect bleeding, vasodilation or constriction, or interact with prescribed medication, including migraine prescriptions. Some even trigger or worsen migraines and that effect is not dose-related or predictable. Those that are more likely to be a concern include butterbur, feverfew, ginkgo biloba, aspirin, and nonsteroidal antiinflammatory drugs.

8. What are the classifications of headaches?

Headaches are classified in several ways: primary, secondary, acute, and chronic.

- Primary headache: an organic cause cannot be identified
- Secondary headache: related to an organic cause (e.g., such as a tumor, aneurysm)
- Acute headache: associated with traumatic injury or medical emergency. It more classically has a sudden, severe onset and may be life-threatening (e.g., ruptured aneurysm, subarachnoid hemorrhage)
- Chronic headache: associated with a history of recurrence. It has a more gradual, progressive onset and the patient can obtain relief with their own measures (e.g., tension, migraine)

9. Does headache pain differ depending on the cause?

Yes. Headaches related to:

- Intracranial bleed are described as "the worst pain I have ever had," or "thunderclap" type onset.
- Vascular spasms (e.g., migraine) are described as "throbbing" or "pulsating."
- Tension are described as "tightness" (like a band is tightened around the head).
- Sinus infection is referred to as pain and a sense of "fullness" around the eyes.
- An ocular cause is described as severe pressure behind or within the eye globe.

10. Talk about symptoms of a subarachnoid hemorrhage.

It is worst at its onset, causing the familiar explanation that it is "like someone hit me with a two by four" (95% to 100%). The distinctive warning "thunderclap" headache (31% to 69%) can occur weeks before, probably from a minor leak, and is sometimes misdiagnosed as a migraine. However, if the patient indicates it is the "worst headache of his/her life," a good follow-up question is "Have you had many other 'worst headaches of your life'?"

11. Discuss epidural/subdural bleeding.

The classic scenario is that it occurs after acute head trauma. An epidural bleed is arterial and symptoms progress rapidly. Subdural bleeds are venous and the presentation is usually slower. The person loses consciousness, becomes lucid, and then the level of consciousness gradually declines. There may be neurologic deficits (6% to 30% have a seizure). Chronic subdural bleeding can manifest a while after the causative incident, especially in the older adult or alcoholics as a result of atrophy.

12. Discuss migraine headaches.

Migraine (from the Greek word *hemikrania*) pain is an acute, stabbing pain usually felt on one side of the head only. (The pain can alternate from one episode to the next, but should remain on the same side during that attack.) One patient has described the pain as "it (the headache) feels like someone is driving a hat pin into my head in the area over my right eye with a large hammer." The current thinking is that hypersensitive nerves fire inappropriately to stimuli that causes inflammation and blood vessel dilation.

13. Describe an aura.

An aura is a sensory warning that comes from the cerebral vasospasms before the onset of the migraine. This often involves visual effects such as a blurring of vision, sparkling multicolored lights in the visual field, or zigzag lines. An individual's aura experience tends to remain the same for each episode and can last up to 30 minutes.

14. List other signs or symptoms that would make me suspect a patient is experiencing a migraine headache.

- History (personal or family) of migraines. (If both parents had migraines, there is a 75% chance that the child will as well.)
- Pain intensifies with climbing stairs
- Photophobia/sensitivity to noise
- Nausea, vomiting
- Numbness of areas of the face, radiating into the arm, hand, fingers

15. Name things that can trigger a migraine.

- Changes in barometric pressure
- Stress
- Pregnancy/hormonal fluctuations (estrogen dropping in the menstrual cycle)
- Foods that contain tyrosamine (e.g., red wine, aged cheeses)
- Foods that contain monosodium glutamate (MSG) (e.g., Chinese food)
- Excessive caffeine intake
- Hypoglycemia (e.g., not eating, duodenal stasis after a heavy meal, or diabetic gastric paresis)

16. The client states she has visual changes from her migraine headache. Do I still need to do a visual acuity because I know the cause?

Yes. Sometimes the client's "self-diagnosis" is wrong. Any vision change warrants a visual acuity assessment.

17. Anything else I should assess for with a migraine besides the routine triage?

Dehydration, particularly if the person has been nauseated or vomiting.

18. Discuss clues I could use to differentiate a tension headache from a migraine.

- Sensation: Tension headaches are a "tight band," nonpulsating, and dull.
- Effect: Tension headaches are bothersome, but are not disabling like migraine headaches. (The National Headache Foundation reports that 53% of migraine sufferers go to bed until the pain resolves.) Tension headaches have no nausea or vomiting.
- Onset: A tension headache is more likely to occur in the later part of the day, migraines after the trigger.
- Treatment: Tension headaches usually lesson with rest, migraines can last for days despite bedrest.

19. Describe cluster headaches.

Cluster headaches are an excruciating, unilateral pain, often accompanied by rhinorrhea and lacrimation. They are nonfamilial and are more common in men. These headaches come in "clusters" or groups, up to a dozen or more a day. The pattern is several headaches a day for several weeks, then remission for several weeks or months, followed by another onset of grouped headaches.

20. Any treatment?

Oxygen relieves 90% within 15 minutes.

21. What is a concern related to patients with chronic daily headaches?

A chronic daily headache is defined as headaches that last longer than 4 hours per day on 15 or more days per month for at least 6 months. These patients (3% of the population) are the one who most frequently use drugs inappropriately as they try to get relief.

22. Talk about rebound headaches.

It is estimated that 1.5% of the population has true rebound headaches, more likely in people with a history of migraine headaches in the family. However, although a little publicized problem, up to 32% of adults create their own rebound phenomena through too many OTC analgesics. It becomes a vicious cycle in which the more analgesics used; the more likely the person will experience a new headache between doses.

There is a newer awareness that this phenomenon is also occurring in children. In one study of pediatric (age 6 to 18) patients with chronic headaches, 22% were using OTC pain relievers as often as 15 to 20 times a week. Interestingly, 1 in 7 were taking the medication without telling a parent.

The maximum recommended frequency for the OTC analgesics is two times a week or nine times a month. Otherwise, the person should be referred for headache prevention and management.

23. Discuss chronic morning headaches.

Chronic morning headaches affect 1 in 13 individuals in the general population. Ohayon (2004) found that they were often a good indicator of both major depressive disorders and insomnia disorders, but not to sleep-related breathing disorders (as previously thought).

24. What will help me distinguish a tension or migraine headache from a headache coming from a more serious etiology?

Tension headaches and migraines tend to be recurrent and similar from one episode to the next. It is always a possibility that the presenting patient is experiencing their first migraine headache ever, but it shouldn't be the automatic initial conclusion. Additionally, consider the age of onset. Migraines most commonly begin before age 30 (usually in the teens or early twenties) and tension headaches usually begin before age 50.

25. Describe symptoms that might help me pursue if the patient's headache is from sinus problems.

- History of a cough or recent upper respiratory infection (70% to 94%)
- Nasal discharge (often green) or nasal congestion (70% to 94%)
- Pain is worse in the morning (no drainage during the night) and improves during the day (compared to tension headache that tends to get worse as the day progresses)
- Headache is worse when bending over, during activity, or coughing (31% to 69%)
- Facial pain, including radiating into the teeth (31% to 69%)
- Fever (31% to 69%)

26. When is there cause to be concerned with a sinus headache?

When there is periorbital cellulitis, ophthalmologic symptoms, or a change in neurologic signs/symptoms. Otherwise treatment is usually outpatient with antibiotics and decongestants.

27. Describe temporal arteritis.

Although relatively infrequent (24 cases per 100,000 people), this inflammation of the arteries' laminal layer is a risk factor for arterial occlusion and blindness. It should be considered in every patient older than 50 who has a headache. Emergent treatment with steroids is required.

28. What symptoms would alert me to further consider temporal arteritis?

The majority have a headache (70% to 94%), with up to a third (6% to 30%) experiencing it unilaterally in the temporal area. Other classic symptoms include visual disturbances (31% to 69%), scalp tenderness, abnormal palpable temporal artery (e.g., feels "cordlike"), and facial pain.

29. What might make me consider the patient's severe headache is from acute, narrow-angle glaucoma?

The headache from this condition can resemble a migraine or temporal arteritis. Other related symptoms to assess for include:

- Tunnel vision or halos around the lights.
- Eyeball will feel hard to palpation.
- Pupils will be fixed and dilated at midpoint.
- History of being in the semidarkness (movie theater) when it started and/or using anticholinergic medications.

30. What might alert me to a headache from carbon monoxide poisoning?

- History of being in an enclosed space in the winter
- Entire family complaining of recurrent headache, dizziness, and nausea that are worse in the morning (after being in the enclosed house all night).
- The family pet is also sick.

31. Talk about bacterial meningitis.

Although a patient with this diagnosis can have a severe headache, the classic symptoms triad is a high fever (70% to 94%), level of consciousness (LOC) changes (31% to 69%), and nuchal rigidity (6% to 30%). I recently had a college student eventually diagnosed with meningitis whose only presenting complaint was a "terrible" headache that acetaminophen (Tylenol) wasn't helping.

Although the Kernig's sign and Brudzinski's sign are classic maneuvers of physical diagnosis for meningitis, they are coming under increasing critical scrutiny for their value early in the course of the disease. In Thomas et al (2002), the Kernig's sign had a sensitivity of 5%, a specificity of 95%, and a positive predictive value of 27%. The Brudzinski's sign had the same performance characteristics as the Kernig's sign.

32. What about a headache that is described as dull, boreing, and unremitting over days or weeks?

It could just be a tension headache, but the patient will need to be evaluated for an intracranial mass lesion or depression.

33. List the symptoms most likely in patients presenting with a primary brain tumor.

- Headache (56%)
- Altered mental status (51%)
- Nausea or vomiting (37%)
- Seizures (37%)
- Visual changes (23%)
- Motor weakness (37%)

34. Why do I get a headache after eating ice cream?

About a third of the general population gets this "brain freeze" that causes a sharp pain around the forehead and eyes (a mini-migraine). The sensation from ingesting cold food rapidly can trigger blood vessel spasms. It is harmless, but you can always cure yourself by eliminating ice cream!

35. What headache would be a level 1 (red, emergent) in a three-tier system?

- Severe headache pain (10 on a 0 to 10 scale)
- Associated signs and symptoms: emesis, weakness, photophobia, pallor, diaphoresis, tachycardia, or tachypnea
- Tried and cannot be relieved with the usual methods of pain management
- Sudden onset of pain that is "worse ever"

36. Who would you rate a level 2 (yellow, urgent) in a three-tier system?

A patient with a headache rated 7 to 8 (0 to 10) without any significant associated symptoms or history. Although the patient is uncomfortable and should be seen as soon as possible, the symptoms are more consistent with a chronic type headache condition, and are not symptomatic of a life-threatening condition.

37. Talk about how that is different in a five-tier triage categorization system.

In a five-tier triage categorization system, the first scenario would also be considered emergent, but would be categorized as a level 2 (level 1 is restricted to patients with an immediate life threat). This patient requires pain relief within 10 minutes.

38. Describe what would be level 3 in a five-tier system.

The second example would be given a level 3 designation. The level 3 patient would require pain relief and two or more resources (e.g., medications for pain and possibly nausea, possible intravenous access, possibly computerized tomography [CT] of the head, lab work). Additionally, the patient's vital signs would be considered.

39. How would you classify a patient who presents to triage with a headache and simply requires a refill of a prescription for a pain medication?

This patient would be a category III (green) in a three-tier system and a category V in a five-tier system.

40. List some nonpharmacologic nursing interventions for headache pain.

- Place in a cool, darkened room
- Apply an ice pack to the forehead or back of the neck
- Distraction/imagery including music, videos, massage

41. What can be done for a patient with chronic headaches?

- Teach the patient to make time for activities that promote a feeling of well being, such as Tai-Chi, yoga, exercise, relaxation exercises, biofeedback.
- Encourage the patient to avoid weather conditions, foods, activities, and situations that are known to precipitate headaches.
- Refer the patient to a headache clinic or neurologist (if indicated). Triptans are usually the first line of treatment for preventing migraines, although other drugs may be prescribed to stabilize blood vessels or regulate serotonin levels.
- Encourage the patient to keep a headache log.
- Suggest that the patient join a support group.

42. I heard Botox injections could be a treatment for migraines.

There have been some promising results with Botox injections for patients who do not get relief from migraines with other treatments or drugs. It appears that it blocks pain messages to the brain. In one study, 80% of the 271 headache patients reported fewer or less painful headaches. The report did not include if they experienced less wrinkles.

43. Tell me more about the use of acupuncture.

In one study, it was shown to work as well as the triptan, Imitrex. In a UK study, after 12 months of the addition of acupuncture to the usual treatment regimen, the headache scores were reduced by 34% in the acupuncture group versus 16% in the control group. Additionally, the acupuncture patients experienced the equivalent of 22 fewer days of headache yearly, used 15% less medication, made 25% fewer general practitioner visits, and took 15% fewer sick days than the control patients. About 10% of UK practitioners incorporate acupuncture in the treatment for the patients with chronic headaches; it may be worthwhile to consider it as a therapeutic option in America.

44. What other alternative therapies are being tried?

- Magnesium: It is suspected that some women, especially those with a menstrual-onset migraine, are deficient in magnesium. Taking 200 to 800mg per day reduced migraines by 42% in one study.

- Riboflavin. In one study, 59% of those taking 400 mg per day for 3 months have fewer and shorter migraines than those given a placebo.
- Coenzyme Q10: Thought to work similar to riboflavin, 60% of those who took 150 mg per day for 3 months had fewer and shorter migraines.
- Peppermint oil: Rubbing this (mixed in an alcohol solution) over the forehead and temples relieved tension headaches.
- Gabapentin (Neurontin) was found in one study to produce statistically significant but clinically modest relief.

Key Points

- Approximately 50% of headaches are some form of a migraine.
- An acute headache with a sudden, severe onset is of the most concern.
- Up to 32% of adults create a rebound headache phenomenon through overuse of OTC analgesics.
- Consider temporal arteritis in every patient over 50 years of age with a headache.
- A sudden change in the characteristics of a chronic headache should be evaluated thoroughly.

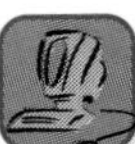

Internet Resources

American Council for Headache Education (ACHE)
www.achenet.org

National Headache Foundation
www.headaches.org

HeadTalk.com. Migraine information site from GlaxoSmithKline.
www.headtalk.com

Robbins Headache Clinic, Northbrook, Illinois (Lawrence Robbins, MD)
www.headachedrugs.com

Bibliography

ACS Committee on Trauma: *Resources for optimal care of the injured patient,* Chicago, Ill, 1999, Author; available at www.facs.org/dept/trauma.

Decker WW, Haro LH: Headache. In Markovchick VJ, Pons PT, editors: *Pons' emergency medicine secrets,* ed 3, Philadelphia, 2003, Hanley & Belfus.

Edlow J, Macnow L: Headache. In Davis MA, Votey SR, Greenough PG, editors: *Greenough's signs and symptoms in emergency medicine: Literature-based approach to emergent conditions,* St Louis, 1999, Mosby.

Gilboy N, Rosenow A, Travers D, et al: *Emergency severity index (ESI),* Des Plaines, Ill, 2003, Emergency Nurses Association.

Jacobs BB, Hoyt KS, editors: *Trauma nursing core course,* ed 5, Des Plaines, Ill, 2000, Emergency Nurses Association.

Jenkins JL, Braen GR: *Manual of emergency medicine,* ed 4, Philadelphia, 2000, Lippincott, Williams & Wilkins.

Jordan KS, editor: *Emergency nursing core curriculum,* ed 5, Emergency Nurses Association. Philadelphia, 2000, WB Saunders, pp. 407-409.

Kappes JN, McNair RS: Headache and visual changes at triage: Do not allow the patient's assumptions to cloud your judgment, *J Emerg Nurs* 29(6):584-586, 2003.

Killian M, editor: *Standards of emergency nursing practice,* ed 4, Des Plaines, Ill, 1999, Emergency Nurses Association.

Newberry L: *Sheehy's emergency nursing: Principles and practice,* St Louis, 2003, Mosby.

Ohayon MM: Prevalence and risk factors of morning headaches in the general population, *Arch Intern Med* 164(1):97-102, 2004.

Robbins L: *Robbin headache clinic presentation: Outpatient management of chronic headache,* Delnor Community Hospital, Geneva, Ill, Feb 20, 2004.

Selfridge-Thomas J: *Emergency nursing: An essential guide for patient care,* Philadelphia, 1997, WB Saunders, pp. 38, 39.

Slovis CM, Wrenn KD, Meador CK: *A little book of emergency medicine rules,* Philadelphia, 2000, Hanley & Belfus.

Spira PJ, Beran RG: Gabapentin in the prophylaxis of chronic daily headaches: A randomized, placebo-controlled study, *Neurology* 61:1753-1759, 2003.

Thomas KE, Hasbun R, Jekel J, Quagliarello VJ: The diagnostic accuracy of Kernig's sign, Brudzinski's sign and nuchal rigidity in adults with suspected meningitis, *Clin Infect Dis* 1(35):46-52, July 2002.

Vickers A, Rees R, Zollman C, Smith C, Ellis N: Acupuncture for chronic headache in primary care: Large, pragmatic, randomized trial, *BMJ* 27(328):744-747, March 2004.

Zimmermann PG: Triage and differential diagosis of patients with headaches, dizziness, low back pain, and rashes: A basic primer, *J Emerg Nurs* 28(3):209-215, 2002.

Chapter 20

Closed Head Injury

Robert D. Herr

1. How common and serious is closed head injury?

Closed head injury causes half of trauma-related deaths and much morbidity. The brain is not as resilient as other tissues. In fact, return to prior functioning happens in only half of patients with severe head injury.

2. Why is head injury so serious?

In a word it is the skull with its bony rigidity and internal irregular surfaces. Sudden skull movement can cause injury to the brain substance or bridging veins. If injury creates bleeding, the skull's inflexibility can cause intracranial pressure to rise. If the pressure approaches arterial pressure, brain blood flow can fall. This creates brain ischemia with neuronal damage or death. Severe pressure rise can lead to herniation of the brain with brain death soon following.

3. What are the types of closed head injury I should look for?

Closed head injuries are either diffuse or focal lesions. Diffuse lesions include concussion and diffuse axonal injury. Focal lesions include depressed skull fractures, intracerebral bleeds, and subdural and epidural hematomas.

4. Describe concussion and diffuse axonal injury.

Concussion results from a jostling of the brain and is manifested by a transient loss of consciousness immediately after closed head injury, generally when the head is moving and strikes an object. The loss of consciousness lasts for a few seconds to minutes. The patient may present at triage with persistent headache and problems with memory, anxiety, insomnia, and dizziness.

Diffuse axonal injury results from a tearing of nerve fibers at the time of impact. It manifests as functional or physiologic abnormality. It results from a spectrum of injury from mild head injury to a prolonged traumatic coma lasting for at least 6 hours.

5. What are focal lesions to watch for?

These include:

- Depressed fractures manifested as scalp bleeding or scalp hematoma. Skull films or head computed tomography (CT) confirm the fracture. Brain contusions are usually hemorrhagic in the brain substance either directly under the area of impact or on the opposite side (so-called contrecoup injury).
- Intracerebral hemorrhage resulting from torn blood vessels. Their presentation can be delayed for days.
- Epidural hematoma, an accumulation of blood between the inner table of the skull and the dura. It is associated with a skull fracture that tears a meningeal artery, usually the middle meningeal.
- Subdural hematoma, an accumulation of blood beneath the dura and overlying the arachnoid and brain. This results from tearing of bridging veins caused by an acceleration-deceleration injury. These can be acute to 2 weeks or more after injury.

6. How do I triage the patient with a closed head injury?

Ask about the mechanism of injury, the time of the injury, the presence of a lucid interval, and prior use of drugs and alcohol. Witnesses are key. Any observer or family can provide information about the patient's condition at baseline and immediately after the injury. The neurologic examination is essential, and the level of consciousness is the single most important factor in neurologically assessing the head-injured patient. The Glasgow Coma Scale (GCS; see Table 20-1) is common and highly reproducible (reliable). A pediatric GCS is also available.

Table 20-1. Glasgow Coma Scale (Adult Version)

Measure	Response	Score
Eye opening	Spontaneously	4
	To verbal command	3
	To pain	2
	No response	1
Verbal	Oriented and converses	5
	Disoriented and converses	4
	Inappropriate words	3
	Incomprehensible sounds	2
	No response	1
Motor	Obeys verbal command	6
	Localizes pain	5
	Flexion-withdrawal	4
	Abnormal flexion (decorticate rigidity)	3
	Extension (decerebrate rigidity)	2
	No response	1

Table 20-1. Glasgow Coma Scale (Infant and Child Versions)—*cont'd*

Activity	Score	Infants	Children
Eye Opening	4	Spontaneous	Spontaneous
	3	To speech or sound	To speech
	2	To painful stimuli	To painful stimuli
	1	None	None
Verbal	5	Appropriate words or sounds, social smile, fixes and follows	Oriented
	4	Cries, but consolable	Confused
	3	Persistently irritable	Inappropriate words
	2	Restless, agitated	Incomprehensible sounds
	1	None	None
Motor	6	Spontaneous movement	Obeys commands
	5	Localizes to pain	Localizes to pain
	4	Withdraws to pain	Withdraws to pain
	3	Abnormal flexion (decorticate)	Abnormal flexion (decorticate)
	2	Abnormal extension (decerebrate)	Abnormal extension (decerebrate)
	1	None	None

7. What does the GCS measure?

The GCS has been unfairly denigrated as "the only test on which your patient can be totally dead and still score a three!" The scale evaluates three aspects of the patient's responsiveness: (a) eye opening, (b) best verbal response, and (c) best motor response.

- Eye Opening
  If the patient does not open eyes by themselves, ask them to open their eyes, then apply noxious stimulation such as vigorous pinching or pressure on the nail beds.
- Verbal Response
  The patient with oriented speech has awareness of name, place, and date. "Disoriented and converses" speech is well articulated but the patient is disoriented. Inappropriate words are those which are random or nonsensical. Incomprehensible speech is moaning or groaning without intelligible words.
- Motor Responses
  The patient who obeys verbal commands can move his limbs readily. Localizing pain means that the patient moves a limb to noxious stimulus to remove it. Flexion-withdrawal means that the patient flexes away from a pain stimulus. An abnormal flexion response is a decorticate response with arms moved toward the body. (HINT: remember that de<u>cor</u>ticate is toward the body's <u>core</u>.) An extensor response is decerebrate with abduction and

internal rotation of the shoulder and pronation of the forearm. No response is hypotonia or flaccidity, which strongly suggests loss of lower brainstem function.

8. What do the GCS scores mean?

The maximum score is 15, the lowest score is 3. Severe head injury is defined as a GCS of 8 or less. Moderate head injury is defined as GCS of 9 to 12, and mild head injury, 13 to 15.

9. What besides the GCS should be assessed?

Record pupil size in millimeters and reactivity to light. A dilating pupil together with a decreasing level of consciousness suggests brain (uncal lobes) herniation with associated oculomotor nerve compression. Because 20% of the "normal" population will have anisocoria (a pupillary inequality of <0.5 mm), it is critical to measure and document pupil size to recognize if the pupil is dilating or is stable.

10. What do I test in the comatose patient to assess level of brain function?

One great test of brainstem function is the corneal reflex. Check it with a wisp of Kleenex or cotton (when applied to the cornea the eye should blink). Intact blink guarantees the pons is intact. The presence or absence of a gag reflex and spontaneous respirations will further assess the status of the lower pons and medulla.

11. How do I recognize a basilar skull fracture?

The diagnosis is primarily clinical—often it is not even detected on head CT. Suspect it when there is hemotympanum or bloody discharge from the ear; retroauricular ecchymosis (Battle sign); periorbital ecchymosis ("raccoon's eyes"); rhinorrhea or otorrhea (which is cerebrospinal fluid dripping) or cranial nerve deficits.

12. What else should I consider at triage?

More than one in twenty patients with severe head injury will have an associated cervical spine fracture. Order cervical spine radiographs for those who are unconscious, have neck pain, evidence of spinal cord injury, or if the mechanism of injury can produce cervical damage.

13. When should I order skull films in adults?

Hardly ever. If the blunt injury is severe enough a brain CT is needed. The CT will show bony abnormalities.

14. When do I go ahead and order a head CT?

Indications include persistent decrease in level of consciousness, neurologic deterioration, or focal neurologic deficit.

15. What lab work should I order at triage?

Minor head injury requires no blood work. All significant head injury should include complete blood cell count, electrolytes, blood glucose, arterial blood gases, urinalysis, ethanol level, and directed toxicologic analysis where indicated. Because brain matter can be released into the circulation and cause coagulopathy, check the partial thromboplastin time, prothrombin time, platelets, and fibrinogen level. Of course, blood for type and crossmatch is routine for severe trauma.

16. What is the "Talk and Deteriorate" Syndrome?

This occurs in one in ten patients with severe head injury whose condition does not warrant immediate aggressive care. These patients speak recognizable words immediately after head injury. Within 48 hours they become confused or have unilateral weakness or both from a severe brain injury.

17. How do I treat this syndrome?

Have the physician order a brain CT scan. If it shows an intracranial hematoma the patient needs immediate surgical decompression. Meanwhile reduce brain edema and intracranial pressure through elevating the head of the bed to 30 degrees, straightening the neck to enhance venous drainage, and having the physician order intravenous (IV) mannitol 1 g/kg. IV furosemide may also be helpful.

18. What should I consider in triaging the child?

The nurse should be familiar with normal stages of neurologic development to assess for deficit, and use an age-appropriate version of the GCS. Of course adult caretakers can be the best reference for their children's normal behavior and developmental milestones. The infant's intracranial pressure can be assessed by palpating the anterior fontanelle. In children, vomiting after head trauma is common and does not predict who has increased intracranial pressure. They may also be diaphoretic, weak, and pale after head injury, then suddenly "snap out of it" with no ill effects. In contrast hypotension is a bad prognostic sign and signals more severe brain injury.

Key Points

- Closed head injury causes a spectrum of injury and considerable long-term disability.
- Use the GCS to assess level of consciousness.
- Although confusion or decreased level of consciousness could be from alcohol or drugs, you should confirm this through blood alcohol levels and toxicologic screens. If the patient does not improve quickly or begins to deteriorate, immediate head CT is indicated. Frequent documentation and serial tracking of neurologic status is important.
- A patient can talk at triage and deteriorate in the treatment area.
- Children require adjustment of the GCS and hypotension is a bad prognostic sign.

Internet Resources

Management of Minor Closed Head Injury in Children
http://www.guideline.gov/summary/summary.aspx?ss=15&doc_id=2272&nbr=1498

Traumatic Emergencies: Part 6 Traumatic Injury and Head Injury
http://www.nursingceu.com/NCEU/courses/06trauma/

Iroquois Memorial Hospital Emergency Department Patient Care Standard for Head Injury
http://www.ena.org/document_share/documents/head_injuries.doc

Guidelines for the Acute Medical Management of Severe Traumatic Brain Injury in Infants, Children, and Adolescents
http://www.ena.org/conferences/annual/2004/handouts/238-c.pdf

Preventing Secondary Brain Injury: Implications for the ED
http://www.ena.org/conferences/annual/2004/handouts/101-c.pdf

Bibliography

Bazarian JJ, Fisher SG, Flesher W, et al: Lateral automobile impacts and the risk of traumatic brain injury, *Ann Emerg Med* 44(2):142-152, 2004.

Cornwell EE: Initial approach to trauma. In Tintinalli JE, Kelen GD, Stapczynski JS, editors: *Emergency medicine,* ed 5, New York, 2000, McGraw-Hill.

Marte E, Baro G, Fifield C: Pediatric trauma. In Tintinalli JE, Ruiz E, Krome R, editors: *Emergency medicine: A comprehensive study guide,* ed 3, New York, 1998, McGraw-Hill.

Rockswold GL: Head injury. In Tintinalli JE, Ruiz E, Krome R, editors: *Emergency medicine: A comprehensive study guide,* ed 3, New York, 1998, McGraw-Hill.

Chapter 21

Dental Pain/Tooth Avulsion

Robert D. Herr

1. What is a toothache?

The classic toothache results from nerve root irritation and pain known as pulpitis. The nerve runs into the innermost part of the dental pulp. This nerve is protected from exposure to air and bacteria by dental enamel and dentin of the normal tooth. At times, a dental filling or crown replaces enamel and dentin worn down or away by dental caries or trauma. If the patient loses a crown, filling, or normal enamel, they experience periodic attacks of sharp, throbbing, aching pain.

If untreated, this pulpitis may progress to periapical abscess. In periapical abscesses, bacteria invade the bone. The patient complains of a sudden onset of constant aching pain. This pain localizes to a single tooth. The pain worsens if the tooth is tapped by a tongue blade. The gum may be tender or swollen. These bacteria are largely anaerobic mouth microbes susceptible to penicillin.

2. When does a toothache involve the root canal?

Root canal is a type of periodontal disease in which the tooth may not be carious. Instead periodontal pockets form around the base of the tooth. The pain of root canal is deeper and more intense.

3. What else causes toothache?

The patient presenting with a toothache should be checked for common disorders that mimic toothache. Toothache of the upper jaw or maxilla could be associated with sinus infections, temporomandibular joint inflammation, parotid gland inflammation, oral ulcerations, or temporal arteritis. Toothaches of the lower jaw or mandible can be associated with disorders of the sublingual salivary gland or oral ulcers.

4. What is dry socket? How is it treated?

A dry socket is pain 2 to 3 days after tooth extraction. It usually affects the mandibular third molars, but may also affect other sockets. It is treated by irrigating the socket with saline until it is clean of debris, then applying an iodoform dressing into the socket.

5. What is dental barotrauma?

Dental barotrauma or barodontalgia is a toothache associated with pressure changes during diving. The mechanism of pain is pressure from air that is trapped under a faulty filling.

6. What are the signs of an emergency?

Any patient in acute pain is at least an urgency. A dental emergency is a patient with a toothache and fever, prostration, or neurologic deficit. These patients have a spreading infection that needs immediate treatment. Another urgency is the patient with fever and swelling of the jaw. Typically the toothache has lasted several days or weeks. This patient may have osteomyelitis. Osteomyelitis requires intravenous (IV) antibiotics and referral to an ear, nose, throat specialist (ENT) for debridement. Fortunately, most toothaches are not emergent and respond to pain treatment and perhaps antibiotics.

7. When does a dentist need to be called?

Dental conditions are rarely emergent enough to warrant immediate dental consult, and only then after evaluation by an emergency physician. Virtually no cases require dental consult ordered at triage.

8. Because toothache patients want pain meds, do I ask the doctor to give drugs to them?

Acute pain usually requires acute treatment with analgesia. However, the patient with a toothache should have probing questions and an examination first. Unfortunately, patients who are seeking opioids for recreational use—or to sell on the street—commonly complain of toothache to get them. For example, one patient alone accounted for over 300 emergency department visits in a single year in Western Washington. Toothache and migraine were her major complaints. Narcotic analgesics were prescribed two-thirds of the time, and kept her coming back for more. This pales in comparison to organized crime, in which a van carrying "professional patients" stops in a city. In one day, the "patients" blanket the EDs to collect prescriptions. Once filled, the prescriptions are worth thousands of dollars in narcotics when each Percocet tablet can fetch $100. I have worked with physicians so "burned" by scammers that they no longer prescribe narcotics.

9. How do I identify a malingerer?

These "malingerers" are difficult to tell from patients who actually have toothache from pulpitis or periapical abscess. The two principles I use to detect scammers are (a) catch them in a lie, or (b) offer a local dental block to relieve toothache.

First, look in their mouth. This gives credence to their complaint and might make for a short visit. An edentulous patient complaining of toothache is at least suspicious for either malingering or a nondental cause of pain (see above). Then ask the patient about their history of dental care and previous analgesics. If possible, call the dentist office, the last ED, or the pharmacy to determine if the history you hear is correct. How many times have I had the pharmacist call me to let me know the patient I just wrote for Vicodin has a history of multiple opioid prescriptions? I just wish I had called before writing the prescription.

Second, see if the patient is more interested in pain relief or getting some pills. Mention that several of the doctors like to inject painful teeth to relieve pain until the patient can be seen by a dentist. Patients truly in pain will be open to anything that helps. Scammers will suddenly decide they are wasting their time and perhaps go down the street.

10. A patient hands me a tooth—what do I do?

A permanent tooth that has been totally knocked out of the bony socket is an emergency. In a patient with good oral hygiene, immediate tooth reimplantation is at least cosmetic, and if done within 30 minutes, has a 90% chance of surviving. After 2 hours the tooth is very unlikely to survive. The following practice will help save the tooth. You or the physician should do the following:

- Bring the patient to the treatment area immediately, to the ENT room if it is available
- Handle the tooth by the crown, not the root. Irrigate debris from the root by spraying saline through an 18-gauge needle. Do not touch the root because you will disrupt the suspensory ligaments needed for the tooth to cement itself back
- Inspect the socket and irrigate with saline sprayed through an 18-gauge bore needle. Any clot should be swabbed free without curetting away the suspensory ligaments in the socket

Insert the tooth into the socket. Have the patient bite down on a gauze placed over the crown to seat the tooth firmly into the socket.

11. Do I worry about primary teeth knocked out?

No. These are usually not reimplanted.

12. What if a patient calls with a tooth knocked out? What do I say?

If the caller can replace the tooth, have them wash it with tap water, handle it by the crown only, and attempt to reimplant it. If this does not work, have the patient come to the ED or call 911. Until they get medical care, have them place the tooth in moist gauze and place it in Hanks solution (Save-a-Tooth, look in first aid kits for this). Saline or milk is a reasonable substitute. If none of this is available, have the patient place the tooth under their tongue. Calling 911 may or may not reduce implantation time. It depends on the training of first responders. If in doubt, driving to the ED may be quicker than calling 911 and waiting for emergency medical services evaluation and transport.

13. How do I handle broken teeth?

A patient with a broken tooth likely has part of the nerve exposed to air. They complain of tooth pain. Touching the tooth hurts as well. Triage considerations include getting radiographs to look for fracture of the alveolar bone surrounding the tooth. A Panorex is best, but requires a Panorex machine. Treatment may include splinting the tooth back into position if the fracture is in the nerve root.

14. How do I triage oral abscesses or canker sores?

Oral abscesses usually result from tooth infection. They present as painful swollen fluctuant areas of the gingival mucosa or base of the tongue. The patient is febrile. If untreated they can cause prostration and sepsis. Treatment depends on location and prompt drainage. Antibiotics are secondary to drainage. The patient with fever, fluctuance, or mouth soreness should be triaged promptly and evaluated thoroughly.

Canker sores are known as aphthous ulcers. They are painful, often recurring sores of the mucous membranes. These may come on during emotional stress or during chemotherapy with certain agents. These should be distinguished from herpes. Herpes occurs with fever, headache, and regional adenopathy. Herpetic lesions occur on the skin outside the mouth; aphthous ulcers are within the mouth.

Because herpes is contagious the patient with mouth ulcers should be triaged with caution. Wear gloves and dispose of the tongue blade promptly. The patient may be given ibuprofen or acetaminophen until a diagnosis is made. Treatment of aphthous ulcers may include mouthwash with one or more ingredients: magnesium antacid (Maalox, Mylanta), diphenhydramine solution (Benadryl), viscous Xylocaine, and/or tetracycline solution. Herpes may be additionally treated with acyclovir.

15. How do I approach the patient with postextraction hemorrhage?

Bleeding is usually self limited. The site of bleeding is identified with suction if needed. Then control bleeding by having the patient bite down on gauze packs. Elevate the head. Measure hematocrit and coagulation, and begin IV fluid bolus if signs of hypovolemia are present. Blood for type and screen is prudent. Severe or persistent bleeding may require emergent consult with ENT or oral surgery for suturing, electrocautery or rarely, direct tie-off of a bleeding artery.

Key Points

- A permanent tooth knocked out should be reimplanted as soon as possible. This can be done at triage.
- Toothache can represent sinus pain, temporomandibular joint (TMJ) dysfunction, or parotid gland inflammation, oral ulcer, oral herpes, temporal arteritis, or malingering.
- The malingerer is more interested in getting a specific narcotic than in getting pain relief.
- Post extraction bleeding should be treated with direct pressure, head elevation, and preparing for cautery or ENT consultation.

Internet Resources

E-medicine Discussion of Toothache
http://www.emedicine.com/aaem/topic452.htm

For Other Topics in Dental Health Care from Abscessed Tooth to Your Relationship With Your Dentist
http://www.ada.org/public/topics/alpha.asp

A Leading Expert on Malingering
http://ourworld.compuserve.com/homepages/Marc_Feldman_2/

Bibliography

Hodgdon A: Toothache and common periodontal problems. In Harwood NA, Wolfson AB, Linden CH, Shepherd SM, Stenklyft PH, editors: *The clinical practice of emergency medicine,* ed 3, Philadelphia, 2001, Lippincott, Williams & Wilkins, pp. 75-78.

Zuckerman LA, Ferrante FM: Nonopioid and opioid analgesics. In Ashburn MA, Rice LJ, editors: *The management of pain,* New York, 1998, Churchill Livingstone, pp. 131-135.

Chapter 22

Ear Pain

Robert D. Herr

Ear pain brings its share of patients (usually children) to the emergency department (ED) triage desk, often on evening or night shift. It is often considered nonemergent because it is as a rule not life-threatening. Yet acute ear pain can be excruciatingly painful to the point of tears. Because the ear canal can be hard to visualize at triage, the full extent of injury or illness can be easily underestimated compared to something as visibly apparent as a rash on the skin. Yet ear pain is much more treatable than a skin condition. Pain relief can be dramatic and the patient can be very grateful.

1. What are the most common causes of ear pain?

Most acute ear pain derives from acute otitis media, also known as "earache." However, acute ear pain can be caused by ear foreign body (including insect or piercing), external otitis media (swimmers ear) and less commonly barotraumas, herpes zoster (shingles), wax impaction, and the common furuncle (boil). Lastly, ear pain can be referred from the jaw and temporomandibular joint (TMJ) or pharynx.

2. What are the most important questions to ask in triage with a primary complaint of "ear pain"?

In addition to the generic triage questions, the type of pain and relationship to ear movement will be important. Include loss of hearing ("muffled" sounds or hearing "through a tunnel,") presence of drainage, previous ear problems, ear pulling, or playing with small items in children. Domestic violence screening can also be significant.

3. What else is key to ask in triage regarding ear pain?

In addition to taking the history, it is crucial to closely examine the skin around the ear, behind the ear, and in the ear. Because the ear canal is both hidden to the patient and family and intrinsically fascinating to children and some adults, it is a treasure to the examiner. My suggestion? Grab the otoscope and look into the ear. The procedure is easy and improves with practice.

4. Describe the technique to use to examine the ear canal with an otoscope.

Make sure you pull back the pinna to straighten the ear canal before inserting the speculum.

5. Any tips for working with children?

Restrain an uncooperative young child by placing him or her supine on a firm surface. Instruct the caregiver or assistant to hold both arms up by the head, embracing the elbow joints on both sides of each arm. Restrain an infant by having the caregiver hold the infant's hands down. Use the lateral side of the same hand that is grasping the otoscope to prevent the child's head from jerking.

6. What is the best size of plastic speculum to use?

Use a plastic speculum that is the largest that will fit in the ear canal. The adult speculum actually begins to work in kids old enough to walk and talk, and is much easier to see through than the smaller child's speculum. In addition, it will make a tight seal and present air from escaping if using a pneumatic bulb.

7. Are there any times you should stop inserting the speculum for examination?

If you see pus or a red boil you might stop there because inserting the speculum will hurt. If the canal is dry or contains wax, go ahead and press the speculum firmly into the canal. Then pull the ear back and press in until the tympanic membrane (TM) can be seen as a white, yellow, or reddish end to the canal. For children under age 3, pull the lower auricle down and out to straighten the ear canal.

8. What am I looking for?

A "normal" ear will have distinct landmarks—the umbo, the short process, and the long handle of the malleus. Look for the narrow cone of the light reflex at 5 o'clock in the right ear and 7 o'clock in the left ear. You will normally see a TM with a pinkish color versus fire red. It is abnormal to see bulging or retraction of the TM. If there is reddish wax occluding the canal, instill Cerumenex. Cerumenex will begin dissolving the wax and enable irrigating or curetting out the wax. Wax must be removed to visualize the TM.

The patient may have a ruptured TM. If the TM is completely ruptured you will be looking past the rim of TM into the middle ear. It looks like a hole. Cerumenex is not used if the TM is ruptured, so a ruptured TM must be distinguished from wax impaction.

9. How will the presence of "tubes" affect what I see?

Tympanoplasty tubes surgically implanted to keep the canal open will reflect back to you as a narrow blue dot. If it is in place, it will prevent the ear from blocking. Because most tubes are simple cylinders they easily come out. Examination may show the tube lying sideways in the canal. There is no cause for alarm as they are intended only for short-term drainage of weeks to months. Longer lasting tubes have flanged ends and are more painful to insert initially so they are not as popular.

10. Describe acute otitis media (AOM).

AOM is the second most common infection in children, peaking around 7 to 18 months. Pain and pressure worsen at night when the child or adult lays down and fluid presses against the eardrum.

11. What would make me suspect AOM in a child?

Because of the age, crying and ear pulling may be the only signs. Is the child fussy? Is there a fever? Is there a history of earache? Patients who have had an earache in the first 6 months of life are more likely than those without to have a recurrence.

Suspect otitis media with ear pulling or ear pain and fever. Treatment can begin with acetaminophen or ibuprofen. After diagnosis the clinician can in most cases give Auralgan, a topical anesthetic that deadens ear pain.

12. What is visualized on otoscope evaluation if it is AOM?

One meta-analysis by Rothman et al shows that the TM in AOM is cloudy, bulging, or clearly immobile. In addition a normal color makes AOM unlikely. An erythematous TM strongly suggests AOM.

13. Talk about foreign bodies in the ear.

Please see Chapter 41. Children may not be able to describe what happened, but ask about a history of playing with cotton, paper, or food such as peas or small beans. The most hazardous things are small batteries that can be found in many toys, talking books, or Grandma's hearing aid. These batteries can be caustic and should be removed soon.

The most annoying ear foreign body is a live insect that cannot find its way out. The patient may scratch or claw at their ear and will not calm down until the insect is removed.

14. What do I look for with ear piercing?

Please see Chapter 42.

15. Talk about external otitis.

External otitis, or "swimmer's ear" is caused by water that accumulates in the ear canals after swimming or showering. This water causes swelling of the skin in the canal and introduces bacterial infection, usually pseudomonas.

- The key history is swimming or showering without draining water from the ear.
- The key finding is intense pain with moving the ear, lack of fever, and an ear canal that is narrowed with yellow or white pus lining it.
- Initial treatment is with analgesics like acetaminophen or ibuprofen and an antibiotic solution like polymyxin-neomycin to eradicate pseudomonas.

16. What is barotrauma?

It is literally pressure change that traumatizes something—usually used to mean damage to the TM. A blow to the ear increases air pressure in the ear canal and can rupture the TM. Or a gradual rise in pressure can cause TM pressure or pain when the Eustachian tube is blocked.

Literally air pressure injury, barotrauma is sudden onset of ear pain from difference in air pressure. The most common cause in most emergency patients is a blow to the side of the head. This hand or foot increases air pressure in the ear canal. It can rupture the TM or cause it to swell and bleed.

Because victims of domestic abuse are reluctant to report it, the triage nurse should carefully inspect the ear and face for bruising or redness that suggests an open hand against the face. Only when confronted directly will someone admit to being assaulted.

17. What could be other causes for barotrauma?

Other settings of barotrauma are changes in air pressure from descent in an airplane or descent underwater while diving. The history is key here. The person will often relate a history of a recent cold, sinus problems, or nasal congestion before the activity. They may relate a history of previous problems "clearing" their ears with pressure change.

18. Describe the otoscope findings for barotrauma, and how are they different than otitis media?

Landmarks are lost in each. Barotrauma shows a ruptured TM with blood in the canal and no pus. Otitis media shows a white or bulging TM. Otitis media can rupture the TM too, but you will see white pus in the canal.

The Valsalva maneuver is not recommended as a diagnostic maneuver. It can forcibly insufflate the middle ear, cause intense pain, and introduce microorganisms into a previously sterile serous otitis that in turn creates infected otitis media.

19. Tell me more about the maneuver to look for TM movement.

Usually this maneuver is done with an otoscope with an attached pneumatic bulb. Some practitioners prefer to gently blow air through the tubing versus squeezing air into the canal. If a light reflex is present, focus on it. Introduce air and observe the TM for movement.

20. Is there anything someone can do to help "unplug" or "pop" their ear?

The first thing is to stop the patient from hurting themselves. Individuals may be noticing the normal and healthy opening and closing of the eustachian tube. If the individual does the nasal Valsalva, they may briefly raise the middle ear pressure and cause the TM to bulge outward. This reduces hearing and causes a plugged feeling. If the patient does the nasal Valsalva again, this perpetuates the full feeling.

If there is a plugged ear from otitis media or allergic rhinitis or otitis externa, the best treatment of plugging is treatment of the underlying cause.

If the ear hurts in the setting of pressure change, then you can help unplug the ear by recommending two gentle maneuvers and then if needed the nasal Valsalva. Place warm compresses over the ear or even a heated teacup. This may equilibrate pressure. If it doesn't, recommend holding the nose shut and swallowing—the internal pressure of this gentle nasal Valsalva forces open the Eustachian tube.

The patient can then be instructed to forcefully perform a nasal Valsalva by holding shut the nose and touching the chin to the chest. If this fails to clear one ear, then recommend that the patient flex the neck toward the opposite side and try the Valsalva again. Flexing the neck will straighten the Eustachian tube on the opposite side and help clear it.

21. What does a patient experience with a herpes zoster infection?

A herpes zoster infection is a vesicular eruption that has pain as its first sign, even days before vesicles appear. The patient is usually over age 40 or immunosuppressed from human immunodeficiency virus (HIV) or antirejection medication. Otologic examination may show small clusters of small clear vesicles in the canal early in the infection. After about a week the vesicles rupture and wound weeping and crusting begins. As with other viral infections the preauricular lymph nodes may be enlarged, but there is no fever. Treatment is usually with acyclovir and oral analgesics.

22. Tell me about wax impaction.

Wax occurs in all ear canals. Wax usually drains out. In some patients, especially the elderly, the wax accumulates in the canal. This alone does not cause pain. However, attempts to clear the wax with a cotton swab can result in pushing the wax against the TM and cause intense pain. Ordinarily the person with excessive wax will recall a history of fullness or itching fullness in the ears, ringing in the ears, or decreased hearing.

23. How is wax impaction dealt with?

Exam shows wax occluding the canal. Although nonimpacted wax can be curetted away by the clinician, impacted wax cannot be curetted without increasing pain and risking rupture of the TM.

Instead, treatment is to loosen the wax with Cerumenex, or mineral oil. Gently wash it away with warmed water. There is special equipment made for this purpose, but a 10-cc syringe and a plastic outer intravenous (IV) catheter (the bigger the cannula the better) works just as well. If irrigation does not reduce pain, the patient may need follow-up with ear, nose, and throat specialist (ENT) for manual wax disimpaction under an operating otoscope.

24. What else causes pain in the ear canal or on the ear?

A common furuncle or boil can be painful. The ear canal does not get more than its share, but the confined space of the canal can make a furuncle especially bothersome.

The ear appears to have a single spot of redness that is exquisitely painful to touch. There is no fever and usually no adenopathy. Treatment is a warm compress and analgesia. The furuncle will resolve in 2 to 3 days. Because this is a staphylococcal infection, it can be easily spread to other locations and other individuals. Advise good handwashing.

25. What causes ear pain that persists for hours after eating?

TMJ syndrome can cause this type of pain. The temporomandibular joint lies just under the skin of the ear canal. Painful arthritis can flare spontaneously or after an episode of usual stress on the joint. TMJ stress occurs from crunching or biting hard food like ice cubes or carrots. It can likely flare from psychological stress causing teeth clenching or grinding (bruxism). Acute TMJ pain can signal a blow to the mandible has occurred and therefore is a sign of potential assault. As in barotrauma and other signs of assault it is well known that victims underreport assault.

26. How can I detect TMJ by quick assessment?

TMJ syndrome hurts when the jaw opens or moves side to side. However, this movement tends to worsen many types of otitis media, otitis externa, and other ear pain. Therefore suspect TMJ when no other causes of pain are found but it hurts when the patient clenches teeth or opens and closes the jaw. Pressure over the TMJ may elicit pain. If trauma is suspected, TMJ films can be done but are usually negative. Treatment is with nonsteroidal anti-inflammatory drugs (NSAIDs) and avoiding eating until the physician can see them.

27. Why does a sore throat cause ear pain?

Inflammation of the pharynx can cause ear pain especially when it occludes the Eustachian tube. This occlusion can cause pressure to build up in the middle ear. The patient will often complain of pharyngitis.

28. What does the throat look like?

The entrance to the Eustachian tube lies above the soft palate and cannot be seen on throat examination, but posterior pharyngeal redness or exudate or swelling suggests it could extend superiorly to the Eustachian tube entrance as well. The usual triage of pharyngitis would apply here along with initial treatment with analgesics.

Key Points

- Ear pain is not life-threatening.
- Ear pain is commonly as a result of acute otitis media, but can be from trauma, infection, and ear foreign body.
- Initial history and examination, especially with the otoscope, can initially distinguish among these entities and suggest initial treatment with analgesics.

Internet Resources

How to Instill Ear Drops
http://nursing.about.com/cs/pharmacology/ht/eardrops.htm

Ear Barotrauma
http://www.shands.org/health/information/article/001064.htm

American Academy of Pediatrics Practice Guideline: Managing Otitis Media With Effusion in Young Children
http://www.aap.org/policy/otitis.htm

Objects or Insects in Ear
http://www.medicinenet.com/objects_or_insects_in_ear/article.htm

Clinical Practice Guidelines for Nurses in Primary Care (Canada): ENT
http://www.hc-sc.gc.ca/fnihb-dgspni/fnihb/ons/nursing/resources/clinical_guidelines/chapter_2.htm

Iowa Health: Wax Blockage
http://www.iowahealth.org/14046.cfm

Eye, Ear, Nose, Throat and Dental Emergency
http://www.nursingceu.com/NCEU/courses/eent-combo/

Bibliography

Koranyi KI: Otitis media and mastoiditis. In Harwood-Nuss A, Wolfson AG, Linden CH, Shepherd SM, Stenklyft PH, editors: *The clinical practice of emergency medicine,* ed 3, Philadelphia, 2001, Lippincott Williams & Wilkins, 1303-1305.

Rothman R, Owens T, Simel DL: Does this child have acute otitis media? *JAMA* 290(12):1633-1640, 2003.

Shah RK, Blevins NH: Otalgia, *Otolaryngol Clin North Am* 36(6):1137-1151, 2003.

Chapter 23

Stiff or Sore Neck

Robert D. Herr

1. How serious can a sore neck be?

Perhaps second only to chest pain, the stiff or sore neck can span a spectrum of maladies from simple muscle strain to the life threats of meningitis or traumatic cervical spinal cord injury.

2. What is most important for me to ask about first?

The first questions to ask are to separate trauma from nontrauma by history.

All motor vehicle crashes (MVC) are at risk for neck trauma. Please see Chapter 45 for further information. Other historical elements at high risk for head injury are diving accidents, skiing accidents, or any setting in which the patient's body and its weight decelerate from contact by the head or neck.

3. Compare that to whiplash.

Most commonly a patient with neck pain after MVC is simple whiplash, a ligament strain, or sprain treated like other sprains. However, some ligamental strain and most fractures are serious enough to create unstable conditions that threaten to harm the spinal cord. Every triage nurse has had or heard of a scenario about a patient walking in with a cervical spine fracture.

4. Talk about the anatomy and physiology related to the spinal cord.

The spinal cord is soft like cooked asparagus and surrounded on all sides by stacked bones. The bones are held in the stack by ligaments. These ligaments are most flexible behind the spinal cord in the area of the spinal lamina. Spinal lamina are flat bones like shingles whose ligaments allow the neck to flex forward, extend backward, and rotate left and right.

5. Are assaults considered trauma?

It has never been reported that fists alone can break a neck, but baseball bats, chairs, and other weapons certainly have. Unless you trust the history that the "fight" was fists only, with no wrestling or body slams, the conservative approach is to consider the potential for c-spine instability and potential spinal cord injury.

6. How do I triage the patient without neck trauma?

The history and vital signs can reveal the cause of neck pain. Onset during sleep suggests muscle spasm from an unusual neck position. Ask about unusual activity or exercise. Many activities such as lifting, gardening, shoveling, or pulling involve neck muscles that become sore. The patient may have to hold the neck in one position as a result of spasm. They may be unable to move the head or neck, called *torticollis.*

Because neck pain is a common symptom of meningitis, ask about fever and headache that accompany meningitis. Take the temperature and inspect skin for petechia that signify acute meningitis. Any elevated temperature above 101.5°F or petechia warrants immediate evaluation by the physician. Further evaluation is mentioned in answer to question 11. It is critical to triage evaluation to consider meningitis before ascribing sore neck to physical exertion or minor trauma. The reason is that patients with new symptoms will often think back to something they might have done to cause these symptoms when in fact they have serious illness unrelated to the activity.

Ask about new medication that can cause neck muscles to cramp, called dystonic torticollis or simply *dystonia.*

7. Talk about dystonic torticollis.

Dystonic torticollis commonly results from the extrapyramidal effects of antipsychotic meds such as haloperidol (Haldol) or antiemetic medication such as droperidol (Inapsine). Patients with this are commonly prescribed benztropine mesylate (Cogentin), diphenhydramine (Benadryl), or Artane to counter these extrapyramidal effects. However, these individuals have probably taken insufficient medication to counter the extrapyramidal effects. It is not unusual for the patient to also have vision problems, such as oculogyric crises.

8. Describe an oculogyric crisis.

It is a spasm of involuntary deviation and fixation of the eyeballs, usually upward, was part of the "dystonic" reaction. It may last for only several minutes or can last for hours.

9. What will be used for treatment of extrapyramidal effects?

The patient with extrapyramidal symptoms responds to Cogentin or Benadryl (50 mg intramuscularly [IM] or intravenously [IV]).

10. What is dystonia (spasmodic torticollis)?

Dystonia is spasm of the cervical musculature that causes the patient to bend the head to one side. The usual cause is psychological stress, but the differential includes unilateral facet dislocation or extrapyramidal syndrome.

11. How do I assess for meningitis?

Assess if the patient has meningismus by asking him or her to touch the chin to the chest. The possibility of meningitis is raised if the patient can't do this or has too much pain to do it. However, only 6% to 30% of patients with meningitis have this "classic" sign early. Assess for other signs or symptoms of meningitis, such as high fever (70% to 94%), headache, decreased level of consciousness (31% to 69%), photophobia, or a petechial or purpuric rash (nonblanching, subcutaneous hemorrhages, especially from *N. meningitidis*).

Note that although the "classic triad" of symptoms is fever, level of consciousness (LOC) changes, and nuchal rigidity, only one third of patients will have all three. Ask also about a history of any known exposure to others with meningitis.

12. What are the Brudzinski sign and the Kernig sign for assessing meningitis?

The Brudzinski sign is when the patient is laid recumbent and you try flexing the neck. It is a positive Brudzinski sign of meningeal irritation if the patient draws up one or both knees. Flexing the hip and then extending the lower leg at the knee test the Kerning's sign. A positive sign is complaining of neck pain and flexing the neck. (Think of the "stiff neck.")

13. Are Brudzinski sign and Kernig sign reliable indicators to use to indicate the patient has meningitis?

Recent studies show that less than 27% of patients with meningitis have these positive signs early in the course of the disease. Although they are "famous" maneuvers for physical diagnosis of meningitis, they have low sensitivity and are actually later signs of irritation. They are no longer considered useful in establishing an early diagnosis of meningitis prior to a lumbar puncture or imaging result. However, if either sign is noted to be positive, the physician should be alerted immediately.

14. What should I always consider with neck swelling?

Airway compromise.

15. When should I suspect airway compromise?

Any time there is neck swelling with pain that is worsening quickly (minutes to hours), trouble with swallowing (drooling), or speech. Stridor is a classic late indication.

16. List some other causes for neck pain or stiffness.

Possible causes include a deep neck space abscess, vascular infection, muscular stress related to overexertion or tension, or a herniated cervical disc.

17. Discuss symptoms that suggest a deep neck space abscess.

Symptoms include neck swelling with pain, suspected airway compromise, or high fever with meningismus. One 57-year-old had a 3-day history of worsening neck swelling, localized erythema, and limited range of motion described as a "stiff neck." His condition was not responding to antibiotics. It turned out his undiagnosed diabetes had contributed to the original "infected hair follicle" becoming a deep neck space abscess.

Studies show plain radiographs of the neck are only 83% sensitive compared to 100% sensitivity for computed tomography (CT) with IV contrast. Other diagnostic tests to consider include white blood cell count (WBC), thyroid studies (T_4) if there is thyroid pain, and serum amylase for suspected mumps.

18. When do I suspect a vascular cause for neck pain?

Any patient with history of IV drug abuse should be ruled out for vascular infection, especially those who use neck veins for IV injection ("pocket shooters").

19. Talk about muscular causes for neck pain.

Muscle pain and stiffness commonly occurs after athletic exertion or in response to stress. The term "pain in the neck" refers to stress-inducing individuals or events that cause us to subconsciously overtax our neck muscles. This can create a painful cycle of muscle tightness that leads to painful spasms that lead to continued muscle tightness.

20. Can this ever be serious?

Neck sprain reduces the range of motion. An individual can "throw out their neck" by dislocating a cervical facet. This can be diagnosed by neck radiograph or by careful neck examination. Generally the patient relocates the cervical facet dislocation in the time between throwing out the neck until he or she seeks medical attention.

21. How is this treated?

The patient benefits taking from anti-inflammatory medication, applying moist heat, and a referral to physical therapy.

22. Describe when I should suspect a herniated cervical disc.

The hallmark is radicular pain. This is sharp lancinating or aching pain in a single dermatome that sometimes shoots down the arm. The C5 nerve root impingement hurts on the forearm, C6 hurts in the radial aspect of the hand, C7 the middle fingers, and the C8 nerve root the ulnar aspect of the hand and forearm. Other symptoms of disc herniation are pain with coughing, sneezing, or going over bumps in the car.

For example, one woman returned to the emergency department (ED) one day after a front-end MVC. She'd been given a tetanus shot in the deltoid muscle, and returned for increased deltoid pain from a "tetanus reaction." On examination the shoulder was nontender to palpation. However, the pain increased when she turned her head to the opposite side, or when I pressed down on her head. She had a C4-5 disc herniation that pinched her C4 nerve root. This innervates the skin over the shoulder and upper arm.

Key Points

- Always first distinguish the traumatic from the nontraumatic "stiff neck" pain.
- Rollover MVCs are the highest risk for neck trauma. A windshield broken by an unrestrained motorist head will cause the most serious spine injury.
- Although common public knowledge as a symptom, only one-third of patients with meningitis have a "stiff neck." Assess also for a high fever, headache, decreased LOC, and petechial rash.
- Brudzinski and Kerning signs are no longer considered reliable early indicators of meningitis.

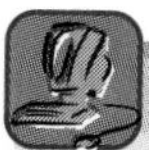

Internet Resources

Fatal Case of Serogroup B Meningococcal Disease
http://www.ena.org/news/CDC-Advisories/SerogroupB.asp

Lumbar Punctures: Principles and Practice
http://www.ena.org/conferences/annual/2004/handouts/capl330-c.pdf

Algorithm for Early Management of Meningococcal Disease in Children
http://www.meningitis.org/index.jsp?page=/content.jsp?sectno=6&subno=3

Early Management of Suspected Bacterial Meningitis and Meningococcal Septicaemiae in Adults
http://www.meningitis.org/index.jsp?page=/content.jsp?sectno=6&subno=3

Early Recognition of Meningitis and Septicaemiae; Vital signs for front-line nurses.
http://www.meningitis.org/index.jsp?page=/content.jsp?sectno=6&subno=3

Bibliography

Broder JS, Hobgood CD: Emergency management of neck masses, Lesson 18, *Crit Decisions Emerg Med* 17(9):11-16, 2003.

Davis MA, Votey SR, Greenough PG: *Signs and symptoms in emergency medicine: Literature-based approach to emergency conditions,* St Louis, 1999, Mosby.

Molitor L: Triage decisions: A 57-year-old man with neck pain and swelling, *J Emerg Nurs* 27(1): 97-98, 2001.

Pennardt AM, Zehner WJ: Paramedic documentation of indicators for cervical spine injury, *Prehospital Disaster Med* 9:40-43, 1994.

Thomas KE, et al: The diagnostic accuracy of Kerning's sign, Brudzinski sign and nuchal rigidity in adults with suspected meningitis, *Clin Infect Dis* 35:46-52, 2002.

Chapter 24

Sore Throat

Robert D. Herr

1. How serious can a sore throat be?

The sore throat that's referred pain from angina can be dangerous, even fatal. The sore throat that's untreated streptococcus can result in rheumatic fever with damage to heart valves. A good triage nurse brings in the angina for immediate treatment, helps diagnose the strep throat, and gets the other 80% of patients seen when it's their turn—all in a day's work. Because most sore throat is from a viral pharyngitis or tonsillitis, a focus of this chapter is on symptomatic treatment of pain and dehydration.

2. How do I identify angina?

Angina is typically a constant pressure or aching pain in the left side of the throat that usually also involves the left chest or left arm. A review of neuroanatomy helps to explain why this happens. The sensation is actually referred pain from myocardia ischemia. Ischemia fires pain receptors in the autonomic sympathetic nervous system of the heart. These stimuli travel to the upper thoracic and cervical sympathetic nerve ganglion, in which they synapse to nerves that enter the spinal cord at these levels. Lying next to these autonomic nerves are somatic sensing nerves from the skin of the neck, left arm, and chest. The body mistakes the pain of cardiac ischemia for pain in these body areas in the process of referred pain.

The angina patient may have had previous angina or active cardiac disease. Their medication list may have nitroglycerin, isosorbide (Isordil), or topical nitrates. The patient without angina or active heart disease is the hardest to diagnose. Few clinical factors reliably identify new angina. The patient who is young or who has obvious pharyngeal exudate, erythema, or new adenopathy does not have angina. Likewise, the patient with significant odynophagia (pain on swallowing) likely has acute pharyngitis, not angina. For those without clear clinical evidence of pharyngitis consider cardiac risk factors such as age, male sex, smoking, hypertension, cholesterol level, family history, and sedentary lifestyle. If you have the slightest suspicion, there is no harm in obtaining an electrocardiogram (ECG) and showing it to the clinician. At least half the time angina correlates with ECG changes.

3. How does strep throat look?

It's hard to clinically distinguish streptococcal infection from a viral pharyngitis. One clue is that bacterial pharyngitis causes fever, throat exudates or erythema, tender cervical lymph nodes, and no cough. In contrast, viral pharyngitis occurs together with a viral illness such as nasal congestion, bronchitis (coughing), myalgias, and/or hoarseness. Every generalization has one major exception. Infectious mononucleosis is the Epstein Barr virus but causes fever, exudative pharyngitis, tender adenopathy, and enlarged liver and spleen. Because clinical distinction is difficult, the strep culture can identify strep usually 2 days later. The strep screen provides information within an hour but doesn't always agree with culture done on the same specimen. Usually the decision about use of strep culture and rapid strep tests at triage depends on emergency room (ER) policy or the suggestion of the clinician you are working with.

4. What if the patient is already taking an antibiotic?

The only patient not testable for strep diagnosis is the patient who's already begun an antibiotic. The antibiotic makes the rapid strep test and strep culture unreliable. The standard of care is to continue such patients on the full 10-day course of an antibiotic.

5. Why does strep throat need treatment?

Antibiotic treatment of streptococcal pharyngitis has been reported to reduce the pain and other symptoms of sore throat by about a day. Antibiotic treatment reduces contagious spread of strep throat after about 24 hours of therapy. About 1% or less of those with untreated Group A strep infection will develop rheumatic fever, and perhaps 2% of those with rheumatic fever will develop rheumatic heart disease. Treatment with a 10-day course of antibiotics can eradicate the infection and prevent rheumatic fever. Children under age 4 have not gotten rheumatic fever, so the benefit of treatment is less clear to them.

6. How contagious is strep and do children need a school or day care excuse?

Sometimes the whole family has strep, including the family dog that's been reported as a carrier of strep that recurs after treatment. School excuse is wise unless the next day is a holiday, even if they are feeling well enough to attend school. After 24 hours of antibiotics, strep throat is not contagious.

7. How do I advise other family members or partners of someone proved to have strep pharyngitis?

Antibiotic therapy can treat strep pharyngitis but cannot reliably prevent it among close contacts. I suggest you advise the strep patient's contacts that if they develop a sore throat that they seek treatment for strep. If those contacts are in front of you and have symptoms then treatment is a good idea.

8. Talk about diphtheria.

Diphtheria is a bacterium that causes bad pharyngitis in those without adequate immunity to it. Recent immigrants may lack primary series of vaccines (it's the D in the DPTH vaccine). Despite guidelines for getting a diphtheria vaccine each decade, many older individuals do not get one. They experience a slow decline in antibodies to diphtheria, and nursing homes are ideal places for outbreak of contagious illness including reports of diphtheria outbreaks. Diphtheria presents as a low-grade fever with flulike malaise and anorexia. The throat shows a gray or white membrane that adheres to the tonsils.

9. Talk about gonococcal pharyngitis.

This can appear as red throat with or without exudate. Because it follows oral sex by 2 to 5 days, a recent sexual history is important. The patient may also have symptoms of gonococcal urethritis, proctitis, or cervicitis.

Throat cultures need to be done on Thayer-Martin plates to detect gonorrhea and treatment requires ceftriaxone.

10. What is thrush?

Thrush is oral candida infection. Candida is a yeast that is present in the environment. It causes infection in infants and in those taking antibiotics or who are immunosuppressed. Candida can extend to the esophagus and cause severe odynophagia. The oral mucosa is red and there are patches of white plaque that appear to be adherent to the red mucosa. These patients are still treated with analgesia and hydration but the medication that helps is nystatin swishes or a fluconazole tablet.

11. What do vesicles mean on the throat or cheek?

Vesicles are a sign of viral infection that together cause more than half of all sore throats. Many of these viruses are untreatable like adenovirus, Coxsackie virus, and others. Herpangina is the name for grayish-white vesicles on the palate of children ages 1 to 7 years who have abrupt fever to 102°F and who may be anorexic with dysphagia and sore throat. These ulcerate and 3 to 4 days later disappear.

Primary herpes virus is treatable with acyclovir. Typically, vesicles appear on the tongue, palate, gingiva, and buccal mucosa. Herpes is very painful with 1- to 3-mm vesicles together with fever and adenopathy. After a day or two, these vesicles leave red-based painful ulcers. It is hard to distinguish these from other viral ulcers (so called aphthous ulcers) at triage.

12. How do I triage the patient with a sore throat?

Each patient needs assessment starting with the ABCs. This includes looking in the mouth to see if there are threats to the airway. One threat may be foreign body including misplaced dentures. Infectious causes include retropharyngeal abscess, peritonsillar abscess, pharyngeal edema from allergic reaction, and diphtheria pseudomembrane. Both types of abscesses can be seen as a protrusion of soft palate forward in a patient with fever. Deep neck space abscess is discussed in Chapter 23. A peritonsillar abscess is a one-sided red and bulging area that pushes the uvula away from midline. Retropharyngeal abscess occurs mostly in children and is symmetric bulging. A lateral neck radiograph shows a widened retropharyngeal space and helps make the diagnosis. Pharyngeal edema is usually painless but stretching tissue can become sore. The most common cause is angioedema from angiotensin-converting enzyme (ACE) inhibitors like Captopril, Enalapril, and Prinivil. However, allergic reaction to anything can cause this.

Immediate airway control including endotracheal intubation may be needed. The airway edema patient may also benefit from an order for antihistamine and injectable corticosteroid. The patient with abscess is also in danger of airway compromise. He should have intravenous (IV), oxygen, monitor and a cardiorespiratory arrest "crash" cart with intubation equipment standing by. The dyspneic patient is considered in the chapter on that complaint.

If the patient has angina symptoms, he needs immediate triage with IV, oxygen, and heart monitoring. They may also require cardioactive medication such as nitroglycerin. The vast majority who do not have angina nevertheless may have a component of dehydration from lack of oral intake. Postural vital signs detect only a fraction of those who are volume depleted, so have a low threshold for recognizing dehydration based on what they are telling you.

If the patient hasn't been able to drink for more than a half-day then they are likely dehydrated. The sooner you help them re-hydrate the faster they can safely leave the emergency department (ED). You have the option of going right to IV isotonic crystalloid such as normal saline boluses, or you can give them a short trial of throat analgesia and oral hydration.

Throat analgesia or oral hydration can change temperature readings and throat swabbing so there is no harm is getting both done quickly and prior to doing the following. The throat swab should be across the posterior pharynx and touch any exudate if possible. Most times this hurts a little. Do what you can to get the patient to open the mouth so you can see the pharynx, depressing the tongue if you need to with a tongue blade. There are various tricks of the trade to get the mouth open wide enough to swab the throat but I can recall patients in whom it's been next to impossible until they got every analgesic and gargle we could offer.

13. What can I give to reduce soreness?

Throat analgesia should have the goal of taking the edge off the pain so that they can drink enough to rehydrate and maintain oral fluid intake. Some EDs offer standing orders for oral analgesia such as viscous lidocaine swish and spit, Cetacaine spray, or a tablet of opioid analgesic such as hydrocodone. The overall best analgesia is warm saltwater gargle because it gets right to the painful area. This works only for those savvy enough to gargle, mostly teens and older. You can add a few teaspoons of salt to a warm cup of tap water, or take normal saline and warm it in a microwave oven. You then ask the patient to gargle and spit. Once they do it with warm water you can advise that they do it with water as hot as their throat can tolerate. This is hotter than their skin can tolerate (if you don't believe me put your finger in your hot coffee or tea next time!). Because they can get scalded (doesn't that finger in your coffee hurt?) it is better that you let them choose what is the hottest they can tolerate. Yes some will say "that didn't do anything to help" so clarify that the goal is to take the edge off the pain to let them take a pill or drink some water.

14. What if the patient is still unable to drink anything?

If they fail the oral hydration trial by just taking sips, I suggest that you move quickly to IV saline hydration. Not only does it make their throat feel better, but hydration will also reduce fever and get them home sooner.

Triage blood work could include a tube for white blood cell (WBC) count and a red top tube for sending a monospot to check for infectious mononucleosis. Blood cultures are indicated only if the patient is having rigors in front of you or the patient is prostrate and septic-appearing. These patients are at risk for a deep neck space infection that can be polymicrobial and culture results can help direct therapy in a day or two.

For fever get an order for an oral antipyretic like acetaminophen or ibuprofen, or for fever and pain get an order for an oral opioid that contains acetaminophen like Vicodin or Percocet.

15. Why are tonsils left in that would have been removed a few decades ago?

Tonsillectomy has risk of bleeding and infection. Those with tonsillectomy still get pharyngitis. Studies show it benefits a smaller number of people than once thought, so it is no longer routinely done. Tonsillectomy is clinically appropriate in those who have three or more severe tonsillitis infections each year for 2 or more years in a row. However, the individual whose infection is persistent and who is missing school or work is also a good candidate for tonsillectomy. The initial approach to the ED patient will be the same with attention to timely assessment and preliminary treatment.

16. What is scarlet fever?

Scarlet fever is widespread skin erythema from Group A streptococcus that releases a substance that reddens skin and causes a sandpaper-feeling rash. As the name implies the individual has a fever. The source in a patient with sore throat is likely a strep pharyngitis. This patient does not require diagnostic tests at triage unless the treating clinician wants confirmation of the visual diagnosis. Treatment is with the same antistreptococcal antibiotics and treatment for pain and fever.

Key Points

- Most sore throats are viral, self-limited, and low acuity.
- Angina can manifest as pressure or aching referred to the neck.
- Strep throat is difficult to distinguish from a virus but triage with rapid strep testing and WBC can help.
- Untreated strep in those age 4 and older can result in rheumatic fever.
- The patient who has already taken an antibiotic against strep has unreliable strep testing so most clinicians would continue the antibiotic for a full 10 days.
- At triage, assess ABCs. Recognize dehydration and begin IV saline if a trial of oral hydration fails.
- Warm saline gargles and/or topical analgesics can reduce pain.

Internet Resources

MedLine Plus Medical Enyclopedia: Sore Throat
http://www.nlm.nih.gov/medlineplus/ency/article/003053.htm

MayoClinic.com: Strep Throat
http://www.mayoclinic.com/invoke.cfm?id=DS00260

Virtual Children's Hospital: Strep Throat/Strep Tonsillitis
http://www.vh.org/pediatric/patient/pediatrics/cqqa/strep.html

Bibliography

Levin W, Wilson GR: Acute infections of the adult pharynx and laryngitis. In Harwood-Nuss A, Wolfson AF, Linden CH, Shepherd SM, Stenklyft PH, editors: *The clinical practice of emergency medicine,* ed 3, Philadelphia, 2001, Lippincott Williams & Wilkins, 94-98.

Todd JK: The sore throat: Pharyngitis and epiglottis, *Infect Dis Clin N Am* 2:1, 1988.

Witt RL: The tonsil and adenoid controversy, *Del Med J* 61(6):289-294, 1989.

Chapter 25

Vision Changes

Rebecca A. Steinmann

1. What types of visual changes am I likely to encounter at triage?

Common visual complaints include blurred vision, double vision (diplopia), decreased visual acuity, decreased visual fields, cloudy or smoky vision, and blindness. The secret to effectively triaging visual changes is to recognize those patients whose signs and symptoms suggest the potential for permanent vision loss (blindness) unless immediate assessment and intervention is expeditiously initiated.

2. What causes visual changes?

Visual changes are usually the result of ocular injury or medical conditions involving the eye. Neurologic conditions such as stroke (sudden trouble seeing in one or both eyes or double vision is one of the warning signs of stroke), head trauma, and increased intracranial pressure (ICP) can also produce visual changes. In general, acute visual changes that affect both eyes suggest a neurologic rather than an ocular dysfunction. Cardiovascular, hematologic, and immunologic disorders are less common precipitators of visual changes.

3. What are the risk factors associated with acute vision loss?

- Age. Although injuries can and do occur in all age groups, the most common disease processes that pose a threat to vision increase with age (glaucoma, central retinal artery occlusion).
- Diabetes
- Cardiovascular disease

4. So what questions will help me identify those patients at risk for permanent vision loss?

First, clarify the visual change: does it affect one or both eyes? Is the visual loss partial or complete? Your focused triage history should include:

- Precipitating events leading to the visual change
- Duration of symptoms (acute, progressive, or chronic)
- Presence of eye pain (PQRST format)
- Presence of systemic symptoms (nausea/vomiting)

- Current and significant past medical history: previous eye surgery/diseases, diabetes, cardiovascular disease
- Tetanus immunization status (eye injuries)
- Current use of corrective lenses (glasses, contact lenses)

5. Is there anything special I should assess when patients complain of visual changes?

Yes, your assessment should include:

- Visual acuity
- Pupillary response
- Appearance of the eye and surrounding structures
- Extraocular movements

6. Does every patient complaining of visual changes really need to have a visual acuity assessment at triage?

With the exception of patients presenting with chemical burns to the eyes (who need to be expedited to the treatment area for immediate eye irrigation), every patient complaining of visual changes should have a visual acuity assessment performed at triage. It is essential to determine the patient's baseline vision on arrival to the emergency department before treatment is initiated to allow meaningful reassessment after treatment is completed and for medico-legal reasons.

7. What's the best way to assess visual acuity?

By having the patient read an eye chart. Various charts are available (Snellen's, E chart, picture chart). Because you're interested in any changes the patient has in their normal vision, assess visual acuity with their corrective lenses on.

- Have the patient stand 20 feet away from the chart.
- Instruct the patient to cover the unaffected eye.
- Have the patient read the letters starting at the top of the chart.
- Record the last line of which the patient can correctly identify at least 50% of the letters, indicating the number of letters missed (right eye 20/40, −2).
- Repeat this by covering the affected eye.
- Repeat one last time by having the patient use both eyes to read the chart.

8. How do I document my findings?

The results of the visual acuity examination are reported as a fraction. The numerator is the distance the patient is standing from the chart (20 feet). The denominator, listed on each line of the eye chart, represents the distance at which the average eye can read that particular line. For example:

With corrective lenses: right eye 20/40, −2
left eye 20/20, −0
both eyes 20/20, −0

9. So what injuries represent a threat to vision?

Accidental eye injury is one of the leading causes of visual impairment with 1,000,000 eye injuries each year in the United States. Injuries associated with vision changes include:

- Chemical burns
- Globe rupture
- Hyphema
- Orbital fractures (with extraocular muscle entrapment)

Eye Injuries Associated With Vision Loss

	Characteristics of Visual Change	Appearance of Eye	Systemic Symptoms
Chemical Burns	Varying degrees of unilateral or bilateral vision loss Photophobia	Opaque-looking cornea Irritation to skin surrounding eye	No
Ruptured globe	Altered light perception Decreased visual acuity	Pupil assumes teardrop shape Extrusion of jelly-like substance from cornea Hyphema may be present	Nausea
Hyphema	Blurred or decreased vision Blood-tinged vision Photophobia	Blood layer at bottom of iris	No
Orbital Fracture	Diplopia Limited upward gaze	Periorbital bruising and edema Crepitus over orbital rim	No

10. How should I manage a patient with chemical burns to the eyes at triage?

If you suspect the patient has chemical burns, your priority should be getting him/her to an area in which the eyes can be immediately irrigated (that usually means back to a treatment room, not triage). Don't waste your time (or the patient's future vision) attempting to obtain a visual acuity or obtaining a detailed history.

Test the conjunctival pH with litmus paper to report the degree of chemical pH change and potential injury if it can be done quickly. Irrigation should be copious and until the pH testing is neutral.

11. What symptoms would suggest a chemical burn in the eye?

Signs/symptoms which suggest chemical burns include:

- History of chemical exposure to the eye
- Visual disturbances

- Photophobia
- Pain
- Tearing
- Irritation to skin surrounding the eye
- Opaque-looking cornea

12. What if I am not sure what the substance is?

It is recommended that any substance that causes burning, stinging, or pain in the eye be considered a "chemical injury" until proven otherwise.

13. What are the signs of a ruptured globe?

A ruptured globe may result from either blunt or penetrating trauma. In the event of penetrating trauma, the patient may arrive with an object still impaled (the object should be secured and stabilized, not removed). Assessment clues that suggest a ruptured globe include:

- Patient complains of altered light perception and decreased visual acuity
- The pupil assumes a teardrop-shape
- A jelly-like substance may be noted extruding from the eye (aqueous or vitreous humor)
- Severe eye pain with nausea

14. What is a hyphema?

A hyphema is a collection of blood (hemorrhage) into the anterior chamber of the eye. The patient is likely to present with a history of blunt trauma to the eye (a fist or tennis ball to the eye). Signs/symptoms include:

- Blurred or decreased vision
- Some patients report "seeing red" or blood-tinged vision (from viewing the world through the layer of blood in the anterior chamber
- Photophobia
- Blood in the anterior chamber
- Deep, aching eye pain

15. Can I detect a hyphema at triage?

Sometimes. A layer of fluid/blood may be visualized at the bottom of the iris when the patient is upright (blood settles at the bottom of the iris as a result of gravity). In patients with light-colored eyes this is usually easily detected. In patients with dark eyes, this layer is extremely difficult to see.

16. What assessment findings suggest an orbital fracture with entrapment of extraocular muscles?

- History of blunt trauma
- Decreased ability to look upward (as a result of entrapment of extraocular muscles in the fracture site)

- Diplopia
- Periorbital bruising and edema
- Sunken eye (enophthalmos)
- Crepitus over the orbital rim
- Numbness/tingling of cheek

17. What urgent medical conditions are associated with permanent loss of vision?

- Central retinal artery occlusion
- Detached retina
- Glaucoma
- Stroke

Medical Conditions Commonly Associated with Vision Loss

Condition	Characteristics of Visual Change	Eye Pain	Appearance of Eye	Systemic Symptoms
Central Retinal Artery Occlusion	Sudden complete loss of vision in one eye	No	Dilated pupil in affected eye	No
Retinal Detachment	Unilateral flashing lights/floaters, cloudy/smoky vision	No, unless caused by eye trauma	Normal	No
Glaucoma	Loss of peripheral vision in affected eye Halos around lights	Severe, sudden, deep ocular pain	Eye appears reddened Cornea is cloudy/hazy Pupil mid-position: fixed to poorly reactive	Intense headache Nausea/ vomiting
Stroke	Total or partial loss of vision in one or both eyes Hemianopsia (visual field defects) Double vision	No	Usually normal May note gaze preference	Weakness/ paresthesia of extremities Speech difficulties

18. What are the signs/symptoms suggestive of central retinal artery occlusion?

- Sudden, complete, painless loss of vision in one eye
- Vision limited to light perception
- Patient description of a shade coming down over the eye
- Dilated pupil in affected eye

19. What causes central retinal artery occlusion?

Central retinal artery occlusion is caused by an embolus (carotid or cardiac), thrombus, or angiospasm. Patients at risk include those with a history of arteriosclerotic disease, atrial fibrillation, diabetes, arteritis, sickle cell disease, and hypertension.

20. How long can the retinal artery be occluded before permanent visual damage occurs?

The retina is deprived of blood as long as the artery is occluded. Visual receptors in the retina will degenerate within 30 to 60 minutes if blood flow is not restored. Retinal circulation must be reestablished within 60 to 90 minutes to prevent permanent loss of vision. Try an initial treatment of breathing into a paper bag to raise the cardiac output (CO) to dilate the carotid artery and to gain some time.

21. What causes a retinal detachment?

Retinal detachment occurs when the sensory layer of the retina is separated from the epithelial layer thus losing its blood supply. In older patients, degenerative changes in either the retina or vitreous body are the most common cause. Direct head trauma and injuries associated with sports activities (racquetball to the eye) account for 15% of all cases.

22. What are the assessment clues of retinal detachment?

- Painless decrease in vision (unless trauma-related)
- Patient complaints of flashing lights, increase in floaters, "swarm of gnats"
- Cloudy/smoky vision
- "Curtain" or "veil" over the visual field
- History of severe myopia (near-sightedness)

23. What causes glaucoma?

The distance between the iris and the cornea through which aqueous humor normally circulates becomes narrowed or blocked resulting in increased intraocular pressure. Blindness occurs when the increased pressure causes damage to the optic nerve resulting in decreased circulation to the retina (glaucoma is the leading cause of blindness in adults).

24. What assessment findings are clues of glaucoma?

- Diminished peripheral vision
- Halos around lights/"tunnel vision"
- Severe, sudden, deep eye pain
- Eye (conjunctiva) appears reddened
- Pupil: mid-position, fixed to poorly reactive
- Globe feels hard
- Cloudy, hazy appearing cornea
- Intense headache

- Nausea and vomiting
- Many will give a history of it starting in the semidarkness (movie theater) and have been on anticholinergic drugs.

25. How do I categorize patients with visual changes?

Your decision regarding the urgency of treatment may well impact the final visual outcome. Regardless of the triage acuity system used in your department, patients with an actual or potential threat to vision (chemical burns to the eyes, ruptured globe, central retinal artery occlusion, retinal detachment, acute glaucoma) require immediate interventions to preserve their sight. In a three-category acuity system, these patients should be categorized as emergent. In a five-category acuity systems such as the Emergency Severity Index (ESI) and the Canadian Triage Acuity System (CTAS), these patients should be categorized as twos.

Key Points

- Patients with visual changes should have visual acuity assessed unless a chemical burn is suspected.
- Patients with acute actual or potential threat to vision should have immediate interventions to preserve their sight.
- Patient's corrective lenses should be in place when visual acuity is assessed.

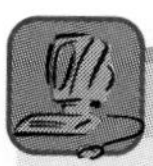

Internet Resources

Emedicinehealth.com: Corneal Flash Burns
http://www.emedicinehealth.com/articles/14433-1.asp

Ocular Injuries from Household Chemicals: Early Signs as Predictors of Recovery
http://www.liebertonline.com/doi/pdf/10.1089/10979330131688250 4

SchoolNurse.com: Eye Injuries: Triage and Prevention
http://www.schoolnurse.com/med_info/Eye_injuries.html

Eye Emergencies
http://www.ena.org/conferences/annual/2004/handouts/capl332-c.pdf

Iroquois Memorial Hospital Emergency Department Patient Care Standard for Eye Injuries
http://www.ena.org/document_share/documents/eye_injuries.doc

The Eyes Have It
http://www.ena.org/conferences/annual/2004/handouts/capl331-c.pdf

Refining Your Skills in Use of the Direct and Panoptic Ophthalmoscopes
http://www.ena.org/conferences/annual/2004/handouts/capl311-c.pdf

Bibliography

Brunette DD: Ophthalmogy. In Marx, JA, editor: *Rosen's emergency medicine: Concepts and clinical practice,* ed 5, St Louis, 2002, Mosby, 908-927.

Dennis WR, Dennis AM: Eye emergencies. In Stone CK, Humphries R, editors: *Current emergency diagnosis and treatment,* ed 5, New York, 2003, Lance Medical Books/McGraw-Hill, 599-625.

Egging D: Ocular emergencies. In Newberry L, editor: *Sheehy's emergency nursing,* ed 5, St Louis, 2003, Mosby, 691-706.

Epifanio PC: Ocular emergencies. In Jordan KS, editor: *Emergency nursing core curriculum,* ed 5, Philadelphia, 2000, WB Saunders, 467-486.

Farina GA, Feliciano A: Sudden visual loss, available: http//:www.emedicine.com/oph/topic271.htm, accessed November 2003.

Gilboy N, Tanabe P, Travers DA, Eitel DR, Wuerz RC: *The emergency severity index implementation handbook,* Des Plaines, Ill, Emergency Nurses Association, 2004.

Grossman VGA: *Eye injuries: Quick reference to triage,* Philadelphia, 1999, Lippincott, 50-51.

Smallwood M: Assessing visual acuity. In Proehl JA, editor: *Emergency nursing procedures,* ed 2, Philadelphia, 1999, WB Saunders, 498-501.

Chapter 26

Shortness of Breath

Maureen Smith

Many people seeking health care do so for the inability to breathe. As the second of the essential opening gambit of patient assessment (i.e., Airway, Breathing, Circulation [ABCs]), it certainly ranks up there in terms of significance. But everyone complaining of an inability to breathe does not necessarily need immediate attention; therefore, the ability to ascertain sick from not sick is essential for proper triage.

1. What are the symptoms of shortness of breath?

Most patients complain of dyspnea, or lack of ability to get enough air, dry cough, and chest tightness. The inability to breathe is very discomforting and stressful, causing many to be anxious and agitated.

2. Name some of the signs of respiratory status.

Two of the five vital signs deal directly with breathing. The respiratory rate and oxygen saturation each give a sense of how well the patient is breathing, although neither indicates how well they are ventilating. Additionally, the heart rate can indicate the level of respiratory distress. Remember, vital signs are important and any abnormality needs to be considered in the context of that patient regarding whether it requires immediate action and/or further assessment, or can wait.

On physical examination, people may have obvious increased work of breathing. Lung sounds often provide a clue to underlying pathology, although may prove misleading. A very smart professor of emergency medicine once told me that lungs are to be seen and not heard. This arose from the myriad of times that lungs sounded awful, but had a normal radiograph; and the clear sounding pulmonary examination being followed by a terribly abnormal chest radiograph.

3. What is the normal breathing pattern?

Most normal breaths involve equal inspiration and expiration at 14 to 20 breaths per minute for adults, with infants breathing up to 44 times a minute.

4. What are some abnormal breathing rates/rhythms?

Tachypnea, hyperventilation, bradypnea, Cheyne-Stokes, ataxic, and obstructive breathing patterns are all indicative of underlying problems.

Tachypnea, or rapid shallow breathing, can be seen in restrictive disease, pleuritic chest pain, or elevated diaphragm. On the other hand, rapid deep breathing of hyperventilation is brought on by anxiety, metabolic acidosis, infarction, and exercise.

Cheyne-Stokes breathing is cyclic, with periods of intermittent apnea between somewhat fast, deep breathing. Causes of this type of pattern include heart failure, acidosis, drug-induced, and strokes.

5. What are the abnormal lung sounds?

Rales, rhonchi, and wheezing are often thought of as hallmarks, but don't forget absent lung sounds and decreased. Stridor and other upper airway noises are often heard during the lung examination, but are radiating from the throat, and can be best heard by auscultating over the neck.

6. What are rales and rhonchi?

Rales are discontinuous noises, or crackles—brief, intermittent, and nonmusical created by fluid in the lung or lung tissue that is collapsed down and popping open (e.g., atelectasis). Rubbing the hair near your ear between your fingers can simulate fine crackles. Normal, healthy individuals can have some rales in the bases on end inspiration, especially following a prolonged period lying down.

Rhonchi are continuous noises made by air movement in the lung being obstructed in some way. Wheezing is a musical quality of higher pitched notes, although rhonchi are lower pitched. Much ado is often made about the distinction between wheezing and rhonchi, but it has no usefulness in diagnosis and they are often used interchangeably.

7. What are some common causes of shortness of breath?

In a world of what seems to be ever increasing cigarette smoking and environmental pollution, chronic obstructive pulmonary disease (COPD) and asthma and myocardial infarctions (MIs) cause shortness of breath and are not decreasing in prevalence. Other causes include pulmonary embolism, pneumonia, bronchitis, pulmonary edema, pneumothorax, allergic reactions, and even anxiety.

8. What signs on quick evaluation/physical examination are worrisome in the dyspneic patient?

Nasal flaring, retractions, accessory muscle use, sweating, posture—such as tripoding, and the "deer in the headlights" look of fear.

9. Does your stethoscope make a difference?

I think that better made stethoscopes allow people to hear more detail on examination. If you are attempting to determine if a person has normal breath sounds versus barely enough air exchange to wheeze or no sounds as in pneumothorax, better equipment can help you make that distinction.

10. What clues are provided by temperature?

Temperature does not in itself determine if the patient with breathing problems needs to be triaged into the emergency department (ED) immediately—unless it is extremely high (e.g., ≥106°F) or low (e.g., ≤94°F), but it does give clues to the diagnosis. An elevation in temperature is often found in cases of pneumonia or bronchitis, but can be high in the common cold. The definition of "fever" in adults varies among health professionals, but above 101°F will work. For neonates, fever includes anything 100.4°F or higher. Keep in mind that teething can cause an elevation in temperature into the 100s, but not over 101°F. Additionally, adults can have temperatures in the low 100s in noninfectious states such as pulmonary embolus and atelectasis.

11. What do heart rate and blood pressure tell us about breathing status?

Tachycardia has many etiologies, but when combined with dyspnea, it changes the differential diagnosis and may require attention sooner than someone with a normal pulse. Resting heart rate is below 100 bpm so remember to ask people what they were doing prior to triage, as they often smoke a last one before entering the ED, which can raise their resting heart rate. Because most people do not like coming to see the doctor and are nervous, they will also have an increased pulse, so use the heart rate along with the history and physical.

Bradycardia by itself is not always abnormal. When the patient complains of dyspnea, chest pain, dizziness, or lightheadedness as well, they probably require further evaluation sooner than later.

Blood pressure, although not a direct measure of lung function, can provide clues to how sick someone is currently. However, keep in mind that hypertension is often a long-standing problem that does not always reflect a recent event.

12. How does respiratory rate help triage patients?

I realize everyone has a rate of 20 (high end of normal, by the way). Tachypnea reflects some underlying abnormality, but not necessarily pulmonary. Someone in metabolic acidosis will breathe faster as will septic patients. If the chief complaint seems to be with breathing, then a respiratory rate in the high 20s or more requires further evaluation.

When someone is not breathing fast enough, it is usually obvious as they have an altered level of consciousness.

13. What is the fifth vital sign?

Although pain is generally considered the fifth vital sign, oxygen saturation is also sometimes called the fifth vital sign. It needs to be checked on almost everyone presenting to be triaged, but especially those with any respiratory complaint—even a cold. Often it is the only abnormal vital sign in someone with the sometimes difficult to diagnose conditions such as pulmonary embolus. Keep in mind that patients with emphysema will often live with saturations in the high 80s to low 90s.

14. Name five general categories of things causing hypoxia/hypoxemia.

Hypoventilation, or not breathing out the by-products of metabolism, usually involves decreased respiratory rate such as heroin abuse. The second cause involves part of the lung receiving typical inspired air without that portion of the lung having blood flow—as in pulmonary embolism. Another etiology involves shunting blood directly from the deoxygenated side to the arterial supply as in ventricular septal defect (VSD). Fourth, the lung may be inflamed or edematous causing diffusion abnormalities. Finally, the environment in which the person was located may have a reduced level of oxygen content (e.g., fire in an enclosed space or high altitude).

15. Is a room air oxygen saturation always necessary?

I find it helps assess patients except those chronically on home oxygen. If people use oxygen continuously outside the hospital, then obtaining a saturation on their typical setting may be helpful, although taking them off oxygen and getting a very low reading is not as useful. This especially is problematic if the person is not in distress (no chest pain or other symptoms with normal vital signs otherwise) and gets moved to the department in front of other, more ill patients, based on a saturation that is probably their baseline. You should, however, get a saturation on their normal oxygen setting and ask them why they require home oxygen.

16. Name some lung pathologies that can cause shortness of breath.

- COPD (Chronic bronchitis, emphysema, asthma)
- Pneumothorax
- Infectious
- Pleural effusion
- Contusion/trauma
- Restrictive (Asbestosis, sarcoid)
- Congenital (Cystic fibrosis, α1-antitrypsin deficiency)

17. What are the most common vital sign abnormalities in pulmonary embolus?

Tachycardia and tachypnea—although both may be normal, of course.

18. How low is the oxygen saturation in pulmonary embolus, if abnormal?

Of course with a large pulmonary embolism (PE) the patient will look sick, with very low saturations to the 70s or 80s and look as if they are dying. They are easier to triage. The smaller PE is often diagnosed on high clinical suspicion with oxygen saturations in the low 90s or high 80s. Combine a chief complaint of short of breath, an O_2 saturation of 90%, and tachycardia and PE is usually on your differential diagnosis list.

19. Does a chest x-ray help diagnose pulmonary embolism?

Not usually, but ordering one as an initial test is standard. Although most commonly normal in PE, chest x-ray may provide alternative diagnoses and establish a baseline.

20. What is COPD?

Chronic obstructive pulmonary disease is a syndrome that includes asthma, chronic bronchitis, and emphysema, which are often found to various degrees in conjunction with each other in older patients, especially smokers.

21. What is the pathology involved in emphysema?

Emphysema involves a breakdown of the alveoli so that the net effect is less surface area over which to exchange oxygen for carbon dioxide—the waste product of metabolism. Because of this decrease in the ability to exchange, these people often have increased levels of carbon dioxide in their blood, hence the name "retainers."

22. Why is oxygen supplementation sometimes a problem for people with emphysema?

If someone retains CO_2 causing higher levels than normal in their bloodstream, their body changes its trigger for breathing. Normally, we breathe when our bodies sense an increase in the amount of by-product of metabolism—CO_2. For example, when you exercise, your tissues utilize increased amounts of oxygen and produce increased amounts of CO_2 causing you to breathe faster and deeper to remove the excess CO_2. If someone's CO_2 level is chronically high, as in emphysema, their body physiology changes, sensing low oxygen as the trigger to breathe. When the oxygen is plentiful, they do not breathe as much causing even more CO_2 to accumulate.

23. What is CO_2 narcosis?

As the CO_2 level in the blood rises, patients become confused, slur their words, and eventually will lose consciousness.

24. How is chronic bronchitis diagnosed?

Although the pathophysiology involves an increased number of mucus-producing cells in the respiratory tree and chronic inflammation, the diagnosis is based on clinical symptoms of chronic cough for greater than 3 months for 2 years or more—the smoker's cough.

25. What is a "pink puffer" versus a "blue bloater"?

Pink puffer refers to the patient with emphysema who shows marked dyspnea, often thin habitus, with pursed lip breathing. On the other hand, a blue bloater usually doesn't feel short of breath, but has a wet cough, CO_2 retention, and rales or rhonchi. Both conditions include wheezing and are often combined in the COPD patient.

26. What is the percentage of smokers who will develop severe COPD?

Only 15% of smokers will develop the severe COPD symptoms, they are the ones we most frequently care for in the emergency departments. Additionally, of all the patients with COPD, about 90% are from smoking.

27. Name some cardiac causes of shortness of breath.

Many times it is difficult to discern which came first, the chest pain or the breathing difficulty. A few of the important cardiac problems that can produce a feeling of shortness of breath (with or without chest pain) include congestive heart failure, coronary artery disease (including angina and MI), pericardial effusion/tamponade, tachycardia (e.g., atrial fibrillation with rapid ventricular response).

28. What is pleuritic chest pain?

Pleuritic chest pain is pain that worsens with inspiration/deep breathing. Because the lung tissue does not have pain-sensing nerves, when lungs are irritated and they contact the inner chest wall the patient will experience pain, such as pleurisy. Other examples of pleuritic chest pain include musculoskeletal conditions, such as costochondritis, which worsens when the chest expands.

29. What are common causes of pleuritic chest pain?

Some of the more frequent ED etiologies of this type of chest pain involve pneumothorax, PE, pericarditis, rib fracture or chest wall contusion, costochondritis, and musculoskeletal (e.g., from frequent coughing).

Of note, as many as 67% of patients with PE, when they complain of chest pain, it is pleuritic. Keep in mind, however, that just because someone says his or her pain changes with breathing, the etiology may still be cardiac.

30. What are some signs of an ill asthmatic (requiring more immediate attention) in triage?

Things to consider as sicker in asthmatics include abnormal vital signs, lots of accessory muscle use/increased work of breathing, looks tired, cyanosis, no wheezing, and looks sick. In an asthmatic that looks like they are sick and you hear no wheezing on physical examination, they need rapid triage and treatment as this is indicative of impending respiratory failure.

31. What happens in the lungs of an asthmatic?

Hyper-reactivity of the airway muscles causes a constriction in response to various stimuli. Additionally, inflammation occurs within the air passages at the bronchiole level. Most commonly this results in an ability to get enough air in, but not easily out, creating positive end expiratory pressure in the alveoli (i.e., air trapping). This is why it is easy to give them a pneumothorax on the ventilator after being intubated.

32. What happens to the lining of the trachea when someone smokes cigarettes?

When someone smokes, the ciliated cells that usually clear the mucous out of your lungs (into your esophagus) are changed into cells more like skin, without cilia (hairlike projections). Therefore, these cells are unable to clear the secretions. Furthermore, the number of mucous producing cells increases, in an attempt to trap and remove the additional impurities in the lungs.

33. What are some risk factors of spontaneous pneumothorax?

Tall, thin, smoking males are typical, as is smoking crack cocaine or having *Pneumocystis carinii* pneumonia (PCP).

34. What is the danger of pneumothorax/hemothorax?

Air or fluid accumulating in the chest cavity may continue until it inhibits lung expansion and cardiac function causing a tension pneumo-/hemothorax. This can be seen by an increasing heart rate, decreasing blood pressure, altered level of consciousness, jugular distension, and tracheal shift away from the affected side.

35. What is the emergent treatment of tension pneumothorax/hemothorax?

Decompression by placing a hole in the chest wall with either a needle or scalpel is needed to relieve the high pressure; followed by a chest tube—the definitive treatment.

36. What conditions in pneumonia increase the mortality/morbidity, requiring admission and more urgent triage evaluation?

Even in this age of numerous antibiotics, people still die of pneumonia. Certain risk factors necessitate admission, including advanced age (actual or apparent greater than 65), hypoxia (saturation less than 90 percent), co-morbidity (e.g., COPD, immunocompromised) and certain social situations. Although not available at the triage desk, multilobar involvement or a white cell count greater than 15 is also indicative of someone needing admission. Of course there is also the gut feeling that this person is sick and won't do well at home.

37. What are some of the ominous signs of someone complaining of severe shortness of breath?

Some of the worrisome signs of someone with imminent respiratory failure include confusion or sleepiness, diaphoresis/sweating (when is the last time you broke out in a sweat just with the effort to breathe?), tripoding (sitting forward with their arms supporting them in a tripod fashion), or the look of fear or expressing feelings of impending doom. Additionally, quiet lungs on examination may be secondary to such a small amount of air exchange that they cannot wheeze.

38. Do all people with pulmonary edema have congestive heart failure (CHF)?

No, pulmonary edema is excess fluid within the lung parenchyma causing impaired diffusion. This fluid originates from excess volume in the pulmonary blood vessels. CHF is a frequent cause but other etiologies include severe hypertension, nonsteroidal anti-inflammatory drug (NSAID) use, salicylate overdose, high altitude, and cocaine or heroin use and re-expansion of the lung. Another cause is adult respiratory disease syndrome (ARDS).

39. Does someone with CHF and pulmonary edema always have peripheral edema?

Right heart failure and diastolic dysfunction cause peripheral edema although left heart failure—the leading cause of right failure—produces pulmonary edema. Many of the patients who have no history of CHF present with pulmonary edema without peripheral edema as they initially experience left-sided heart failure.

40. What physical examination findings are worrisome in patients with possible CHF?

As always, increased work of breathing and hypoxia are signs of significant pulmonary compromise. Additionally, rales are often heard throughout the lung fields, not just in the bases; or, no lung sounds in one or both bases. Lack of lung sounds may be from pleural effusion—fluid within the chest cavity.

41. What are some etiologies of fluid in the chest cavity?

Various conditions may result in fluid in the chest cavity. Pleural effusions may be transudative or exudative and include CHF, cancer, renal failure, anasarca, and infections, such as pneumonia and tuberculosis. Often a sample of the fluid must be obtained to determine the etiology. If large enough, the fluid may compromise breathing and needs to be drained (via thoracentesis) to improve lung expansion.

Another cause is trauma, either to the lungs, chest wall, heart, or blood vessels, resulting in blood loss into the chest cavity. These almost always require a chest tube.

42. Does everyone with pulmonary edema require a diuretic, such as furosemide?

If the cause of the pulmonary edema is not primarily excess vascular volume, then giving a diuretic is not the solution, and, may cause the patient's condition to worsen. Knowing the etiology of the edema is the best method for determining proper treatment.

43. Name some causes of chest pain and shortness of breath not resulting from cardiac or lung problems.

Although the underlying pathology is not cardiopulmonary, the symptoms of chest pain and shortness of breath can be severe and the outcome poor. Some of these other etiologies include sickle cell anemia—acute chest syndrome, anaphylaxis/angioedema, aspirated foreign body, laryngotracheobronchitis (croup)/bacterial tracheitis/pharyngitis, metabolic acidosis, sepsis, and air embolism. Additionally, hyperventilation and anxiety can cause breathing problems.

44. What causes cyanosis?

Cyanosis may be as a result of a reduced delivery of oxygen to tissue from decreased blood flow, severe anemia, or a change in the hemoglobin oxygen binding properties. The pulse oximeter measures oxyhemoglobin in the blood using light wave absorption. Impaired perfusion (hypotension, hypothermia), fluorescent lighting, nail polish—especially blue, and abnormal hemoglobin, all affect the accuracy and effectiveness of pulse oximetry.

45. Which abnormal hemoglobins affect oxygen saturation readings?

Carboxyhemoglobin is read as oxyhemoglobin by pulse oximeters causing normal readings in the cyanotic patient. On the other hand, methemoglobin lowers the readings. Additionally, cyanide does not allow the oxygen to be released from the red cell, which causes tissue hypoxia with normal pulse oximetry readings.

46. What is the most common form of cyanotic congenital heart disease?

Ventricular septal defects compromise 30% to 40% of all congenital heart defects. Most get diagnosed in the first week (50%), with most of the remaining found over the first year. Congenital heart defects are basically divided into cyanotic or not. Cyanosis in this case is caused by the mixing of deoxygenated blood with the arterial blood through the VSD. The treatment available in the ED is oxygen. If undiagnosed, an echocardiogram (ECC) is needed to assess the defect.

47. What is an air embolism?

Undissolved intravascular air in either the arterial or venous system is an air embolism. This is something people always worry about when they see air bubbles in the intravenous (IV) tubing connected to their IV.

48. What quantity of air is considered fatal in air embolism?

Approximately 100 to 300 mL of air is necessary to be harmful. In dog models, 40% mortality was associated with 0.5 to 1.0 mL/kg of air, which corresponds to as little as 50 mL of air.

49. What would be the most common history on presentation to triage of an arterial gas embolism?

Recent diving (SCUBA or free) would be the most frequent cause of air embolism usually presenting within 10 minutes of surfacing, but presentations may be delayed. People often present with dyspnea or altered level of consciousness. Arterial gas embolism may also follow intrathoracic trauma, pressurized gas inhalation, or a venous gas embolism via a patent foramen ovale. Arterial gas embolisms most commonly travel to the cerebral arterial system, causing stroke, coronary arteries causing infarct/ischemia, and spinal arteries causing paralysis.

50. What can cause venous gas embolisms?

Any injury to a vein, central lines (including patient on hemodialysis), chest trauma (blunt or penetrating), high-pressure mechanical ventilation, and many surgical procedures are all risk factors for venous gas embolisms (VGEs).

51. What are the signs and symptoms of VGE?

Patients will complain of nonspecific symptoms including sudden onset of dyspnea, chest pain, and a sense of impending doom or unconsciousness. Additionally, signs of VGE are sudden wheezing, rapid shallow breathing, and unexplained drop in oxygen saturation and P_{CO_2}.

52. What things do you consider in a patient with unilateral low or absent lung sounds?

Unilaterally absent breath sounds are indicative of pneumothorax, hemothorax (or other fluid in the thorax), pleural effusion, or consolidation.

Key Points

- Nasal flaring, retractions, accessory muscle use, sweating, tripoding posture, and the "deer in the headlights" look of fear are worrisome signs in the dyspneic patient.
- Tachypnea reflects some underlying abnormality, but not necessarily pulmonary.
- An asthmatic that looks sick and has no audible wheezing needs rapid triage and treatment as this is indicative of impending respiratory failure.
- Absence of wheezing in the COPD or asthma patient in respiratory distress means severely obstructed airways. These patients have such a small amount of air exchange that they cannot wheeze.
- Do not trust the pulse oximeter alone to assess the respiratory status because it does not measure the carbon dioxide. It can read normal in the cyanotic patient.
- In patients with emphysema, do not withhold oxygen for fear of blunting the respiratory drive; the hypoxia should be corrected first.

Internet Resources

Iroquois Memorial Hospital Emergency Department Patient Care Standard for Respiratory Distress
http://www.ena.org/document_share/documents/respiratory_distress.doc

Respiratory Emergency: Breathing, Choking, Drowning and Carbon Monoxide Emergencies
http://www.nursingceu.com/NCEU/courses/respiratory-combo/

"I can't breathe!" Respiratory Problems in the ED
http://www.enw.org/Can'tBreathe.htm

Dyspnea Is a Common Symptom of Lung, Breast Cancer
http://www.cancernetwork.com/journals/oncnews/n9809ll.htm

Emergency Management of Myasthenia Gravis: Important information for the patient, family, emergency medical technician, nurse, and emergency department personnel.
http://www.myasthenia.org/information/EmergencyMgmt.htm

Carbon Monoxide
http://www.enw.org/Research-CO.htm

Emergency Medicine: Asthma/COPD/Dyspnea
http://medi-smart.com/emer_asthma.htm

Bibliography

Emerman C: The patient with chronic obstructive pulmonary disease or asthma. In Herr RD, Cydulka R, editors: *Emergency care of the compromised patient,* Philadelphia, 1994, Lippincott, Williams & Wilkins, 1385-1392.

Stone CK, Waters DS: Dyspnea. In Harwood-Nuss A, Wolfson AB, Linden CH, Shepherd SM, Stenklyft PH, editors. *The clinical practice of emergency medicine,* ed 3, Philadelphia, 2001, Lippincott, Williams & Wilkins, 16-21.

Chapter 27

Chest Pain

Jin H. Han

1. What are the different causes of chest pain?

Chest pain can originate from the cardiovascular, pulmonary, gastrointestinal, or musculoskeletal systems, making diagnosis very difficult. However, our goal in triaging chest pain patients in the emergency department is to rule out the diagnoses with the highest mortality and morbidity.

Causes of Chest Pain

Cardiovascular	Pulmonary	Gastrointestinal	Musculoskeletal
Acute coronary syndromes	Pulmonary embolism	Esophageal perforation	Costochondritis
Aortic dissection	Pneumothorax	Esophageal spasms	Rib fracture
Pericarditis	Pneumomediastinum	Esophageal food impaction	Shingles
Myocarditis	Pneumonia	Gastroesophageal reflux disease	
	Pleuritis	Esophagitis	
		Peptic ulcer disease	
		Cholecystitis	
		Pancreatitis	

2. Which causes of chest pain are potentially lethal?

We are most concerned about the most lethal diagnoses first, rather than the most common. Acute coronary syndromes, aortic dissection, pulmonary embolism, pneumothorax, and esophageal perforation are potentially life-threatening causes of chest pain. Patients with myocarditis, pericarditis, and pneumonia can also have potentially poor outcomes.

3. Which patient is most urgent from my initial across-the-room glance?

Any patient appearing uncomfortable, pale, diaphoretic, clammy, cyanotic, or acutely ill should be evaluated immediately.

4. List vital sign abnormalities that are worrisome in a patient with chest pain.

- Tachycardia
- Tachypnea
- Hypoxia
- Hypotension
- Hypertension (systolic blood pressure >180, diastolic blood pressure >110)

5. Discuss important physical assessments in all chest pain patients.

A focused examination could include:

- Assessment of pulse rate and rhythm.
- Attempt auscultation of abnormal heart sounds such as murmurs, gallops, or pericardial rubs. However, these findings are often difficult to hear in the loud emergency department (ED) environment.
- Assess for breath sound symmetry and auscultate for wheezes, rales, or rhonchi.
- Look for tracheal deviation (especially if the patient is dyspneic with the chest pain) and/or the presence of jugular venous distension.

6. Indicate some important questions to ask for patients with chest pain.

The description of the chest pain is key in helping to determine the source of pain. I use the PPQRST mnemonic:

- What are the **P**alliating and **P**recipitating factors? Does it happen at rest or exertion? Does lying down, exertion, or swallowing make it worse? Does rest or sitting forward make it better?
- What is the **Q**uality of the chest pain? Is it sharp, pleuritic, dull, tearing, squeezing, or crushing?
- Does the pain **R**adiate? Does it travel to the jaw, neck, shoulder, arms, or back?
- How **S**evere is the pain? Ask the patient to rate the pain from 1 to 10. The initial score can be used as a baseline. Subsequent pain scores can be used to assess after a therapy has been given.
- What is **T**emporal nature of the pain? Does it last for several seconds or minutes or hours? Is it intermittent or constant?

7. List other questions I should ask in obtaining a history.

Ask about:

- Associated symptoms: nausea, diaphoresis, shortness of breath, feeling faint
- Fevers, coughs, or recent upper respiratory infections
- History of similar chest pain in the past or previous acute myocardial infarctions
- Recent trauma

8. Describe the minimum workup for a chest pain patient.

Along with vital signs, a thorough history, and physical examination, most patients should have a chest x-ray and an electrocardiogram (ECG) performed.

A complete blood cell count (CBC), electrolytes, and serum markers for myocyte injury such as troponin, CPK, and CPK-MB are sometimes part of a standing protocol for triage of chest pain.

9. What is one thing every triage nurse should remember when evaluating chest pain?

Very few patients read the textbook! More often than not, the clinical presentations will be atypical.

10. Should I mount the rhythm strip if I put a patient on a monitor?

Policies vary, but many institutions require at least one mounted strip with the interpretation for any patient placed on a monitor. Some also encourage baseline measurements (e.g., P-R interval, etc.).

11. Are emergency medical services (EMS) systems having providers fax in the electrocardiograms (EKGs) obtained in the field?

Again policies vary. Some do activate the catheter lab only after the patient arrives; others have used them as the basis for activation and found a 15- to 30-minute time savings. Regardless, if the EKGs are faxed, there needs to be a procedure in place to insure they are noted and reviewed in a timely fashion.

12. How should I handle a phone call from a person having chest pain?

Tell them to call 911. In one study they found that the median time for the patient to arrive at the emergency department was 5.7 hours. Those who called 911 arrived in 90 minutes. Those who took themselves to the ED (11%) took 2 to 3 times longer and those who called their physician (26%) took 3 to 4 times longer.

13. Why does it take people so long to come in?

The individual must decide there is a problem and that help is needed. One study looking at the reasons patients delayed seeking care with chest pain refutes many common perceptions. Those who delayed the longest were:

- Women (see Chapter 14)
- History of past medical problems (hypertension, diabetes, heart disease)
- Fewer years of education (<12 years)
- Lower income (<$20,000/yr)
- Older (>65 years)
- African American

14. Discuss nurse-initiated triage protocols.

- A growing trend is symptom-driven initial triage and treatment standing orders that allow essential first-line diagnosis and treatment to begin. Chest pain is one of the most frequent patient complaints for a protocol. For instance in Memorial Regional Hospital (Hollywood, Fla), the nurse initiates labs, x-ray, EKG, oxygen, aspirin, and nitroglycerin for visceral chest pain, and a chest radiograph, EKG, and pulse oximetry for pleuritic chest pain. In Cape Cod Hospital (Mass), the ST Elevation Caremap requires the ED nurse to recognize ST elevation (or depression) on the EKG and notify the physician. For further discussion, see Chapter 8.

CARDIAC

15. What is ischemic heart disease?

Ischemic heart disease is a spectrum of cardiac diseases in which myocardial oxygen demand exceeds supply and range from stable angina to acute myocardial infarction (AMI). The most common cause of decreased oxygen supply is coronary artery disease (CAD) secondary to atherosclerosis. Decreased oxygen supply may also be secondary to vasospasm or decreased oxygen carrying capacity of the blood, as seen in anemia.

16. Why should I worry about ischemic heart disease?

Cardiovascular disease is the leading cause of death in the United States (500,000 deaths per year). Half of these deaths occur before they arrive to the ED.

17. What is stable angina?

Stable angina is a pattern of chest pain that is very typical for the patient. These patients live with chest pain on a regular basis. The amount of exertion required to elicit chest pain, length of chest pain, and the method of relief are usually constant. Any change in these patterns may be indicative of acute coronary syndrome (ACS).

18. What is acute coronary syndrome?

ACS is a spectrum of CAD, consisting of unstable angina and AMI. The distinction between these two diagnoses is based on whether or not the ischemic myocardium has infarcted. An infarction is when the heart muscle cells (myocytes) die.

19. Describe what precipitates ACS.

In stable angina, the atherosclerotic plaque is stable. When it ruptures, it becomes unstable, causing a cascade of events resulting in platelet aggregation and fibrin deposition. As a result, worsening coronary artery stenosis or complete occlusion occurs.

20. What is unstable angina?

Once a coronary artery stenosis worsens or becomes completely occluded, the oxygen supply becomes limited to the heart. The myocardium becomes ischemic and chest pain occurs. Unstable angina occurs when no damage occurs to the myocardium. New onset-angina (lasting greater than 20 minutes and causing moderate physical impairment), angina at rest, and changing pattern of angina are indicative of unstable angina.

21. What is acute myocardial infarction (AMI)?

After a half hour of myocardial ischemia, myocyte necrosis occurs. Once the myocardium becomes irreversibly damaged, the patient has suffered an AMI. Cardiac biomarkers are subsequently released into the bloodstream. Elevations in these cardiac markers can be the only differentiating factor between unstable angina and AMI when the EKG is nondiagnostic.

22. Name risk factors for CAD.

- Male
- Age greater than 65 years old
- Hypertension
- Diabetes mellitus
- Smoking
- Family history as defined as a first degree relative having an AMI whose age is less than 55 years old if the relative is a male and 65 years old if the relative is a female
- Hypercholesteremia
- Chronic renal insufficiency
- Previous history atherosclerotic disease such as CAD, peripheral vascular disease, or cerebrovascular accident

23. Should I be reassured if the patient has no risk factors?

No, up to 50% of ACS patients may not have any known risk factors.

24. How quickly should the EKG be obtained when ACS or AMI is suspected?

An EKG should be obtained within 5 to 10 minutes of patient arrival.

25. Tell me how busy EDs are meeting this time line. We often have no treatment rooms open.

A growing trend is EKG rooms by triage for anyone with chest pain, a strong cardiac history, or many risk factors. One hospital has a nurse practitioner from the cardiology service read the technician-acquired EKG, and then follows up with the ED attending physician for abnormal results. In addition, initial labs are drawn and a saline lock inserted. Those with a normal EKG and no other presenting symptoms of an AMI are sent back to the waiting room.

Those with presenting symptoms such as diaphoresis, nausea, shortness of breath, and lightheadedness are still seen immediately even if their EKG appears normal.

Others have used a "fast track" room or even a "family room" for this purpose with the technician taking the obtained EKG to the ED physician for interpretation.

26. What are cardiac biomarkers?

Serial measurements of cardiac biomarkers have become the mainstay of diagnosis when the EKG is nondiagnostic. Elevations in cardiac biomarkers are indicative of myocardial necrosis. The cardiac biomarkers used are myoglobin, creatinine-kinase MB isoenzyme, troponin T, and troponin I.

27. Is the first set of cardiac biomarkers enough to rule out an AMI?

No. Initial sensitivities are poor and should not be the sole criteria for ruling out AMI. It may take several hours for cardiac biomarkers to become detectable in the serum. Serial cardiac biomarker measurements are more sensitive.

28. Explain the difference between an ST-elevation myocardial infarction (STEMI) and non-ST elevation myocardial infarction (NSTEMI).

There are two main classifications of AMIs, which are distinguishable by electrocardiographic criteria. STEMIs have ST-segment elevations greater than 1 mm in at least two contiguous leads or a left bundle branch block. Reciprocal ST-depressions are usually present and Q waves will develop.

Non-STEMIs may have ST-segment depressions, T-wave inversions, or hyperacute T-waves. However, the EKG may be normal in many NSTEMI patients.

29. What are the EKG findings for unstable angina?

The EKG findings in unstable angina are the same as those found in NSTEMI. Again, the distinction between NSTEMI and unstable angina can only be made retrospectively in nondiagnostic EKGs by the use of cardiac markers.

30. How useful is the EKG as a definitive indication of AMI?

Only 50% of EKGs are diagnostic for AMI. However, ST-segment elevations are specific for AMI, but can be elevated in other conditions such as acute pericarditis. EKG changes are important for risk stratification. Patients with ST-segment deviations have the highest risk for death.

31. State the classic symptoms consistent with ACS.

- Description: Tight, pressure-like, or crushing sensation located in the substernal region, the left side of the chest, or to the back. The pain may be precipitated or exacerbated by exertion.

- Duration: Usually lasts for several minutes or hours.
- Radiation: The pain may radiate into the shoulder, arms, neck, or jaw.
- Associated symptoms: Shortness of breath, nausea, vomiting, weakness, lightheadedness, dizziness, and diaphoresis.

32. What are atypical symptoms of chest pain?

- Description: Pleuritic, sharp, or stabbing precipitated by positional change and local pressure.
- Location: Can be shoulder, neck, or back.
- Duration: Lasting several seconds or greater than 24 hours are atypical features.

The presence of these features moderately decreases the likelihood of ACS, but should not be the sole basis for excluding this diagnosis. Specific patient groups are prone to asymptomatic presentations.

33. Which patients are prone to atypical presentations of ACS?

The older adult, diabetics, females, nonwhites, patients with dementia, congestive heart failure (CHF), and previous strokes have been found to have atypical presentations or no chest pain. See Chapter 14.

In the older adult, shortness of breath is the most common complaint in patients with ACS and they can present with just syncope or nonspecific constitutional symptoms, such as feeling weak. Approximately 40% of older adult patients diagnosed with AMI did not complain of any chest pain and 50% had no evidence of ischemia or infarction on their presenting EKG. In a small percentage of older adult patients, cerebrovascular accident and mental status changes will be the primary manifestation of AMI.

34. Tell me something to use that will help remember the atypical presentations of AMI in the older adult.

The mnemonic GRANDFATHERS
General malaise
Refers to a gastrointestinal complaint
Altered mental status
Neurologic deficits
Dyspnea
Falls or **F**lu symptoms
Atypical chest pain
Trouble walking
Hypotension
Exhaustion
Reverse in functional status
Syncope or presyncope

35. Can AMI occur in the young patient (less than 40 years old)?

Yes. Approximately 8% of all AMI occur in patients under 40 years of age.

36. How are AMIs in the younger population different from the older population?

These patients tend to have higher prevalence of smoking, family history of CAD, or hyperlipidemia. These patients usually have single-vessel disease. Because they are relatively healthy, their prognosis is better than their older counterparts.

37. Can I use reproducible chest pain to differentiate between a costochondritis and ACS?

One study found 20% of AMI patients had reproducible chest pain. The presence of reproducible pain does not exclude the diagnosis ACS.

38. Is ACS confirmed when the pain goes away with nitroglycerin?

No. Response to nitroglycerin should not affect your suspicion for ACS in any way. Nitroglycerin can also relax the esophageal smooth muscle so patients with esophageal spasms will have chest pain relief when given nitroglycerin. Conversely, a patient with myocardial ischemia may not have any response to nitroglycerin. In one study of 459 patients, it showed no prognostic or diagnostic value in patients who presented with chest pain to the ED.

39. Can cocaine and amphetamines use cause ACS?

Yes, because both drugs can induce vasospasm. Vasospasm may occur in the absence of pre-existing CAD. Chronic cocaine and amphetamine use may also cause premature atherosclerosis.

40. What is Prinzmetal's angina?

Prinzmetal's angina is a rare variant of angina that is caused by coronary artery vasospasm. There may be underlying atherosclerosis but the coronary arteries can sometimes be normal. The chest pain usually occurs at night and a prolonged attack may cause MI, arrhythmias, and sudden death. An EKG will show ST-elevations.

41. Is it important to provide an initial aspirin?

Yes. Aspirin is a cost-effective antiplatelet aggregation therapy that improves AMI mortality with little risk to the patient. Any patient with chest pain should get an aspirin if no contraindications exist.

42. Discuss nitroglycerin.

Nitroglycerin can be given to reduce pain. However, caution must be taken in patients with inferior wall AMIs. A large proportion of these patients may have a right ventricular AMI also. Patients with right ventricular AMIs are preload-dependent. Because nitroglycerin reduces preload through venous dilation, patients with right ventricular infarctions may become hypotensive.

43. Talk about other drugs that might be indicated.

- Beta-blockers have also shown to improve mortality in AMI patients.
- Morphine can be given to further relieve pain and anxiety.
- High-risk patients can receive glycoprotein IIb-IIIa inhibitors and clopidogrel. Like aspirin, they prevent platelet aggregation, but through different pathways.

44. What is an aortic dissection?

An aortic dissection is when blood breaks through the intimal wall and dissects along the planes of the aortic wall at the level of the media. The dissection can extend longitudinally and circumferentially, causing pain. The majority of aortic dissections originate near the aortic valve, in which the greatest stress to the aortic wall exists.

45. How frequent are aortic dissections?

Aortic dissections are relatively rare events when compared to ACS. The frequency is estimated to be between 5 and 30 occurrences per 1 million cases.

46. Describe the pain associated with aortic dissection.

Chest pain will be present if the proximal aorta is involved, but the pain can occur in the back, abdomen, or lower extremities. The pain begins abruptly and is excruciating in the vast majority of cases. However, the "classic" description of "ripping" or "tearing" pain is present in only 50% of the cases.

47. Is aortic dissection lethal?

The mortality rate is extremely high. If untreated, approximately 33% of patients die within the first 24 hours, 50% die within 48 hours, and the 2-week mortality rate approaches 75%.

48. Why don't we catch aortic dissection earlier?

The signs and symptoms of aortic dissections are nonspecific and the diagnosis may be elusive. As a result, approximately 38% of the cases are missed on initial evaluation.

49. What are the risk factors for aortic dissection?

- Age (peak age is 60 to 70 years)
- Hypertension (50%, although 30% are normotensive)
- Male
- Any condition that weakens the aortic wall

50. What are the physical findings (besides the pain) that can be important for a patient with a suspected aortic dissection?

- Chest pain with neurologic deficits
- Significant differentials between the blood pressure and pulses in both arms. They occur only 20% of the time but are from occlusions of the innominate or subclavian arteries.
- Aortic regurgitation murmur (heard during diastole in the left upper sternal border)
- Signs/symptoms of limb ischemia

51. What are the diagnostic tests to anticipate for a suspected aortic dissection?

- No laboratory test can accurately screen for an aortic dissection.
- Cardiac enzymes (rule out concurrent AMI)
- Electrolytes, bicarbonate, blood urea nitrogen (BUN), and creatinine (assess for renal function)
- Type and screen (if the patient is hypotensive or shocky)
- Chest x-ray (60% have a widened mediastinum)
- EKG (nonspecific ST-segment and T-wave changes are most common)
- Computed tomography (CT) of the chest (or transesophageal echocardiogram [ECC])

52. What is acute pericarditis?

Pericarditis is inflammation of the pericardium.

53. What symptoms are consistent with acute pericarditis?

Most patients with acute pericarditis will present with substernal chest pain that is sharp and pleuritic. The chest pain can radiate to the back or the trapezius ridge. The pain may be improved by sitting forward. A recent history of viral symptoms such as fever, myalgias, malaise, anorexia, or fatigue may be present.

54. Elaborate on the causes of acute pericarditis.

In the majority of cases, the etiology of acute pericarditis is unknown. Enteroviruses such as Coxsackie virus are thought to be one of the more common viral etiologies of acute pericarditis. Other causes include HIV+; tuberculosis; collagen, vascular, and rheumatic disorders; and drug use.

55. Describe the physical findings that are suggestive of acute pericarditis.

The presence of a pericardial rub in two to three phases may be present. It is best appreciated when the patient is sitting forward and in full expiration. The stethoscope diaphragm should be placed at the left lower sternal border. The pericardial rub may be intermittent and transient in nature, and is often mistaken for a murmur.

56. Discuss the electrocardiographic changes noted in acute pericarditis.

EKG changes are typically seen in four stages and last up to 4 months. Stage one is the most characteristic and usually occurs during the acute phase of symptoms. Diffuse concave ST-segment elevation will be seen with PR depression. PR depression is specific for acute pericarditis and can be present in all leads except in $_{A}V_{R}$ and V_1. This phase may last up to 2 weeks.

57. What is pericardial tamponade?

Normally, the pericardial space holds 20 mL of fluid. When pericardial fluid rapidly accumulates, ventricular filling is impaired, and cardiac output is decreased. When the amount of pericardial fluid becomes large enough, hemodynamic instability can occur.

58. Are there specific causes of acute pericarditis that are more likely to cause pericardial tamponade?

Yes. Pericardial tamponade is uncommon in idiopathic and post-MI pericarditis. However, it is more frequent in patients with bacterial, malignant, or tuberculous pericarditis.

59. State the symptoms of pericardial tamponade.

The patient may complain of chest pain or tightness, shortness of breath, orthopnea, and weakness.

60. Describe the physical findings of pericardial tamponade.

The classical findings of pericardial tamponade are muffled heart sounds, hypotension, and jugular venous distension. However, these findings are not usually found until significant tamponade has occurred. Pulsus paradoxus as defined as a systolic blood pressure decrease of greater than 10 mm Hg after inspiration may exist, but it can be seen in other illnesses.

61. What is myocarditis?

Myocarditis is inflammation of the heart muscle.

62. Talk about the causes of myocarditis.

The causes of myocarditis are numerous and in many cases are unknown. A large variety of infections, drugs, toxins, and systemic illnesses may cause myocarditis. Viral etiologies are common in younger patients. Enteroviruses such as Coxsackie virus are frequent causes in the western hemisphere.

63. Discuss the incidence and prevalence of myocarditis.

The incidence and prevalence of myocarditis is largely unknown, because many patients are asymptomatic. Most of what we know come from postmortem studies. It is a major cause of death in patients under 40 years of age.

64. What are the symptoms of myocarditis?

Acute onset of chest pain is usual and may be mistaken for AMI. Because viruses are major causes, the patient may have preceding upper respiratory or gastrointestinal illnesses. These illnesses are usually associated with fever, malaise, skeletal myalgia, and anorexia.

65. Indicate the physical findings of myocarditis.

There are no key physical findings that distinguish myocarditis from other illnesses. The patients may have manifestations of congestive heart failure in advanced cases.

PULMONARY

66. What is a pulmonary embolism?

A pulmonary embolism (PE) is a blood clot that migrates to the pulmonary arteries.

67. Where do these blood clots come from?

Over 90% of all PEs come from lower extremity deep vein thrombosis.

68. Is the Homans' sign the most accurate indication of a deep vein thrombosis?

No. The Homans' sign is present in only 10% of deep vein thrombosis (DVT) cases, and many patients have a false positive. The most classic sign is unilateral leg swelling, although up to 69% of DVT patients have a normal examination.

69. Should I be worried about patients having a PE?

Yes. It is estimated that the incidence is more than 1 in 1,000 per year in the United States, and it is the third most common cause of death. Mortality is greater than 15% in the first month of diagnosis, attributed to being difficult to detect. The clinical presentation is often nonspecific or absent.

70. Tell me the classic risk factors of pulmonary embolism.

Virchow's triad, which consists of venous stasis, intimal damage, and hypercoagulable states. Patients with a previous history of DVT or PE have a 15- to 30-fold increased risk of having a PE.

71. List other contributing factors.

The more significant risks include:
- Obesity
- Smoking
- Hypertension
- Birth control pills and hormone replacement therapy (especially in smokers and older women (>50 years old)
- Long-haul airplane travel in coach seating is frequently blamed, but this is a rare cause

72. Do all patients with PEs have these risk factors?

No, 10% to 15% of patients with PE have no risk factors.

73. List the classic symptoms of PE.

The classical triad is chest pain, dyspnea, and hemoptysis, but they are present in less than 20% of the cases and many healthy patients are asymptomatic. The sudden-onset chest pain is usually described as sharp and pleuritic. Syncope may be the only complaint, especially in the older adult.

74. Name important physical findings in patients with PE.

Although the physical examination is often insensitive and nonspecific, be alert for:
- Tachycardia and tachypnea
- Hypoxia
- Fever (40%)

It is easy to see why it is difficult to differentiate from an infectious cause. Pneumonia is the most common misdiagnosis in autopsy-proven cases of PE.

75. Doesn't the presence of chest wall tenderness rule out a PE?

No, the presence of chest wall tenderness is common in PE. In fact, the presence of chest wall tenderness in the absence of any trauma should increase your suspicion of a PE!

76. Indicate what tests I should anticipate in a patient with a suspected PE?

A chest x-ray and EKG to diagnose other potential causes. The chest x-ray is often normal or nondiagnostic. If the D-dimer is positive or the suspicion of

PE is relatively high, patients should get either ventilation-perfusion scan (V/Q scan) or a computer tomography pulmonary angiogram (CT-PA).

77. Shouldn't I get a STAT arterial blood gas?

Arterial blood gases (ABGs) are not very useful and are used to measure A-a gradient. This is the difference in oxygen concentration between alveolar air (calculated from inspired oxygen corrected for expired CO_2, "A") and arterial oxygenation "a." This gradient is higher in those with PE because PE shunts some deoxygenated pulmonary artery to other pulmonary vessels in which it doesn't oxygenate. This shunt of oxygen poor blood lowers the overall arterial blood oxygenation sampled by ABG usually drawn at an artery in the arm or wrist. Unfortunately relying on increased A-a gradient alone will miss patients with PE.

78. What is a spontaneous pneumothorax?

A pneumothorax is a partial or total lung collapse with potentially serious hemodynamic and respiratory consequences. They occur without any obvious provocation.

79. Who is more prone to getting a spontaneous pneumothorax?

Males, smokers, and patients with underlying lung disease such as emphysema.

80. Discuss the symptoms of a spontaneous pneumothorax.

The symptoms are dependent on the size of the pneumothorax and the rate of development. Sudden onset, pleuritic chest pain is present in more than 95% of the cases, usually on the side of the pneumothorax. Dyspnea may be present and is indicative of a larger pneumothorax.

81. List classic physical findings of spontaneous pneumothorax.

Some findings are absent in small pneumothoraces. Classic findings include:
- Decreased breath sounds (approximately 85%)
- Tachypnea
- Tachycardia
- Hypoxia
- Hyperresonance (33%)

Careful attention should be made to trachea position and blood pressure. Tracheal shift and hypotension are indicative of a tension pneumothorax and need to be treated emergently.

82. How is a spontaneous pneumothorax diagnosed?

Chest x-ray is the primary means of diagnosis, but is sensitive only 80% of the time. The chest x-ray should be performed in an upright position and comparing end-inspiratory and end-expiratory films may be useful.

83. Discuss the treatment of spontaneous pneumothorax.

Tube thoracostomy is usually required in most cases, but a conservative management may be performed in patients with small pneumothoraces. If the patient is unstable, perform immediate needle decompression by inserting a 14-gauge intravenous (IV) catheter in the second intercostal space (at the mid-clavicular line).

84. What is pneumonia?

Pneumonia is an infection of the lower airways, causing a triad of fever, cough, and hypoxia. The chest pain is usually pleuritic and sharp; the cough is usually productive; and decreased breath sounds, rales, or rhonchi can be auscultation over the affected lobes.

GASTROINTESTINAL

85. What is Boerhaave's syndrome?

Boerhaave's syndrome is a full thickness esophageal perforation caused by increased intra-esophageal pressure.

86. Tell me about the usual cause of Boerhaave's syndrome.

Forced emesis causes 75% of the cases; alcohol ingestion is frequently the root cause of the emesis.

87. Describe the symptoms of esophageal perforation.

Severe and unrelenting pain can occur in the chest, neck, or abdomen and this pain may radiate to the back and shoulders. Swallowing typically worsens the pain.

88. List the physical findings of esophageal perforation.

- The physical findings depend on the degree of the perforation and the time elapsed.
- The patient appears uncomfortable and ill.
- Fever, tachypnea, and tachycardia are usually present.
- Subcutaneous emphysema may be palpable in the soft tissues of the neck.
- Mediastinal emphysema may be detected during cardiac auscultation (Hammon's crunch).
- Decreased breath sounds may be auscultated because over half of these patients will develop a pleural effusion.

89. What are esophageal dysmotility disorders?

This is a broad category of esophageal diseases characterized by excessive, uncoordinated contraction of the esophageal smooth muscle. It usually begins in the fifth decade of life.

90. Talk about symptoms of esophageal dysmotility disorders.

Chest pain is the most frequent complaint and usually occurs with rest. The pain is described as a dull and achy sensation, which can last for hours. Stress or ingestion of hot and cold liquids may precipitate esophageal dysmotility. Esophageal spasms can be relieved with nitroglycerin, making it difficult to distinguish with ACS.

91. Are esophageal dysmotility disorders life-threatening?

No. However, because these patients may be indistinguishable from ACS, they should be promptly and thoroughly evaluated.

92. What is gastroesophageal reflux disease?

Gastroesophageal reflux disease (GERD) causes chest pain that is burning and gnawing. The pain is usually worsened when lying down. The patient may describe an acidic taste in the mouth.

93. What is peptic ulcer disease?

Patients with peptic ulcer disease will describe a dull and gnawing pain in the mid-epigastric region. Patients are often awakened from sleep. Food may improve or worsen symptoms. Antacids will relieve the pain.

94. Should I be reassured if the patient's symptoms resolve with antacids or a GI cocktail?

Therapeutic response to antacids may occur in patients with myocardial ischemia because of placebo effect.

MUSCULOSKELETAL

95. What about musculoskeletal chest pain?

Musculoskeletal chest pain is a common cause of chest pain. Pain is often well localized, sharp, reproducible, and movement makes it worse. However, in the absence of any recent trauma or precipitating event, other etiologies of chest pain should be considered. In is important to remember that AMI and pulmonary emboli can present with pain that appears to be musculoskeletal in nature.

Key Points

- Patients don't read the textbook: many presentations are atypical.
- Only 50% of EKGs are diagnostic for AMI.
- Up to 50% of patients with ACS have no risk factors.
- Reproducible chest wall pain does not rule out the diagnosis of ACS.
- Relief with nitroglycerin is not diagnostic for cardiac pain.
- Chest wall tenderness, without a history of trauma, should raise the suspicion of a PE.

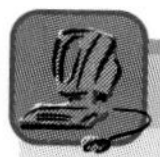

Internet Resources

Management of Chest Pain Suggestive of Ischemia
http://www1.va.gov/cardiology/docs/TimeisLifenewchestpain.doc

Emergency Nursing Record: Chest Pain Complaints (Prototype)
http://www.tsystem.com/pdf/18chest.pdf

Detecting High-Risk Patients With Chest Pain: Douglas Speake and Colleagues Discuss Nurse Detection of High-Risk Patients With Cardiac Chest Pain Using the Manchester Triage System (Clinical)
http://static.highbeam.com/e/emergencynurse/september012003/detectinghighriskpatients withchestpaindouglasspeak/

Chest Pain Units in Emergency Departments
http://www.acep.org/1,4718,0.html

Differential Diagnosis of Chest Pain
http://www.ena.org/conferences/annual/2004/handouts/224-c.pdf

Cardiac Labs—Just What is a "Cardiac Panel"?
http://www.ena.org/conferences/annual/2004/handouts/323-c.pdf

CHEST PAIN/SOB—Presumed Cardiac in Nature
http://www.ena.org/document_share/documents/ani-mhs-7-02.doc

Iroquois Memorial Hospital Emergency Department Patient Care Standard (PCS)
For Chest Pain (suspect cardiac origin)
http://www.ena.org/document_share/documents/chest_pain.doc

Iroquois Memorial Hospital Emergency Department Chest Pain Protocol (suspected cardiac)
http://www.ena.org/document_share/documents/chests_pain_protocol.pdf

Don't Let Time Run Out! Chest Pain Evaluations
http://www.ena.org/conferences/annual/2004/handouts/215-c.pdf

Bibliography

Canto JG, et al: Prevalence, clinical characteristics, and mortality among patients with myocardial infarction presenting without chest pain, *JAMA* 283:3223-3229, 2000.

Dunmire SM: Pulmonary embolism. In Harwood-Nuss A, editor: *The clinical practice of emergency medicine,* ed 3, Philadelphia, 2001, Lippincott, Williams & Wilkins, 753-756.

Goldhaber SZ, et al: Acute pulmonary embolism. Part I: Epidemiology, pathophysiology, and diagnosis, *Circulation* 108:2726-2729, 2003.

Knaut AL, et al: Aortic emergencies, *Emerg Med Clin N Am* 21:817-845, 2003.

Mendelson MH: Esophageal emergencies. In Tintinalli JE, editor: *Emergency medicine: A comprehensive study guide,* ed 5, Philadelphia, 2000, McGraw-Hill, 523-529.

Oakley CM: Myocarditis, pericarditis, and other pericardial diseases, *Heart* 84:449-454, 2000.

Panju AA, et al: The rational clinical examination: Is this patient having a myocardial infarction? *JAMA* 280:1256-1263, 1998.

Pratt FD, et al: Acute pericarditis and pericarditis and tamponade. In Harwood-Nuss A, editor: *The clinical practice of emergency medicine,* ed 3, Philadelphia, 2001, Lippincott, Williams & Wilkins, 704-707.

Young WF, et al: Spontaneous and iatrogenic pneumothorax. In Tintinalli JE, editor: *Emergency medicine: A comprehensive study guide,* ed 5, Philadelphia, 2000, McGraw-Hill, 471-474.

Chapter 28

Cough

Patricia M. Campbell

When a patient presents at triage with the chief complaint of "cough" the initial history and triage nursing assessment is instrumental in differentiating the life-threatening or emergent conditions from those that are less urgent. The cough reflex plays an important role in the body by clearing the airway of secretions or foreign bodies. It is a protective mechanism and is not harmful in its own right. Patients usually present for medical care when the cough is persistent, painful, interferes with activities of daily living, or is associated with other symptoms. This chapter presents information for the triage nurse to assist in the initial assessment of patients who present with a complaint of a cough.

1. What are the most important goals at triage when a patient presents with a cough?

- Identify life-threatening conditions
- Obtain a concise history
- Prevent the spread of infectious disease

2. How do you define a chronic versus acute cough?

An acute cough is defined as lasting less than 3 weeks and is usually associated with a brief upper/lower respiratory illness. However, life-threatening conditions, such as congestive heart failure (CHF), pericardial tamponade or pulmonary embolism (PE) are all associated with an acute cough.

A chronic cough usually is defined as a cough lasting more than 6 to 8 weeks.

3. What are the common causes of acute cough?

The most common causes of an acute cough are upper respiratory infections, allergies, sinusitis, environmental irritants, aspiration, and acute exacerbations of chronic illnesses such as asthma or chronic obstructive lung disease. Lower respiratory tract infections such as pneumonia can also cause an acute cough. PE and other life-threatening conditions such as CHF, aortic aneurysm, and airway obstruction can also present with a cough.

4. What are the most common causes of chronic cough?

The most common causes of a chronic cough include postnasal drip (PNDS), gastroesophageal reflux (GERD), asthma, eosinophilic bronchitis, or angiotensin-converting enzyme (ACE) inhibitors. Other causes of chronic cough include lung cancer, heart failure, mitral stenosis, sarcoidosis, chronic pulmonary disease (CPD), tuberculosis, smoking, and psychogenic cough. Aspiration associated with GERD can also cause a chronic cough. Determining the length of time the patient has had the cough and a focused triage history to include additional signs and symptoms will help determine the cause of the cough.

5. What are some other causes of cough?

Medications. Medications such as the ACE inhibitors are associated with a dry persistent cough. The cough is irritating to the patient and resolves within a few weeks after the medication is discontinued.

Psychogenic. Psychogenic cough is a diagnosis of exclusion. It most frequently occurs in patients under the age of 18. It has been associated with fear of rejection and school phobias. Although this diagnosis would not be made in the emergency department (ED), patients may present with this diagnosis in their history.

6. During the triage process, is there a mnemonic to remind me of the specific questions I should ask about cough?

There are several mnemonics used in triage for history taking. These can be used for any complaint that presents in triage. They are as follows:

PQRST

- **P**rovokes—what provokes the symptoms (better/worse)
- **Q**uality—what does it feel like
- **R**adiation—where is the pain and does it radiate?
- **S**everity—rate it on the pain scale—1 to 10
- **T**ime—how long have you had this? Has it ever happened before?
- **T**reatment—prior to arrival

OLD CART

- **O**nset of symptoms
- **L**ocation of the problem
- **D**uration of symptoms
- **C**haracteristics
- **A**ggravating factors
- **R**elieving factors
- **T**reatment administered before arrival

7. Why is it important to determine when the cough started?

Determining when the cough started will provide information about the duration of the cough and whether it is acute or chronic. It will also provide information on the circumstances surrounding the cough such as:

- Allergens
- Travel
- New medication
- Exposure to infectious disease

8. How should the cough be described?

The following terms are often used to describe a cough:

- Nonproductive—short, dry cough that does not produce sputum
- Productive—loose, longer duration, audible secretions, productive of sputum
- Brassy —nonproductive, hoarse, strident quality
- Wheezy—tight cough with audible wheezing associated with asthma
- Barky cough—described as a "barking seal" and associated with croup
- Whooping cough—a distinctive long and deep cough followed by a quick inhalation causing a whooping sound—associated with Pertussis

9. What other symptoms associated with a cough may help identify the cause of the cough?

Associated symptoms assist in determining the cause of the cough. The following are common symptoms associated with specific etiologies of cough:

- A cough associated with an infectious process will often have accompanying symptoms such as a fever, sore throat, pleuritic chest pain, shortness of breath, nausea/vomiting, and malaise.
- CHF may present with a cough that may or may not be productive of sputum.
- A chronic cough associated with night sweats, weight loss and a history of exposure to tuberculosis or high risk environmental situation for tuberculosis (homeless, prisons, Indian reservations, close living quarters, travel) may be indicative of tuberculosis.
- A cough associated with asthma or an allergic reaction can be tight, with or without wheezing, shortness of breath.
- Patients with end-stage renal disease with the complaint of cough may have cardiac tamponade, congestive heart failure, or fluid overload.
- Hemoptysis can present with lung cancer, tuberculosis, trauma, or infection.
- A cough that usually occurs during the day in the upright position, and is associated with hoarseness, dysphagia, sore throat, heartburn, sour taste, or regurgitation, may be associated with gastric reflux disease (GRD) and micro-aspiration.

10. List some considerations related to the answer about what makes the cough better or worse.

- Is it associated with allergies (environmental, animal, etc.)?
- Positioning—is the cough worse when you lie down versus sitting up?
- Are there environmental irritants at home or in the workplace?
- Is it associated with a new medication?

11. Why should the nurse ask about recent exposure to infectious diseases?

Exposure to an infectious disease, in addition to other signs and symptoms may indicate an infectious process. Questions to ask in triage include:
- Are other family members ill with the same symptoms?
- Do work associates or other close contacts have the same symptoms?
- Does the child attend day care where other children may be ill?
- Is there a travel history to an area with a respiratory epidemic (e.g., China during the SARS infection)?

12. List considerations to include related to treatment prior to arrival.

- Over-the-counter medications
- Prescription medications
- Herbal remedies
- Alternative medication
- Inquire when the treatment was started and the duration. What were the results of the treatment?

13. When a patient reveals he smokes, what else should I ask and why?

Ask someone who smokes (including marijuana and cigar smoking) how many per day and for how many years. Most smokers have a chronic cough—often productive of sputum and usually worse in the morning on rising. Ask if the cough they have now is different from their usual "smoker's cough."

14. If an infant presents to triage with a cough, what should I be concerned about?

Common causes of cough in an infant include the following:
- Aspiration of foreign body
- Obstructed airway
- Congenital malformations
- Respiratory infection

15. What are the common causes of chronic cough in children?

The most common causes of cough in the pediatric population are age-related. In the infant population (birth to 18 months) the most common causes are:
- Cough-variant asthma
- Aberrant innominate artery
- Congenital malformations

Ages 18 months to 6 years:
- Cough-variant asthma
- Sinusitis

Ages 6 years to 16 years:
- Cough-variant asthma
- Psychogenic cough

16. What are some other causes of cough in the pediatric population?

There are many other causes of cough in the pediatric population:

- Postnasal drip
- GERD
- Secondhand smoke/irritants
- Allergies

17. Why should I ask if the child's immunizations are up to date?

When a child presents with a cough, it is important to determine what immunizations the child has received and if they are up to date.

18. What should I do at triage for all patients with a cough?

When patients present at triage, a nursing assessment must be done. It is important to avoid focusing on the one symptom of "cough." A complete assessment will prevent overlooking a potentially life-threatening condition. The triage assessment should be focused, concise, and designed to differentiate and identify high acuity from low acuity patients.

- Primary assessment—evaluate airway, breathing, and circulation (ABCs)
  - Evaluate airway for patency, adequate breathing, and oxygenation (obtain a pulse oximetry reading).
  - Evaluate circulation—ensure there are no signs of shock or altered circulatory status.
  - Apply oxygen if needed.
  - Evaluate level of consciousness.
- Secondary assessment
  - Respiratory Assessment. Listen to breath sounds—do you hear wheezing, rales, rhonchi, tight breath sounds, stridor, etc.? Observe the chest for normal/abnormal movement—is the patient using accessory muscles, is chest wall movement symmetrical? Evaluate the pulse oximetry reading.
  - Cardiac Assessment. Listen to heart tones—evaluate the rate, rhythm, quality. Determine the presence of extra heart sounds, gallop, murmur, or rub.
  - Record Vital Signs
    - Respiratory assessment—record the respiratory rate, quality, pulse oximetry reading
    - Cardiac assessment— record the cardiac rate, quality, regular/irregular, heart tones, presence of murmur, gallop, extra heart sounds, rub
    - Check temperature
  - Record nursing observations
  - Observe for the presence of a rash. If a rash is present, identify the location and pattern of the rash on the body.
    - Prevention of the spread of infectious disease. If there is suspicion of an infectious disease (respiratory infection, common cold, flu, etc.) precautions should be initiated at triage to prevent the spread of infectious disease to staff and other patients.

- A simple surgical mask should be placed over the mouth and nose of every patient who presents with a cough and a possible infectious disease, if they can tolerate it. The use of the mask is very beneficial in preventing the spread of disease to other patients in the waiting room and in the ED.
- Instruct the patient to cover his/her mouth and nose when sneezing or coughing to prevent the spread of respiratory droplets into the air and on surfaces. Tissues should be available to all patients in the triage area.
- Isolate the patient—placing the patient with a suspected infectious disease who is actively coughing in an isolation room can be very effective in preventing the spread of the illness to others in the waiting room.

19. What equipment should be present at the nursing triage station specifically for patients who complain of a cough?

- Mask—surgical (for all patients with a cough or respiratory infection)
- N-95 mask (for use by the ED staff/triage)
- Large facial tissues
- Alcohol-based hand cleaner
- Sink with soap and water
- Trash container
- Gloves
- Oxygen and equipment
- Pulse oximetry
- Surface cleaner approved for hospital surface cleaning
- Isolation room

20. What equipment should be available to patients in the emergency waiting room to prevent the spread of infectious disease?

Patients who are waiting in the waiting room should be instructed to use the available resources that should be available. Providing multiple "stations" with ample tissues, trash container, and hand cleaner, will assist in promoting proper disposal of potentially infectious tissues, trash, and hand cleaning following each use of tissues.

- Facial tissues
- Trash container for the tissues
- Hand cleaner next to the trash container and tissues

Additionally, educational materials such as wall posters can be distributed throughout the emergency waiting area to educate patients on the importance of covering their mouth and nose when sneezing/coughing, hand washing/cleaning, and proper disposal of infectious materials.

21. What tests and diagnostic studies can be ordered in triage to expedite the assessment and treatment of the patient?

You should follow the triage guidelines in your facility regarding the initiation of diagnostic tests in the triage area. However, many EDs have protocols for the triage nurses to order tests to facilitate the assessment and treatment of patients.

The following are common tests ordered in the initial evaluation of the patient with cough, but should be guided by the complete history and accompanying symptoms:

- Chest radiograph—PA & Lateral
- Sputum C&S/Gram stain
- Complete blood cell count
- Blood cultures (two sets in adults, one set in children)
- electrocardiogram (EKG; if CHF, PE suspected)

22. What life-threatening conditions present with the complaint of cough?

- PE
- Obstructed airway
- Acute exacerbation of asthma
- Pericardial tamponade
- CHF
- Pulmonary edema

23. What additional signs and symptoms in addition to cough may signal a severe illness?

A cough can be a presenting symptom of an underlying life-threatening event such as pulmonary edema, acute exacerbation of asthma, PE, or CHF. Any patient presenting to the triage area with the following symptoms should be immediately taken to the treatment area and assessed by the emergency practitioner.

- Shortness of breath (asthma, congestive heart failure, pulmonary embolism)
- Blood in sputum (bronchitis, pneumonia, lung cancer, epistaxis, violent coughing/irritation, PE)
- Chest pain (congestive heart failure, PE, myocardial infarction)
- Pink, frothy sputum (CHF/PE)
- Severe wheezing/dyspnea (asthma, airway obstruction, severe allergic reaction)
- Rash (infectious disease)
- High fever (infectious disease)
- Lethargy or altered level of consciousness (infectious disease, sepsis, shock)
- Abnormal vital signs—high fever, tachypnea, dyspnea, tachycardia, low pulse oximetry readings

24. What complications can occur with severe coughing?

- Hemoptysis
- Chest/rib pain
- Abdominal pain (muscular)
- Vomiting
- Fatigue/sleeplessness
- Incontinence

Key Points

Initial triage goals when evaluating a patient with a cough:

- Identify life-threatening conditions
- Obtain a concise history
- Prevent the spread of infectious disease

Life-threatening conditions associated with a cough:

- PE
- Obstructed airway
- Acute exacerbation of asthma
- Pericardial tamponade
- CHF
- Pulmonary edema
- Angioedema

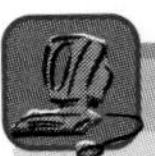

Internet Resources

Iroquois Memorial Hospital Emergency Department Patient Care Standard for

Respiratory Distress
http://www.ena.org/document_share/documents/respiratory_distress.doc

Update on Influenza A (H5N1) and SARS: Interim Recommendations for Enhanced U.S. Surveillance, Testing, and Infection Control
http://www.ena.org/news/CDC-Advisories/UpdateOnInfluenza.asp

Bibliography

Irwin RS, Madison JM: A persistently troublesome cough, *Am J Resp Crit Care Med* 165:1469-1474, 2002.

Irwin RS, Richter JE: Gastroesophageal reflux and chronic cough, *Am J Gastroenterol* 95(8 suppl):S9-S14, 2000.

Lawler WR: An office approach to the diagnosis of chronic cough, *Am Fam Physician* 58:2015-2022, 1998.

Morice AH, Kastelik JA: Chronic cough in adults, *Thorax* 58:901-907, 2003.

Oman KS, Koziol-McLain J, Scheetz L: *Emergency nursing secrets*, Philadelphia, 2001, Hanley & Belfus.

Spiro C: Evaluating chronic cough, *Clin Rev* 13(10):52-57, 2003.

Section IV

Abdominal Complaints

Chapter 29

Nausea and Vomiting

Mary Ellen Wilson and Marylou S. Moeller

1. What is most important to remember with a patient complaint of nausea?

Nausea is a disruptive, preoccupying, and distressful symptom to patients, but it is not a disease condition in itself. Treatment is directed at relieving the cause. Obtain a good history and rule out the worst-case scenario etiology.

2. Should the triage nurse just focus on the gastrointestinal (GI) system?

No. Other common causes of nausea include:

- Infection in another part of body: flu, otitis media
- Pregnancy
- Problems with balance/equilibrium: motion sickness
- Anxiety/psychologic issues
- Certain drugs: antibiotics
- Problems in abdomen: appendicitis
- Systemic conditions: diabetes mellitus, chronic renal failure, cancer

3. What are the key factors to obtain specifically related to nausea/vomiting?

- Associated signs and symptoms. For instance, pain, fever, jaundice, bowel habits, duration, neurologic symptoms, cardiac risk factors, and/or pregnancy
- Relationship of nausea in regard to eating or vomiting
- Food eaten in the previous 6 hours
- Characteristics of the emesis (color/consistency, projectile)

4. Why establish the relationship of the onset of nausea and/or vomiting?

The timing of the onset can be helpful in diagnosing. Generally:

- Pain preceding vomiting is suggestive of a surgical process, whereas vomiting before pain is more typical of a nonsurgical condition.
- Nausea and vomiting that occurs simultaneously with the onset of pain is associated with torsion, ectopic, ureteral colic, or bowel obstruction.
- Epigastric pain relieved by vomiting is more likely to be caused by an intragastric pathology.
- Late onset nausea and vomiting is often seen in infectious processes, as the disease progresses, such as pelvic inflammatory disease (PID).

5. Why should I ask about the timing of the emesis related to eating?

Vomiting that is:
- Soon after a meal is common with gastric outlet obstruction (peptic ulcer disease)
- After a fatty meal is common with cholecystitis
- Food eaten more than 6 hours earlier is common of gastric retention (diabetic gastric paresis)

6. How does the proficient triage nurse determine the degree of urgency?

- Severity of pain
- Number of emesis
- Presence of and degree of dehydration (see Chapter 30)
- Concurrent medical conditions

7. Any specific guidelines?

The Canadian Emergency Department Triage and Acuity Scale (CTAS) lists:
Level 2/Emergent (≤15 minutes)
Lethargy with h/o of vomiting
History of poor feeding
History of vomiting with any signs/symptoms of dehydration
Level 3, Urgent (≤30 minutes)
Any vomiting in a child age <2 years
Level 4, Less Urgent (≤1 hour)
Vomiting without any s/s of dehydration
Age >2 years

8. Compare that with the Manchester Triage Group's guidelines.

In this five-level triage system, any signs of dehydration or presence of persistent vomiting would result in the person placed at triage Level 3 (Urgent, 60 minutes). Vomiting at all or a "recent" (within 1 week) problem makes the person a Level 4 (Standard, 120 minutes).

9. How do the characteristics of the emesis vary depending on the cause?

Vomiting blood is always a concern and "bumps up" the patient to a higher acuity. Coffee ground emesis signals it has been exposed to the digestive juices. In:
- Acute gastritis: vomit is usually stomach contents mixed with a little bile.
- Biliary or ureteral colic: the vomit is usually bilious.
- Sympathetic nervous system involvement, such as acute testicular torsion—the patient with retch frequently but actually vomits only a small amount.
- Intestinal obstruction: the vomit is first gastric contents, then bilious, and then progresses to brown feculent material.

10. What is the most common ailment producing nausea and vomiting?

Gastroenteritis. However, do not let the condition's common presentation lull anyone into complacency. Based on the presenting symptoms, the patient can be urgent.

11. What are the most common agents that produce bacterial food poisoning?

Staphylococcus, Clostridium perfringens, and *Salmonella* species. There is a growing awareness that unsuspected food contamination occurs more often than commonly considered. Imported hot sauce that was not refrigerated after opening, drug-resistant salmonella contaminated ground beef, scallions, and alfalfa sprouts were all identified recently as sources. Food-borne infection can be decreased by up to 50% with good hand washing before food preparation.

12. What is the typical history of symptoms related to food poisoning?

The patient usually has nausea, vomiting, diarrhea, low-grade fever, and crampy abdominal pain. A history suggestive of food poisoning is the presence of similar symptoms in other family members or others who ingested the same food or water, presence of blood in the stools, and recent travel to underdeveloped countries or mountainous regions.

13. Isn't food poisoning harmless?

In one study there was a significant risk of food-borne illness effects (especially *Salmonella* and *Campylobacter*) on longer-term mortality. Some of the longer-term complications included endocarditis, abscesses, vasculitis, intestinal perforation, and complications of surgery. Food poisoning should not be taken lightly, especially in a patient who is already compromised from other factors.

14. What key history factor will rule out the nausea that commonly accompanies a myocardial ischemia?

Absolute distinction is impossible with history alone. An immediate electrocardiogram (EKG) can help distinguish acute myocardial ischemia in patients with cardiac risk factors or history of cardiac ischemia.

15. I know nausea is a common side effect of many drugs. Any other medication consideration with nausea/vomiting?

Rule out digoxin (Lanoxin) toxicity (if appropriate). Although the normal therapeutic range is 0.5 to 2.0 ng/mL, it can be toxic at the high end of normal (1.8 or 1.9), especially for older adult patients. Early signs of digoxin toxicity are anorexia, nausea/vomiting, and weakness. The "classic" signs of bradycardia, yellow/green halos, and confusion are actually late signs of toxicity.

16. What condition would be considered in a pregnant woman of less than 20 weeks' gestation?

Hyperemesis gravidarum.

17. I know an appendicitis presentation often has nausea and vomiting. What else should I look for in the classic scenario?

- Anorexia (70% to 94%)
- Abdominal tenderness (70% to 94%)
- Nausea and vomiting (31% to 69%). The nausea/vomiting will often present before the appendicitis pain.
- Consider in a child who is limping or won't walk
- Consider in scrotal pain without signs of renal colic or other genital complaints

18. What is gastroesophageal reflux disease (GERD)?

Acidic gastric contents that are refluxed into the esophagus cause the classic heartburn. Although it is estimated that 35% to 50% of our population reports some degree of "heartburn," GERD (in comparison) tends to be chronic and relapsing.

19. Why are we concerned about this minor problem?

The reflux acid contributes to esophageal cancer. In addition, there is increasing awareness that it can be aspirated into the trachea. This can cause coughing, chest tightness, and/or wheezing.

20. Can GERD really influence wheezing?

As many as 75% of adults with asthma may also have GERD and several studies have shown a decrease in asthma symptoms when it is properly treated. In another study, 59% of children with asthma also had GERD and greater than 50% had improvement in the asthma symptoms when treated. In addition, it can lead to sleep disturbances.

21. Name some common causes of GERD.

Anything that relaxes the lower esophageal sphincter (LES) or increases the intra-abdominal pressures can result in GERD.

Foods that Relax the Lower Esophageal Sphincter (LES)	Stomach-Irritating Foods	Medicines that Relax the LES*	Medications that Irritate Gastric Mucosa	Others
Chocolate	Citrus fruits	Theophylline	NSAIDs*	Smoking
Peppermint	Spicy foods	Anticholinergics	Tetracycline	Coffee
High-fat foods	Tomatoes	Progesterone	Quinidine	Caffeine
		Calcium channel blockers		Alcohol
		Alpha-adrenergic agents		
		Diazepam		

**LES*, lower esophageal sphincter; *NSAIDs*, nonsteroidal anti-inflammatory drugs.

22. List other causes that contribute to GERD.

Lifestyle, such as obesity, heavy large meals, tight abdominal clothing, and age
Pregnancy (decrease gastric motility and increase gastric acid production)

23. Do infants experience gastric esophageal reflux?

Most definitely; we just tend to refer to them as "wet burps." It usually recedes by the age of 9 months. Concern is warranted if there is poor growth, weight loss, or a refusal to eat.

24. Tell me symptoms of gastric esophageal reflux in infants and children.

INFANTS	CHILDREN
Spitting up	Heartburn
Vomiting	Frequent chest or abdominal pain
Coughing	Regurgitating and belching acid
Irritability	Sour or bitter taste in the mouth
Blood in stools	Salty tasting saliva
	Hoarseness
	Sore throat
	Coughing

25. Discuss the difference in vomiting between children and adults.

Children have a lower vomiting threshold and will dehydrate more quickly. Telephone triage author Valerie Grossman indicates immediate care is needed if there is persistent vomiting for more than:

- 18 hours in patients older than 6 years
- 12 hours in children less than 6 years
- 8 hours since the last void

26. I do phone triage. When do I encourage the home use of ipecac for children?

The American Academy of Pediatrics (AAP) no longer recommends keeping a home supply of syrup of ipecac to induce vomiting in children who have ingested poisonous substances. It should only be administered on the advice of a physician or poison control center (800-222-1222). It is not effective in removing harmful substances from the stomach, was being used inappropriately, can lead to lethargy, and can compromise diagnosis and treatment.

27. Are there any anti-emetics that are appropriate to give at triage?

Depending on the patient's symptoms and standing orders, promethazine hydrochloride (Phenergan) is a relatively low risk drug to give at triage.

28. Give an example of a standing order for nausea/vomiting.

Memorial Regional Hospital in Hollywood, Fla
Source: Melinda Stibal, RN BSHC, ED/Trauma Administrative Director
Phenergan 12.5 mg intravenous (IV) every 30 minutes × 2 p.r.n. for nausea
If severe vomiting or dehydration:

- Complete blood cell count, SMA_7
- Urine pregnancy (for all premenopausal women)
- Saline lock

29. List some home care instructions for children with nausea/vomiting.

Infants:

- 1 teaspoon Pedialyte (Lytren, Infalyte, KAO-Lectrolte) every 5 minutes and increase as tolerated.
- If the infant drinks juice, introduce 1 teaspoon every 5 minutes. Do not give juice if diarrhea is present.
- If breast feeding, and infant vomits 3 or more times, offer breast for 4 to 5 minutes every 30 to 60 minutes, and offer rehydration fluids between breast feeds of 1 teaspoon every 5 to 15 minutes.

Children:

- Avoid eating or drinking for 1 to 2 hours after vomiting
- Drink 1 tablespoon every 5 minutes for 4 hours (fruit juice diluted with water, weak tea with sugar, clear broth, gelatin, flavored ice. After 4 hours without vomiting, the amount of fluids offered may increase.

- Avoid milk for 12 to 24 hours after vomiting subsides.
- Slowly introduce the BRATT diet (banana, rice, applesauce, tea, toast) and then normal foods.

30. What are some of the more common home remedies?

- Saltine crackers, hard candy, bread, tea and ginger, and carbonated soda pop. The carbonation ("fizz") should be allowed to dissipate as the bubbles irritate the GI system.
- The ten most commonly used herbal preparations used are ginger, chamomile, lavender, cinnamon, garlic, cola-nut drinks, peppermint/spearmint, cloves, nutmeg, and sweet fennel.
- Acupressure. Based on the acupuncture concept of "life energy" flowing along meridians, pressure on specific areas releases the blockages through specific stimulation. For nausea:
  - Press about one third of the way down from the shoulder to the elbow, at the bottom of the deltoid muscle.
  - Press three finger-widths up the arm from the wrist crease on both the palm side and backside of the forearm.

Key Points

- History is important: Ask accompanying signs/symptoms, frequency, characteristics, and s/s of dehydration.
- Pain before vomiting suggests a surgical process; vomiting before pain is more typical of a nonsurgical condition.
- Digoxin toxicity (at a high level of the "normal range" in the older adult) can cause nausea and vomiting (like the "flu").

Bibliography

Armenteros R: Acupress: *The pain relief of acupuncture without the needle,* Harbor Press, 1996, Thera Research Consultants.

Beckman JS: Food poisoning. In Markovchick VJ, Pons PT, editors: *Pons' emergency medicine secrets,* ed 3, Philadelphia, 2001, Hanley & Belfus.

Blum R, et al: *Nausea and vomiting: Overview, challenges, practical treatments and new perspectives,* Philadelphia, 2000, Whurr Publishers Ltd.

Briggs JK: *Telephone triage protocols for nurses,* ed 2, Philadelphia, 2002, Lippincott, Williams & Wilkins.

Canadian Emergency Department Triage and Acuity Scale Implementation Guidelines, *J Can Assoc Emerg Physicians* 1:3, Oct 1999.

Char E, Wong J: Abdominal pain. In Davis MA, Votey SR, Greenough PJ, editors: *Greenough's signs and symptoms in emergency medicine: Literature-based approach to emergency conditions,* St Louis, 1999, Mosby.

Dahlberg NP, et al: Differential diagnosis of abdominal pain in women of childbearing age, *Adv Nurse Pract* 12(1):40-45, 2004.

Grossman VGA: *Quick reference to triage*, ed 2, Philadelphia, 2003, Lippincott, Williams & Wilkins.

Helms M, et al: Short and long-term mortality associated with food-borne bacterial gastrointestinal infections: Registry based study, *BMJ* 325:357-359, 2003.

Jordan K, editor: *Emergency nursing core curriculum*, ed 5, Philadelphia, 2000, WB Saunders.

Karp J: Nausea and vomiting. In Markovchick VJ, Pons PT, editors. *Pons' emergency medicine secrets*, ed 3, Philadelphia, 2003, Hanley & Belfus.

Khoshoo V, Le T, Haydel RM Jr, Landry L, Nelson C: Role of gastroesophageal reflux in older children with persistent asthma, *Chest* 123(4):1008-1013, 2003.

Mackway-Jones K: *Emergency triage, Manchester Triage Group*, London, 1997, BMJ Publishing Group.

Moble-Boetani JC, et al: *Escherichia coli* 0157 and *Salmonella* infections associated with sprouts in California, 1996-1998, *Ann Intern Med* 21(135):239-247, 2001.

Moellman JJ, Bocock JM: Acute pelvic pain. In Hamilton GC, Sanders AB, Strange GR, Trott AT, editors: *Trott's emergency medicine: An approach to clinical problem-solving*, ed 2, St Louis, 2003, WB Saunders.

Newberry L, editor: *Sheehy's emergency nursing principles and practice*, ed 5, St Louis, 2003, Mosby.

Outbreak of multi-drug resistant *Salmonella*, Newport—United States, January-April 2002, *MMWR* 28(51):545-548, 2002.

Purcell TB: Abdominal pain. In Markovchick VJ, Pons PT, editors: *Pons' emergency medicine secrets*, ed 3, Philadelphia, 2003, Hanley & Belfus.

Chapter 30

Diarrhea and Dehydration

Polly Gerber Zimmermann

1. What is essential to ask in the history of someone with diarrhea?

- Frequency and amount
- Characteristics and consistency of stool
- Presence of blood in stool (bright red, black tarry)
- Recent food (and fluid) ingestion
- Previous abdominal surgeries
- Antibiotic use
- Pets at home
- Nocturnal symptoms (rare with functional disease)
- Presence of vomiting
- The risk of dehydration is always higher if there is vomiting *and* diarrhea.

2. Name something besides digested blood that causes stool to turn black.

- Bismuth from Pepto-Bismol
- Ferrous sulfate (iron)

3. Define "mild-to-moderate" diarrhea.

Five or fewer unformed stools a day without fever, blood, significant cramps, pain, nausea, or vomiting.

4. Apply some objective criteria for "frequent" diarrhea to triage categories.

The Canadian Emergency Department Triage and Acuity Scale (CTAS) defines "frequent vomiting or stools" as either ten or more episodes vomiting in the previous 24 hours or five or more bowel movements per day for 2 or more days. If signs of dehydration are present the person should be a Level 2 (≤15 minutes) and a Level 3 (≤30 minutes) if there are no signs of dehydration.

5. Any other definitions?

Julie K Briggs' Telephone Triage Protocols book (2002) defines it as:

- An adult with diarrhea for >5 days or every 30 to 60 minutes for >6 hours should seek medical care within 24 hours.

- A child with diarrhea every hour for >8 hours or >3 diarrhea stools in 24 hours in a child younger than 1 month should seek medical care within 2 to 4 hours.
- A child with diarrhea for >3 days or diarrhea although receiving antibiotic therapy should seek medical care within 24 hours.

Valerie Grossman's book on telephone triage indicates immediate care should be taken if there is persistent vomiting or profuse diarrhea more than:
- 18 hours in patients older than 6 years of age
- 12 hours in children less than 6 years of age
- 8 hours since the last void

6. What helps to rule-out or rule-in "food poisoning"?

- Presence of similar symptoms in other family members or others who ingested the same food or water
- Recent travel to underdeveloped countries or to mountainous regions

7. Define gastroenteritis.

The majority (60%) of gastroenteritis is viral and the enterotoxins produced affect the adenosine monophosphate pump on the gut mucosa. True gastroenteritis has watery diarrhea (with hyperactive bowel sounds) and is usually self-limiting. There is often an accompanying mild, crampy lower abdominal pain that improves with defecation.

8. How about diarrhea from a bacterial infection?

Bacterial infections, such as the three most common examples of *Shigella, Campylobacter,* or *Salmonella,* are responsible for about 20% of the "gastroenteritis." Antibiotics are usually not needed. Some initial differentiations include:
- The patient is more toxic looking.
- There is bloody, mucoid stool (because they invade the mucosa).
- There is a history of oral-fecal contamination (meat, poultry, raw eggs). In addition, chicks, turtles, and rodents carry salmonella.

9. When would I suspect diarrhea is caused from *Clostridium difficile*?

C. difficile is the most common cause of nosocomial infectious diarrhea. The toxins are produced that damage the mucosal lining. Untreated, it leads to pseudomembranous colitis. The risk factors are hospitalization, surgery, and recent (defined at within 8 weeks) antibiotics. The stool's overpowering foul smell is the tip-off for most nurses. Classic signs and symptoms include:
- Frequent (six or more watery stools/36 hours) watery stool
- "Barn odor"
- Green to grossly bloody stool
- Fever
- Abdominal pain

10. Discuss "traveler's diarrhea."

Also known as Montezuma's revenge, diarrhea while traveling in underdeveloped countries is usually caused by enterotoxigenic *Escherichia coli.* Besides fluid replacement, treatment can include bismuth subsalicylate (Pepto-Bismol) to help reduce the number of unformed stools by 50% or loperamide (Imodium), which reduces diarrhea by 80%. Pepto-Bismol can be taken prophylactically (two tablets four times daily) but should not be taken by patients on anticoagulants, salicylates, or who have an allergy to salicylates.

11. What is the difference between fluid volume deficit and dehydration?

Fluid volume deficit (FVD) results when water and electrolytes are lost in an isotonic fashion. Dehydration refers to a loss of water alone (leaving the patient with a sodium excess). However, in practice, the terms are often used interchangeably.

12. Talk about signs of mild FVD.

Mild (3% to 5%) symptoms are mild tachycardia and thirst. An aviation industry "secret" is that another early sign of dehydration is fatigue. Because you lose 8 ounces of water for every hour of flight, airline flight personnel have learned to drink plenty of fluids.

13. Describe the signs of moderate FVD (5% to 10%) for children.

- Weight (1 lb equals 500 mL)
- Sunken anterior fontanel
- No tears
- Capillary refill more than 2 to 3 seconds
- Dry mucous membranes
- Skin turgor
- Decrease in the number of diapers/amout of voiding

Children must lose at least 25% of their fluid volume to have hypotension as a result of their ability to vasoconstrict.

14. Which indicator is the most sensitive for fluid balance in any patient?

Weight

15. Discuss assessing skin turgor.

In a healthy person, pinched skin will immediately fall back to its normal position when released. The skin in patients with FVD may remain elevated for several seconds, or at least flatten more slowly. Skin turgor begins to diminish in children after 3% to 5% of the body weight is lost, but it can also be affected by the child's nutritional state, race, or complexion. It is most useful when it is used as a sequential assessment.

16. Where is the best location to assess skin turgor?

Alterations in skin elasticity are less marked in the sternum, inner aspect of the thighs, or the forehead. In children, the abdominal area or medial aspects of the thighs are also used. However, regardless of location, skin turgor has limited value in persons older than 55 to 60 years as a result of age-related decrease in skin elasticity.

17. How helpful is it to depend on sunken eyes as an assessment?

Sunken eyes (as a result of decreased intraocular fluid) are a valid indicator in all ages. However, this sign is not present until severe fluid and electrolyte deficiency occurs (> 10%).

18. Any guidelines available for triage levels related to FVD?

The CTAS lists:

Level 2/Emergent (≤15 minutes)

- Lethargy
- History of poor feeding
- History of diarrhea/vomiting with any signs/symptoms (s/s) of dehydration
- Less than six wet diapers/day or no urine for >6 to 8 hours
- No urine for >12 hours in older children

Level 3, Urgent (≤30 minutes)

- Any vomiting/diarrhea in any child age <2

Level 4, Less Urgent (≤1 hour)

- Vomiting and/or diarrhea present but
- No s/s dehydration
- Age >2 years

19. Compare that with the Manchester Triage Group's guidelines.

Any signs of dehydration or presence of persistent vomiting result is the person being triaged at Level 3 (Urgent, 60 minutes). Vomiting at all or a "recent" (within 1 week) problem makes the person a Level 4 (Standard, 120 minutes).

20. Any other objective criteria?

Julie Briggs (2002) prescribes for telephone triage that a child should seek medical care within 2 to 4 hours if:

- No urine for >8 hours in child younger than 1 year
- No urine >12 hours in child older than 1 year
- Crying without tears

21. Tell me how to assess for moderate (5% to 10%) FVD in an adult.

- Tongue furrows

- Mucous membranes—if the patient is a mouth breather, look where the gum and mucous membranes meet; that remains moist in hydrated individuals regardless of the breathing pattern
- Tachycardia—defined as an increase in the heart rate of ≥15 to 20 beats or above 120 beats per minute; an increase in the normal heart rate of >30 is a very specific indication for dehydration
- Systolic blood pressure falls >25 mm Hg and diastolic falls by >10 mm Hg
- Vein filling
- Orthostatic vital sign changes

The adult must have a fluid volume deficit of 1,500 mL before exhibiting hypotension.

22. Describe how to use tongue furrows as a part of the assessment.

Tongue furrows are unaffected by mouth breathing or age. In a healthy person, the tongue has one longitudinal furrow. With a fluid volume deficit, additional longitudinal furrows are noted and the tongue is smaller (as a result of fluid loss).

23. Discuss using "vein filling" or jugular vein assessment.

Changes in fluid volume are reliably reflected in the filling of the jugular neck veins, provided the assessment is done correctly and the patient is not in heart failure. Use the right side because the right internal jugular vein is nearly a direct conduit to the right atrium. The left internal jugular vein, in comparison, can have the brachycephalic vein compressed by the aortic knob, which results in false elevation.

Position the patient at a 45-degree angle: the venous distention should not extend higher than 2 cm above the sternal angle. Flat neck veins indicate a decreased plasma volume. Neck veins distended to the angle of the jaw indicate elevated venous pressure.

24. Any other related test to vein filling?

The rate and degree of filling of the small veins in the foot can be a sensitive test for the older adult, if they do not have peripheral vascular disease or cardiac failure. A dorsal foot vein can be occluded by finger pressure at a distal point and emptied of its blood by stroking proximally with another finger. In a well-hydrated patient, the vein will fill instantly when the pressure is released. In a volume-depleted patient, the vein will fill slowly, over a period longer than 3 seconds.

25. How do you take orthostatic vital signs?

Sources vary but an increase of 10 to 20 beats in pulse and a decrease of 10 to 20 in the systolic blood pressure reading with position change from lying to standing (waiting at least 1 minute between position changes) is considered positive. This is because the body is already maximally compensated with vasoconstriction for the dehydration.

26. Are positive orthostatic vital signs always an accurate indication of fluid volume deficit or dehydration?

One study found that a blood pressure drop of 20 mm Hg was only 29% sensitivity and 81% specific for ≥5% fluid deficit. In normal hydrated patients ≥65 years, there were false positive orthostatic vital signs >25% of the time. Consider the results more reliable if the patient is also experiencing other symptoms, such as a sensation of thirst, dizziness (especially immediately after a position change), and/or parched mucous membranes.

27. What else, besides age, could affect orthostatic readings?

Medications. They include antihypertensives (alpha-adrenergic blockers, beta blockers, calcium channel blockers), aminoglycosides, anticonvulsants, tranquilizers, and vasodilators.

28. Is there any other simple test I could do to further explore a patient's hydration status?

An early sign of dehydration (and dementia) is the decreased ability to focus. Ask the client to name as many fruits or colors or animals as possible within 1 minute. The person should be able to name at least 15. An alternative version is to name the days of the week backwards.

29. Talk about geriatric considerations regarding fluid balance.

The elderly are at a particular risk because of the physiologic changes associated with aging. These include a decrease in total body water (6%), thirst sensation, glomerular filtration (46% by age 90), and ability to concentrate the urine. As a result, the elderly are less able to respond to stresses and fluid and electrolyte alteration frequently accompany acute illness.

30. What is one of the best indications in the history of an older adult person's recent fluid intake?

Their recent food intake.

31. Why is FVD so concerning in hospitalized geriatric patients?

Dehydration was one of the four independent baseline risk factors for development of delirium in hospitalized elders. (Vision impairment, severe illness, and cognitive impairments were the other three.) In one study, 25% of the medical patients aged 70 or older developed delirium during their hospital stay.

32. What labs should I consider to help determine fluid volume deficit/dehydration?

- Elevated blood urea nitrogen and the blood urea nitrogen (BUN)/Creatinine (CR) ratio >18:1.

- Elevated hematocrit (if there has been no blood loss).
- Elevated urine specific gravity and ketones.

33. Give some considerations about the urine specimen for specific gravity.

Fresh urine specimens at room temperature are best. Refrigerated samples may have a false reading. In addition, heavy molecules, such as the presence of glucose, albumin, or radio-contrast dye, will cause a false specific gravity elevation.

34. What would I expect for a specific gravity in a volume-depleted patient who has healthy kidneys?

A urine specific gravity (SG) of more than 1.020. The person should be "holding"/conserving fluid to keep the urine adequately dilute and below that number. Urine ketones of 2+ or greater suggest a starvation ketosis.

35. Explain the BUN/Cr ratio.

Normally the BUN/Cr ratio is approximately 10:1. If the ratio increases in favor of the BUN, hypovolemia may be present. If both the BUN and Cr levels rise (with the 10:1 ratio intact), the problem is more likely intrinsic renal disease, although it may also be seen when fluid volume depletion results in reduction in the glomerular filtration rate.

36. Is parenteral fluid replacement always the best treatment for dehydrated pediatric patients?

No, enteral rehydration is the best, especially if the dehydration is mild. It is the most similar to the way fluids are normally processed. Researchers did a meta-analysis of 16 studies that rehydrated children with gastroenteritis through nasogastric/enteral means. The children who received enteral rehydration had significantly briefer hospital stays and the weight gain at discharge was similar to the children who had intravenous (IV) hydration.

37. What about moderate/severe FVD?

Adults can be rehydrated with a rapid infusion of IV 0.9% NaCl or LR solution 1 to 2 liters per hour (if there is normal kidney and cardiovascular function). Children are rehydrated with an initial infusion of 20 mg/kg.

38. Is using Jell-O mixed in water or sports drinks recommended for infants?

No. These do not contain enough sodium and the sugar content can make diarrhea worse.

39. I work at a clinic. How should I handle requests for antidiarrheal medications?

Diarrhea is the body's natural way of getting rid of toxins. Don't stop it immediately. If it persists more than 6 hours and/or you are concerned about dehydration, then medication can be added. Use a bulk, absorbant laxative, such as Metamucil (ground psyllium seeds). It absorbs water in the gut lumen. To absorb toxins and provide some binding effects, add over-the-counter antidiarrheal medications, such as Amphojel, Kaopectate, and Pepto-Bismol.

Key Points

- Tongue furrows are unaffected by mouth breathing. There will be additional longitudinal furrows if the person is dehydrated.
- A pulse of ≥120 beats per minute (bpm) is highly indicative of dehydration.
- FVD is indicated by urine SG higher than 1.020 and/or a BUN/Cr ratio >18:1.
- After diarrhea of 6 hours, use a bulk absorbant laxative (to absorb water) and Pepto-Bismol to absorb toxins.
- Do not use Jell-O water to rehydrate children.

Internet Resources

Canadian Association of Emergency Physicians
www.caep.ca

Emergency Medicine Journal Online
www.emj.bmjjournals.com

Bibliography

Briggs JK: *Telephone triage protocols for nurses,* ed 2, Philadelphia, 2002, Lippincott.

Buttaravoli P, Stair T: *Minor emergencies: Splinters to fractures,* St Louis, 2000, Mosby.

Canadian Emergency Department Triage and Acuity Scale Implementation Guidelines, *J Can Assoc Emerg Physicians* 1:3, 1999.

Decastro J: Age-related changes in natural spontaneous fluid ingestion and thirst in humans, *J Gerontol* 47:321, 1992.

Grossman VGA: *Quick reference to triage,* ed 2, Philadelphia, 2003, Lippincott.

Inouye S, Viscoli C, Horwitz R, Hurst L, Tinetti M: A predictive model for delirium in hospitalized elderly medical patients based on admission characteristics, *Ann Intern Med* 119:474, 1993.

Mackway-Jones K: *Emergency triage: Manchester Triage Group,* London, 1997, BMJ Publishing Group.

Mentes J, Buckwalter K: Getting back to basics: Maintaining hydration to prevent acute confusion in frail elderly, *J Gerontol Nursing* 23(10):48-51, 1997.

Metheny N: *Fluid and electrolyte balance: Nursing considerations,* ed 4, Philadelphia, 2000, Lippincott.

Chapter 31

Acute Abdomen and Peritonitis

Polly Gerber Zimmermann

1. What is peritonitis?

Peritonitis is a chemical or bacterial invasion from infection or perforation into the normal sterile peritoneal cavity with a resulting inflammatory response that can lead to death.

2. Why do some patients have a localized pain and some have a generalized pain?

It will depend on the cause and the current progression of the condition. Initially the patient is likely to have visceral pain (deep, dull, poorly localized). As the inflammation progresses to the parietal peritoneum, the pain becomes better localized to the involved organs. The sharp, constant, intense (somatic) pain is sometimes referred to as localized peritonitis. One female patient described the sensation as "worse than having a baby." Visceral pain superseded by somatic pain often signals a need for surgical intervention.

When there is perforation, 70% to 94% have a severe sudden localized onset, then a brief period of being pain free, followed by a gradual generalized worsening of the pain. The perforation releases pressure and provides the temporary "improvement" until the more global response of the entire peritoneal surface becomes sensitive from the irritating material. This is referred to as generalized peritonitis. Always suspect peritonitis if a pain becomes generalized after it was well localized.

3. List some factors that may affect the classic patterns.

- Children are less likely to localize intra-abdominally, and serious pathology is usually diffuse with generalized peritonitis.
- Older adults are more likely to have an atypical presentation as a result of their age-related depressed immune system.
- Patients with type II diabetes mellitus may have muted pain as a result of neuropathy.
- Any medication (such as steroids, recent chemotherapy) or co-morbidity (such as human immunodeficiency virus [HIV+]) that suppresses the immune system can blunt the presentation.

4. Children are so hard to assess. Any tips?

Ask the child to point to where it hurts. If they point to the navel and look well, it is probably psychogenic and nothing serious. If the child points anywhere besides the navel and looks ill, explore further. For further discussion, see Chapter 11.

5. Discuss causes of peritonitis.

The etiology of peritonitis can be a result of anything that causes an infection, perforation, or chemical irritation. Examples include:

- Pancreatitis, with its bloody exudate from the self-digesting pancreas
- Perforated gastric ulcer
- Ruptured ovarian cyst
- Diverticulitis
- Penetrating abdominal trauma
- Infection from peritoneal dialysis

6. How can the triage nurse determine the cause of a patient's suspected peritonitis?

The triage nurse doesn't determine the cause of possible peritonitis. All that matters is that the patient has an "acute abdomen" and needs emergent or urgent definitive care.

7. List some classic signs or symptoms to signal an "acute abdomen."

- *"Boardlike" or rigid abdomen (31% to 69%).* The abdomen is firm or hard to palpation from the muscle spasms as a result of the irritant.
- *Position.* The person's automatic position of comfort is to lie rigidly still or assume a fetal position. Both positions minimize the movement of the muscles and lessen the irritated peritoneum. A rule-of-thumb: if someone with abdominal pain appears well and/or comfortable and moves easily, the person probably does not have peritonitis.
- *Right Shoulder Tip Pain.* Any abdominal pain with right shoulder tip pain could be the free air from the perforation irritating the phrenic nerve in the diaphragm.

In addition, look for indications of an acute infection (fever, malaise) or shock (rapid pulse, decrease in blood pressure).

8. How about vomiting?

The general guideline is pain that precedes vomiting is suggestive of a surgical process, whereas vomiting before pain is more typical of a nonsurgical condition. Typically anorexia, nausea, and vomiting are directly proportional to the severity and extent of peritoneal irritation.

9. Which vital sign is associated most closely with the degree of peritonitis?

Tachycardia. The initial pulse is less important than serial observations. As the condition progresses, there will be more third spacing with hypotonic/absent bowel sounds and signs of shock.

10. What are some general guidelines in evaluating the severity of abdominal pain from the Canadian Emergency Department Triage and Acuity Scale?

The *Canadian Emergency Department Triage and Acuity Scale (CTAS)* gives these guidelines for their five-tier triage system:

Level 1 (immediate):	Shock states
Level 2 (≤15 minutes):	Acute onset Over age 50 with visceral abdominal pain Associated signs and symptoms Abnormal vital signs
Level 3 (≤30 minutes):	Crampy, intermittent, or sharp brief pains No associated signs and symptoms Normal vital signs Abdominal trauma (even if mild discomfort)
Level 2 (≤1 hour):	Moderate abdominal pain (4 to 7 on a 0 to 10 scale) Normal vital signs
Level 1 (≤2 hours):	Mild abdominal pain (<4 on a 0 to 10 scale) Chronic, recurring Normal vital signs

11. Give me the guidelines from the Manchester Triage Group.

The Manchester Triage Group's Emergency Triage placements:

Level 1 (immediate):	"Life-threat," such as shock
Level 2 (very urgent, target time 10 minutes):	Severe abdominal pain Pain radiating to the back
Level 3 (urgent, target time 60 minutes):	Moderate abdominal pain Presence of shoulder tip pain
Level 4 (standard, target time 120 minutes):	Mild abdominal pain Any history of a "recent problem"
Level 5 (not urgent, target time 240 minutes):	Mild abdominal pain No history of a "recent problem"

"Recent" is defined as within 1 week. For further discussion of these systems, see the section of five-tier triage systems.

12. Name some classic physical assessments I can do to help make the determination.

All of these positive physical assessments are a result of the irritated peritoneum.

- *Positive rebound tenderness (Blumberg's sign):* Normally there is more discomfort when pressing inward on the abdomen, with relief on releasing the pressure. With rebound tenderness the discomfort is worse when the hand is lifted, rather than during the direct pressure. In addition, there will be tensing ("guarding") with palpation.
- *Kehr's sign:* Abdominal pain accompanied by left shoulder tip pain.
- *Rovsing's sign:* Palpation of the left lower quadrant results in pain in the right lower quadrant.
- *Hop test:* Hopping on one foot intensifies the pain. A similar version is the heel jar/Markle test. The patient stands on the tiptoes with knees straight and forcibly drops both heels to the floor. If the patient is unable to perform this action, the practitioner can hit a hand against the patient's heel.

13. Will anything else work for assessing someone who is in obvious distress? These seem harsh if you know the patient is already wincing.

Ask the patient to cough. This generally supplies adequate peritoneal motion to give a positive test.

14. Is it essential to withhold all analgesics until a firm diagnosis is made?

This is one of the "rules" that is changing. Some studies show controlling the pain with morphine did not have deleterious effects on preoperative diagnostic accuracy (Pace and Burke, 1996; Thomas et al, 2003; Vermeulen et al, 1999). Three major specialty organizations recommend changing the practice of routinely withholding analgesia during the diagnostic work-up. In addition, a more comfortable patient is able to cooperate better with the examination. Just be sure that there has been a surgical consult and any necessary consent forms are signed first.

15. Tell me these organizations' recommendations.

- The 2004 American Pain Society (APS) guidelines state pain should be treated as the investigation proceeds and withholding all analgesia is rarely justified.
- The American College of Emergency Physicians' (ACEP) clinical policy statement (1999) encourages early pain relief in stable patients with nontraumatic acute abdominal pain.
- The Canadian Association of Emergency Physicians' (1994) consensus statement indicates that there is "no justification to not relieve the (abdominal) pain immediately. Judicious IV opioid titration used to relieve most of the pain but not leave the patient somnolent is not only humane but, in fact, allows a better abdominal examination."

16. Are there any other conditions that could mimic peritonitis?

- *Diabetic ketoacidosis (DKA):* DKA is the first manifestation in 20% to 30% of the new cases of type 1 diabetes mellitus. Type 1 is probably caused by a virus in susceptible individuals (ask about a history of flu in the previous weeks) so there is sudden onset of this new condition. The accumulating acid causing the abdominal pain is often why treatment was sought. NOTE: For a quick rule-out: check for high blood glucose, ketones in the urine, and note if any Kussmaul respirations.

- *Black Widow (Latrodectus) Spider Bite:* The black widow spider's bite is neurotoxic. Within 30 minutes to 2 hours after the bite, severe local muscle pain and spasms begin. It progresses to the abdomen with muscle fasciculations in 3 to 4 hours after the bite. NOTE: For a quick rule-out: ask about a history of a recent exposure. Black widow spiders reside in dark, cool places, particularly woodpiles.

Key Points

- The hop/heel jar test/Markle test is sensitive for peritoneal/lower abdominal pathology.
- Have the patient cough, instead of palpating for rebound tenderness, if the patient is in severe discomfort.
- Serial tachycardia is the most indicative vital sign for worsening peritonitis.
- It is no longer a "rule" that analgesics must always be held during the diagnostic work-up.

Internet Resources

Canadian Association of Emergency Physicians
www.caep.ca

British Medical Journals
www.bmj.bmjjournals.com

American Pain Society
http://www.ampainsoc.org/

American College of Emergency Physicians
http://www.acep.org/

Bibliography

American Pain Society: *Principles of analgesic use in the treatment of acute pain and cancer pain,* ed 5, Glenview, Ill, 2004, American Pain Society.

Bickley LS, Hoekelman RA: *Bates' pocket guide to physical examination and history taking,* ed 3, Philadelphia, 2000, Lippincott.

Canadian Association of Emergency Physicians: *Canadian Emergency Department Triage and Acuity Scale: Implementation guidelines,* 1(3 suppl), 1999.

Char E, Wong J: Abdominal pain. In Davis MA, Votey SR, Greenough PG, editors: *Greenough's signs and symptoms in emergency medicine: Literature-based approach to emergent conditions,* St Louis, 1999, Mosby, 1-22.

Mackway-Jones K: *Emergency triage: Manchester Triage Group,* London, 1997, BMJ Publishing Group.

Pace S, Burke TF: Intravenous morphine for early pain relief in patients, with acute abdominal pain, *J Acad Emerg Med* 3:1086-1092, 1996.

Pasero C: Pain in the emergency department: Withholding pain medication is not justified, *Am J Nurs* 103(7):73-74, 2003.

Purcell TB: Abdominal pain. In Markovchick VJ, Pons PT: *Pons' emergency medicine secrets,* ed 3, Philadelphia, 2003, Hanley & Belfus, 54-57.

Seidel HM, Ball JW, Dains JE, Benedict GW: *Mosby's physical examination handbook,* ed 4, St Louis, 1999, Mosby.

Thomas SH, William S, Cheema F, et al: Effects of morphine analgesia on diagnostic accuracy in emergency department patients with abdominal pain: A prospective, randomized trial, *J Am Coll Surg* 196(1):18-31, 2003.

Vermeulen B, Morabia A, Unger PF, et al: Acute appendicitis: Influence of early pain relief on the accuracy of clinical and US findings in the decision to operate—a randomized trial, *Radiology* 210(3):639-643, 1999.

Zimmermann PG: Tips to manage pain more effectively, *J Emerg Nurs* 30(5):470-472, 2004.

Zimmermann PG: Triaging lower abdominal pain, *RN* 65(12):52-58, 2002.

Chapter 32

Upper Abdominal Presentations

Darcy Egging

1. How common is the complaint of abdominal pain?

Annually there are nearly 5 million patients who present to emergency departments (EDs) across the country with the complaint of abdominal pain. Approximately 30% of these patients will not have a specific diagnosis when they leave the ED.

2. What major organs are located in the upper abdomen?

Characteristic location of abdominal pain

Right Upper Quadrant	Left Upper Quadrant
Gallbladder and biliary tract	Gastritis
Hepatitis	Diverticulitis
Hepatic abscess	Pancreatitis
Peptic ulcer	Splenic: enlargement, rupture, infarction, aneurysm
Pancreatitis	Renal pain
Retrocecal appendicitis	Herpes zoster
Renal pain	Myocardial ischemia
Herpes zoster	Pneumonia
Myocardial ischemia	
Pericarditis	
Pneumonia	

3. What information should be obtained while triaging a patient with abdominal pain?

As with all triage, identify any airway-breathing-circulation-disability (ABCD) threat, and then proceed in a systematic approach to avoid missing key elements. Associated symptoms to ask are included in the following table:

Description of Pain	Associated Symptoms
Provoking factors (what makes it better or worse?)	Fever
Quality of pain (dull, sharp, burning, intermittent, constant)	Anorexia
Region/radiation	Nausea, vomiting, diarrhea, constipation
Severity of pain (0 to 10)	Chest pain
Time (onset, duration)	Difficulty breathing
Treatment (what has the patient tried at home to alleviate the pain?)	Genitourinary symptoms
	Menstrual history

Specific questions could include:

- When did the patient last eat and what did they eat?
- Does food help or hurt?
- The number, quality, and quantity of each emesis or diarrheal stool.

4. What should I look for in a patient with right upper quadrant pain?

- Is the pain constant or intermittent? When did it start?
- What were they doing when the pain started?

Consider gallbladder problem if after eating (especially a fatty meal), lasts 15 minutes to hours, and is an acute, colicky, severe pain (70% to 94%).

Triage five-tier system: 3

Triage three-tier system: urgent

5. What are other symptoms that would make me suspect gallbladder disease?

Other common co-existing symptoms include:

- Pain radiating to the right shoulder/subscapular
- Nausea/vomiting (31% to 69%)
- Jaundice (if the obstruction causes the bilirubin to rise 3× the normal)
- Some of the "Fs" (fat, forty fair, fertile, female, flatulent)

Gallbladder disease is often associated with dehydration (dieting, nothing by mouth [NPO] from surgery, etc.).

6. Can children have acute gallbladder disease?

Although not a typical presentation, children as young as 2 months have had gallbladder disease. There is a rising incidence in adolescent girls. Children at high risk are those with hemolytic diseases, a history of parenteral nutrition, pregnant adolescents, morbid obesity, cystic fibrosis, and a family history.

7. What physical assessment techniques help assess gallbladder disease?

Murphy's sign. A positive sign when palpating the liver's edge, underneath the right costal margin, is a sharp increase in the tenderness with a sudden stop ("arrest") of respiration/inspiratory effort. The fingertips are irritating the inflamed (normally not palpable) gallbladder. See also Chapter 33.

8. What should I consider with severe left upper quadrant pain?

Pain from pancreatitis is left upper quadrant (LUQ) or epigastric (70% to 94%) and/or radiates to the back (6% to 30%) as a result of the retroperitoneal location. Ask the patient about the two leading causes, alcohol intake and a history of cholelithiasis gallbladder stones (70% of the cases).
Triage category in five-tier system: 2 or 3 depending on pain levels and vital signs
Triage category in three-tier system: emergent or urgent depending on the vital signs

9. List other symptoms of pancreatitis.

- The pain is sudden, sharp, "boreing," severe, intense. (Many times the initial impression is biliary colic.)
- The pain improves if the patient sits up and leans forward.
- Severely nauseated/usually vomiting (70% to 94%)
- Abdominal tenderness (70% to 94%)
- Appears acutely ill

Pancreatitis produces elevated serum amylase (specificity 70% to 95%) and lipase levels (70% to 95%), three to five or more times normal values, 70% to 94% of the time. Serum amylase rises first, but clears quickly; urine amylase can be detected up to a week.

10. What complications should I consider with suspected pancreatitis?

- Hypovolemia. Up to 6 L of fluid can third-space around the pancreas.
- Hypoxemia. Up to 30% have a latent hypoxemia (not detected unless a pulse oximeter reading is taken) and need supplemental oxygen.
- Hypocalcemia (40% to 75%). Usually latent and minor enough to avoid tetany.

11. List considerations for an older adult patient presenting with abdominal pain.

- Older adult patients may have decreased pain perception, therefore never assume that the pain is not severe.
- Always consider that pain in the upper abdomen in the older adult patient maybe an atypical cardiac presentation.
- Consider vertebral etiology or aneurysm with upper abdominal pain that is boring to the back (but no other symptoms that would suggest an abdominal complaint).

12. What do I consider with boreing epigastric pain?

Peptic Ulcer Disease (PUD). Classic signs and symptoms include:

- Gnawing or burning sensation or dyspepsia in the epigastrium (that can radiate to the back), which lasts for minutes intermittent with asymptomatic periods
- Relief with food or antacids. (There may be a history of weight gain.)
- Nausea with occasional vomiting (40%)

Patients with duodenal ulcers may report a reduction in pain after eating; patient with gastric ulcers tend to experience more intense pain after eating, which is a result of increased gastric acids. However, 31% to 69% have a "silent" ulcer without symptoms except for hematemesis or melena.

Triage five-tier system: 3

Triage three-tier system: Urgent

13. What risk factors may increase the likelihood of ulcer formation?

- Smoking (by inhibiting bicarbonate ion production)
- Aspirin or nonsteroidal anti-inflammatory drugs (NSAIDs) inhibit prostaglandin synthesis (decreasing mucous and bicarbonate production allowing ulcer formation). Of those who take NSAIDs for more than 1 year without prophylactic protection, 2% to 4% will have gastrointestinal (GI) complaints. This risk has found to exist even in the newer COX-2 inhibitors (such as celecoxib, Celebrex).

14. How common is peptic ulcer disease?

It is 10% of all ED abdominal pain and the major cause of GI bleeding in adolescents. In those with PUD, 10% will perforate.

15. Compare PUD to erosive gastritis.

Gastritis is related to overindulgence (food, alcohol), drugs (NSAIDs), stress, or a hiatal hernia. Gastritis can be differentiated from PUD by:

- History (presence of irritants)
- Milder pain, present only with palpation (PUD is constant, severe)
- No relief with eating (PUD is relieved with food)
- Self-limiting (PUD is repetitive)

16. What should I assess next with upper abdominal pain but no tenderness?

Examine the chest for lung involvement. A chest film may be needed to rule out pneumonia, pulmonary infarction, or pleural effusions.

Consider cardiac if the patient is in an age/gender group in which coronary artery disease is prevalent. Always have a higher index of suspicion for cardiac rather than gastrointestinal in the older adult. Err on the side of "overreacting."

Triage five-tier system: 2 or 3 depending on the patient presentation

Triage three-tier system: Emergent or urgent

17. What are potential causes for a patient presenting with hematemesis?

PUD (60% of all cases), erosive gastritis and esophagitis, esophageal and gastric varices, and Mallory-Weiss syndrome. Alcohol abuse is strongly associated with PUD, erosive gastritis, and esophageal varices. Consider unmentioned past hematemesis or occult melena in patients who are hypotensive, tachycardic, weak, or confused.
Triage five-tier system: 2 or 3
Triage three-tier system: emergent or urgent

18. When assessing hematemesis, what questions should be asked?

- What is the quality and quantity of bleeding?
- Is the bleeding bright red or like coffee grounds in appearance?

Streaking may be seen with severe vomiting caused by the breaking of capillaries.
Triage five-tier system: 2 or 3
Triage three-tier system: emergent or urgent

19. A 25-year-old woman presents with a 2-week history of vomiting. What questions should the triage nurse ask?

Don't forget the obvious: any female of childbearing age must be questioned about her menstrual cycle. Ask about the timing of vomiting: is it only in the morning? Does it resolve after time? What makes it better or worse?

A quick pregnancy check should be performed prior to the million-dollar workup; it may be morning sickness. Remember that 50% of pregnant women with nausea and vomiting will experience it only in the morning, although 30% will experience it throughout the entire day. If the symptoms are severe, hyperemesis gravidarum should be considered.
Triage five-tier system: 3 or 4
Triage three-tier system: urgent or nonurgent

20. A 12-year-old presents with fever, abdominal pain, and vomiting and urinating more than usual. What questions should the triage nurse ask?

Many times the pediatric patient who presents with severe abdominal pain, vomiting, fever, and decreased level of consciousness is an undiagnosed diabetic.

- Ask about an increase in thirst and fluid intake.
- Dip the urine for glucose or ketones.
- Draw labs for chemistry and glucose.

Triage five-tier system: 2 or 3
Triage three-tier system: emergency or urgent

21. What should I consider in a patient with the "flu" and a yellow hue?

Hepatitis begins with a prodromal phase of viral symptoms with fever (70% to 94%) and nausea/vomiting (31% to 69%) before the icteric state. Only 31% to

69% become jaundice (bilirubin must be three times the normal value), but any patient that presents with jaundice should trigger a suspicion of liver involvement.

Ask about recent drug intake. In two studies, 35% to 38% of the hospitalized patients with acute liver failure were a result of taking two to three times the maximum dose of acetaminophen (4 g/day). Acetaminophen and idiosyncrasy drug reactions have replaced viral hepatitis as the most frequent cause of acute liver failure. If the jaundice is accompanied by acute abdominal pain and RUQ pain, consider gallbladder disease. This patient will need a complete work-up.
Triage five-tier system: 3
Triage three-tier system: urgent

22. How should I proceed with a 7-year-old patient with a history of recurrent abdominal pain who walks into the triage area eating French fries?

This is one of the most difficult cases to assess. Have a high index of suspicion to ensure that nothing is missed. Obtain a thorough history. Explore the pattern of pain (including timing and duration), and any new problems. For example, stress may be the cause if the pain started when the school year began.

Children between the ages of 7 and 12 many times present with psychosomatic symptoms triggered by psychologic factors. Unexplained episodes of recurrent, generalized abdominal pain can occur in 10% of school-age children. However, do not be lulled into thinking that any child who cannot define their pain is having psychosocial pain. Consider bullying or domestic violence. The worst-case scenario should always be thought of prior to considering pain as psychosomatic. See also Chapter 33.
Triage five-tier: 3 or 4
Triage three-tier: emergent or nonurgent

23. What should I suspect for a 2-year-old patient with bloating and LUQ colicky pain that is worse when the child bends over?

The differential diagnosis can be quite extensive; in this case however the clue is colicky pain with worsening of symptoms when bending over. This is usually associated with gas entrapment.

Pain associated with gas entrapment can range from mild to severe and described as a mobile pain, that is, pain starting in one area and travels. The pain of gas entrapment is usually aggravated by flexion of the leg on the side in which the pain is located (because of compression of the bowel). Ask about what relieves the pain: usually the pain will subside when flatus is passed. It can be difficult to ascertain this information from a small child. The parent may be able to give the information needed.
Triage five-tier system: 3 or 4
Triage three-tier system: nonurgent or emergent

24. A 13-year-old presents with left lower chest pain after running into his open locker door. How does this relate to a chapter on upper abdominal pain?

Any patient with lower chest wall trauma must be examined for the potential of abdominal trauma. The spleen and liver are relatively protected by the lower rib cage; any injury to those areas make abdominal trauma highly probable. The spleen is in close proximity to ribs 7 to 10, which makes it vulnerable to injury. It is important to assess the abdomen with anyone who presents with lower chest trauma.
Triage five-tier system: 3, possibly 2 if hemodynamically compromised
Triage three-tier system: urgent or emergent

Key Points

- All abdominal pain could be a surgical case; initially keep the patient NPO.
- Older adult patients may have decreased pain perception; therefore never assume that the pain is not severe.
- Always consider that pain in the upper abdomen in the older adult patient may be an atypical cardiac presentation.
- If your patient appears ill, he is ill.
- Abdominal pain may be a symptom of an extra-abdominal presentation, look beyond the obvious.

Internet Resources

NursingCEU.com: Abdominal Pain and Abdominal Emergency
http://www.nursingceu.com/NCEU/courses/01bemis/

Management of Upper Abdominal Solid Organ Injuries
http://www.findarticles.com/p/articles/mi_m0FSL/is_n5_v63/ai_19034155

Abdominal Trauma: A Major Cause of Morbidity and Mortality
http://nsweb.nursingspectrum.com/ce/ce346.htm

Who Gets Gallstones and Gallbladder Disease?
http://www.umm.edu/patiented/articles/who_gets_gallstones_gallbladder_disease_000010_4.htm

MediFocus MedCenter—Chronic Pancreatitis
http://www.crashcards.com/Medifocus%20Guides/chronicpancreatitisGS007.htm

The Patient with Pancreatitis
http://nsweb.nursingspectrum.com/ce/ce110.htm

Peptic Ulcer Disease
http://www.vnh.org/FSManual/05/02bPepticUlcer.html

NSAIDs and Peptic Ulcers
http://digestive.niddk.nih.gov/diseases/pubs/nsaids/

EM guidemap—Upper GI bleed
http://emguidemaps.homestead.com/files/gibleedupper.html

A Five-Year-Old Boy with Hematemesis
http://www.courses.ahc.umn.edu/pharmacy/5880/case_studies/stress_ulcers.htm

Bibliography

American College of Emergency Physicians: *Clinical policy: Critical issues for the initial evaluation and management of patients presenting with a chief complaint of nontraumatic acute abdominal pain,* 2000, available: www.acep.org.

Chan F, Hung LCT, Suen BY, et al: Celecoxib versus Diclofenac and Omeprazole in reducing the risk of recurrent ulcer bleeding in patients with arthritis, *N Engl J Med* 347(26):2104-2110, 2002.

Char E, Wong J: Abdominal pain. In Davis MA, Votey SR, and Greenough PG, editors: *Greenough's signs and symptoms in emergency medicine: Literature-based approach to emergent conditions,* St Louis, 1999, Mosby.

Gallagher EJ: Acute abdominal pain. In Tintinalli JE, Kelen GD, Stapczynski JS, editors: *Emergency medicine: A comprehensive study guide,* ed 5, New York, 2000, McGraw-Hill, 497-515.

Grossman VG: Abdominal pain. In Grossman VG, editor: *Quick reference to triage,* Philadelphia, 1999, Lippincott, 19-21.

Mason JD: The evaluation of acute abdominal pain in children, *Emerg Med Clin North Am* 14(3):629-643, 1996.

Metheny NM: *Fluid and electrolyte balance: Nursing considerations,* ed 4, Philadelphia, 2000, Lippincott.

Miltenburg DM, Schaffer R, Breslin T, Brandt ML: Changing indications for pediatric cholecystectomy, *Pediatrics* 105(6):1250-1253, 2000.

Montoney JM: Abdominal injuries. In McQuillian KA, Truter K, Von Rueden RJ, Hartsock M, Flynn B, Whalen E, editors: *Resuscitation through rehabilitation,* ed 3, Philadelpha, 2002, WB Saunders, 591-619.

Ostapowicz G, Fontana RJ, Schiedt FV, et al: Results of a prospective study of acute liver failure in 17 tertiary care centers in the United States, *Ann Intern Med* 137(12): 947-954, 2002.

Overton DT: Gastrointestinal bleeding. In Tintinalli JE, Kelen GD, Stapczynski JS, editors: *Emergency medicine: A comprehensive study guide,* ed 5, New York, 2002, McGraw-Hill, 520-522.

Rodriquez M, Thom AM: The diabetic child and diabetic ketoacidosis. In Tintinalli JE, Kelen GD, Stapczynski JS, editors: *Emergency medicine: A comprehensive study guide,* ed 5, New York, 2000, McGraw-Hill, 854-855.

Sanson TG, O'Keefe KP: Evaluation of abdominal pain in the elderly, *Emerg Med Clin N Am* 14(3):615-627, 1996.

Seller RH: Abdominal pain in children. In Seller RH, editor: *Differential diagnosis of common complaints,* ed 3, Philadelphia, 1996, WB Saunders, 18-27.

Seller RH: Belching, bloating and flatulence. In Seller RH, editor: *Differential diagnosis of common complaints,* ed 3, Philadelphia, 1996, WB Saunders, 44-50.

Thomas D, Fletcher L: Abdominal problems. In Dunphy LM, Winland-Brown JE, editors: *Primary care: The art and science of advanced practice nursing,* Philadelphia, 2001, FA Davis, 557-657.

van de Ven CJM: Nausea and vomiting in early pregnancy. In Pearlman MD, Tintinalli JE, editors: *Emergency care of the woman,* New York, 1998, McGraw-Hill, 49-56.

Chapter 33

Lower Abdominal Pain

Joan Somes and Polly Gerber Zimmermann

1. What helps determine if the abdominal pain is serious?

There are three types of abdominal pain that help determine acuity: visceral, somatic, and referred. Visceral pain is caused by the stretching of nerve fibers. It causes a crampy, colicky, gaseous, and intermittent pain. The pain is diffuse and patients are usually restless. Somatic pain occurs when chemicals or bacteria irritate the peritoneum and frequently occurs after visceral pain. It is sharp, constant, localized pain that movement exacerbates (so the patient lies as still as possible). As a whole, central pain (in an organ or body cavity) is more serious than peripheral pain (e.g., skin, eye).

2. What is referred pain?

Referred pain is felt at a distance from the area of the disease process. Some classic causes and referred sites include:

- Kidney (renal colic): One-sided lower abdominal pain radiating to groin/scrotum
- Shoulder tip pain: Peritonitis/free air irritating the phrenic nerve in the diaphragm
- Aorta (dissection/rupture): Back
- Small bowel/ascending colon: Periumbilical
- Descending colon: Suprapubic/low back

3. What questions should be the focus in the history for lower abdominal pain?

Besides a complete description of the pain (PQRST) (see Chapters 3 and 6), obtain a thorough history including:

- Onset, location, referral
- Associated symptoms (especially fever, nausea/vomiting, presence of blood)
- Prior medical and surgical histories
- History of similar episodes
- Current medications

4. How can I accurately describe the amount of vomitus or bleeding?

Try using household measurements to pin down the amount. Start with a larger amount and narrow it down, such as: "A cup? Half a cup? A tablespoon?" etc. Ask if the vomiting is associated with nausea, or as a result of coughing so hard the person vomits.

5. Give examples of questions to ask to get more specific information.

Nausea

- Does nausea effect intake of fluid or foods or do foods affect the nausea?
- How soon after eating does the nausea or vomiting occur?
- Is the nausea constant or intermittent (comes in waves)?

Bowel Movements

- When was the last one and was it normal? If not normal, what was different?
- Have bowel movements (BMs) been loose, soft, or hard? Explosive?
- What color was the stool? Any blood? Floating? Mucus? Undigested food?
- If blood, was it mixed within the stool, or just on the outside of the stool?
- How does it smell? Different than usual? (Anyone who smelled bloody stool or *Clostridium difficile* won't forget.)
- How does this compare with the normal bowel function?
- Passing gas?
- Used any stool softeners, enemas, or other adjuncts to move the bowels?
- Anything been placed into the rectum for medical or recreational purposes?
- Are symptoms affecting normal life? Can they still go to work?
- Weight changed by 10 lbs in the last month?

6. What other, non-GI questions would be helpful to ask?

- What's been going on in the patient's life?
- Recent coughing and/or sore throat? Infections of the chest and throat can lead to painful swollen lymph tissue in the abdomen.
- Recent activity? Too many sit-ups or heavy lifting can cause abdominal soreness.
- Co-existing urinary symptoms
- History of trauma (of any magnitude)

7. Why ask about trauma? Wouldn't that be obvious?

Bleeding into the abdomen can go undetected because patients:

- Do not mention a minor motor vehicle crash (MVC) because they are unaware of the significant force applied to their abdominal organs from an improperly applied, or no, seatbelt.
- Forget about something hitting them in the abdomen or a fall unless they have other resulting problems at the time.
- Underestimate the force of an incident, such as a small child jumping onto their abdomen during "horseplay."

8. Describe the first step, inspection, in the physical assessment of the abdomen.

- *Gait.* Patients with inflamed organs/peritonitis will have a stiff walk, limp, or lay rigidly still; patients with colic writhe. Patients moving about easily usually do not have a significant abdominal pathology. See Chapter 31.
- *Distention?*
- *Bruising?*
- *Unusual scars, distention, rashes, marks, redness, tubes/catheters?*

9. What are the five Fs that can cause generalized abdominal distention?

Fat, fluid, feces, flatus, and fetus

10. I can never tell if the patient is distended or obese.

Distention, usually caused by flatus, will have no flank bulging, will feel "tight," and have tympany on percussion. Obesity has adipose at the flank, normal percussion, and a "sunken" looking umbilicus.

11. Give some example of bruising that could signify internal bleeding.

- Flank bruising (Grey-Turner sign) can indicate retroperitoneal bleeding.
- Periumbilical bruising (Cullen's sign) implies an intraperitoneal bleed.
- Bruising across the lap area can signal injuries from a seatbelt.

12. Talk about the second step in physical assessment, auscultation.

It is becoming standard practice to listen in the center of the abdomen just to hear if there are any sounds at all because sound travels across the abdomen. Place the stethoscope slightly to the right and below the umbilicus; the ileocecal valve area (right lower quadrant) is also a good place to listen. Normal bowel sounds is 5 to 35 irregular clicks and gurgles per minutes, each lasting about one-half second to several seconds, with occasional borborygmi (rushes of air or "growling").

13. Discuss the technique for the third step of physical assessment, percussion.

Hyperextend the middle finger of one hand and press the distal phalanx and joint firmly on the body surface. Avoid the contact of the other part of the hand or it will deaden the resulting sound. Lightly tap with a snapping (quick, sharp) motion of the wrist from the (partially flexed) finger on the other hand. Practice on a pouched-out cheek to hear tympany; on a thigh for the dullness sound.

14. What are normal percussion findings?

Percuss all four quadrants, the liver span, and the spleen span. Tympany predominates, even more so in children. There is dullness over organs and solid masses.

The upper border of the liver is at the 5th to 7th intercostal space; the lower border is at/slightly below the costal margin (rib cage). Young children and some adults may have a normal liver edge 2 to 3 cm below the right costal margin. The spleen span is normally perceived as dullness from the 6th to 10th intercostal spaces on the left midaxillary line.

15. Discuss how to perform the fourth step of physical assessment, palpation.

Use the palmar surfaces of the fingers and initially palpate all quadrants, but avoid "trouble spots" (tender). First lightly palpate up to 1 cm, and then do a deeper palpation (up to 3 inches) moving the fingers back and forth over abdominal contents. Palpate all four quadrants and the liver and spleen edges. Do not palpate an enlarged spleen. Normal findings are a soft, nontender abdomen that does not tense up or resist.

16. What should I do if there is tenderness?

Note any "guarding," an almost involuntary tensing of the muscles. Then test for rebound tenderness (press deeply with a quick release). Normally there should be less pain when the pressure is released; positive rebound tenderness indicating an underlying pathology is an increase in the pain sensation when the pressure is released.

17. Some people seem to resist palpation as a result of fear or ticklishness.

- Position the patient with a pillow under the knees and a small pillow under the head.
- Ask the patient to breathe slowly through the mouth.
- Place your whole hand flush on the surface prior to starting the palpation.
- Use distraction.
- Try the small bell of the stethoscope for initial pressure because people associate it with listening and so will endure pressure from it.
- Place their hand underneath yours, especially if a child. This gives them a sense of control.

18. What can I do when deep palpation is difficult from obesity or muscular resistance?

Use two hands, with one on top of the other. Exert pressure with the outside hand while concentrating on the sensation with the inside hand.

19. Give examples of standing triage orders for a patient with lower abdominal pain:

Memorial Regional Hospital (Hollywood, Fla)
Source, Melinda Stibal, RN BSHC, Administrative Director Emergency/Trauma Services

- Complete blood cell count (CBC)
- Urinalysis
- Serum qualitative pregnancy test if pregnancy status is unknown (all premenopausal women)
- Quantitative beta human chorionic gonadotropin (HCG) if patient is known to be pregnant and the patient is less than 16 weeks pregnant by dates

Glens Falls Hospital (Glens Falls, NY) and Saratoga Hospital (Saratoga Springs, NY)
Source: Connie Tucker, RN CEN, Emergency Department Supervisor

- CBC
- $Chem_7$

- Amylase
- Urinalysis
- Saline lock, 0.9% intravenous (IV) infusion if orthostatic
- Keep nothing by mouth (NPO)
- Prepare supplies for stool Hemoccult
- If female of child-bearing age: urine pregnancy, place on pelvic exam stretcher

Christus Santa Rose Hospital (San Antonio, Tx)
Source: Kevin Trainor, RN CEN, Emergency Department/Trauma Nurse Manager
For upper, persistent abdominal pain, either sex

If >35 years	Electrocardiogram (EKG), SMA7, CBC, Liver Panel, Lipase
	Urine dip
	Kidney, ureter, and bladder (KUB) flat and upright if vomiting and no BM for 12 to 24 hours
Low abdominal pain: males	CBC
	Dip U/A, micro if positive
	KUB flat and upright if vomiting and no BM for 12 to 24 hours
Low abdominal pain: menstruating female	CBC, HCG
	Catheterize, dip U/A with micro if positive

20. Talk about what might signal "shingles."

Shingles (herpes zoster, varicella) is the chicken pox virus reactivated, usually during a period of physiologic or psychologic stress. Up to 66% of the cases are in patients about 50 years of age or older because the childhood immunity has worn off. The classic presentation is one-sided, severe stabbing pain along a dermatome with vesicular eruptions. It is highly contagious by respiratory route before the vesicles appear dry and crusted (with incubation period of about 2 weeks). Mask the patient if there is any suspicion.

21. Do ulcers cause pain in the lower abdomen?

A crampy pain can occur if the ulcer bleeds, as blood is irritating to the bowel.

22. Discuss symptoms of an abdominal aortic aneurysm.

Abdominal aortic aneurysm (AAA) is a painless dilation of the aorta secondary to weakening of all layers of the aortic wall. If it leaks or dissects (the intima tears leading to a separation in the vessel wall layers), there is intense abdominal pain (70% to 94%) that can be confused with the pain of a renal stone. The classic description is a "tearing" or "ripping" pain that radiates to the back (aorta), leg (iliac artery), or kidney (renal artery). There can be a pulsatile abdominal mass (70% to 94%), an abdominal bruit (6% to 30%), with peripheral embolization (less than 5%) causing ischemic lower extremities.

23. Describe the problem of the presentation of appendicitis.

Although appendicitis occurs in 6% of the population, it is difficult to diagnose because patients present at different points over the typical course, which can be up to 48 hours. Half of the 700,000 cases of suspected appendicitis in the United States each year lack the usual symptoms of fever and right lower quadrant (RLQ) pain. An atypical presentation is more likely in:

- Children under age 2 or adults over age 50 (only fever and nonspecific abdominal pain)
- Patients with diabetes ("blunted pain")
- Pregnancy (Pain is higher in the abdomen as a result of the upward migration of internal organs. One out of every 2,200 pregnant women will develop appendicitis.)

24. What are the "classic" signs of appendicitis?

70% to 94%	Crampy (sometimes colicky, vs. steady) pain that starts in the middle of the abdomen (periumbilical) and moves (over 12 to 48 hours) to the RLQ (McBurney's point—4 to 6 cm from the iliac crest).
	Anorexia
31% to 69%	Nausea and vomiting (although not severe)
	Low-grade fever (100.4°F, 38°C)
	Rebound tenderness (Blumberg's sign)
	Pain in the left lower quadrant (LLQ) when palpating the RLQ (Rovsing's sign)
6% to 30%	Diarrhea
	Psoas sign
	Obturator sign

25. Describe the psoas sign and obturator sign.

The psoas sign or obturator sign is only positive 6% to 30% of the time, but a positive response is highly suggestive of appendicitis.

- *Psoas sign (positive iliopsoas muscle test).* There is RLQ pain when a patient lying on the left side has the right hip extended. This stretches the right iliopsoas muscle. If the appendix is posterior in the abdominal cavity, it lies against this muscle. Stretching the muscle causes increased pain in the inflamed appendix.
- *Obturator sign (positive obturator muscle test).* There is hypogastric pain when a supine patient's right flexed hip is rotated inward. This stretches the obturator muscle and increases pain if the appendix lies against the muscle.

26. What other physical assessments can I do for a suspected appendicitis?

- *Markle sign* (heel jar/heel drop) is positive in 74% of patients with appendicitis. Abdominal pain is produced when the patient stands on tiptoes and allows both heels to hit the floor with a thump. If the patient is too sick to perform the test, the examiner can hit the heel with their hand.

- *Aaron's sign* is when palpation of McBurney's point causes pain by the child's heart or stomach.
- *Cutaneous hyperesthesia* is an abnormally acute sensitivity to touch. At a series of points down the abdomen, gently pick up a fold of skin between the thumb and index finger without pinching it. Positive finding is if there is localized pain to all or part of the right lower quadrant.

27. What is the key concern with appendicitis?

A key concern is to get treatment before it ruptures. Perforation occurs in up to 20% of all patients, and is reported to occur in 50% of patients younger than 3 and older than 50.

28. Is there an appendicitis rule-out pathway?

Ziegler (2004) developed this clinical path:

- If there are signs/symptoms (s/s) consistent with appendicitis: appendectomy
- Equivocal presentations: computed tomography (CT) or ultrasound, IV hydration, and observe for 4 hours.
- Reexamine after 4 hours: surgery or another 4 hours observation period
- All patients either had surgery or discharge after 2 observation periods.

Of 356 children, a retrospective analysis of the protocol indicated a good sensitivity (99%), specificity (92%) with positive (95%) and negative (99%) predictive values.

In 2004, the Food and Drug Administration (FDA) approved a new diagnostic technique, NeutroSpec.

29. Discuss LLQ pain related to diverticulitis.

Diverticulosis (small outpouchings in the large intestine) occurs in 40% of the U.S. population over the age of 40 and two thirds of the population by age 85. It only becomes a problem in the 10% to 35% that develop the inflammation of diverticulitis. The classic sign and symptom is LLQ pain (70% to 94%): "the left-sided appendicitis".

30. Describe signs and symptoms of bowel obstruction.

The abdominal pain (present 95% to 100%) of small bowel obstructions are caused by adhesions (50%), incarcerated or strangulated hernias (15%), or neoplasms (15%). Other classic signs and symptoms (each present 70% to 94% of the time) include:

- Nausea
- Vomiting
- Bloating
- Abdominal distention and tenderness

31. Describe classic abnormal findings that signal a large intestine obstruction.

- *Altered bowel sounds.* Bowel sounds could be hyperactive, hypoactive or absent.
- *A "rush" or "tinkling" (higher-pitched frequency) of air that coincides with an abrupt, severe spasmodic pain "cramp."* (Frequently referred to the umbilicus.)
- *Obstipation.* Inability to pass flatus for more than 8 hours despite feeling a need.

32. Compare these symptoms to those with a small bowel obstruction.

Bowel sounds can initially remain "normal" in a small bowel obstruction because the auscultation is of the large intestine's activity. Since the obstruction is so high, the contents come up instead of going down. Classic symptoms include the following:

- Severe vomiting with feculent odor
- History of abdominal surgery
- Diffuse or periumbilical discomfort
- Symptoms that are worse with eating and relieved by vomiting

33. Talk about constipation history and symptoms.

- Small amounts of hard stool less than 3 times per week
- No stool for 5 or more days
- Blood streaked stool

The patient will often report a crampy pain after eating, and a "loaded" descending colon can be palpated. There can be liquid stool passing around the obstructing solid stool.

34. Describe the signs and symptoms of hernia incarceration.

Hernias are usually not a problem unless they become incarcerated (about 10%). When the abdominal contents cannot be returned to the abdomen; strangulation (blood compromise to the entrapped contents) can occur. Although the male:female ratio of hernias is 4:1; the incarceration rate is higher in females.

The patient will have a history of an "abdominal mass" that comes and goes, but now the mass is now tender and tense. The pain is initially sudden, especially after lifting something, but progresses rapidly to the pain of ischemic bowel and peritonitis.

35. Discuss symptoms of an infarcted bowel.

The patient with infarcted bowel will classically be an older person as a result of sluggish mesenteric circulation. The pain is crampy and poorly localized.

36. Distinguish inflammatory bowel disease and irritable bowel syndrome.

Inflammatory bowel disease (IBD) covers both ulcerative colitis in the large intestine and Crohn's disease in the small and large intestines. Both are chronic recurring inflammations.

Irritable bowel syndrome (IBS) (17% of gastrointestinal problems) is as a result of abnormal intestinal motility and increased perception of sensation with constipation and diarrhea.

It is not serious. Treatment consists of regular dietary bulk, newer drugs (Zelnorm, Lotronex), peppermint oil (as a calcium channel blocker), and probiotic therapy.

37. Is IBS an adult disease?

That was the common assumption for many years. However, in one study, 6% of middle school and 14% of high school children met the diagnostic criteria for IBS.

38. Discuss the role of food intolerance

IBS may be related to food intolerance, such as lactose (dairy) or celiac (non-tropical sprue), which is sensitivity to gluten in grains. It is now thought to be 10 times more common than previously believed, e.g., 1 in 133 individuals (compared to 1 in 10,000) or 3 million Americans. Some believe IBS may often be misdiagnosed celiac.

39. What are the causes of low abdominal pain specific to children?

- Intestinal colic (2 to 3 weeks to 3 months).
- Volvulus (1 month). A malrotation or twisting of the intestines.
- Intussusception. The bowel telescopes on itself leading to mesenteric vessel obstruction.

40. Are there other common etiologies that will cause abdominal pain?

- An abscess or hematoma against the psoas muscle
- Withdrawal from narcotics
- Electrolyte imbalance
- Sickle cell crisis
- Exposures to, or ingestion of, poisons (heavy metals, organophosphates)
- Black widow spider bites
- Toxic shock syndrome
- Diabetic ketoacidosis (DKA) (Up to 46% of patients with DKA experience abdominal pain. It is more likely with a history of alcohol or cocaine abuse.)

41. What helps determine whether the pain is a functional problem or an acute process?

Abdominal pain is functional 95% of the time if:

- The patient is older than age 5.
- The pain has a duration of longer than 3 months.
- The abdominal pain is intermittent.

42. Have any contributing factors been found related to recurrent abdominal pain in children or adolescents?

Recurrent abdominal pain (RAP) is defined as at least three pain episodes that span at least 3 months and affect daily living. Compo et al (2004) found they had a high prevalence of anxiety (79%), depressive disorders (43%), and disruptive disorders (24%). It is estimated that children today have stress levels as high as the "psychiatric" children had in the 1930s.

43. Give some objective guidelines in determining the triage acuity in the five-level Canadian Triage and Acuity Scale.

Level 2 (≤15 minutes)
- Visceral with associated s/s & abnormal vital signs
- Severe pain (patient rating 8 to 10 out of 10)
- Signs of dehydration

Level 3 (≤30 minutes)
- Crampy, intermittent, sharp brief pain, and normal vital signs
- Severe (patient rating 8 to 10 out of 10)
- Gastrointestinal (GI) bleed that is not actively bleeding

Level 4 (≤1 hour)
- Acute pain, moderate intensity (4 to 7 out of 10)
- A child in "no acute distress"

Level 5 (≤2 hours)
- Chronic or recurring mild pain (<4) with normal vital signs

44. Compare that to the five-level triage of the Manchester Triage Group.

Level 2 (very urgent, 10 minutes)
- Severe pain
- Pain radiating to the back
- Acutely passing blood

Level 3 (urgent, 60 minutes)
- Moderate pain
- Shoulder tip pain
- Possible pregnancy
- Black or red currant stools
- Persistent vomiting
- Visible abdominal mass
- Child inconsolable by parents
- Inappropriate history in a child

Level 4 (standard, 120 minutes)
- Any vomiting
- "Recent" (within the last week) problem

45. How can I determine the etiology of lower abdominal pain in triage?

Triage isn't there to diagnose. The important role of triage is to determine the acuity of the patient's pain and prioritize accordingly for more diagnostic work-up and treatment.

46. What is the most common discharge diagnosis for patients presenting with lower abdominal pain that is not gynecologic or urinary based?

"Abdominal pain-etiology unknown." However, a current, obvious serious etiology has been ruled out in 33% to 69% of all emergency department (ED) abdominal pain.

47. What are the most common ED diagnoses for abdominal pain?

Gastroenteritis and appendicitis.

48. What are the most commonly missed surgical causes for all ED abdominal pain?

Appendicitis and acute intestinal obstruction.

49. What are the most common diagnoses for abdominal pain in the older adult?

Appendicitis and diverticulitis.

50. Why should I be more concerned about abdominal pain in the older adult?

About 33% to 39% of patients older than 65 admitted for abdominal pain need surgery. The manifestation is often blunted and the conditions can progress rapidly. The most common of the diagnosis are cholecystitis, intestinal obstruction, and appendicitis.

51. What are clues that the cause of a patient's abdominal pain may be surgical?

- Pain preceding vomiting (vs. vomiting, then pain).
- Severe pain that persists for 6 or more hours.

52. What should always be considered in lower abdominal pain in an adult male?

Testicular problems

53. What diagnosis do many patients with abdominal pain fear they have?

Cancer, but colon cancer usually has no pain. More common symptoms are rectal bleeding and/or "ribbon" stool.

Key Points

- Use pain type and rating, vital sign abnormality, s/s of dehydration, bleeding, and onset to help determine the triage acuity.
- 70% to 94% of patients with appendicitis have abdominal pain and anorexia.
- Pain more than 6 hours or occurring before vomiting is indicative of a potential surgical pathology.
- 33% to 39% of patients older than 65 admitted for abdominal pain need surgery.

Internet Resources

Situs Inversus
http://emedicine.com/radio/topic639.htm

Abdominal Pain in Older Adult Persons
http://www.emedicine.com/emerg/topic931.htm

Appendicitis, Acute
http://www.emedicine.com/emerg/topic41.htm

Constipation
http://www.emedicine.com/emerg/topic111.htm

Obstruction, Small Bowel
http://www.emedicine.com/emerg/topic66.htm

Inflammatory Bowel Disease
http://www.emedicine.com/emerg/topic106.htm

Triaging Lower Abdominal Pain
http://rnweb.com/rnweb/article/articleDetail.jsp?id=118602

Abdominal Pain and Abdominal Emergency
http://www.nursingceu.com/NCEU/courses/01bemis/

Abdominal Pain
http://www.rnceus.com/triage/trabdom.html

Bibliography

Bemis PA: *Clinical practice guide of emergency care: The ultimate core curriculum,* 2000, Cocoa Beach Learning Systems, available at www.CocoaBeachLearning.com; accessed June 4, 2004.

Bickley LS, Szilagyi PG: *Bates' guide to physical examination and history taking,* ed 8, Philadelphia, 2003, Lippincott.

Bowman M, Baxt W: *Office emergencies,* Philadelphia, 2003, WB Saunders.

Burke M, Laramie J: *Primary care of the older adult: A multidisciplinary approach,* St Louis, 2000, Mosby.

Camp JV, et al: Recurrent abdominal pain, anxiety, and depression in primary care, *Pediatrics* 113:817-824, 2004.

Canadian Association of Emergency Physicians: Canadian Emergency Department Triage and Acuity Scale Implementation Guidelines, *J Can Assoc Emerg Physicians* 1(3 suppl), 1999.

Char E, Wong J: Abdominal pain. In Davis MA, Voey SR, Greenough PG: *Greenough's signs and symptoms in emergency medicine: Literature-based approach to emergent conditions,* St Louis, 1999, Mosby.

Dowds P: Surgical emergencies. In Dolan B, Holt L. *Holt's accident and emergency theory into practice,* London, 2000, Harcourt Publishers Limited.

Emergency Nurses Association: *Emergency core curriculum,* ed 5, New York, 2000, WB Saunders.

Fasano A, Berti I, et al: Prevalence of celiac disease in at-risk and not-at-risk groups in the United States: A large multicenter study, *Arch Intern Med* 163(3):286, 2003.

Holmes HN: *3-Minute assessment,* Philadelphia, 2003, Lippincott.

Mackway-Jones K: *Emergency triage: Manchester Triage Group,* London, 1997, BMJ Publishing Group.

Purcell TB: Abdominal pain. In Markovchick VJ, Pons PT: *Pons' emergency medicine secrets,* ed 3, Philadelphia, 2003, Hanley & Belfus.

Rosen P, Barkin R, Hayden S, Schaider J, Wolf R: *The 5 Minute emergency medicine consult,* Philadelphia, 1999, Lippincott, Williams & Wilkins.

Shaw M: *Assessment made incredibly easy,* New York, 1998, Springhouse.

Tintinalli J, Gabor K, Stapczynski JS: *Emergency medicine: A comprehensive study guide,* ed 6, New York, 2004, McGraw-Hill.

Umpierrez G, Freire A: Abdominal pain in patients with hyperglycemic crises, *J Crit Care* 17(1):63-67, 2002.

Wilhelm A: *Situs inversus,* available at http://www.eMedicine.com/radio/topic639.htm, accessed April 22, 2003.

Ziegler MM: The diagnosis of appendicitis: An evolving paradigm, *Pediatrics* 113:130-132, 2004.

Zimmermann PG: Triaging lower abdominal pain, *RN* 65(12):53-58, 2002.

Chapter 34

Gynecologic-Related Abdominal Pain

Darleen A. Williams and Polly Gerber Zimmermann

1. Why do you have a focus on this subject?

Abdominal pain accounts for up to 5% of all emergency department (ED) visits, with pelvic pain occurring in 7% to 20% of those patients. It is one of the most ED common complaints in women.

2. Is there a quick and easy way to remember all the things I need to ask in triage relevant to a complaint of female-related abdominal pain?

There are multiple mnemonics that can be easily adapted. One example:

S Signs and symptoms (including the duration and any previous history of the same or similar illnesses)

Chief complaint in the patient's own words

A Allergies to any medications and latex

M Medications, doses and frequencies, for prescriptions, over-the-counter (OTC), herbals and home remedies. Taken anyone else's medications to treat?

P Past medical history, including reproductive history
Regular medical doctor or health care provider?

L Last time the patient ate, urine and bowel status (I&O)

E Events surrounding their illness
Partner having any of the same symptoms?

3. How can I ask the patient about sexual history in an appropriate and sensitive manner?

Awareness is a start. It can be easy for others to overhear. Certain techniques will increase the likelihood of honesty and minimize the possibility of confidentiality breaches.

- Ask anyone accompanying the patient to wait in the waiting room while the necessary private information is obtained. Do it automatically. The patient can always initiate the request for the person to stay.

- Take the patient to another area. Accompany the patient to the restroom or x-ray.
- Look directly at the person, get close (in their personal space) and speak quietly, in low tones. People tend to mimic your tone in their answer.
- Remain nonjudgmental, matter-of-fact, with a sensitive demeanor. One expert recommends asking everyone, "Do you have sex with men, women, or both?" Simply refer to their "partner" without stating a specific gender. Some patients are offended if the term "significant other" is used as society attaches this term with homosexuality.

4. How can I obtain an accurate answer about being "sexually active"?

Many people are not familiar with the meaning of our standard clinical phrasing. One woman answered, "No, I just lie there." Try more direct phrasing, "Do you have sex?"

5. I find many women seem vague in their answers about any aspect of sexual history.

The key is often to keep probing.

- *LMP:* Last *normal* menstrual period?
- *History of sexually transmitted disease (STD):* Was both she and her partner treated? Was the complete course of medication taken?
- *Birth control:* What is the method? If a barrier method, is it *every* sexual encounter? If an oral pill, was *every* pill taken? Any new medications (such as antibiotics) that may affect its effectiveness?
- *Sexual activity:* How often? How many partners? When was the last intercourse?

6. Why is a description of the vaginal discharge helpful?

Ask not only about discharge, but labia/vagina itching and irritation. A description helps determine the causative organism.

- Bacterial: thin, homogenous, gray-to-white.
- *Trichomonas:* profuse, frothy, greenish. It may be accompanied by vague, mild abdominal symptoms.
- *Candida:* thick, white discharge resembling cottage cheese.

7. What else should I consider if the woman has discharge that sounds like it could be candida?

It is a normal flora that has some "overgrowth." Contributing factors include tight/nonporous clothing (including wet bathing suits in the summer), contraceptives (which alter vaginal mucus), immunosuppression, or broad-spectrum antibiotics. However, also consider the possibility of undiagnosed diabetes mellitus (especially in older women).

8. What else should I ask if the complaint is of vulvar pruritus, erythema, or edema?

Contact vulvovaginitis may result for an allergic or chemical reaction to using common products, such as feminine hygiene sprays, douches, bubble bath, dyed toilet paper, dyed underwear, and/or scented tampons/pads. Ask about use of these products.

9. When do I need to rule out pregnancy?

Any female patient between 11 and 55 years old who is sexually active (especially if having unprotected sex) should be suspected of being pregnant until proven otherwise.

Pregnancy can occur even after a tubal ligation or while the woman is on birth control pills. Of pregnancies occurring after bilateral tubal ligation (BTL), 30% to 40% will be ectopic. Do not automatically assume a negative answer is correct. Denial is a powerful force. Psychiatrists indicate that many mothers of the "dumpster babies" literally detach and deny the entire pregnancy.

10. How accurate are home pregnancy tests?

In one study, investigators tested the accuracy in 18 different home pregnancy tests. Rarely were the positive tests falsely positive, but negative tests were often falsely negative. Accuracy improved when allowing an extended 10 minutes read time.

11. Women sometimes demand a hospital pregnancy test. This is not an emergency.

It probably is not life- or limb-threatening. It is, however, an indication of what a pregnancy could psychologically mean to this patient. Ask about that "crisis."

12. Give some guidelines in establishing a triage category.

- Level of pain.
- Type of pain. Visceral with associated signs/symptoms is usually more serious than crampy, intermittent, sharp brief pain (e.g., somatic).
- Referral pattern. Although pelvic referral patterns are not as constant and predictable as abdominal ones, some general ones are:
  - Ovarian: T10, pain to the infraumbilical region
  - Fallopian and uterine: T11, T12 pain to the lower abdomen and inguinal regions
  - Inferior uterine, vaginal, and perineal (sacral roots: pain to the sacral area, buttocks, and suprapubic region).
- Vital signs (normal/abnormal)
- Vaginal bleeding (Present? Amount? Clots?)
- Discharge (How is this discharge different from the "ordinary" discharge?)
- Lesions/sores?

- *Possible pregnancy* (≥20 weeks?)
- *Associated symptoms including itching, burning, dysuria, painful bowel movements*

See Chapter 33 for further discussion.

13. Anything more specific related to vaginal discharge?

Consider some of the criteria for ranking urgency suggested by Briggs' Telephone Triage Protocols:

Seek medical care within 2 to 4 hrs:
- Severe pelvic pain that interferes with activity
- Temperature >102°F (>38.9°C), increased pain, chills, shakes, or vomiting
- Foul-smelling vaginal discharge, pain, itching, or history of recent trauma, rape, surgery, pregnancy, or abortion
- Last menstrual period >6 weeks ago, abdominal pain, suspicion of pregnancy

Seek medical care within 24 hours:
- Itching interferes with activity
- Temperature >100°F (>37.8°C)
- Foul odor and large amount of discharge
- Green, brown, or white cottage cheese-like discharge
- Exposure to venereal disease or other STD and request for an examination
- Painful sores or irritation on labia or vagina
- History of one ovary and of childbearing age
- Tampon in place and unable to remove

Call for a primary care provider appointment (after 24 hours OK):
- Frequent use of scented feminine hygiene products
- Pain during or after intercourse
- Past Papanicolaou (Pap) smear >1 year ago
- Small amount of clear, white, or yellow discharge
- Recent prolonged sexual activity

14. Why is it important to confirm the demographics?

Female abdominal pain patients have a high frequency of infectious causes and the EDs may need to follow up (different antibiotic, etc.). In addition, most states have regulatory requirements for reporting some culture results.

15. Name the classic signs and symptoms of pelvic inflammatory disease.

Pelvic inflammatory disease (PID) is an acute syndrome caused by the spread of microorganisms from the vagina and cervix to reproductive organs. Overall, patients with PID look "sick." Frequency of the occurrence of common signs and symptoms are:

95% to 100%	Lower abdominal or pelvic pain
	Constant dull, aching pain
	Poorly localized (usually bilateral)
	Worse with activity ("PID shuffle")
	Cervical movement tenderness

70% to 94%	Vaginal discharge (thick)
	Lower abdominal tenderness to palpation
6% to 30%	Abnormal vaginal bleeding
	Urinary symptoms

16. Just exactly what is the "PID shuffle"?

The reason for the shuffling gait (usually bent over, with the hands "splinting" the abdomen) is directly related to pelvic inflammation, usually secondary to an STD. This ambulation minimizes movement of the irritated pelvic cavity.

17. Indicate key history/background information that would make PID likely.

- New or multiple sexual partners
- Frequent intercourse (at least a history of sexual activity)
- Recent insertion of an intrauterine device (IUD)
- Previous PID or STD
- Lower socioeconomic status
- Younger age (age 15 to 19)
- History of smoking
- Vaginal douching

18. What other conditions should be considered when PID is suspected?

Of all patients admitted to the hospital for PID, 25% are found to have other conditions, including ectopic pregnancy and acute appendicitis. It is possible to have both PID and pregnancy, so consider an ectopic pregnancy if the pain is sharp and/or localized.

19. What information is important to teach before discharge?

Complete the treatment for PID and prevention. The risk of infertility is 11% with a single episode of PID, 54% with three or more PID infections. Aspects to emphasize include:

- Identifying and treating or referring all sexual partners.
- Avoiding all sexual contact with the partners until all parties have finished treatment (or 2 weeks).
- Use condoms with all future sexual contacts to avoid further infections, including human immunodeficiency virus (HIV).
- STD education.

20. List symptoms that might indicate dysmenorrhea is causing the pain.

Although most women do not go for medical help with this complaint, it is possible when the typical symptoms change with a perimenopausal or an inexperienced young female.

- *Type of pain: crampy, low abdominal pain.* The pain may be referred to the back or legs.

- *Time of pain.* The pain is within 24 hours before or with the onset of the menstrual period.
- *Associated hormonal signs/symptoms.* These include breast tenderness, nausea, or headache.

21. Distinguish dysmenorrhea from mittelschmerz or PID.

Mittelschmerz is a local irritation caused by the release of blood, follicular fluid, prostaglandins, and increased fallopian tube peristalsis during ovulation. Classic symptoms include:

- Pain is sudden, and one-sided (PID is usually bilateral)
- Midcycle (days 12 to 16)
- Unassociated with any other systemic complaints
- Last less than 8 hours
- No discharge (70% to 94% of patients with PID have discharge)

22. When should mittelschmerz not be a consideration in triage?

If there is:

- Vaginal bleeding/spotting (rule out [r/o] ectopic)
- History of birth control pills (BCP) (because they prevent ovulation)
- A general sick appearance

It addition, the patient must be assessed for the possibility of PID (can be unilateral) and/or an appendicitis if the pain is right lower quadrant (RLQ).

23. Define endometriosis.

Endometrial cells are outside the uterus and react to the cyclic hormonal change. Signs and symptoms include dysmenorrhea/episodic pelvic pain, dysuria/hematuria, and dyspareunia (labia, vagina, or pelvic pain during or after sexual intercourse).

24. What is a "risin" and is it contagious?

"Risin" is frequently used to describe the presence of an elevated infected area. Common causes include Bartholin's abscess (often from *Escherichia coli* and *Neisseria gonorrhoeae*), genital herpes, or genital warts. Wear gloves and practice good handwashing with direct contact.

25. List the most common causes of pelvic pain in the prepubertal patient.

Vaginal foreign body, urinary tract infection, or sexual abuse. Malodorous vaginal discharge is suggestive of a foreign body.

26. Give a rule to guide assessment in an older adult, postmenopausal woman with pelvic pain.

The "atypical is typical." Particularly in the older adult, the pain may be referred (because of complex innervation of the pelvic structures) and not related to a pelvic pathology.

27. Discuss chronic pelvic pain.

Chronic pelvic pain is defined as pain, in the same location, that lasts longer than 4 to 6 months. One third of cases are as a result of adhesions secondary to infection, one-third is as a result of endometriosis, and one-third is of unknown cause.

Key Points

- Ask personal questions by facing the patient directly in their "personal space" and speaking in low terms to prevent inadvertent overhearing.
- Despite a "PID shuffle," 25% of women with these symptoms have other conditions. Consider the possibility of ectopic pregnancy and acute appendicitis.
- Mittelschmerz should not be considered if there is vaginal bleeding (r/o ectopic), history of BCP, or a "sick" appearance.
- Common causes of pelvic pain in the prepubertal patient are a vaginal foreign body, urinary tract infection, or sexual abuse.

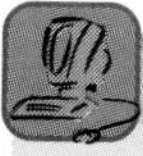

Internet Resources

Nursing Spectrum: Ectopic Pregnancy
http://nsweb.nursingspectrum.com/ce/ce77.htm

Abdominal Pain and Abdominal Emergency
http://www.nursingceu.com/RCEU/courses/01bemis/

Abdominal Pain
http://www.rnceus.com/triage/trabdom.html

Pediatric and Adolescent Gynecology for the ED Nurse Practitioner
http://www.ena.org/conferences/annual/2004/handouts/capl233-c.pdf

Abdominal Pain—Pathway to Excellence
http://www.ena.org/conferences/annual/2004/handouts/220-c.pdf

Bibliography

Briggs JK: *Telephone triage protocols for nurses,* ed 2, Philadelphia, 2002, Lippincott.

Broderick KB: Sexually transmitted diseases. In Markovchick VJ, Pons PT: *Pons' emergency medicine secrets,* ed 3, Philadelphia, 2003, Hanley & Belfus.

Buttaravoli P, Stair T: *Minor emergencies: Splinters to fractures,* St Louis, 2000, Mosby.

Canadian Association of Emergency Physicians: Canadian Emergency Department Triage and Acuity Scale (CTAS) Implementation guidelines, *J Can Assoc Emerg Physicians* 1(3 suppl), 1999.

Char E, Wong J: Abdominal pain. In Davis MA, Votey SR, Greenough P, editors: *Signs and symptoms in emergency medicine: Literature-based approach to emergent conditions,* St Louis, 1999, Mosby.

Cole LA: Accuracy of home pregnancy tests at the time of missed menses, *Am J Obstet Gynecol* 190:100-105, 2004.

Emergency Nurses Association: *Position statement: Patients with spontaneous abortions in the emergency department,* Des Plaines, Ill, 2000, Author.

Jenkin JL, Braen GR: *Manual of emergency medicine,* ed 4, Philadelphia, 2000, Lippincott, Williams & Wilkins.

Jordan K: *Emergency nursing core curriculum,* ed 5, Philadelphia, 2000, WB Saunders.

Lowdermilk D, Perry S: *Maternity and women's health care,* ed 8, St Louis, 2004, Mosby.

McNair R (President): The nature of the beast: Comprehensive triage and patient flow workshop, Triage First, Inc. Fairview, NC, available at www.triagefirst.com.

Moellman JJ, Bocock JM : Acute pelvic pain. In Hamilton GC, Sanders AB, Stragne GR, Trott AT: *Trott's emergency medicine: An approach to clinical problem-solving,* ed 2, St Louis, 2003, WB Saunders.

Newberry L: *Sheehy's emergency nursing principles and practice,* ed 5, St Louis, 2003, Mosby.

Trott AT: Pelvic inflammatory disease. In Markovchick VJ, Pons PT: *Pons' emergency medicine secrets,* ed 3, Philadelphia, 2003, Hanley & Belfus.

Zimmermann PG: Triaging lower abdominal pain, *RN* 65(12):53-58, 2002.

Chapter 35

Male Genital Pain

Susanne A. Quallich

1. Are there "red flag" conditions that require emergent or urgent intervention?

Yes. These include:

- Sudden onset of acute testicular pain
- Cellulitic or necrotic changes to the skin of the scrotum, penis, perineal region
- An erection lasting >60 minutes after cessation of sexual activity
- Inability to advance the foreskin
- Inability to urinate, especially if accompanied by perineal (prostatic) complaints
- New, painful mass in the scrotum

2. Are there any specific guidelines for a relevant history and evaluation of pain to the male genitalia?

- Duration of the current complaint
- History of previous such complaints
- Pattern and location of pain (acute vs. gradual radiation?)
- Presence of any constitutional symptoms
- Urethral discharge or dysuria
- History of trauma, mechanism of injury
- Avulsion of any genital structures

3. Classify the patterns of male genital pain.

Prostatic pain	Pain directly from prostate uncommon Acute inflammation: may cause discomfort or fullness to perineal and/or rectal area Possible lumbosacral backache Can cause dysuria, frequency, urgency
Epididymal pain	As a result of acute infection Pain in scrotum Begins as pain in groin or left quadrant (LQ) abdomen Can reach costal angle and mimic stone pain Inflammation of testicle possible
Testicular pain	Very severe, felt locally Can radiate along spermatic cord to lower abdomen and/or costovertebral angle Varicocele can cause dull ache that worsens after heavy exercise (see Chapter 36)

4. I heard the term "penile fracture." What does this mean?

A penile fracture is the result of trauma during intercourse that causes a rupture to the tunica albuginea of one of the paired corpora cavernosa of the penis. The patient will present with a history of a lateral buckling of the penis and a "snap" heard during intercourse, typically when the woman is in the superior position. If a man presents acutely after a penile fracture, there may be blood at the meatus or ecchymosis to the penis or scrotum. With time, he may complain of decreased and/or painful erections and a palpable scar.

5. Have you heard of a "testicular rupture"?

This is a rupture of the thick tunica albuginea that covers the testicle, and can occur as the result of blunt trauma to the scrotum/testicles. The incidence may be as high as 50% (Rosenstein & McAninch, 2004). Risk factors include sports injuries and assault. Definitive evaluation is performed surgically; pertinent assessment would include establishing the mechanism of injury and length of time since the injury.

6. What makes Fournier's gangrene an emergency?

This is a progressive necrotizing fasciitis of the genitals and perineum, usually caused by a combination of aerobic and anaerobic organisms. It can rapidly progress to involve the entire perineal area, abdominal wall, and buttocks.

The patient may recall a prodromal period of generalized discomfort, followed by erythema and edema to the affected areas. Often there are also constitutional complaints of fever, chills, nausea, and vomiting, and the patient may progress to frank sepsis.

Fournier's gangrene is most commonly seen in males in their sixth decade. Risk factors for its development include poor personal hygiene, phimosis, diabetes, alcoholism, malnutrition, chemotherapy or radiation treatment, perirectal or perianal infections, and local trauma to the genitals or perineal area (such as surgery).

7. What is prostatitis and why is it painful?

This is an acute or chronic infection of the prostate gland itself. The prostate becomes infected because bacteria ascend from the urethra (there is a reflux of infected urine into the prostatic ducts) and less commonly by direct extension and migration via the lymphatic and vascular system. Prostatitis can be very painful, as a result of a distortion of the gland itself, and because it may be associated with acute cystitis and the swollen gland may result in urinary retention.

8. What is a typical patient history with prostatitis?

There can be a variety of presenting symptoms. If it is acute prostatitis, the patient may present with a febrile illness, low back and perineal pain, urinary urgency and frequency, nocturia, dysuria, and complaints of muscle and joint aches. His urine may smell strong, be cloudy, and there may be gross hematuria. Chronic prostatitis manifests as recurrent episodes of irritative symptoms of dysuria, nocturia, frequency, urgency, and possibly inadequately treated episodes of acute prostatitis.

9. Is urgent treatment needed if a patient is diagnosed with a spermatocele?

No. A spermatocele is a mass in the head of the epididymis that contains fluid and sperm. It is typically painless.

10. Discuss a patient complaint of pain to his penis and a constant erection.

Priapism is a prolonged erection that occurs in the absence of sexual stimulation or that remains after ejaculation. The penis does not have to be 100% erect to be considered priapism; the defining factor being that it remains after the cessation of sexual activity. The complaint of pain depends on the length of the time the penis has remained erect (pain usually does not occur until after 6 to 8 hours). Your patient may also provide a history of the use of injectable erotogenic agents (such as Caverject), sickle cell disease, or a history of similar episodes in the past that resolved painlessly after a couple of hours.

11. What should I do about priapism?

It is vital to establish as accurately as possible the duration of the erection. Priapism requires immediate treatment, and often requires evaluation by a urologist.

12. Describe Peyronie's disease.

Although the precise cause of Peyronie's disease is not known, current belief regarding its etiology is that the plaque formation results after disordered wound healing (Levine & Elterman, 1997). The plaque is present in the tunica albuginea of the corpora cavernosa, which leads to shortening and curvature of the shaft of the penis. The quality of the erection distal to the plaque is poor and prevents adequate penetration during sexual activity.

13. Phimosis and paraphimosis: which one needs urgent treatment?

Phimosis is seen in males who are uncircumcised. The patient will often present with a history of progressive difficulty retracting the foreskin and may complain of pain when retracting or attempting to retract the foreskin. Physical examination may show the opening of the foreskin to be contracted to the point where the actual opening is quite small, putting the patient at risk for urinary obstruction.

Paraphimosis is also seen in males who are uncircumcised; it is the inability to advance the foreskin to its normal position over the glans after it has been retracted. The patient may present with complaints of pain, swelling, and possible discoloration of the glans; examination of the penis will reveal a foreskin that cannot be advanced or can be advanced only with difficulty. The shaft of the penis and glans may be tender, swollen, and painful on palpation. Paraphimosis is a *urologic emergency*, as arterial occlusion and necrosis of the glans and distal urethra may result if the paraphimosis is not reduced.

14. Are sexually transmitted diseases in the male a cause of pain?

Sometimes. There are many ways in which a sexually transmitted disease (STD) can present in the male patient (see chart). The presentation is typically more occult than in the female, and does not always cause pain or discomfort.

Sexually Transmitted Disease	Clinical Presentation in the Male
Chancroid	Tender ulcer with deep undermined border, may be soft or indurated; friable base with ragged edges; purulent exudate possible; painful lymphadenopathy
Chlamydia	Scant mucoid or mucopurulent urethral discharge; may be accompanied by mild dysuria and urethral itching
Genital Herpes Simplex	First episode: fluid-filled painful vesicles that may coalesce, with erythema to surrounding skin that eventually rupture, resulting in painful ulcerative lesions with erythematous edges; tender adenopathy, fever, dysuria also common. Lesions typically last 2 to 3 weeks, possibly up to 6 weeks. Recurrences: prodromal pain, burning, tingling at site in which vesicles will erupt with shorter course of constitutional symptoms; lesions usually resolve after 7 to 10 days
Genital Warts (Human Papillomavirus)	Soft, fleshy, exophytic lesions with raised granular surface; commonly seen on glans and prepuce; also present as small papular lesions on the skin or nonhealing penile lesion(s) Majority of lesions are subclinical and can be detected by using 3% to 5% acetic acid
Gonorrhea	Urethral discharge may be yellowish or gray-brown, purulent, and accompanied by itching and dysuria; may be accompanied by epididymal or testicular pain; asymptomatic in 5% to 10% of cases; rare superficial lesions to the penile shaft
Nongonococcal urethritis	Mild to moderate, clear or white urethral discharge; or thin mucoid urethral discharge; accompanied by mild dysuria and urethral itching
Pediculosis pubis	Severe pruritus; observation of ectoparasites on hair and/or skin in the genital area
Scabies	Papular or linear burrow-like lesions
Syphilis	Primary: solitary, painless, nontender and rubbery ulcer (chancre), superficial or deep, with indurated edge and no exudate Secondary: papulosquamous or maculopapular rash that is indicative of systemic infection
Trichomoniasis	Usually asymptomatic, may cause urethritis

15. Describe the presentation of a patient with testicular torsion.

The patient will give a history of acute and sudden onset of pain that localizes to the affected testicle and the pain may have woke him up from sleep. The pain may radiate to the inguinal areas or abdomen and is often accompanied by abdominal discomfort, nausea, and vomiting.

Scrotal swelling may be apparent on physical examination, particularly on the affected side. The classic physical findings are the affected testicle being somewhat elevated and with a somewhat horizontal lie. Other scrotal structures may be difficult to assess as a result of edema.

A less typical presentation is that of gradual onset of testicular pain. There may also be a history that is consistent with spontaneous torsion/detorsion of the spermatic cord and testicle.

Testicular torsion is most commonly seen in early puberty, as a result of the rapid growth of the testes. The resulting loss of blood flow to the affected testicle will result in swelling, tissue necrosis and may potentially affect future fertility (if the remaining testicle is unable to compensate).

16. Do patients with testicular tumors always present with pain?

Not usually. The patient may provide a history of a painless swelling of the testicle or a distinct nodule noted on self-examination. There may have been some minor trauma to the affected side that initiated the onset of pain and/or swelling. The testicle may have gradually enlarged over time, with some associated heaviness. Patients will rarely complain of acute pain as their presenting symptom, but rather a dull ache or heaviness that localizes to the affected side.

17. My patient is complaining of scrotal pain and says that he feels "worms" in his scrotum. What could this be?

It sounds like your patient is trying to describe a varicocele: a palpable or visible dilation of the vessels of the pampiniform plexus in the scrotum. If the varicocele is large enough, there may be resulting scrotal swelling that is noticeable to the patient, along with a bluish discoloration beneath the scrotal skin, and it may be visible during inspection ("bag of worms").

18. Can a patient get an infection in his epididymis?

Yes, unless he has had a vasectomy, and it can be quite painful. It is caused by the spread of an infection from the bladder, prostate, or urethra. Uncircumcised men, men with indwelling catheters, benign prostatic hypertrophy (BPH), recent genitourinary (GU) instrumentation, or prostatic surgery create a risk for epididymitis. If epididymitis is left unrecognized and untreated, it can progress to an abscess or chronic infection, with resulting fibrosis, chronic scrotal pain, and infertility.

19. How does the patient with epididymitis usually present?

- History of a sudden onset (over 24 to 48 hours)
- Painful swelling in the scrotum, which can be unilateral or bilateral.
- Pain may decrease with elevation of the scrotum (Plehn's sign), although this is not diagnostic.
- Associated urethral discharge, fever, and complaints of urethritis, cystitis, or prostatitis are possible.

On physical exam, the patient will find sitting uncomfortable and his pain will localize to the affected epididymis with palpation, which will be swollen and indurated. The spermatic cord may be tender and swollen as well, and pain may radiate to the inguinal canal and/or flank.

20. Is it possible to have an infection in a testicle?

Yes, especially if your patient has been diagnosed with epididymitis. Orchitis is caused by the extension of an infection from the epididymis to the testicle itself, and rarely exists independent of epididymitis. Pain will also localize to the affected testicle, and it may not be possible to distinguish the separation between the epididymis and testicle as a result of inflammation.

The risks and causative organisms are the same as for epididymitis. Viral orchitis may occur as sequelae of mumps, and occurs in up to 30% of prepubertal male patients with mumps.

21. Does balanitis cause penile pain?

The patient with balanitis may present with a combination of symptoms that include not only pain to the glans of the penis but edema, dysuria, urethral discharge, and a history of a discharge from between the foreskin and glans; there may be a cracked appearance to the prepuce. Balanitis is seen only in uncircumcised males; this inflammation is caused by a *Candida albicans* infection. Men with poorly controlled diabetes mellitus are at particular risk for balanitis.

22. My patient states that he has "a large, painful bag of water" in his scrotum.

He is describing a hydrocele—a collection of fluid between the layers of the tunica vaginalis that surround the testicle or fluid along the spermatic cord, and it may be large enough to completely encompass the testicle. Hydroceles are not usually painful, but there may be associated heaviness or discomfort during specific activities, such as prolonged sitting or bicycle riding.

23. Are there other conditions that will cause a male patient to present with complaints of genital pain?

Yes. The most common is a kidney stone, which can lead to pain that radiates to the spermatic cord and/or testicle on the affected side. There can also be complaints of pain to the urethra as the stone is passed.

An inguinal hernia can lead to complaints of pain that may extend to the scrotum on the affected side, particularly with changes to intraabdominal pressure.

24. Is there anything else I might expect if a patient is vague about the cause of his penile or genital pain?

Your patient may be embarrassed to admit that he has a:

- Penile or scrotal piercing that might be painful or possibly infected.
- Penile tourniquet injury as the result of some sort of ring (such as those used with vacuum erection devices) or string tied around the base of the penis.
- "Zipper entrapment," particularly of the foreskin.

25. What must be considered in a male with a urinary tract infection?

STD. Delay obtaining a urine specimen until a culture can be obtained.

Key Points

- In the case of genital trauma, establish the mechanism of injury.
- Any conditions that cause ischemia to the genitals are urologic emergencies.
- Pain to a male genital structure will often cause pain to adjacent structures.
- Evaluation of pain to the scrotal structures should involve a physical examination as rapidly as possible, as subsequent swelling will obscure individual structures.

Internet Resources

American Urological Association: UrologyHealth.org
http://www.urologyhealth.org

American Urological Association Clinical Guidelines
http://www.auanet.org/guidelines/

The Merck Manual of Medical Information—Second Home Edition, Online Version, Men's Health Issues: Penile and Testicular Disorders
http://www.merck.com/mmhe/sec21/ch238/ch238a.html

Prostate Disorders
http://www.merck.com/mmhe/sec21/ch239/ch239a.html

Sexual Dysfunction
http://www.merck.com/mmhe/sec21/ch240/ch240a.html

Bibliography

Batstone G, Doble A, Batstone D: Chronic prostatitis, *Curr Opin Urol* 13(1):23-29, 2003.

Burgher SW: Acute scrotal pain, *Emerg Med Clin North Am* 16:781-808, 1998.

Montague DK, Jarow J, Broderick GA, et al: American Urological Association guidelines on the management of priapism, *J Urol* 170(4):1318-1324, 2003.

Levine LA, Elterman L: Peyronie's disease and its medical management. In Hellstrom WJG, editor: *Male infertility and sexual dysfunction,* New York, 1997, Springer, 474-475.

Rosenstein D, McAninch JW: Urologic emergencies, *Med Clin N Am* 88(2):495, 2004.

Chapter 36

Pregnancy Considerations

Darleen A. Williams

1. So, just what is considered "childbearing" age?

The age ranges given vary but, in general, it is accepted that a female can become pregnant any time from 11 to 55 years old. The Manchester Triage Group defines "possible pregnancy" as any woman whose normal menstruation is late or any woman of childbearing age that is having unprotected sex.

2. What should the triage nurse obtain about a patient's reproductive history?

- Currently pregnant?
- History of multiple pregnancies?
- History of sexually transmitted diseases?
- Gravida, Parity, Abortions (GPA)?

3. Elaborate on the meaning of the patient's GPA.

Gravida is the total number of pregnancies a woman has had.

Parity is the number of pregnancies in which the fetus actually reached a viable gestational age.

Abortion is any termination of the pregnancy, either spontaneous or elective. The common use for the term is only an elective termination of a pregnancy and patients may become defensive or insulted with the question without explanation.

4. How can I quickly and easily estimate how far along the patient is with a pregnancy?

Nägele's rule: identify the first day of the patient's last menses, add 7 days then subtract 3 months for estimated date of birth (EDB). Of course, accuracy of the results is dependent on the information the patient gives you. The terminology traditionally used to express this had been EDC (estimated date of confinement), but has now evolved to the more accurate "EDB."

5. Is there any other way?

- Measure the fundal height (the distance in centimeters from the symphysis pubis to the top of the pregnant uterus). The rough estimate of a pregnancy is 2 weeks less and more than the number. For instance, if the fundal height is 32 cm; a rough estimate is 30 to 34 weeks.
- Use an obstetric (OB) wheel.

6. As the triage nurse, how do I determine if the patient's presenting complaint is related to her pregnancy?

To establish if the patient's complaint is related to their pregnancy, the emergency nurse must be aware of the related physiologic changes. The table below lists some of the normal changes that are expected during pregnancy.

Category	Change
Respiratory	Resting respiratory rate increases with oxygen consumption by 20%. Minute volume is up by 50% and the Pco_2 will be low, a normal respiratory alkalosis secondary to hyperventilation.
Cardiac	Total circulating blood volume will increase approximately 30%. Cardiac output will increase by 30% to 40% by the 27th week and resting heart rate will increase 15 to 20 beats over the nonpregnant state.
Gastrointestinal	Increased time in gastric emptying caused by smooth muscle relaxation. Increased constipation caused by decreased peristalsis. Increased hormonal levels will relax sphincter and increase the risk of aspiration.
General	Dilutional anemia secondary to increased circulating volume and increased iron usage by the mother and the fetus.

If the patient's complaint or symptoms is not a physiologic change associated with the pregnancy, consider that the problem may arise independent of the pregnancy (but still may affect the pregnancy).

7. How do I not miss any of the important information related to pain?

Mnemonics are an easy way to remember important concepts. Adapt the PQRST mnemonic to the pregnant patient.

Provokes or causes the **P**roblem/**P**ain? Signs of labor, including abdominal pain, backache, or increased vaginal pressure?

Quality Description? Associated symptoms such as nausea, vomiting, vaginal bleeding, or discharge?

Region: Where is the discomfort? Does it radiate? To the back? Across the low abdomen? Patient's shoulder?

Severity: What number would the patient give this on the 1 to 10 scale? Evaluate the pain level with each set of vital signs.

Timing. Is the discomfort constant or intermittent? Contraction intervals? Length of contractions?

8. Are there any other mnemonics that can be used to evaluate the patient's complaint?

Adapt CIAMPEDS from the Emergency Nurses Association's Emergency Nurse Pediatric Course (ENPC) course.

Chief complaint. Why are they here today? The triage nurse needs to determine this although not necessarily addressing all the somatic complaints the patient may be experiencing related to a normal pregnancy.

Isolation. Has the patient been exposed to any communicable diseases recently? Is she immunocompromised? **I**mmunizations: Has this patient received the "usual shots" growing up?

Allergies. Medications? Latex allergy? Blood type? Rh negative?

Medications. Prescribed? Over-the-counter (OTC), herbal products, or home remedies?

Past medical history. Reproductive history and this current pregnancy? Prenatal care? More than one fetus?

Event(s). What led the patient to come to the emergency department (ED) at this time? Any mechanisms of illness or injury?

Diet and "**D**iapers." Urine and bowel movement (I&O)? Any gastrointestinal (GI) or genitourinary (GU) signs or symptoms?

Signs and symptoms of ruptured membranes? If the patient's membranes have ruptured, use the TACO mnemonic to assess (see below).

9. What do the letters of TACO for ruptured membranes stand for?

Time of rupture
Amount (estimated)
Color of secretions
Odor (none or foul)

10. Why are urinary symptoms included when taking the history of a pregnant woman?

Early in the pregnancy, a urinary tract infection (UTI) can cause miscarriage.

In the third trimester, frequent urination/dribbling can actually be a leaking amniotic fluid.

11. At what gestational age can fetal heart tones be heard?

At about the 12th to 13th week of pregnancy, fetal heart tones (FHTs) may be heard if the nurse uses a Doppler low on the patient's abdomen just above her symphysis pubis and pushes firmly. FHT may still be present even if there is initially difficulty in hearing them. Patient position, extraneous noise, and amount of body tissue can all contribute to this being a difficult assessment, especially in triage.

12. Should I listen to FHTs in triage?

Although ascertaining FHTs is a very important component of the pregnant patient's assessment, it may not be feasible to perform this assessment in triage. Instead determine if there has been any fetal movement. Ask the patient when the last time was her baby moved or kicked.

13. What is a normal FHT range?

The acceptable range is considered 120 to 160 beats per minute (bpm). If too low, check the mother's pulse. If the rates are the same, you are hearing the mother's, not the fetal, heartbeat. If the fetal rate is less than 120 bpm, immediately notify the physician.

14. Give an example of triage categories related to pregnancy.

Manchester Triage Group

Level 1 (immediate):	Airway, breathing, circulation (ABC) instability Exsanguinating hemorrhage Presenting fetal parts Prolapsed umbilical cord Currently seizing
Level 2 (very urgent) (10 minutes):	Severe pain History of seizures within the last 6 hours (rule out eclampsia) In active labor (frequent, regular painful contractions) Heavy blood loss Any blood loss >24 weeks pregnant
Level 3 (urgent) (60 minutes):	Moderate pain Shoulder tip pain Inappropriate history History of recent trauma High blood pressure (by history or currently)

Level 4 (standard) (120 minutes):	Any pain Warmth by touch >99.5°F (>37.5°C)
Canadian Triage and Acuity Scale (CTAS)	
Level 2 (emergent) (≤15 minutes):	Vaginal bleeding and lower abdominal pain Abnormal vital signs ≥20 weeks gestation
Level 3 (urgent) (≤30 minutes):	Mild pain (≤4 out of 10) and bleeding not severe First trimester (last menstrual period [LMP] ≥4 weeks) and/or previously positive beta human chorionic gonadotropin (HCG) with normal vital signs

15. Define "severe bleeding." That can be hard to assess.

The Manchester Triage Group defines it as the presence of large clots, constant blood flow, and a history of using a large number of peri-pads.

16. Give examples of some standing triage orders related to pregnancy.

Memorial Regional Hospital (Hollywood, Fla)
Melinda Stibal, RN BSHC; Administrative Director, Emergency/Trauma
For lower abdominal pain and/or vaginal bleeding:

- Complete blood cell count (CBC)
- Urinalysis (U/A)
- Serum qualitative pregnancy test if pregnancy status unknown (all premenopausal women)
- Beta HCG if patient known to be pregnant and the patient is <16 weeks by date
- Group and Rh if vaginal bleeding *and* suspected to be pregnant
- Fetal heart tones if gestational age >12 weeks

Saratoga Hospital (Saratoga Falls, NY) and Glens Falls Hospital, Glens Falls, NY
Conni Tucker, RN CEN; ED Supervisor
For patients with suspected ectopic pregnancy:

- Initiate two large-bore intravenous lines (IVs) with normal saline
- CBC
- Beta HCG
- Clot for type and cross

17. Are there any problems specific to the pregnant patient that the triage nurse should be aware of?

The following table gives a brief description of the potential complications associated with pregnancy.

Complications	Signs and Symptoms
Premature labor	Contractions occurring more often than every 10 minutes lasting more than 1 hour. These contractions *do not* have to be painful ("tightness") and may be noticed in the low abdominal area or low back. There may or may not be any vaginal discharge. Membranes do not have to rupture.
Ectopic pregnancy	Moderate to severe pelvic pain (Kehr's sign [shoulder pain] if ruptured), usually with bleeding (see below).
Abortion	Either spontaneous or elective termination of the pregnancy before the fetus is viable is considered an abortion. As a result of technology today the viability of a fetus can be ascertained as early as around 21 weeks.
Pregnancy-induced hypertension (PIH)	Also called toxemia and includes preeclampsia and eclampsia. Preeclampsia is characterized by hypertension, edema, and proteinuria. The patient has eclampsia if seizures begin. This is a medical emergency.
Placenta previa	Classic signs are bright red painless bleeding late in the pregnancy with *no* contractions.
Abruptio placentae	Occurs during the last trimester when the placenta separates from the uterine wall. Classic symptoms are a firm or hard uterus, severe abdominal pain, and dark red vaginal bleeding (80%).
HELLP syndrome	Hemolysis, elevated liver enzymes, and low platelets (HELLP). It is associated with PIH (10%).

18. Why is ectopic pregnancy a concern?

One in 60 pregnancies in the U.S. is ectopic; the incidence has increased four times since 1980. It is the leading cause of maternal death in the first trimester. An ectopic pregnancy must be ruled out if an early pregnancy produces:

- Vaginal bleeding
- Pelvic pain
- Syncope

19. Can you give the incidences of the most common signs and symptoms of ectopic pregnancy?

70% to 94%	Pelvic or abdominal pain (unilateral, lower quadrant)
	Vaginal spotting
31% to 69%	Amenorrhea
	Dizziness
5% to 30%	Nausea/vomiting
	Asymptomatic

20. Discuss the causes of an ectopic pregnancy.

History of pelvic inflammatory disease (PID). More than 50% of women who have an ectopic pregnancy have a history of PID. After an initial episode of PID, the risk of an ectopic pregnancy increases fivefold to sevenfold.

Presence of an intrauterine device (IUD). If pregnancy does occur, the relative risk of an ectopic pregnancy may be as high as 1.5 to 2.8 times the normal population.

Previous tubal surgery/ligation. The failure rate of a tubal ligation is as high as 36 per 1,000; 30% to 40% of pregnancies occurring after ligation are ectopic.

Previous ectopic pregnancy. Women with one previous ectopic pregnancy have a greater than 10% of a repeat ectopic pregnancy with each subsequent pregnancy.

21. Who is most at risk for preeclampsia and eclampsia?

- Pregnancy that is more than 20 weeks up to 3 days after the delivery
- Patient age less than 20 (primiparous) or more than 40 years old (multiparous)
- Family history
- Co-morbidities of diabetes, obesity, multiple gestation, or preexisting hypertension
- Lower socioeconomic group

The cause is still not fully understood, and no known prevention exists. It occurs in 5% to 10% of all pregnancies and early detection is the best approach. (The triage nurse can screen for PIH by taking the blood pressure and dipping the urine for protein with pregnant women after the 20th week.)

22. Describe some signs or symptoms a woman with preeclampsia might have.

- Swelling of the hands, face, or legs
- Headache
- Visual disturbances
- Altered mental status
- Hyperreflexia

23. What blood pressure measurements are used to screen for preeclampsia?

Hypertension is diagnosed at a lower pressure in preeclampsia than other situations: blood pressure of 140/90 or an increase of 30/15 from the baseline. Treatment is required for blood pressure of 160/110 or higher, accompanied by proteinuria. (Generalized edema is no longer recognized by many authorities as a required accompanying symptom for preeclampsia.)

24. What should I consider in a pregnant woman who has experienced trauma?

Any trauma, whether mild, moderate, or severe, is a risk factor for abruption. Usually women greater than 24 weeks of gestation are monitored afterward for uterine irritability and fetal distress.

25. What are classic distinguishers between placenta abruption (abruptio placentae) and placenta previa?

- The pain with placenta abruption is severe; placenta previa is painless.
- The vaginal bleeding with placenta abruption is dark red; the bleeding with placenta previa is bright red.

26. What should I do when a woman in the third trimester is lying on her back and experiences hypotension and tachycardia?

Position the woman in a left side-lying position to aid blood return.

27. If bruising is seen on a pregnant woman, what should I further investigate?

The potential for domestic violence: 4% to 8% of pregnant women are abused. If abused during pregnancy, the woman is at a three times higher risk to be a victim of attempted or completed homicide.

28. Am I required to report it if I suspect my pregnant patient has been using recreational substances?

The legal requirements to report even suspected incidences vary from state to state. Many experts believe the best approach is to not advocate for laws requiring punitive measures. This practice has not shown to make a difference in the woman's drug use, but often does result in her seeking less prenatal care.

29. What signals an imminent delivery?

The desire to push with (or especially between) her contractions. Transport the patient by stretcher to an appropriate area of the department.

30. What is essential for me to ask an obviously pregnant woman who walks through the doors and shouts, "The baby is coming now!"

- When are you due? (e.g., is the baby term or premature?)
- Is your bag of water intact? (If it was broken, what color was the water to rule out meconium staining.)
- How many babies are you expecting? (To prepare in case there will be two or more.)
- What drugs have you taken in the last 4 hours? (Will this delivered infant be depressed?)

31. Who is the priority for emergency care: the pregnant patient or the unborn child?

Although each of us has our own personal and professional opinion regarding this, in general, the accepted practice has been that what is good for the mother is good for the baby. Thankfully these kinds of decisions will not need to be made in triage, and there are adequate resources to care for both in ordinary circumstances.

32. Should I automatically assign all pregnant patients a higher triage level, as we are really dealing with two patients and not just one?

No. The acuity level assigned to the patient in triage should be assigned based on the patient's current needs and not solely on a preexisting history or condition. The fact that the patient is pregnant can be a contributing factor in your decision, but only after you have done your primary and abbreviated secondary assessment. Concern is usually raised when the complaint is either pregnancy related or systemic.

Key Points

- Ask TACO for ruptured membranes (T: time of rupture, A: estimated amount, C: color of secretions, O: any foul odor noted).
- Consider an ectopic pregnancy as a possibility for childbearing female who has one-sided severe low abdominal pain 2 weeks after the LMP.
- Be concerned if a pregnant woman more than 20 weeks has urinary symptoms, low back pain, hypertension, vaginal bleeding, edema, or seizures.
- Assess FHT every ED visit (after the 12th to 13th week); ask about fetal movement in triage.

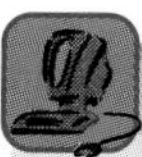

Internet Resources

Ectopic Pregnancy
http://nsweb.nursingspectrum.com/ce/ce77.htm

Pregnancy, Eclampsia
http://www.emedicine.com/emerg/topic796.htm

Pregnancy, Hyperemesis Gravidarum
http://www.emedicine.com/emerg/topic479.htm

Pregnancy, Preeclampsia
http://www.emedicine.com/emerg/topic480.htm

Pregnancy, Trauma
http://www.emedicine.com/emerg/topic484.htm

Placenta Previa
http://www.emedicine.com/emerg/topic427.htm

Abortion, Complete
http://www.emedicine.com/emerg/topic3.htm

Abortion, Complications
http://www.emedicine.com/emerg/topic4.htm

Abortion, Incomplete
http://www.emedicine.com/emerg/topic5.htm

Abortion, Inevitable
http://www.emedicine.com/emerg/topic6.htm

Abruptio Placentae
http://www.emedicine.com/emerg/topic12.htm

Bibliography

Abbott JT: Ectopic pregnancy. In Markovchick VJ, Pons PT: *Pons' emergency medicine secrets,* ed 3, Philadelphia, 2003, Hanley & Belfus.

Canadian Association of Emergency Physicians: Canadian Emergency Department Triage and Acuity Scale Implementation Guidelines, *J Can Assoc Emerg Physicians* 1(3 suppl), 1999.

Emergency Nurses Association: Position statement: Patients with spontaneous abortions in the emergency department, available at ena.org, accessed Apr 1, 2005.

Howell JM: Third-trimester vaginal bleeding. In Markovchick VJ, Pons PT, editors: *Pons' emergency medicine secrets,* ed 3, Philadelphia, 2003, Hanley & Belfus.

Jones RO: Childbirth. In Markovchick VJ, Pons PT, editors: *Pons' emergency medicine secrets,* ed 3, Philadelphia, 2003, Hanley & Belfus.

Jordan K: *Emergency nursing core curriculum,* ed 5, Philadelphia, 2000, WB Saunders.

Louden M, Uner A: Hypertension. In Davis MA, Votey SR, Greenough PG, editors: *Greenough's signs and symptoms in emergency medicine: Literature-based approach to emergent conditions,* St Louis, 1999, Mosby.

Lowdermilk D, Perry S: Maternity & women's health care, ed 8, St Louis, 2004, Mosby.

Mackway-Jones K: *Emergency triage: Manchester Triage Group,* London, 1997, BMJ Publishing.

McFarlane J, et al: Abuse during pregnancy and femicide: Urgent implications for women's health, *Obstet Gynecol* 100:27-36, 2002.

Moellman JJ, Bocock JM: Acute pelvic pain. In Hamilton GC, Sanders AB, Strange GR, Trott AT, editors: *Trott's emergency medicine: An approach to clinical problem-solving,* ed 2, St Louis, 2003, WB Saunders.

Newberry L: *Sheehy's emergency nursing principles and practice,* ed 5, St Louis, 2003, Mosby.

Rickets V: Vaginal bleeding. In Davis MA, Votey SR, Greenough PG: *Greenough's signs and symptoms in emergency medicine: Literature-based approach to emergent conditions,* St Louis, 1999, Mosby.

Van Hare RS: Preeclampsia and eclampsia. In Markovchick VJ, Pons PT, editors: *Pons' Emergency Medicine Secrets,* ed 3, St Louis, 2003, Mosby.

Chapter 37

Dysuria

Susanne A. Quallich

1. What exactly is dysuria?

Dysuria is burning, pain, or discomfort on urination. Women present more frequently with the complaint as a result of their shorter urethral length.

2. A patient with a complaint of dysuria does not seem in urgent need of evaluation and treatment. What am I missing?

Although it seems like a simple complaint, dysuria can be an indicator of other serious conditions:

- Renal or bladder carcinoma.
- Ureteral obstruction.
- A secondary infection from anatomic abnormality.
- A secondary infection from abnormality of function, including postmenopausal status or prostatic hypertrophy.
- Mechanical causes, such as recent genitourinary (GU) instrumentation or catheter placement.
- Indicator of other systemic conditions, such as diabetes mellitus, renal calculi, or depression.

3. What are the structures that can contribute to a complaint of dysuria?

Basically any and all structures of the GU tract can contribute to dysuria.

4. So the physical examination with dysuria should include all the GU structures?

The physical examination should definitely include all the GU structures, and an abdominal exam, male and female genital examination, and pelvic examination (women) or rectal examination (men).

5. Are there specific nerve pathways that contribute to bladder sensation and pain?

The bladder receives afferent and efferent innervation from both the autonomic and somatic nervous system. Parasympathetic innervation arises from 2nd to 4th sacral segments and projects to pelvic plexus. Sympathetic control originates at T10 to L2. Somatic innervation originates S2 to S3, and travels via the pudendal nerve to external urethral sphincter, and permits the sensation of fullness, inflammation, or pain depending on the specific pathway.

Damage or other pathologies that impact these areas of the spine (herniated disc, spinal stenosis, degenerative changes to the vertebrae, or metastatic disease) can result in changes to bladder function and/or sensation. Diseases that result in neuropathies (such as diabetes mellitus or multiple sclerosis) can contribute to the dysfunction of bladder sensation and function.

6. How does the patient's description of dysuria contribute to making the diagnosis?

The timing of pain with urination matters. External pain (pain as the urine passes over the labia) can indicate inflammatory vaginal or meatal causes, although pain when beginning the urine stream can indicate that the urethra is irritated, such as with a sexually transmitted disease (STD). Pain felt internally is more likely as a result of irritation of the bladder.

7. What is the most common cause of dysuria?

The urinary tract infection (UTI) is the most common cause for dysuria. UTIs are the second most common bacterial disease and the most common source of bacteremia in older adults. Onset is typically sudden and without other constitutional symptoms. The most common pathogen causing acute, uncomplicated UTIs is *Escherichia coli.*

8. Are there specific risk factors for developing a UTI?

Yes. The risk factors for the development of a UTI are well established. They include:

- Increasing age
- Recent sexual intercourse
- A history of prior UTI
- Use of a diaphragm or cervical cap
- Anatomic abnormalities

9. What symptoms should I expect when evaluating a patient with a UTI?

The patient is likely to have a variety of complaints including pain, hesitancy, urgency, frequency and discomfort on urination, and he or she may also describe bladder fullness. There is usually a negative history of fever, chills, or other constitutional symptoms. There may be a color change to urine or the presence of a strong odor.

Both men and women should be asked about their risk for STDs. The patient should also be asked about any herbal, homeopathic, or vaginal hygiene remedies that have been tried since symptom onset. Female patients should be asked about associated vaginal symptoms; male patients should be queried symptoms related to the enlargement of the prostate.

10. Are there exceptions?

About half of all people with significant bacteriuria have no symptoms or have nonspecific signs, such as fatigue/lethargic (30%) or anorexia or cognitive change in the older adult. Geriatric experts indicate the most common symptom in patients with dementia is a change in behavior, particularly a new-onset of restlessness. In a child, consider the possibility with a presentation of malaise, rectal pain, or new onset of enuresis.

11. Should I just depend on a urine dipstick to determine if a patient has a UTI?

In one study of UTIs, the urine dipstick was positive for nitrate, leukocytes, or bacteria only 31% to 69% of the time. Nitrate will be positive if the organism is gram-negative because of the enzyme produced. However, gram-positive and yeast bacteria do not contain the converting enzyme. Overall, a urine dipstick that is positive for leukocyte esterase test and a positive nitrite test provides a high sensitivity and specificity for infection.

12. Will lab work or imaging studies help me evaluate dysuria?

A simple urinalysis will confirm the presence of a UTI: some combination of hematuria, pyuria, or bacteriuria will be observed. There is debate regarding whether the specimen must be a clean catch specimen. In women whose symptoms suggest uncomplicated UTI, a culture of $\geq 10^2$ CFU/mL is indicative of cystitis (Bent & Saint, 2003). Urine cultures should be considered when there is a recurrent UTI, refractory UTI, or the patient who appears toxic. Complete blood cell count (CBC) and electrolytes should be drawn based on the overall clinical presentation and comorbidities.

13. Can you give an example of triage protocols for suspected UTIs?

Memorial Regional Hospital, Hollywood, Fla
Source: Melinda Stibal, RN BSHC, Administrative Director for Emergency/Trauma
Suspected UTI without fever
- Urinalysis (U/A) (clean catch/catheter if bleeding)
- Urine pregnancy (for all premenopausal women)

Suspected Pyelonephritis
- U/A (clean catch/catheter)
- Urine culture and sensitivity (C&S)
- Urine Pregnancy (for all premenopausal women)
- Saline lock
- Acetaminophen (Tylenol) 650 mg PO for temperature >100.5°F (38°C)

14. What should I consider in a young teenager who presents with UTI symptoms?

UTIs traditionally have an increased incidence in women who are sexually active and/or pregnant. Ask about the teenager's sexual activity.

15. When I do phone triage, should I be skeptical when I have female patients who call and say, "I have a UTI again."?

Twenty percent to 30% of women who have UTIs have recurrent episodes. In one study, about half of the women in the study were able to accurately self-diagnose at least one UTI in the following year.

16. Do we still recommend cranberry juice as a preventive measure?

There is evidence that cranberry juice is effective in reducing recurrent UTIs. It is believed the resulting acidic environment prevents germ growth.

17. What makes a UTI "complicated"?

This is defined as a UTI in a context that increases the likelihood of treatment failure or recurrent infection. This includes patients with abnormalities of GU anatomy, functional abnormalities, and/or diabetes. Other risk factors for a complicated UTI include: male gender, pregnancy, extreme older or young age, or immunocompromised status. A complicated UTI can also be indicated when multiple organisms are present on culture.

18. What distinctions would make me suspect pyelonephritis?

This is a bacterial infection of the renal pelvis and parenchyma, typically caused by *E. coli* ascending from the lower urinary tract. Risk factors include vesicoureteral reflux, neurogenic bladder, stone disease of any part of the GU tract, immunosuppression, and diabetes mellitus. Although UTI and cystitis can have back pain, cystitis is more typically a low back pain whereas the pain of pyelonephritis typically localizes to the costovertebral angle (CVA) on the side of the infected kidney or "flank pain." This classic unilateral CVA tenderness is not exacerbated by movement, as musculoskeletal back pain typically does. The onset can be sudden or insidious. The patient will appear ill, with fever, chills, tachycardia, nausea, and vomiting in addition to the lower urinary tract symptoms.

19. How do I test for CVA tenderness?

The examiner's hand is placed over the opposite side CVA and lightly tapped on top of it by the examiner's other hand making a fist. The patient should feel a thud, but no pain. Reverse the hands and repeat on the opposite side.

20. Will lab work and imaging studies help me assess the severity of pyelonephritis?

Lab work can help in determining how ill the patient is. CBC can show leukocytosis, often with a shift to the left. A urinalysis will usually show leukocytosis, red blood cells (RBCs), protein, and bacteria. A urine culture will be positive, and with heavy growth. Blood cultures may be necessary, depending on the patient's overall presentation. Imaging studies should be considered if the patient appears ill or does not respond to initial outpatient management.

21. What would distinguish renal or ureteral colic?

Classic symptoms for kidney stones include these key, unique distinctions:

- Sudden onset of severe unilateral "flank" pain that often radiates to the testicle or vulva
- Restlessness, "writhing" unable to find a comfortable spot; pacing
- Diaphoresis

In addition, there is often a history of kidney stones (50% have recurrences), male, intermittent symptoms, history of dehydration, and microscopic or gross hematuria.

22. What is interstitial cystitis?

Interstitial cystitis (IC) is poorly understood entity with a suspected cause related to autoimmune, allergic or infectious components. Patients with IC suffer from a variety of chronic symptoms and negative urine cultures in addition to dysuria. Patients may report up to 40 trips to the bathroom in 24 hours. IC is much more prevalent in women, and some authors estimate the nationwide prevalence of IC among females to be approximately one in five (Parsons et al., 2002). There are periods of remission and flare-up throughout a patient's lifetime. Most patients visit an average of five physicians and wait up to four years before the correct diagnosis is made.

23. How does the presentation of interstitial cystitis differ from other dysuria complaints?

In addition to complaints of dysuria, patients will usually describe a history of irritative voiding symptoms: urinary urgency, frequency, and pain. There may also be complaints of suprapubic pain, dyspareunia, and chronic pelvic pain. Symptoms may worsen in the week prior to menstruation, and have often been present for a period of several months or years. A urinalysis will eliminate a UTI as the cause of these complaints. In order to diagnose IC, all other potential etiologies should be ruled out. Confirmation of diagnosis is via bladder appearance on cystoscopy.

24. Should I consider an STD in a male with dysuria?

Yes. The male's longer urethra makes them less likely to acquire a routine *E. coli* UTI. Chlamydia, herpes simplex, gonorrhea, nongonococcal urethritis, and trichomoniasis can all cause dysuria in men. He will need the appropriate cultures.

25. What is urethral syndrome?

This is an acute urethral pain syndrome in men or women, usually due from *Chlamydia trachomatis* or *Neisseria gonorrhoeae*. The female patient may present with vaginal discharge or bleeding and more gradual symptom onset (compared with the abrupt onset of symptoms in acute cystitis) and may report a new sexual partner. Men may have complaints of dysuria that cannot be localized to a specific part of urination (such as initiation of the urinary stream) and there may or may not be a urethral discharge. Whereas pyuria usually is present on microscopic examination, bacteriuria is not present and the presence of hematuria is variable. Pelvic examination is indicated if the diagnosis of cystitis is not straightforward or if vaginitis or acute urethral syndrome is suspected.

26. Are there other pain syndromes that include dysuria?

Yes. See the table below.

Genitourinary Pain Syndromes	Description
Painful bladder syndrome	Complaints of suprapubic pain are related to bladder filling, and it may be associated with other symptoms. There are complaints of increased daytime and nighttime frequency, in the absence of proven urinary infection or other pathology.
Pelvic pain syndrome	This includes persistent or recurrent episodic pain associated with symptoms similar to UTI. This may include complaints of sexual dysfunction, bowel, or gynecologic dysfunction in the absence of proven pathology.
Perineal pain syndrome	Persistent or recurrent episodic perineal pain is related to urinary voiding, or with symptoms similar to UTI. This can include such diverse etiologies as prostatodynia and interstitial cystitis. There may be associated complaints of sexual dysfunction (male or female).
Scrotal pain syndrome	Persistent or episodic scrotal pain of varying degree that may be associated with symptoms similar to UTI. There may also be complaints of sexual or erectile dysfunction.
Urethral pain syndrome	Describes recurrent episodic urethral pain usually present while voiding, and in the absence of proven infection or other disease process.
Vulvar pain syndrome	Persistent or recurrent episodic vaginal pain is associated with symptoms similar to a UTI. There may be complaints of sexual dysfunction.

27. Are women at risk for noninfectious dysuria?

Yes. Noninfectious causes of dysuria in women include:

- Urethral syndrome
- Urethral trauma during sexual intercourse, such as the "honeymooners' UTI"
- Sensitivity to scented feminine protection items, creams, sprays, or toilet paper
- Activities that represent prolonged perineal pressure, such as cycling

28. Can vaginitis cause dysuria?

Vaginitis can certainly contribute to dysuria. It can be accompanied by irritation to adjacent structures (such as the urethra) and vaginal discharge and vulvar irritation.

Specific types of vaginitis, such as those caused by *Candida albicans*, *Trichomonas vaginalis*, *Chlamydia trachomatis*, and *Neisseria gonorrhoeae* have all been cited as causes of dysuria secondary to gynecologic infections (Zeger & Holt, 2003).

29. Are there unusual presentations for dysuria?

The most unusual presentations, although rare, are often caused by objects that are inserted into the urethra, and possibly retained, causing dysuria. Even if an object is removed, dysuria may result as a result of urethral trauma. In these cases, the urinalysis will be negative, or with microscopic hematuria as a result of the trauma.

Key Points

- Dysuria may be an indicator of more serious disease.
- Timing of pain with urination can help establish a diagnosis.
- Obstruction of any portion of the urinary tract often results in dysuria.

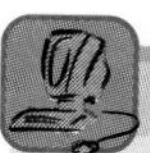

Internet Resources

American Urological Association Online Patient Information Resource
http://www.urologyhealth.org

The Merck Manual—Second Home Edition
http://www.merck.com/mrkshared/mmanual_home2/home.jsp

Medline Plus Medical Encyclopedia: Urination—Painful
http://www.nlm.nih.gov/medlineplus/ency/article/003145.htm

Bibliography

Batstone G, Doble A, Batstone D: Chronic prostatitis, *Curr Opin Urol* 13(1):23-29, 2003.

Bent S, Saint S: The optimal use of diagnostic testing in women with acute uncomplicated cystitis, *Dis Mon* 49(2):83-98, 2003.

Gupta K, Hooton TM, Roberts PL, et al: Patient-initiated treatment of uncomplicated recurrent urinary tract infections in young women, *Ann Intern Med* 135(1):9-16, 2001.

Huang ES, Stafford RS: National patterns in the treatment of urinary tract infections in women by ambulatory care physicians, *Arch Intern Med* 162(2):41-47, 2002.

Kontiokari T, Sundquist KJ, Nuutinen M, et al: Randomized trial of cranberry-lingonberry juice and Lactobacillus GG drink for the prevention of urinary tract infections in women, *BMJ* 322(7302): 1571, 2001.

Parsons CL, Dell J, Stanford EJ, et al: Increased prevalence of interstitial cystitis: Previously unrecognized urologic and gynecologic cases identified using a new symptom questionnaire and intervesical potassium sensitivity, *Urology* 60(4):573-578, 2002.

Zeger W, Holt K: Gynecologic infections, *Emerg Med Clin North* Am 21(3):631-648, 2003.

Section V

Orthopedics

Chapter 38

Low Back Pain

Polly Gerber Zimmermann

1. How common is low back pain?

It is estimated that 80% of adults in the United States have low back pain at least once during their life, with 40% having sciatic nerve irritation. Low back pain rarely indicates a serious disorder, but it is a major cause of disability and costs.

2. Elaborate on what is meant by low back pain's disability and cost.

Low back pain is responsible for more lost working hours than any other medical condition, particularly in hospital workers. Low back pain accounts for one-third of all workers' compensation costs, with an average cost of $8,000 per claim.

3. Why is low back pain such a common complaint?

The lumbar region is an inherently weak structural area that bears most of the body's weight. In addition, the nerve roots are vulnerable to injury, disease, or aging. Most cases of low back pain are musculoskeletal causes or lumbar disc disease.

4. List risk factors for low back pain.

Risk factors include any action that causes repetitive overuse, undue strain, or acceleration of the normal degeneration from aging of the spine. Some specific examples include:

- Lack of muscle tone (especially abdominal muscles)
- Excessive weight
- Poor posture
- Smoking (Nicotine decreases circulation to the discs)
- Emotional stress
- Occupations requiring heavy lifting, vibration, or prolonged periods of sitting

5. What specific actions might result in low back pain?

The most common cause is a mechanical strain of the paravertebral muscles. Activities that can cause this include:

- Continued bending at the waist
- Lifting below the knees
- Lifting above the shoulder
- Twisting at the waist while lifting

6. Isn't the real cause just improper body mechanics?

Research in the past 35 years shows that using correct body mechanics or training for lifting, *by themselves*, have consistently failed to reduce job-related injuries. The past body mechanic studies were flawed and fail to account for the balance, shape, or unpredictability of routine patient-care situations. The force on the musculoskeletal system is often beyond reasonable limits when some patient lifting is done manually, rather than with mechanical aids, regardless of the technique used.

Besides, not all back strain comes from lifting. Nurses spend 20% to 30% of their time bent forward or with the trunk twisted while performing routine nursing activities as changing a patient or administering medications.

7. List the classic history for triaging low back pain related to muscle strain.

- *Gradual onset.* Most muscular acute low back pain is caused by undue stress and appears later, after the injury, as the paravertebral muscle spasms.
- *Pain is dull and poorly localized,* usually from the sciatic nerve inflammation.
- *Pain does not travel below the knee.*
- *No point tenderness over the spinous processes of the lumbar vertebrae.* However, there may be point tenderness to firm palpation or percussion over the sacroiliac joint, especially if the pain is on that side.
- *Negative (–) straight-leg raising test.*

8. Describe the straight-leg raise test.

The examiner asks the patient to lie supine with the hips and knees extended. The examiner then slowly raises one relaxed leg, with the knee extended, until back pain occurs. Then the examiner dorsiflexes the foot. A normal finding is no pain or mild back pain. Mild discomfort behind the knee from tight hamstring muscles is not significant.

An abnormal finding (e.g., + straight-leg raising test) is a sharp pain that radiates down the leg to below the knee when the straight leg is flexed at the hip more than 30 degrees. Foot dorsiflexion may also bring on the sharp pain as a result of the additional stretch on the sciatic nerves caused by the passive dorsiflexion of the foot. A positive crossed straight-leg raising test occurs when the elevation of the uninvolved leg causes pain to radiate down the involved leg. This is a sensitive, specific sign for disc herniation.

9. Name classic key distinguishers to indicate disc involvement.

- *Sudden, sharp, well-localized pain.* The pain is usually at the maximum severity within a minute of onset.
- *Pain worsens with coughing, Valsalva maneuver, truck flexion, or prolonged sitting or standing.*
- *The pain radiates below the knee.* A limp may be evident if there is sciatic nerve impairment. Unlike muscular pain, the radiating leg pain from a disc is equal to or overshadows the back pain.
- *Positive (+) straight-leg raising test.*

10. Are there any other physical assessment tests?

Heel-toe walking may cause severe pain in the affected leg or back. There can be a weakness in the ankle or great toe dorsiflexion (drooping of the big toe and inability to heel walk).

An additional test is to have the patient clasp one knee firmly flexed against the abdomen while carefully lowering the other extended leg and thigh over the edge of the table. This action hyperextends that leg at the hip. If pain exists on the hyperextended side, the client has sacroiliac disease.

11. What are the "red flags" of low back pain?

- New or evolving neurologic symptoms
- Direct trauma to the back
- An inability to walk (versus difficulty walking because of the pain)
- Cauda equina syndrome (central herniation of the disc)
- Fever with a bloodstream infection, history of IV drug abuse, or a spinal epidural abscess

12. Describe cauda equina syndrome.

There is compression on several nerve roots below the spinal cord in which multiple nerve roots leave the cord and pass through the sacral foramina, an obvious cause for concern. Classic symptoms of this neurologic problem include:

- *Severe or progressing neurologic deficit.* This includes motor weakness and numbness of the perineum and perianal area.
- *New, recent onset of bladder or bowel dysfunction.* Initially it is most often urinary retention, increased frequency, or overflow incontinence. Bowel dysfunction (if seen) is usually later.
- *Saddle anesthesia (bilateral buttock numbness).*

13. What trauma can result in serious back injuries?

Concern is raised if the individual:

- Experienced a direct blow to the back

- Falls and lands on the feet from a height of 5 feet or more (the shock is absorbed up the spine)
- Does heavy lifting with a history of osteoporosis or in an older person

14. What are the unusual causes (the "zebras") of low back pain?

- *Tumors and infections.* Pain from these causes is more severe at nighttime and when supine (normal muscular pain improves with rest), and/or the pain is present for more than a month without relief from nonsteroidal antiinflammatory drugs (NSAIDs).
- *Abdominal aortic aneurysms (especially in patients >80 years).* This pain is constant without change from movement. A lateral radiograph of the abdomen will demonstrate calcified aneurysm (80%), but the definitive test is to find a pulsatile mass or identify on computed tomography (CT) scan an aortic width of 6 cm or more. Emergency surgery is indicated.

15. State factors that could make these "zebras" more likely.

Other contributing factors could include:

- Age (>50 and <20 years)
- Intravenous drug abuse
- History of cancer, unexplained weight loss, or back surgery
- Recent fever/chills
- Immunosuppression

16. We have a patient who frequently presents to the emergency department requesting narcotics for the severe low back pain. Is there any way of assessing the true need?

Complaints of back pain comprised more than half of the patients in one emergency department's managed program for "heavy users" who requested narcotics. If suspicious that a patient's pain is psychosomatic or nonorganic try:

- *To watch the gait without the patient being aware.* The patient should move as cautiously as when being watched.
- *The axial loading test.* Press down gently on the head of the standing patient. This should not cause significant musculoskeletal back pain: be suspicious if the patient claims it does.
- *The rotation test.* Have the patient stand with his/her arms at the side. Hold the wrists next to the hips and turn the body from side to side. The maneuver passively rotates the shoulders, truck and pelvis as a unit, but creates the illusion that the spinal rotation is being tested. In fact, the maneuver is not altering the spinal axis at all so any patient complaint of related back pain should be suspect.

17. What are the recommendations for diagnosing low back pain?

Atlas and Nardin (2003) point out that a patient's history and physical examination usually provide clues to the uncommon, but potentially serious, causes of low back pain. Diagnostic testing should not be a routine part of the initial evaluation unless a red flag is present.

18. What can I say when the patient wants an x-ray "just to be sure"?

In one study, only 1 out of 2,500 radiographs was positive for a clinically unsuspected finding in patients <50 years of age who were complaining of back pain. Yet a typical lumbar radiograph series provides the gonadal dose equivalent to daily chest radiographs for 6 years! In addition, many adults have an unknown, but lifelong, radiographic anomaly that is not responsible for the current symptoms. Besides there is the cost: In the United States, approximately $1 billion per year on is spent lumbosacral spine films.

In my experience, sharing this information with the patient helps them to accept the advisability of waiting. They are also more receptive if I point out that the response is *not* "never," but "if there is no improvement in a week or so."

19. Give an example of standing triage orders for low back pain.

Christus Santa Rose Hospital (San Antonio, Tx)

Source: Kevin Trainor, RN CEN; Emergency and Trauma Services Nurse Manager

≤55 years atraumatic	Dip urinalysis (U/A), wait for MD orders
>55 years either sex regardless of trauma	Dip U/A, lumbosacral (L/S) spine x-ray

20. What are the recommendations for initial routine treatment?

Atlas and Nardin (2003) recommend activity modification, nonnarcotic analgesics, and education for patients without significant neurological impairment. Additional diagnostic tests and treatment options are pursued if there is no improvement in 2 to 4 weeks.

21. What over-the-counter medications are usually given for low back pain?

The NSAIDs are the most effective over-the-counter (OTC) analgesic for musculoskeletal pain. See Chapter 6 for further discussion.

22. Discuss whether muscle relaxant drugs should be routinely used for all patients with low back pain.

An analysis of 14 studies found that muscle relaxants, such as cyclobenzaprine (Flexeril) have a modest value if used during the first few days of treatment. However, side effects are common and may outweigh the benefits for some patients.

23. Why isn't more aggressive initial treatment indicated?

Various studies differ in the exact results. Overall around 50% to 70% of patients with low back pain improve in 1 week, 80% by 2 weeks, and most (90%) have improved by 1 month. Even when there was a disc herniation with neuropathy, 90% to 95% improved without surgery. The key determinant is if any initial neurologic deficit is *stable.*

24. List teaching for low back pain.

- *Bed rest may be initially indicated for 2 days for moderate-to-severe discomfort* if the spasms increase when upright, but should not be recommended for more than 4 days.
  - Raise the head of the bed 30 degrees
  - Lie with the knees flexed. Use a pillow underneath the knees if on the back, or between the knees if on the side
  - Avoid lying on the stomach
- *Activity restrictions for mild-to-moderate discomfort.* Avoid heavy lifting (usually defined as ≥20 pounds), prolonged sitting, or high heels
- *Apply ice for 20 to 30 minutes per hour for the first 24 hours*
- *Change positions frequently*
- *Listen to music* One study found patients with herniated discs or recent back surgery who listened to relaxing music 25 minutes a day had significantly lower pain levels.

25. Should lumbar belt support be recommended for all patients?

There is no reduction in self-reported back pain or disability claims for back pain associated with either the self-reported use of back belts or with store policies mandating workers use the belts.

26. Are backpacks ever an issue?

Up to 46% of school-age children get backaches, and it is attributed to excess weight in the backpack (typically 20 to 40 pounds). (Others advocate that poor muscular conditioning is also a significant contributor.) The Consumer Product Safety Commission estimates that there are 6,512 ED visits/year from injuries related to book bags.

Proper use of backpacks includes:
- Holding no more than 15% of the body weight
- Using both shoulder straps
- Applying the waist strap

There are newer ergonomic styles; whether they are "cool" enough for widespread use is still to be determined.

27. Patients often ask about the benefit of chiropractors. Is there scientific-based information to give them?

One-third of the patients with low back pain seek chiropractic care for relief. Studies suggest that results are comparable and the patients are more satisfied with the chiropractic care. This is attributed to the fact that chiropractors are more likely to explain their treatment and to advise them about self-care.

28. We're considering a "back class" for our institution's employees to lessen back injury. What helps reduce work-related back injuries?

A literature review shows that education, body mechanics training, and mechanical devices are important aspects of a back injury prevention program. Additional impact is achieved with a specially trained lift team. Lifting must be viewed as a skill involving specialized training and mandated use of mechanical equipment. One hospital had a 69% decrease in reported back injuries (and a year's savings of $45,817) after instituting a lift team (Hefti et al, 2003).

Key Points

- Red flags for low back pain are evolving neurologic deficit, direct trauma to the back, an inability to walk, cauda equina syndrome, or signs/symptoms of infection, metastasis, or AAA.
- Muscular pain (compared to pain from a disc) tends to be more gradual in onset, poorly localized, does not radiate below the knee, and does not have spinal point tenderness.
- Positive straight leg raising test signals disc involvement.
- Routine diagnostic x-rays for acute low back pain is not recommended. The overwhelming majority of patients improve without aggressive interventions, such as surgery.

Internet Resources

NursingCEU.com: Back Pain
http://www.nursingceu.com/NCEU/courses/05bemis/

Sample Implementation Action Plan: Dod/VA Low Back Pain Guideline
http://www.rand.org/publications/MR/MR1267/mr1267.appg.pdf

Emergency Nurses Association Center for Advanced Practice Nursing: Diagnosis and Management of Acute Low Back Pain
http://www.ena.org/conferences/annual/2004/handouts/CAPL341-C.pdf

Bibliography

Atlas SJ, Nardin RA: Evaluation and treatment of low back pain: An evidence-based approach to clinical care, *Muscle Nerve* 27:265-284, 2003.

Browning R: Cyclobenzaprine and back pain: A meta-analysis, *Arch Intern Med* 161:1613-1620, 2001.

Buttaravoli P, Stair T: *Minor emergencies: Splinters to fractures,* St Louis, 2001, Mosby.

Edlich RF, Woodard CR, Haines MJ: Disabling back injuries in nursing personnel, *J Emerg Nurs* 27:150-155, 2001.

Hefti KS, Farnham RJ, Docken L, et al: Back injury prevention: A lift team success story, *AAOHN J* 51(6):246-251, 2003.

Hertzman-Miller RP, Morgenstern H, Hurwitz EL, et al: Comparing the satisfaction of low back pain patients randomized to receive medical or chiropractic care: Results from the UCLA low-back pain study, *Am J Public Health* 92 (10):1628-1633, 2002.

Hockberger RS: Low back pain. In Markovchick VJ, Pons PT: *Pons' emergency medicine secrets,* ed 3, Philadelphia, 2003, Hanley & Belfus.

Hurwitz EL, Morgenstern H, Harber P, et al: A randomized trial of medical care with and without medical therapy and chiropractic care with and without physical modalities for patients with low back pain: 6-month follow-up outcomes from the UCLA low back pain study, *Spine* 28(14):1625-1626, 2003.

Nelson A, Fragala G, Menzel N: Myths and facts about back injuries in nursing, *Am J Nurs* 103(2):32-41, 2003.

Ramos NE: How heavy is your backpack? *Chicago Sun Times*, Sept 2, 2003, p. 42.

Weitz M: Back pain, lower. In Davis MA, Votey SR, Greenough PG: *Greenough's signs and symptoms in emergency medicine: Literature-based approach to emergent conditions,* St Louis, 1999, Mosby.

Zimmermann PG: Triage and differential diagnosis of patients with headaches, dizziness, low back pain, and rashes: A basic primer, *J Emerg Nurs* 28(3):209-215, 2002.

Chapter 39

Extremity Trauma

Robert W. Stein, III

"Sticks and stones may break bones, but slips and falls can hurt too."

—*Anonymous Triage Nurse*

1. What are the steps in triaging a patient with an extremity injury?

There are six basic components to triaging an extremity injury. They are the same steps involved in triaging any illness or injury. The components are (1) primary survey, (2) history, (3) secondary survey (a limited and focused physical assessment), (4) differential diagnosis or considering the worst-case scenario, (5) initial treatment, and (6) prioritization. If advanced triage protocols exist to start treatments, they would comprise a seventh step in extremity injury triage. All six or seven steps ought to be completed in no more than 5 minutes. Triage is about accuracy, but it is also about speed.

2. Why is taking a history important for an obvious extremity injury? Shouldn't I just focus in on the presenting complaint?

Focusing on the presenting complaint can often lead you to miss the forest for the trees. Simply asking, "what happened?" can gain valuable information that may significantly change how you prioritize a patient's care. For example, focusing only on the broken ankle of a 70-year-old woman might cause you to miss that a syncopal episode preceded the fall.

3. Beyond routine triage questions, what questions should I ask for an extremity injury?

- Time, force, and mechanism of injury
- Activity at the time of the injury (certain activities are associated with specific injuries, such as inline skaters with a Colles fracture)
- "Did you hear anything?"
- Position of the extremity when injured. (e.g., "Did the foot turn inward or outward?" for an ankle injury; "Was the hand outstretched?" for a hand injury).
- Previous injury to the extremity
- End the history interview with: "Is there anything else that I should know about?"

4. Why do I need to ask what they "heard"?

Frequently patients with fractures or torn ligaments will hear an audible "pop" when the accident occurs. This, along with an immediate loss of function suggests a disruption of a ligament.

5. Ok, what next?

Check jewelry. Edema results from every injury. At this point, stop and remove any rings or jewelry they may be wearing. Patients may be resistant because of fear of pain, sentimentality, or a lack of understanding that any swelling may get worse. Even if a ring has to be cut off, the earlier you get to it the easier it will be.

6. Tell me how to easily remove a ring.

- Elevate the extremity (this also works for toe rings).
- Apply ice for a few minutes. The ice may help decrease some of the swelling, but it really works great to help reduce the discomfort.
- Apply a lubricant jelly or hand lotion.
- Grab the ring (use a gauze sponge if needed) and rotate it distally.
- As you spin the ring, push any distal edema proximally underneath the ring.

If this does not work, try wrapping the digits tightly with dental floss from the distal end, threading the floss underneath the ring. However, this procedure can take 45 minutes. In the end, the ring may need to be cut off with a ring-cutter.

7. Why do I care if there was a previous injury to the extremity?

The patient has an increased risk of recurrence in that extremity.

8. What is included in a secondary survey for an extremity injury?

- A secondary survey is a *limited* and *focused* physical assessment of the injured extremity.
- Evaluate the extremity function. For hands, assess functionality by determining whether they can touch their thumb to each of their fingers. For lower extremity injuries use weight-bearing capacity
- Check the motor function of radial, ulnar, and median nerves.
  - Radial nerve: dorsiflexes wrist, extends thumb
  - Medial nerve: flexes thumb (thumb touches fifth finger)
  - Ulnar nerve: spreads fingers (test strength in abduction of fifth digit and second digit)
- Grossly note the range of motion (full, limited, or none).
- Assess the joint immediately above and below the area of tenderness.
- Verify pulses to the injured extremity.

9. What should I consider if I note swelling on the dorsum of the hand?

Palmar-side injury. Most of the palmar lymphatics drain to the dorsum of the hand.

10. What do I look for in assessing the extremity's neurovascular condition?

Major points to consider are the "Six Ps" of pain, pallor, paresthesia, paresis, pulselessness, and polar. Some sources use pressure of the compartment as a "P" (normal is 0 to 8 mm Hg; 30 to 40 mm Hg indicate compartment syndrome). Each finding and its significance in the triage setting are summarized in the following table.

The "Six Ps" of Extremity Assessment

Finding	Significance
Pain	Assess for the location and the severity of pain. Evaluate whether the pain reported is consistent with apparent severity of the injury. Pain that is disproportionate to the severity of the injury may be indicative of vascular impairment.
Pallor	Assess the color of the extremity. Pallor, cyanosis, or delayed capillary refill. Pallor may be indicative of vascular impairment.
Paresthesia	Assess for any numbness or tingling. Paresthesia may indicate neurologic impairment.
Paresis	Assess for any weakness or loss of muscle tone. Paresis may be indicative of neuromuscular impairment.
Pulselessness	An absent/nonpalpable pulse in an injured extremity is an emergent finding.
Polar	Assess the temperature of the extremity, especially in comparison with the opposing noninjured extremity. A cold extremity may indicate vascular impairment. A hot extremity may suggest an infectious process.

11. Which "P" is the most sensitive?

Paresthesia or the "pins and needles" sensation we all feel when our arm "falls asleep." The nerve is affected before circulation loss of pulse. Paralysis is a late finding.

12. How do I test digit sensation?

Check two-point discrimination on the volar pad. The points should be 5 mm apart and aligned longitudinally.

13. Describe the Allen test.

The Allen test verifies patency of the radial and ulnar arteries. This is often done before a radial arterial blood gas (ABG) but can also be used for a circulation assessment. Occlude both and have the patient open and close the hand five or six times. The hand should blanch. Release the ulnar artery and the blanching should resolve within 3 to 5 seconds. Repeat the test, using the radial artery.

14. Sometimes it is hard to determine if there is a new problem because of the patient's chronic conditions.

The possibility of diagnosed or undiagnosed co-morbid conditions such as diabetes, peripheral vascular disease, arthritis, and others will have an effect on your findings. Always make comparisons with the opposite side extremity.

Any *unilateral* positive finding is significant. Consider upgrading the triage category to "emergent" for immediate definitive treatment.

15. Should I worry when the patient says it is worse today than when it was injured yesterday?

No, the typical course from the resulting inflammation's swelling and pain peaks about 1 day after the injury.

16. What are classic signs of a fracture versus a sprain/strain/ligament injury?

- Inability to bear weight both immediately after the injury and in the initial physical examination is classic, although there are exceptions. (Weight bearing is defined as the ability to transfer weight twice onto each leg, a total of four steps, regardless of limping.)
- Bony point tenderness to palpation, versus a global "entire" extremity pain.

X-rays are typically taken, regardless, if there is other distracting painful injuries, altered sensorium, history of bone disease, or intoxication.

17. You mentioned differential diagnosis as coming next. I thought only physicians and mid-level providers did that.

Physicians and mid-level providers will establish a differential diagnosis in determining what diagnostics to order to confirm or rule out their differential diagnosis. However, those in a triage role must consider what might be wrong with the patient as well, considering the probable and the worst-case scenario for each injury to guide initial treatment, triage prioritization, and which advanced triage protocols to utilize. The following table summarizes "probable" and "worst-case" scenarios for common extremity injuries.

Probable and Worst-Case Injury Scenarios

Probable Injury	Worst-Case Injury
Superficial laceration	Lacerated nerve/tendon or retained foreign body
Contusion	Sprain/strain
Sprain/strain	Nondisplaced fracture
Nondisplaced fracture	Displaced fracture
Displaced fracture/dislocation	Compound fracture
First-degree burn	Second-degree burn
Second-degree burn	Third-degree or circumferential burn

18. Tell me about compartment syndrome.

Compartment syndrome is a condition in which the elevated intracompartmental pressure within a confined myofascial compartment compromises the neurovascular function of tissues. The capillary perfusion is reduced below a level necessary for tissue viability. Causes are typically restrictive external pressure (e.g., cast) and internal edema, bleeding, intravenous (IV) infiltration, etc. Early recognition is important to avoid permanent damage. Ischemia can occur within 4 to 12 hours.

19. List what is important to document on an extremity injury.

- Chief complaint, time, and mechanism of injury, using the patient's wording
- Areas of tenderness, noting diffuse, and/or pinpoint pain
- The "Six Ps"
- Bruising, swelling, deformity, or breaks in skin integrity
- Range of motion and functionality of the injured extremity

20. Sometimes the patient does not make any sense. What do I do now?

Unfortunately, patients are not taught how to help us. Some patients will complain of vague, diffuse, or wildly exaggerated pain, such as just repeating "It's a bad injury!" Different patients respond to injury differently, but we all have the same physiology.

- Trust your assessment.
- Calm the hysterical patient who wildly complains about everything, but has no physical findings.
- Worry about the quiet patient who does not complain much, but has a significant degree of bruising and swelling.
- Do not be fooled by the old wives tale of "you cannot walk on a broken bone." Indeed, you *can.*

21. Give some examples of assigned triage levels related to the patient's presentation.

In the Canadian Triage and Acuity Scale (CTAS):
Level 3 (urgent, ≤30 minutes)

- Fractures, dislocations, sprains
- Severe pain (8 to 10 out of 10)
- Stable vital signs

Level 4 (less urgent, ≤1 hour)

- Minor fractures or sprains requiring investigation or intervention
- Moderate pain (4 to 7 out of 10)
- Stable vital signs

Level 5 (nonurgent, ≤2 hours)

- Minor sprains, overuse syndrome requiring minor analgesics

The Manchester Triage Group
Level 2 (very urgent, 10 minutes)

- Severe pain
- Distal vascular compromise

Level 3 (urgent, 60 minutes)
- New neurologic signs/symptoms (s/s)
- Moderate pain
- Inappropriate history

Level 4 (standard, 120 minutes)
- Any local inflammation or infections
- Any pain
- Recent injury (within 7 days)

22. With so many possibilities, how do I determine the patient's final diagnosis in triage?

You don't. Guide your actions based on your differential diagnosis. Initial treatment of most extremity injuries is the same regardless of what the final diagnosis may be.

Initial Treatments in Triage

Symptom	Initial Treatment	Tip
Pain	Medicate per protocol.	If the injury might require surgical intervention, withhold oral pain medication and raise the triage priority to allow for parental administration.
Bleeding	Apply a bandage.	Moistened saline gauze under a dressing will make its removal easier and less painful.
Burns	Apply cool saline dressing.	NOTE: "Cool," but not "cold" saline dressings. Applying ice or cold saline will constrict the blood flow and potentially further extend the size and/or degree of the burn. Calculate the percent of the burn area using the "Rule of Nines." Any patient with burns >15% should be moved to the treatment area for possible transfer to a burn center (see Chapter 43).
Swelling	Ice, compression, and elevation.	Remember the mnemonic "ICE." If circulation is impaired as evidenced by pallor or pulselessness, do not "ICE" and raise the triage priority to emergent.
Deformity	Apply a splint.	Splint in whatever position you find the extremity in. Do not attempt to straighten the extremity or reduce a fracture/dislocation in triage.
Weakness	Consider severity and potential cause.	If symptom is found alone, it may indicate a more serious condition. Consider raising the triage priority to urgent or higher.

23. What is usually included in advanced triage orders/protocols for extremity trauma?

- Ice (protected with a towel to prevent frostbite)
- Splint and/or dressings as needed
- Analgesia (usually nonsteroidal anti-inflammatory drugs [NSAIDs] are given rather than narcotics)
- Pregnancy testing (if an x-ray is anticipated and the woman is of childbearing age)
- X-rays
- Tetanus immunization update

24. When are x-rays a particular priority?

- *Fingers and hands:* They are so vital it is best to get an x-ray. Hand injuries account for 75% of all partially disabling injuries. For isolated finger injuries, order an x-ray of the finger only.
- *Obvious dislocations.* Dislocations are easier to reduce the sooner you get to them and reduction provides significant and immediate pain relief.

25. Give examples of some standing triage orders/protocols.

St. Joseph Medical Center (Towson, Md)
Source: Vicki Blucher, RN BSN CEN, ED Clinical Educator
In addition to routine assessment and treatment (e.g., ice, elevate)

- Nurse orders radiograph for any injury to the "glove or sock" region (e.g., area includes distal radius and ulna to metacarpal region and from the malleolus region distal to the metatarsal area).
- Nurse orders x-ray for any patient with a possible foreign body (glass, metal, etc.).

Dartmouth-Hitchcock Medical Center (Lebanon, NH)
Source: Jean A. Proehl, RN MN CEN CCRN, Emergency CNS
Nurse orders x-ray if there is a recent extremity injury with:

- Deformity
- Bony instability
- Crepitus
- Point tenderness
- Ecchymosis
- Severe swelling
- Moderate to severe pain in the hip, thigh, or foot with weight-bearing
- Any penetrating injury to a joint area
- Foreign body present or suspected

Toes/Fingers: Order only the involved digit if all s/s are distal to the web space, but an entire foot/hand if any involvement proximal to the web space.

Foot: Use Ottawa Ankle Rules. Calcaneus films may be ordered for isolated heel pain after a fall from a height where the patient landed on the heels. (See Question 26.)

Knee: Use Ottawa Knee Rules. (See Question 28.)

Elbow: Order when there is pain associated with limitations/loss of supination/pronation/extension. However, children <5 years of age with suspected radial head subluxation (Nursemaid's elbow) do not require x-rays.

Hip/Pelvis: History of fall with hip pain, externally rotated and/or shortened extremity, unable to bear weight

Source: Pediatric Triage Guidelines by Kathleen Murphy

X-rays may be ordered of the bones listed below if there is:

- Point tenderness or a clear deformity of the limb with significant swelling and decreased range of motion
- History of trauma to the specific area less than 48 hours before arrival at the emergency department.
  - Clavicle
  - Shoulder
  - Humerus
  - Elbow
  - Forearm
  - Wrist
  - Hand
  - Finger
  - Knee
  - Tibia/fibula
  - Ankle
  - Foot
- The following x-ray studies are not ordered without first consulting with the attending physician:
  - Spine
  - Scapula
  - Skull
  - Facial bones
  - Soft tissue of the neck
  - Chest
  - Ribs
  - Abdomen
  - Hip
  - Femur

26. Discuss the Ottawa Ankle Rules.

The Ottawa Ankle Rules (1996) guide which patients were most likely to have a fracture, indicating when to order an x-ray and when an x-ray is likely to be negative. They are summarized in the table below. Anatomic landmarks used in the Ottawa Ankle Rules are illustrated in the following figure.

Ottawa Ankle Rules

Order an ankle x-ray if you find pain in the malleolar zone, and
Bone tenderness at the posterior edge or tip of the lateral malleolus, or
Bone tenderness at the posterior edge or tip of the medial malleolus, or
Inability to bear weight

Order a foot x-ray if you find pain in the midfoot, and
Bone tenderness at the base of the fifth metatarsal, or
Bone tenderness at the navicular, or
Inability to bear weight

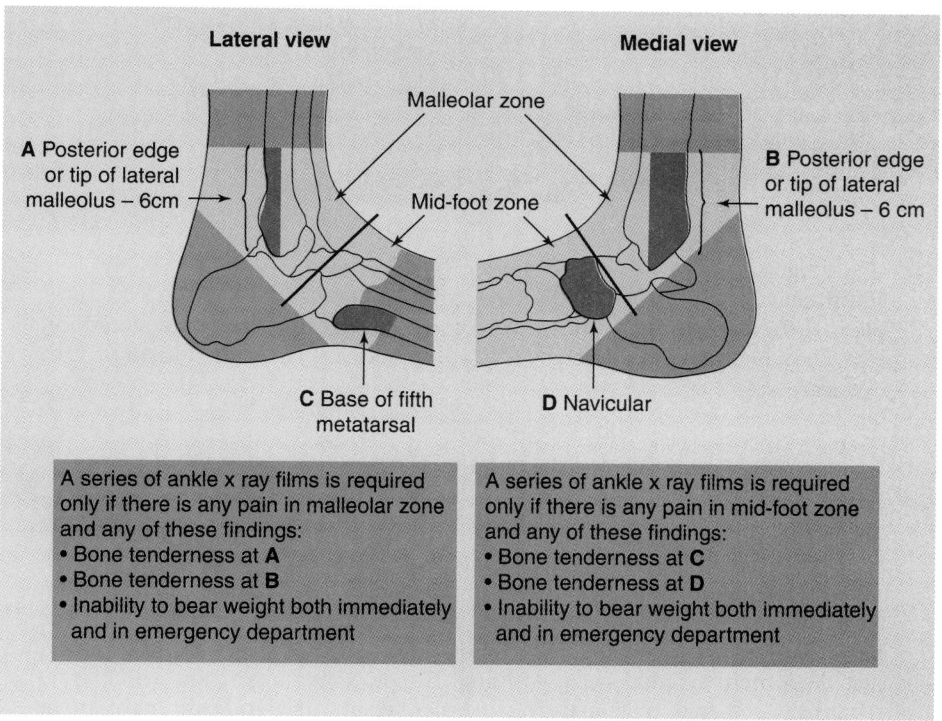
Lateral view
Medial view
Malleolar zone
Mid-foot zone
A Posterior edge or tip of lateral malleolus – 6cm
B Posterior edge or tip of lateral malleolus – 6 cm
C Base of fifth metatarsal
D Navicular
A series of ankle x ray films is required only if there is any pain in malleolar zone and any of these findings:
• Bone tenderness at A
• Bone tenderness at B
• Inability to bear weight both immediately and in emergency department
A series of ankle x ray films is required only if there is any pain in mid-foot zone and any of these findings:
• Bone tenderness at C
• Bone tenderness at D
• Inability to bear weight both immediately and in emergency department

Anatomy of the Ottawa Ankle Rules.
From Stiell I, Wells G, Laupacis A, et al: Multicentre trial to introduce the Ottawa Ankle Rules for use of radiography in acute ankle injuries, Br Med J 311:594-597, 1995.

27. Why do we need these Rules? Isn't it best to just x-ray all ankles?

Less than 15% of patients with blunt ankle trauma have a clinically significant fracture. (They may still need immobilization, etc. for their sprains.) Using the rules has been shown to be a safe way to reduce unnecessary radiation and cost.

28. What about the Ottawa Knee Rules? How do they compare to the Pittsburgh Decision Rules?

A follow-up study led to the development of the Ottawa Knee Rules. A 1999 study showed that the "Pittsburgh Decision Rules" were slightly more accurate. While the Ottawa Knee Rules were developed first, the Pittsburgh Decision Rules are a better choice and far easier to use in a triage setting. The following table provides a comparison of the Ottawa and Pittsburgh rules.

Comparison of Ottawa Knee Rules and Pittsburgh Decision Rules

Ottawa Knee Rules	Pittsburgh Decision Rules
Order a knee x-ray if you find . . .	
Age over 55 years, or Isolated patella tenderness, or Tenderness at the head of the fibula, or Inability to flex the knee 90 degrees, or Inability to walk four weight-bearing steps	History of blunt trauma or a fall, and Age younger than 12 or older than 50 years, or Inability to walk four weight-bearing steps

29. Describe a boxer's fracture.

The fracture of the fourth or fifth metacarpal is referred to as a "boxer's fracture" because the mechanism of the injury is most often from punching a face, door, etc. There is classic significant swelling and deformity over the fourth or fifth metacarpal.

30. Discuss when to order a wrist x-ray and when to order a hand x-ray.

Frequently an x-ray of the hand or wrist will show enough of both areas to allow for a large margin of error. An ordered hand x-ray when the injury is actually in the wrist (or vice versa), will often still show enough of the wrist to make a diagnosis. Fracture of the scaphoid bone is one major exception: it can be seen only in a wrist x-ray. The scaphoid bone, also referred to as the navicular bone, is on the medial side of the wrist proximal to the thumb and just distal of the radial head. Although small, it has important articulating surfaces. A missed navicular fracture can result in significant permanent impairment of the wrist.

31. How can I assess for a possible navicular fracture?

Have the patient raise their thumb in the traditional "hitch hiker" position. A small dimpled area will appear proximal to the thumb and just distal to the head of the radius called the "snuff box." If your patient has point tenderness in that dimpled area, suspect a navicular fracture and order an x-ray of the wrist.

32. Tell me more about a Colles' fracture.

A more obvious wrist injury is called a "Colles' fracture"; this is a fracture of the distal end of the radius. The fracture most often occurs from a fall where the patient stretches out their hand to break their fall. It results in a characteristic bowing of the distal forearm.

33. What might clue me to a major tendon or joint injury in the hand?

A variation in the normal posture of the hand at rest. Normally, with the wrist in slight extension, the resting fingers "cascade," e.g., a progressively more flexed position from the index finger to the small finger.

34. Are high-pressure injection injuries serious? The wound looks small.

These injuries (from paint guns, grease guns, or hydraulic lines) may initially seem innocuous, with a limited involvement. However, up to 70% of such injuries result in some form of amputation and an average of 7 months' lost work time.

35. What about a bite to the hand?

Bites are a high risk for infection: human and animal bites carry the same risk. Antibiotics are essential. See also Chapters 40 and 49 for further discussion.

36. Should I routinely do an x-ray for an injured toe?

Generally, it is of little benefit to x-ray a toe injury, as the treatment will be the same regardless of whether a fracture exists or not (buddy-tape). The only exception is injuries to the great toe and toes with obvious deformity.

37. Any final thoughts about ordering an x-ray?

- Do not forget about speed. There is little point in ordering an x-ray from triage if there is room available in the treatment area.
- Consider the role of customer satisfaction. Many patients feel a "need" for an x-ray regardless. One physician discusses it with the patients, and has even shown them the book where it indicates that x-ray is not needed. If the patients continue to insist, he indicates they will have to sign a release saying they will not hold him responsible for any complications (including brain damage) that they might experience from the radiation exposure of what he believes is an unnecessary x-ray. Most acquiesce. If they sign the form, he orders the x-ray.

38. Any last words of wisdom?

See the following table for a quick reference when faced with triaging a patient with an extremity injury.

Summary of Extremity Triage Steps

Step	Assessment	Data	Action
1	Primary Assessment	Assess airway, breathing, circulation (ABCs).	Triage compromised patients directly to the treatment area.
2	History	Determine mechanism and force of injury.	Determine area for focused assessment. Triage seriously ill patients immediately to the treatment area.
3	Secondary Assessment	Focused assessment of isolated extremity injury.	Document findings.
4	Differential Diagnosis	Apply assessment findings to determine probable injury and worst-case injury.	Consider need for immediate definitive treatment to avoid deterioration or impairment.
5	Initial Treatment	Provide initial stabilizing treatment.	Stop whatever brought the patient to you.
6	Prioritization	Apply triage acuity score.	If the triage score does not "feel" right: Reconsider your assessment. Consider need for immediate definitive treatment to avoid deterioration or impairment.
7	Advanced Triage	Implement advanced triage protocols.	Initiate diagnostic work up based on assessment and protocols.

Key Points

- *Unilateral* extremity findings are significant.
- Assess for the six "Ps." Paresthesia is the most sensitive.
- Key clues for a need for x-ray is inability to bear weight and pinpoint tenderness. Use the Ottawa Ankle Rules and the Pittsburgh Decision Rules (for knees).
- Check the palmar side of the hand for injury when there is swelling on the dorsum side.

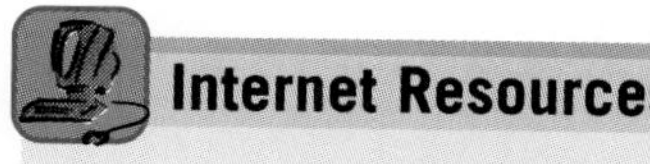

Internet Resources

Canadian Association of Emergency Physicians
www.caep.ca

Emergency Medicine Journal Online
http://emj.bmjjournals.com

American Academy of Family Physicians—Pitfalls in the Radiologic Evaluation of Extremity Trauma: Part II. The Lower Extremity
http://www.aafp.org/afp/980315ap/shearman.html

American Academy of Family Physicians—Pitfalls in the Radiologic Evaluation of Extremity Trauma: Part I. The Upper Extremity
http://www.aafp.org/afp/980301ap/shearman.html

Bibliography

Blucher V: X-ray protocols (Managers Forum), *J Emerg Nurs* 31(1):93, 2005.

Buttaravoli P, Stair T: *Minor emergencies: Splinters to fractures,* St Louis, 2000, Mosby.

Canadian Association of Emergency Physicians: Canadian Emergency Department Triage and Acuity Scale: Implementation guidelines, *J Can Assoc Emerg Physicians* 1(3 suppl), 1999.

Fiessler F, Szucs P, Kec R, Richman PB: Can nurses appropriately utilize the Ottawa Ankle Rule? An implementation trial, *Acad Emerg Med* 9:455a, 2002.

Fry M: Triage nurses order x-rays for patients with isolated distal limb injuries: A 12-month ED study, *J Emerg Nurs* 27(1):17-22, 2001.

Harrahill M: A quick examination of the lower extremity, *J Emerg Nurs* 26(6):631-632, 2000.

Kec RM, Richman PB, Szucs PA, et al: Can emergency department triage nurses appropriately utilize the Ottawa Knee Rules to order radiographs? An implementation trial, *Acad Emerg Med* 10:146-150, 2003.

Kohn MA: Hand injuries and infections. In Markovchick VJ, Pons PT, editors: *Pons' emergency medicine secrets,* ed 3, Philadelphia, 2003, Hanley & Belfus.

Mackway-Jones K: *Emergency triage: Manchester Triage Group,* London, 1997, BMJ Publishing.

Maher AB, et al, editors: *Orthopedic nursing,* ed 2, Philadelphia, 1998, WB Saunders.

Murphy KA: *Pediatric triage guidelines,* St Louis, 1997, Mosby.

Newberry L, editor. *Sheehy's emergency nursing principles and practice,* ed 5, St Louis, 2003, Mosby.

Proehl JA: Radiograph protocols (Managers Forum), *J Emerg Nurs* 31(1):93-94, 2005.

Robertson J: The Ottawa Knee Rules accurately identified fractures in children with knee injuries, *Evidence Based Nurs* 7:24, 2004.

Rourke K: An orthopedic nurse practitioner's practical guide to evaluating knee injuries, *J Emerg Nurs* 29(4):366-372, 2003.

Seaburg DC, Jackson R: Clinical decision rule for knee radiographs, *Am J Emerg Med* 12:541-543, 1994.

Stiell IG, McKnight RD, Greenberg GH, et al: Implementation of the Ottawa Ankle Rules, *JAMA* 271: 827-832, 1994.

Stiell IG, Greenberg GH, Wells GA, et al: Prospective validation of a decision rule for use of radiography in acute knee injury, *JAMA* 275:611-615, 1996.

Tandeter HB, Shvartzman P, Stevens MA: Acute knee injuries: Use of decision rules for selective radiographic ordering, *Am Fam Physician* 60:2599-2608, 1999.

Zimmermann P: Guiding principles at triage: Advice for new triage nurses, *J Emerg Nurs* 28(1):24-33, 2002.

Section VI

Wounds

Chapter 40

Lacerations and Puncture Wounds

Mary E. Fecht Gramley and Polly Gerber Zimmermann

1. Define common wound classifications.

- Laceration: A tear in the skin.
- Puncture wounds: A piercing.
- Abrasion: The epithelial layer is removed by means of friction. The epidermis may also be denuded, e.g., "road rash."
- Avulsion: Loss (or flap) of the full thickness of the skin layers.
- Degloving: Pulling or tearing away of deeper tissues (including tendons and ligaments) from the bony structures.
- Abscess: Localized collection of pus and debris underneath or between the skin layers.
- Bites: Human or animals.

2. How do I remember all of the important steps for wound management?

Escobar, Tiller, and Harwood-Nuss (2003) recommend the mnemonic LACERATE:

Look
Anesthetize
Clip and Clean
Equipment
Repair
Assess results
Tetanus
Educate

3. What is important to include in the history and physical assessment of a laceration (after airway, breathing, circulation [ABCs] are stable) specific to wounds?

- Mechanism of injury?
- How did the injury happen?
- Any possibility of a retained foreign body?
- Time of injury?
- Circumstances surrounding the injury (job-related?)
- Length and depth of the laceration in centimeters?
- Amount and character of bleeding present and if bleeding is currently controlled?

- Presence of or potential for contamination?
- Functional deficits of the injured part (assess circulation, sensation, and movement) beyond the laceration?
- Description of the appearance of the laceration, (e.g., gaping, linear, jagged edges, avulsed, flap present)?
- Occupation/normal use of the area?
- Need to notify authorities (domestic violence, animal bite, etc.)?
- See also Chapter 39 for further discussion.

4. What laceration/wound presentations "raise the red flag" for a high risk for complications?

- Human and animal bites.
- Degloving injury (soft tissue pulled away from the bony structures).
- Avulsion injuries (loss of segments of tissue).
- Extending across flexor or extensor surfaces or joints.
- In areas of high use or tension.
- Accompanied by a functional disability.
- With deep tissues exposed (e.g., tendons).
- In the lower body extremities.
- Puncture wounds.
- Wounds from a crush injury.
- Eye structure involvement.
- Presence of an impaled object.
- Lip involvement (may have unrecognized tooth fragments).
- Contaminated wounds.
- Co-existing patient factors that contribute to delayed wound healing (diabetes, drugs, immunosuppression).

5. I work in an occupational health clinic. What considerations will help me to know whether this laceration will require stitches?

- Can the wound edges be approximated?
- Depth/size of wound?
- Location? (area of movement, joint, high risk of damage to underlying tissue, desire to minimize scaring)
- Is the bleeding controlled?
- Risk of complication, including delay in wound healing, injury to underlying structures or any "red flag"?

6. Any other recommendations for knowing when treatment is needed?

Call an ambulance when there is:

- Large gaping wound
- Partial or complete amputation
- Deep wound to the head, back of mouth or throat, chest, neck, genitals, or abdomen
- Pulsating or squirting blood
- Visible bone

Seek medical care within 2 to 4 hours when there is:

- Gaping, split, jagged, or deep wound located around the eye, face, or joint
- Inability to move or limited movement of the injured part
- History of diabetes
- Persistent bleeding after 10 minutes of direct pressure
- Foreign body in wound
- Laceration through the eyelid, lip border, or eyebrow

7. How are lacerations categorized at triage in a three-level system?

Level 1 (red)	Life-threatening hemorrhage
Level 2 (yellow)	Bleeding that is difficult to control
	Injury across a joint or vital structure (eye globe)
	Associated with other injuries
Level 3 (green):	Simple laceration

8. In five-tier systems?

In the various five-level triage systems, Level 1 is life-threatening, systemic injuries to Level 5 with the least acuity/complexity. The applicable levels specific to common laceration/puncture wound presentations include:

Emergency Severity Index (ESI)

Level 4:	Simple laceration, vital signs (VS) stable
Level 3:	More complex laceration requiring culture, x-ray, etc. (≥2 resources)
Level 2:	Concurrent traumatic injuries that would place the individual at risk for deterioration, requiring three or more resources (IVs, medication, tests, etc.)

Canadian Triage and Acuity Scale (CTAS)

Level 4 less urgent (≤1 hour):	Laceration requiring investigation/intervention
	Stable vital signs
	Moderate pain (4 to 7 out of 10)
Level 5 nonurgent (≤2 hours):	Laceration not requiring closure but only cleansing, splinting, minor analgesics, and/or immunization.

Manchester Triage Group

Level 2 very urgent (10 minutes):	Severe pain (8 to 10 out of 10)
	Distal vascular compromise
Level 3 urgent (60 minutes):	Moderate pain (7 to 10 out of 10)
	Inappropriate history (alleged mechanism does not explain the apparent injury)
	Uncontrollable minor hemorrhage
	New neuro signs/symptoms
Level 4 standard (120 minutes):	Any pain
	Local inflammation
	Local infection
	Recent injury

9. What patient factors could result in a delay in wound healing?

- Long-term steroid therapy
- Anticoagulant administration
- Hepatic compromise
- Poor nutritional state
- Immunosuppression (HIV+, splenectomy)
- Compromised vascular supply (diabetes, smoking, atherosclerosis)
- Long-term medications that slow collagen formation (phenytoin [Dilantin])
- Advanced age

10. Give examples of contaminated wounds.

- Full-thickness bites (human or animal)
- Wounds of the perineum or axilla
- Exposed to contaminated water (ponds)
- Exposed to fecal material (barnyard)

11. What causes wounds to get infected?

- Infection results when the skin barrier to infection is broken and bacteria contamination in the tissue wound edges exceeds the body's capability of containing it.
- The extent of the wound edge contamination (e.g., more than 10 to the sixth power of bacteria per gram)

OR

- The organism is particularly virulent or releases dangerous substances that destroy tissue or disable immune mediators, such as in necrotizing fasciitis, bacillus anthracis (anthrax), or clostridium tetani ("tetanus")
- The colonization threshold is reduced

12. What would increase the likelihood of bacterial colonization?

- A retained foreign body
- Certain kinds of clay found in dirt in the wound (common in industrial or farming accidents)
- A crush injury with devitalized tissue
- Poor vascularity from causes such as smoking or diabetes

13. Anything I can do to help control bleeding and swelling for a small laceration in the mouth?

Have the patient suck on an ice cube or flavored ice.

14. What are appropriate solutions for cleaning the skin?

Scrub the wound with a fine-pore sponge or gauze and a nonionic surfactant. This could include:

- Shur-Clens

- Normal saline
- One percent iodophor solution. This concentration is not toxic to tissue and is as effective as 10% iodophor solution in killing *Staphylococcus aureus*

No one solution has been shown to be superior.

15. What about tap water?

Riyat and Wuinton (1997) found that tap water (preferably running) was as effective for initial cleansing of wounds as other commercial products.

16. Any solution that is not recommended for routine wound cleansing?

Chlorhexidine (Hibiclens) and 10% iodophor (Betadine) kill bacteria, but also injure wound defenses. Use only on the skin around the wound, not the wound itself.

Hydrogen peroxide (3%) damages tissues by hemolyzing erythrocytes, occluding local microvasculatature, and releasing gas that causes crepitus and tissue distortion. It loses its ability to destroy bacteria once it is in contact with blood or pus.

17. Are routine prophylactic antibiotics the best method to prevent wound infection?

No, although prophylaxis may be needed for grossly contaminated wounds. High-pressure mechanical irrigation remains the best way to decrease the chance of wound infection. Possibilities include

- 19-gauge syringe attached to a 35- or 12-mL syringe
- Disposable irrigation sets (Zero-Wet)

There is no evidence that one apparatus is superior, although a mechanical devise is usually preferred for a contaminated or dirty, extensive wound. Irrigate by placing the needle perpendicular to the wound, as close as possible to the surface.

18. How much should I irrigate?

Copious. One guide is 60 mL per cm of wound length.

19. Why aren't prophylactic antibiotics given in addition, just to be safe?

Simple lacerations less than 8 hours old will become infected at a rate of 6% both with and without antibiotic prophylaxis.

20. Should I shave the area?

Shaving hair results in higher wound bacterial counts and increased rates of infection. If the hair is excessive, cut it with scissors. Never shave the eyebrows as they may not grow back and are used as a landmark.

21. What is the maximum time usually allowed from the time the injury occurred until the wound must be closed?

Most physicians want to perform wound closure only 8 to 10 hours after injury, as closure after 8 hours has a higher rate of infection. Lacerations more than 24 hours old are not closed, with several exceptions.

22. Tell me the exceptions.

- Face: blood supply and infection resistance is so good that primary closure can be done regardless of the wound's age.
- Scalp.
- Areas that are cosmetically insignificant but the injury could involve disability if left open, such as large lacerations close to joints.

23. Give examples of laceration standing orders.

Iroquois Memorial Hospital (Watseka, Ill)
Source: Abbey Purvis, RN CEN; ED Director
Wound >8 hours old, ask physician about culture prior to cleaning
Clean wound with Shur-Clens and irrigate with at least 200 mL normal saline
Steri-strip closure (ordered by physician) may be done by a nurse

Memorial Regional Hospital (Hollywood, Fla)
Source: Melinda Stibal, RN BSHC, Administrative Director, Emergency/Trauma
Clean wound with normal saline
X-ray injured area if indicated to rule out foreign body or suspected fracture
Administer tetanus diphtheria (Td) 0.5mL IM (if appropriate)

24. Our clinic policies allow us to apply sterile, microporous tape (such as Steri-Strips). Tell me the steps.

- "Tape" is appropriate for well-approximated wound edges that have minimal skin tension. It results in less scaring than sutures.
- Apply benzoin or similar type of solution to skin beforehand to aid adherence.
- Pull the wound edges together but do not overlap the skin edges.
- Do not apply topical antibiotic ointment.
- Apply the strips with space between the strips.
- Leave the strips on till they fall off naturally.

25. Can we also apply the adhesive "glue"?

This type of closure is best for small, linear wounds that have minimal tension (areas in which 5-0 or 6-0 sutures would be appropriate). This method has less bacterial count than sutured wounds and obvious patient comfort.

- The adhesive bonding (2-Octyl cyanoacrylate [DERMABOND]) dries fast in seconds.
- Apply a protective coat of petroleum jelly and dab any excess immediately to prevent it from going into undesired area.

- Loosen the bond with petroleum jelly or antibiotic ointment if it accidentally dries on an undesired area, such as the eyelid being glued shut.
- Apply three separate thin layers of glue for maximum strength.
- Do not apply antibiotic ointment as it weakens (dissolves) the adhesive.
- Teach the patient to keep the area dry. The material sloughs off in 5 to 10 days.

26. Why are Steri-Strips applied across the wound after it is stitched or "glued"?

As reinforcement because the wound does not regain full tensile strength for a considerable time.

27. What medications are used for anesthesia associated with wounds?

- Lidocaine (Xylocaine)
- Lidocaine with epinephrine for high vascularity areas: Lidocaine with epinephrine causes vasoconstriction and is useful to reduce actively bleeding wounds, such as in the scalp. Traditionally it has been avoided for the digits, penis, nose, and ears, but studies have failed to show harm from use on these areas.
- Viscous lidocaine for abrasion to minimize pain during cleansing.
- See Chapter 6 for further discussion of topical anesthetics, including TAC, LET, and EMLA.

28. Why do some practitioners add sodium bicarbonate to the lidocaine?

Lidocaine injections can be made more comfortable by either warming the lidocaine to 37°C (place it in the blanket warmer) or by buffering it with sodium bicarbonate as a 10:1 solution of 10 mL 1% lidocaine and 1 mEq/mL (3 mL of 4.2%) sodium bicarbonate. This buffering reduces the shelf life of lidocaine to a few days.

29. Discuss stapling.

Compared to suturing, stapling is faster, less painful, has a lower level of tissue reactivity, and a higher resistance to infection. The drawbacks of staples include wound edges may be more difficult to approximate, staples may catch on clothing, and staples on visible areas of the upper body give a "Frankenstein" appearance some individuals may not want. Provide the same wound care instructions as stitches. (No magnetic resonance imaging (MRI) should be done until the staples are removed.)

30. Talk about how the selection of suture material is made.

Sutures with absorbable material are used on mucous membranes or deeper lacerations that require suturing the subcutaneous tissue, muscle, or fascia. Nonabsorbables are used to close the skin layers.

Suture size ranges from 0-0 (very thick) to extremely fine (6-0). The more commonly used sizes in the emergency department are 3-0 to 6-0.

Size of the needle also varies (30-gauge advisable) and can be straight or curved.

The smaller the suture and needle and the less time suture is left in, the smaller the scar will be.

31. Can nurses suture?

Yes, as long as they have completed a program that has proper training, supervision, and demonstrated competency and it falls within the state statutes. Joint Commission of Accreditation for Healthcare Organizations (JCAHO) accepts this scope of expanded practice.

Departments that allow nurses or military medics to suture usually still have the physician apply the topical liquid skin adhesive, staples, and/or sutures on the face, hands, or joint.

32. When is the wound the weakest?

Three days after the injury. After the initial blood clot, the fibroblasts stimulate growth for 2 to 3 days, with remodeling after day 5. Initial scar tissue is fragile and bleeds easily.

33. What types of dressings are recommended?

Three layers:

- Nonadhering type of material (e.g., Telfa, Adaptic) next to the wound
- Absorbant material for the intermediate layer, such as gauze pads
- Protective top layer (e.g., Kerlix, Kling, elastic net) or a transparent dressing (Tegaderm, Op-site)

34. How long should a wound have a dressing?

Dressings should be used for a minimum of 48 hours to protect the healing wound.

35. Isn't it best to leave wounds "open to air" to prevent infection?

No, the dressing allows a moist scab to develop. This promotes healing by allowing the epidermal cells to migrate 40% faster. One study also found wound pain was reduced in a moist healing environment.

36. When should sutures and staples be removed?

The location guidelines are indicated, considering the type of suture material and injury. Nonabsorbable sutures should be removed as soon as epithelization occurs to minimize scarring.

Type of tissue sutured	*Suggested removal time frame*
Eyelid, eyebrow, lip, face, ear	3 to 5 days
Scalp, trunk, hands, feet	7 to 10 days
Arms, legs	10 to 14 days
Sutures over joint areas	14 days

37. How about staples?

Staples follow the same guidelines as sutures.

38. Review when and what tetanus immunizations are given.

- Simple, clean, minor wounds in a patient who has never been immunized against tetanus: immunization schedule started with administration of tetanus toxoid 0.5 mL IM.
- Contaminated or infection-prone wound: human tetanus immune globulin 250 to 500 U in addition.
- Simple, clean, minor laceration with a history of having been immunized against tetanus within the past 5 to 10 years: no need for a tetanus booster.
- If it has been more than 10 years since the last tetanus booster: tetanus toxoid 0.5 mL. For adults, the booster may be a combination of diphtheria/tetanus toxoid.
- Contaminated wound in an individual who has not had an immunization in the past 5 years: tetanus toxoid 0.5mL IM.
- Contaminated wounds in the individual who has not had a primary set of tetanus immunizations (think immigrant) and who has not been immunized within the past 10 years: both tetanus toxoid 0.5 mL and tetanus immune globulin 250 to 500 U.

39. In the occupational clinic in which I work, employees often request to receive the tetanus immunization "just to be sure." Is that advisable?

No. Besides the pain, expense, and documentation work, some individuals will become hyperimmune to tetanus from too frequent immunizations. Subsequent tetanus immunization causes the arm to become painfully swollen for several days and is the usual source of a "tetanus allergy." (The other possible cause of tetanus allergy is a hypersensitivity to past preparations that used horse serum. All current preparations are now human-derived.)

40. What are the important discharge instructions to include besides the typical wound/infection instructions?

- Elevate to limit edema
- May shower without increasing the chance of infection but avoid public or polluted water (swimming pools, ocean)
- Wear sunscreen for 6 months because the scar has the potential for hyperpigmentation

41. Why should I teach the patient with an abrasion to clean the wound and change the dressing every 24 hours?

Removing the old dressing can remove tissue coagulum and eschar. This cleans the wound of debris that retards migration of fibroblasts and promotes healing.

42. How can I prevent cosmetic tattooing in a "road rash" abrasion?

Eliminate all retained foreign material before healing begins. Enhance patient comfort by anesthetizing with viscous lidocaine and dressing with silver sulfadiazine. Consider a toothbrush for scrubbing.

43. Why is a puncture wound a concern? It looks small.

A puncture wound results in a narrow, deep wound with minimal bleeding. It will close early, is difficult to clean, and may contain a foreign body. They are tetanus-prone by definition. Infection occurs in 11% to 15% of puncture wounds.

44. How about punctures on the bottom of the foot?

Wounds over the metatarsal-phalangeal joints warrant special attention because the injury is usually from weight bearing on a sharp object. The force can result in deep penetration to the bone (0.4% to 0.6% of all punctures). About half of infected plantar puncture wounds will contain a foreign body (usually a piece of fabric).

45. When is an x-ray useful for a patient with a potential imbedded foreign body?

Glass (larger than 2 mm), metal, and gravel (larger than 1 mm) can be visualized on radiographs. Woods, plastics, and some aluminum products are not visible on x-rays.

Key Points

- Human and animal bites are contaminated and at high risk for complications, such as infections.
- Control bleeding and pain with a mouth laceration by having the patient suck an ice cube or flavored ice.
- Shaving hair around the laceration is not recommended. Never shave eyebrows.
- Wounds should be closed within 8 hours. Wounds are not closed after 24 hours except for the face, scalp, or a region in which scarring from not suturing is insignificant.
- Dressings allow a moist healing environment that enhances epithelization.

Internet Resources

Iroquois Memorial Hospital Emergency Department Patient Care Standard for Surface Trauma
http://www.ena.org/document_share/documents/surface_trauma.doc

MedicineNet.com: Cuts, Scrapes, and Puncture Wounds
http://www.medicinenet.com/cuts_scrapes_and_puncture_wounds/article.htm

NCEMI.org: Puncture Wounds
http://www.ncemi.org/cse/cse1015.htm

Ethicon, Inc.: Dermabond
http://www.jnjgateway.com/public/USENG/7011DERMABOND_Topical_Skin_Adhesive_2_Octyl_Cyanoacrylate.pdf

Bibliography

American College of Surgeons, Committee on Trauma: *Resources for optimal care of the injured patient,* Chicago, 1999, American College of Surgeons, 14-16, 27-30.

Briggs JK: *Telephone triage protocols for nurses,* ed 2, Philadelphia, 2002, Lippincott, Williams & Wilkins.

Canadian Association of Emergency Physicians: Canadian Emergency Department Triage and Acuity Scale Implementation Guidelines, *J Can Assoc Emerg Physicians* 1(3 suppl), 1999.

Emergency Nurses Association: *Course in advanced trauma nursing (CATN II), Ch 8: Host defense systems,* ed 2, Dubuque, 2003, Kendall/Hunt Publishing, 229.

Escobar JI, Bryce RT, Harwood-Nuss AL: Wound management. In Markovchick VJ, Pons PT, editors: *Pons' emergency medicine secrets,* ed 3, Philadelphia, 2003, Hanley & Belfus.

Gilboy N, Rosenau A, Travers D, et al: *Emergency severity index (ESI).* Des Plaines, Ill, 2003, Emergency Nurses Association, 6-9, 12-33.

Herr RD, Zimmermann PG: Wound management. In Sheehy SB, Lenehan GP, editors: *Lenehan's manual of emergency care,* ed 5, St Louis, 1999, Mosby.

Hill NA: Suturing (Managers Forum), *J Emerg Nurs* 26(5):495, 2000.

Holt L: Wound care. In Dolan B, Holt L, editors: *Holt's accident and emergency theory into practice,* London, 2000, Harcourt.

Jacobs BB, Hoyt KS, editors: *Trauma nursing core course,* ed 5, Des Plaines, Ill, 2000, Emergency Nurses Association, 192.

Jenkins JL, Braen GR: *Manual of emergency medicine,* ed 4, Philadelphia, 2000, Lippincott, Williams & Wilkins.

Jordan KS, editor: *Emergency nursing core curriculum,* ed 5, Philadelphia, 2000, WB Saunders, 218-220, 665-666, 669-670.

Killian M, editor: *Standards of emergency nursing practice,* ed 4, Des Plaines, Ill, 1999, Emergency Nurses Association, 10-17, 19-28, 43-49.

Mackway-Jones K: *Emergency triage: Manchester Triage Group,* London, 1997, BMJ Publishing.

Newberry L: *Sheehy's emergency nursing: Principles and practice,* St Louis, 2003, Mosby, 145-146, 255, 370, 701.

Proehl JA: *Emergency nursing procedures,* ed 2, Philadelphia, 1999, WB Saunders, 446-476.

Riyat MS, Quinton DN: Tap water as a wound cleansing agent in A & E, *J Accident Emerg Med* 14:165-166, 1997.

Selfridge-Thomas J: *Emergency nursing: An essential guide for patient care,* Philadelphia, 1997, WB Saunders, 154.

Chapter 41

Foreign Bodies

Robert D. Herr

1. What types of foreign bodies are most common?

The answer is most meaningful by age group. Children play with food and toys. Their driving curiosity and lack of inhibition leads to seeing what will happen through putting both in nearly every available orifice. Things get stuck.

Young adults acquire foreign bodies through jewelry piercing the ear, nose, tongue, nipple, navel, and genitals. When these become infected, torn, or painful they may become emergencies and require removal. Please see Chapter 42.

Older patients have implanted foreign bodies such as cardiac pacemakers, subcutaneous catheters, vascular stents, prosthetic valves, corneal implants, joint replacements, and so on. The variety of implants continues to grow. The overriding principle is that any foreign body can become infected from migration of skin organisms such as *Staphylococcus epidermidis* or through blood-borne organisms such as *S. aureus*. Patients may present with fever, pain, or component malfunction that suggests infected implant. The discussion of each is beyond the scope of this chapter. However, it is important to preserve function of the implant through noting it. Some implants cannot survive magnetic resonance imaging (MRI) scanning; others require prophylactic antibiotics prior to incision and drainage (I&D) of abscess to prevent staphylococcus seeding of the implant. Lastly, mechanical heart valves need anticoagulation assessed and can cause embolic stroke as valve clotting if it is inadequate.

2. How do I approach foreign bodies differently depending on body site?

Airway foreign body is emergent. Assess for stridorous breathing, hoarseness, and coughing. Assess the lungs for diminished breath sounds that could indicate an obstructed mainstem bronchus or smaller bronchus. Mouth inspection can reveal parts of the foreign body such as pieces of balloon or parts of a denture. Get an order for plain radiograph. One pearl is that objects in the larynx look on edge on the posteroanterior (PA) or anteroposterior (AP) neck film, whereas those in the esophagus are flat on the same film.

Once the airway, breathing, and circulation (ABCs) have been cleared, the triage nurse can ask in a supportive empathetic manner what happened and what the object might be. The individual might localize the foreign body to a particular orifice. Preverbal children will point or scratch to help reveal the orifice. Sometimes it is a parental complaint of blood coming from an ear, nose, anus, or vagina that reveals where the foreign body is. I had one girl brought for increasing bad breath (halitosis) over weeks. Inspection revealed a blue spot up one nostril. With help of forceps I removed a gauze pad-sized piece of blue foam from the nostril. "Wow" the mom said, "that's from the cushion we threw away a month ago." Sometimes halitosis is the only sign of a nasal foreign body—so take a look during triage.

It is difficult at triage to inspect the anus or vagina, and vaginal exam in girls may require general anesthesia. Options at triage are to get an order for plain radiograph that may reveal the foreign body.

The history can reveal what object the individual was playing with or eating that might be the foreign body, especially if it got "lost."

The biggest challenge is the older person who is so embarrassed about lost objects in the rectum or vagina that they won't talk about it at triage. Again a plain film of the pelvis can paint the picture that's worth a thousand seconds of trying to get words. One man couldn't bring himself to tell me what he had "up there." When the radiograph showed a light bulb up his rectum we immediately focused on what to do about it.

3. How do I approach the swallowed foreign body, including button (disc) batteries?

Swallowed objects usually pass without problem and can be triaged to a lower level. The big exception is the button battery from Grandma's hearing aid or from the family garage door opener. If these lodge in the esophagus their current can burn through the esophagus and lead to mediastinitis within 6 hours. Get an order for a chest and/or abdominal film to see where the battery might be. If it is esophageal, prepare for quick endoscopic removal with need for IV and transfer to a gastrointestinal (GI) lab.

Patients with esophageal foreign body that's not a battery may have endoscopic removal or a period of waiting to see if it passes into the stomach.

Although most objects that make it to the stomach can be passed in the stool without injury to the intestine, there are notable exceptions. Open safety pins and other objects that can perforate bowel may be safer to remove than to let pass. That's why history and radiographic visualization are so important to get in the triage process.

Lastly, consider lead objects like shot or fishing sinkers can release lead. Anticipate an order for a lead level and for possible endoscopic retrieval if the lead level is high or rising.

4. How do I approach the fishhook embedded in the skin?

Like any impaled object its best to control any bleeding with direct pressure and elevation, then stabilize the object until the clinician can remove it. If it is a small hook and piercing only skin, it can be safely removed by at least three methods.

- The most elegant method is to unstick the barb by pressing in and forward on the hook, then pulling back on the hook to pop it out. The best way to pull back on the hook is by placing a small string around the curve of the hook and pulling with the string parallel to the shank of the hook. Pull back quickly after the barb is freed.
- The second method is to push forward the barb through the skin, cut off the barb with metal cutters and pull out the hook. I find it hard to push the barb through the skin and harder to cut it painlessly; usually local anesthetic helps.
- The third method is to directly incise the skin and remove the hook. This requires local anesthetic or you have a very unhappy patient.

5. How do I approach a large embedded foreign body such as a nail from a nail gun or pressurized paint or other chemical gun?

Detecting it is crucial. One construction worker presented with headache the day after using a nail gun. He had a beard and there was no entry wound visible anywhere. The astute triage nurse got an order for a skull film (one of the few times a skull film is helpful) and it showed—you guessed it—a 4-inch nail in the brain.

Nails are like other impaled objects. Once bleeding is controlled the object should be stabilized and not removed because it could be tamponading a bleed. One tip is that removal in the operating room is required for any object that fractures bone or contacts brain or bowel or other important organ. The reason is that even though the nail could be pulled out safely, the object introduced bacteria from skin and perhaps pieces of clothing. To restore function and prevent infection the surgeon needs to give good wound debridement and cleaning.

Pressurized paint or chemical guns can inject foreign material long distances under the skin. The injectants follow tendon sheaths and other tissue planes. Even a needle-prick sized entry hole can hide several ounces of injectant. The hand injury patient should be assessed for pain and range of motion of all digits close to the injecting hole. Such patients frequently need the operating room (OR) for incision and debridement of injectant. The key is to obtain the history, alert the clinician, and prepare for an order to send the patient to the OR.

6. How do I approach a nasal foreign body?

If the object cannot be pulled out with forceps, have the patient cover the other nostril and gently blow through the affected nostril.

7. How do I approach the ear foreign body, including insects?

One study of 698 ear foreign bodies showed emergency department (ED) removal succeeded 77% of the time. Failures occurred with spherical foreign bodies, objects lodged against the tympanic membrane, and objects in the canal for more than 24 hours. Failures of removal in the ED were referred to the otolaryngologist who used otomicroscopy for an 85% success rate.

Insects can be washed out with warm water if you place an Angiocath sheath on a syringe like you would use for cleaning a cerumen impaction. Even better is to get an order for lidocaine. This can paralyze the insect and wash it out.

8. How do I approach rectal or vaginal foreign bodies?

These cause alarm and the patient may be very emotional, yet embarrassed to admit what happened. Plain radiograph can help identify glass and metal, and also vibrators by revealing their batteries. You can reassure the patient that nothing has been invented that cannot be found and removed, and that there is little you have not seen before. Now you have to avoid exclamation when you see the radiograph or hear the real story!

Prepare for the clinician to perform an anoscopy or pelvic examination depending on the situation. Pelvic examination in girls may require general anesthesia and therefore transfer to the OR. Rectal objects are hard to remove if they are jagged because edges lodge against rectal folds. Likewise they are hard to remove if they are smooth because removal is resisted by suction from the bowel above the foreign body. One tip is to prepare to have the clinician ask for a Foley catheter to insert to the side of the smooth object and beyond the object to break the suction and permit retrieval. Of course prepare for further orders because many larger objects will require the colonoscopy suite or the OR with a surgeon. You can remind the patient what he/she can now appreciate: the rectum is biologically designed to hold something inside rather than to easily expel it. Consider also that assault is one possibility for how objects get into rectums and vaginas. Ask questions in a supportive way and be cognizant of other signs of abuse, especially in situations like these in which clinicians may be enthralled with the technical challenges of foreign body retrieval rather than asking how the body actually got there in the first place.

Key Points

- Foreign bodies can be cosmetic as in piercing, therapeutic as in implants, and accidental. This chapter focuses on accidental.
- A nonjudgmental history is key; a plain radiograph is even better.
- Swallowed button batteries are emergencies, other objects that do not pass the esophagus into the stomach after a few hours need removal.
- Nails and paint guns may have deeper injury that requires the OR to debride.
- Ear foreign bodies can be removed by direct visualization in three fourths of the cases.
- Referral to ear, nose, and throat specialist (ENT) may be needed especially with spherical objects, delayed presentation, and objects lodged against the tympanic membrane.
- Rectal and vaginal foreign bodies may be manifestations of assault.

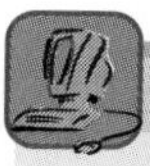

Internet Resources

Emedicine.com: Foreign Bodies, Trachea
http://www.emedicine.com/EMERG/topic751.htm

Emedicine.com: Pediatrics, Foreign Body Ingestion
http://www.emedicine.com/emerg/topic379.htm

Virtual Children's Hospital: Pediatrics Foreign Body
http://www.vh.org/pediatric/patient/pediatrics/cqqa/foreignbody.html

Medline Plus: Foreign Body in the Nose
http://www.nlm.nih.gov/medlineplus/ency/article/000037.htm

Bibliography

Duncan M, Wong RK: Esophageal emergencies: Things that will wake you from a sound sleep, *Gastroenterol Clin North Am* 32(4):1035-1052, 2003.

Hadfield-Law L: Body piercing: Issues for A&E nurses, *Accid Emerg Nurs* 9(1):14-19, 2001.

Lao J, Bostwick HE, Berezin S, et al: Esophageal food impaction in children, *Pediatr Emerg Care* 19(6): 402-407, 2003.

Schulze SL, Kerschner J, Beste D: Pediatric external auditory canal foreign bodies: A review of 698 cases, *Otolaryngol Head Neck Surg* 127(1):73-78, 2002.

Settle LL: Foreign-body ingestion. In Harwood-Nuss A, Wolfson AG, Linden CH, et al, editors: *The clinical practice of emergency medicine,* ed 3, Philadelphia, 2001, Lippincott Williams & Wilkins, 1261-1262.

Chapter 42

Piercings (Voluntary)

Jared Strote

1. What and where are body piercings?

Simply put, body piercings are jewelry placed through the skin of various body parts. Piercings can and are placed literally everywhere throughout the body. The most common sites include the ear, eyebrow, nose, lip, tongue, nipple, navel, and genitals.

2. How common is body piercing?

In the United States, some estimates of female ear piercing approach 80% to 90%. There are no prevalence data for other body piercings, but the numbers are certainly on the rise as the practice becomes more mainstream. One study in a New York college found 42% of males and 60% of females had at least one body piercing.

3. How are piercings performed?

Body piercing is usually done without anesthesia or preprocedure antibiotics. Most often, a hollow 12- to 18-gauge needle is placed through the piercing site either with or without the jewelry attached. The jewelry is then passed through. Piercing guns that automate the process are falling into disfavor as they are difficult to sterilize. The jewelry used depends on the site and may need to be bigger for the first few weeks to accommodate swelling. Aftercare usually involves weeks of cleaning with antiseptic solution and strict hygiene.

4. Why do people get piercings?

There is a long history of body piercing in humans, in almost every society dating back to the beginnings of recorded history. Its significance varies widely in history from fashion to politics to rites of passage to religious meanings.

More recently, piercings have been done as an act of rebellion against mainstream culture and even more recently still as part of a fashion or aesthetic trend or for sexual practices. It also has been described as a means of self-empowerment after a traumatic experience. In any case, given its universally intimate and personal significance, clinicians should take care not to judge those with piercings or treat them any differently than those without.

5. How common are complications from piercings?

As piercing clinicians are generally not licensed or regulated and patients will often perform the procedure on themselves, rates vary greatly. Furthermore, complications vary by site, materials used, and aftercare hygiene. Under any circumstances, however, complications are common. One survey of family clinicians in the United Kingdom found that 95% had treated a piercing-related complication. Other surveys and studies show rates as high as 17% to 35% of all piercings, although only a fraction of these seek medical care, many often returning to their clinician for advice or self-treating at home.

6. What are the common complications?

There is almost always inflammation during the healing period, caused by the local trauma of the piercing itself. Tender, inflamed nearby lymph nodes are also common and usually benign. Immediate or delayed bleeding can occur, usually self-limiting or easily arrested with pressure.

Delayed complications include allergic contact dermatitis (usually from nickel jewelry), jewelry that becomes embedded in the tissue, and cyst, scar, or keloid formation. The most common medically urgent delayed complication is local infection, either with cellulitis or abscess formation. This can occur in up to 10% to 25% of piercings but are usually self-limiting. Local trauma from piercings catching on other objects (e.g., torn ear lobes) can also occur.

Rarely, more significant infections occur with reports of endocarditis, sepsis, and toxic shock syndrome. Additionally, when a nonsterile technique is used, viral transmission is a risk, including Hepatitis B and C and human immunodeficiency virus (HIV).

Other complications specific to different piercing sites are discussed below.

7. Why do piercing infections occur?

Piercing infections occur for a variety of reasons but almost always involve skin pathogens, usually either *Staphylococcus* or *Streptococcus* species. The procedure itself provides a portal of entry for bacteria into the tissues; initial nonsterile technique can dramatically increase the initial risk. The trauma and subsequent inflammation decrease blood flow to the area and immune system capability although the tissue exposure continues. Piercing aftercare, designed to decrease inflammation and keep the exposed tissue as clean and bacteria-free as possible, is often done incompletely or not at all.

Retained foreign bodies can increase the risk as does any disease process or medication that causes systemic immunosuppression. When piercings become embedded, abscess formation can occur as there is no outflow tract for drainage.

8. How long do piercings take to heal?

This depends on the site. The tongue and labia minora heal most quickly (3 to 6 weeks). Other genital piercings take 2 weeks to 2 months. And most facial piercings and nipples heal between 6 weeks and 6 months. The navel can take up to 1 year to be completely healed, usually because tight clothing worn over the piercing slows tissue recovery.

During the period of healing, the area around the piercing can be mildly warm, red, and swollen just adjacent to the site. Discharge can occur with normal healing although it should be clear and not thick or white.

9. How can I tell the difference between normal healing, allergic dermatitis, and infection?

Each of these presents similarly along a spectrum of symptomatology. Normal healing occurs in the time frame outlined above. Redness, warmth, tenderness, and inflammation is limited to a small area surrounding the piercing and there should be no systemic symptoms like fever or chills.

Allergic dermatitis most often presents as a reaction to brass or nickel jewelry and often occurs when the stainless steel jewelry used in the initial piercing is replaced some time later. It is very localized to only areas directly in contact with the jewelry. Redness, pruritus, and tenderness are common. Usually there is no significant warmth or swelling.

Infection can occur at any time once the piercing has occurred but occurs more frequently soon afterward. Swelling, redness, warmth, and tenderness are more pronounced and can spread from the piercing site both by lymphangitic streaking and widely as a cellulitis. Drainage can be thick, white, and foul-smelling. Symptoms may increase rapidly. There also may be associated systemic symptoms or a fluctuant area in which abscess formation has begun.

10. What emergent piercing complications need to be addressed acutely?

Few piercing complications evolve into truly emergent situations. As with all triaged patients, airway, breathing, and circulation (ABCs) must be addressed first and foremost and resuscitation begun if appropriate. Patients with aspirated mouth jewelry or tongue swelling should be immediately treated with oxygen, intravenous (IV) access, monitoring, and airway control. Systemically ill patients from disseminated infection should likewise be immediately stabilized and monitored. Persistent bleeding can often be controlled with direct pressure.

More commonly, piercings will need to be removed acutely after trauma to a pierced area. Early removal is important to avoid having the jewelry embedded in the tissue or create a constriction. Removal also becomes increasingly difficult as swelling progresses and is often necessary under any circumstance for proper radiographic imaging of affected areas.

Piercings should not be immediately removed in the case of infection. As with all puncture wounds, the risk of abscess formation is high when the open route of drainage is closed.

11. How do I remove piercings?

Barbells usually have one end that unscrews with counterclockwise turning. Common ear and nose jewelry often have backings that need to be squeezed and then pulled. Hoops are often held closed by pressure; these need only be pulled apart perpendicular to the jewelry at the connecting point.

12. What triage difficulties are unique to piercings?

Patients are often reluctant to talk about piercing-related medical problems, either because of their intimate location, their personal significance, or a sense of shame or embarrassment. Again sensitivity and a nonjudgmental approach is important to get a complete history.

Piercings are also often visually inaccessible without disrobing, so initial focused physical examination may not be possible.

13. What history is particularly important to piercing-related medical complaints?

A history of the piercing event is important. How long ago did it happen? Who performed it (the patient, a friend, a clinician)? What techniques/materials were used (antiseptic, autoclaved jewelry and piercing tools, nickel or surgical steel)? What aftercare was performed (frequent cleanings, antiseptic rinsing, moving the jewelry to decrease chance of abscess formation). Has the patient been self-treating with antibiotics or other medicines?

Other than that, history of similar complications or increased risks of infection (e.g., diabetes, immunocompromise) should be assessed given its commonness as a piercing complication.

14. What immunization history is important to piercings?

Every patient with a recent piercing should be asked about tetanus and hepatitis immunization history. Tetanus should be updated if a booster has not been received in the last 10 years or in the last 5 years if a nonsterile instrument was used for the piercing.

15. What complications are specific to ear piercing?

Ear piercing has a higher incidence of cosmetic disfiguring as a result of the more extreme inflammatory response of ear cartilage. Tearing of the ear lobe also occurs.

16. What complications are specific to genital piercing?

Urethral stricture or other injury can occur, obstructing or disturbing urinary flow. Other documented complications include priapism, paraphimosis, and recurrent condyloma acuminatum.

Genital piercings are notable for the complications they can inflict on others. Trauma to the vagina, mouth, and anus occur and should be treated like any other trauma.

17. What complications are specific to tongue and lip piercing?

Perhaps the most life-threatening complications can occur with oral piercing. Most worrisome is local edema, excessive bleeding, or aspiration leading to a potential airway loss. Any patient with difficulty breathing or controlling his secretions needs to be treated immediately. Aspiration is also a risk for those with nasal piercings or partners of genitally pierced patients.

Other less emergent but more common complications include tooth chipping, gum breakdown, and hypersalivation.

18. What complications are specific to nipple piercing?

Defibrillation during cardiac arrest can cause severe burns if nipple rings are not removed before shocking. There is one case report of a hormonal change as a result of constant nipple stimulation leading to breast milk production. Aspiration from nursing infants or restriction of breast-feeding can also occur.

19. Do parents need to be informed of minor's piercing-related injury?

Unlike pregnancy-related medical visits, treatment for piercing complications requires parental approval if the patient is under 18 and not emancipated. In most states, piercings themselves do not require a parent's consent. This can lead to situations in which a piercing-related medical condition is the first a parent hears of the patient's piercing, requiring extra sensitivity by the clinician.

20. Are piercing-related injuries reportable?

At this time, piercing-related injuries are not reportable. Some states are considering more stringent licensing and monitoring of piercing clinicians, which may involve reporting of piercing-related complications at some point in the future.

Key Points

- Piercing aftercare includes hygiene and cleaning with antiseptic.
- Complications include inflammation, bleeding, and local infection 10% to 25% of the time.
- Rare complications are endocarditis, sepsis, and toxic shock syndrome.
- Infectious organisms are mostly *Staphylococcus* and *Streptococcus* species.
- Normal healing of pierced sites can take up to 6 months or longer if there is repeated trauma to the site.
- It is important to distinguish inflammation from allergic dermatitis or infection.

Internet Resources

WebMD: Piercings Prone to Problems
http://aolsvc.health.webmd.aol.com/content/article/25/3606_1145

Security World.com: The Safety of Tattoos and Piercing
http://www.securityworld.com/library/health/tatoos.html

MayoClinic.com: Tattoos and piercings: What to Know Before You Go Under the Needle
http://www.mayoclinic.com/invoke.cfm?id=MC00020

Journal of Antimicrobial Chemotherapy: Antibiotic Prophylaxis, Body Piercing, and Infective Endocarditis
http://jac.oupjournals.org/cgi/content/full/53/2/123

Pennsylvania Medical Society: "Poke and Stick" Parties Pose Serious Health Risks to Teens
http://www.pamedsoc.org/Template.cfm?Section=CPH&template=/ContentManagement/ContentDisplay.cfm&ContentID=7984

Bibliography

Anderson W, et al: The urologist's guide to genital piercing, *Int Braz J Urol* 91(3):245-251, 2003.

Folz B, et al: Jewelry-induced diseases of the head and neck, *Ann Plast Surg* 49:264-271, 2002.

Koenig L, et al: Body piercing: Medical concerns with cutting edge fashion, *J Gen Int Med* 14:379-385, 1999.

Mayers L, et al: Prevalence of body art (body piercing and tatooing) in university undergraduates and incidence of medical complications, *Mayo Clin Proc* 77:29-34, 2002.

Samantha S, et al: Infectious complications of body piercing, *Clin Infect Dis* 26:735-740, 1998.

Stirn A: Body piercing: Medical consequences and psychological motivations. *Lancet* 361:1205-1215, 2003.

Chapter 43

Burns

Dona Martin Laing

1. How can I help get this burn patient transferred, ASAP?

There are 1.25 to 2 million burn injuries a year. All emergency care facilities can initiate successful burn resuscitation. Transfer is a later concern.

2. What are the environmental agents responsible for burns?

- Thermal (heat, flames)
- Chemical (acid, alkali)
- Electrical (lightning strikes, ultraviolet)

3. What types of patients should I expect from thermal flame incidents?

The most likely patients are the children less than 14 years of age and adults over age 65. Children have a hard time recognizing danger or difficulty escaping. The elderly also may find it hard to escape and they often have concurrent health care issues.

4. What are the most common causes of thermal burns?

Scalds and hot substances account for 58% and fire and flame for 34%.

5. What are important assessment questions I should ask my patient with a thermal burn?

- How did the injury occur?
- What was the source of injury?
- Were you in an enclosed space?
- Was smoke involved?

6. Why is it important to ask about concurrent injuries that are common with burns?

Assume all burn patients have associated injuries until proven otherwise. Many concurrent injuries occur as the result of falls or jumps, being struck by falling objects, thrown by explosive forces, or penetrating injuries from the burning structure's shards.

7. How can I help prevent further burn injury to my patient?

The number one intervention is to stop the burning process. Remove all clothing; it harbors heat—elastic waistbands can be especially harmful. Remove all jewelry, metal retains heat. Additionally, rings, watches, and bracelets can act as tourniquets as edema formation occurs.

8. I understand that inhalation injury is an enormous concern with thermal burns.

Patients involved in flame events in closed spaces take in less than 21% O_2. This leads to arterial hypoxemia from the unavailability of oxygen or the inhalation of toxic substances. Debris accumulates in the lungs and can result in obstruction, atelectasis, or pneumonia.

9. Discuss airway injury.

The lower airway can be burned by inhalation of steam, but direct burns of this region are fairly uncommon. However the upper airway is susceptible to burns from direct transfer of heat and from steam inhalation. The lower airway is more often injured through inhalation of toxic fumes and the inert products of incomplete combustion are extremely injurious. Annually, greater than 50% of burn deaths are attributed to inhalation injuries.

10. Can I expect most burn patients to present with acute respiratory symptoms?

It can take from 12 to 36 hours for signs to appear. A rule of thumb is, the earlier the symptoms appear the worse the actual injury. Alerting signs and symptoms for prophylactic intubation (prior to the onset of airway edema) include:

- Singed facial hairs
- Hypoxemia
- Carbonaceous sputum
- History of being in a confined space
- Change in the patient's voice
- Decreased level of consciousness (LOC)
- Dyspnea
- Circumferential burns of the trunk

11. Does the sequence of assessment change for patients with burns?

"I" for "Inspect the back" is at the very end of the assessment list. But burn patients could be lying on smoldering clothes or chemically soaked clothing. "I" should come out of sequence. Also, be sure and inspect the axilla and groin for burning clothing.

12. List the standard interventions for burns.

- Stop the burning process and confirm airway
- Give 100% O_2 via non-rebreather

- Auscultate breath sounds
- Consider positive end expiratory pressure (PEEP) and continuous positive airway pressure (CPAP) for alveolar inflation
- Palpate peripheral pulses
- Doppler distal pulses if not palpable
- Initiate two large-bore IVs with warmed fluids, usually lactated Ringers
- Assess extremities for sensory function and neurovascular compromise
- Advocate for pain medication (intravenous [IV] route)
- Because edema formation is an issue throughout the body in severe burns, urinary catheterization, and gastric tube insertion should not be delayed
- For burns <10% cool saline dressing
- For burns >10% clean dry dressing
- Keep patient warm

Additionally:

- Assist with escharotomies
- Elevate burned extremities to the level of the heart
- Perform burn care per your institution's protocol
- Provide psychosocial support
- Prepare for admission, transfer, or direct admit to the operating room
- Monitor arterial blood gases (ABGs)
- Titrate IVs to optimal urine output of 70 to 100 mL per hour, in adults
- Assess urine for myoglobin
- Monitor cardiac rate and rhythm
- Monitor for compartment syndrome

13. What is important to include in a burn patient's ongoing care?

- Monitor pulmonary status
- Monitor urine output
- Assess peripheral circulation
- Assess edema progression

14. Why must an ABG be obtained prior to relying on pulse oximetry?

Pulse oximetry monitors are unable to differentiate between oxygen and carbon monoxide.

Carbon monoxide binds to the O_2 binding sites on hemoglobin, reducing the O_2 carrying capacity. Because it binds with myoglobin, carbon monoxide can also affect cardiac muscle directly, leading to hemorrhage or necrosis.

15. How do I estimate the percentage of burn?

Only partial-thickness and full-thickness burns are included when calculating total body surface area (TBSA). The Rule of Nines is an easy to remember, common guide that divides major portions of the body into 9% or 18% sections and is considered adequate for initial assessment. The other frequently used guide for TBSA affected is the Lund-Browder chart. It is considered more accurate because the patient's age, in proportion to relative body-size area, is taken into account.

The palm of the patient's extended hand, including the fingers, is equal to 1% of body surface area for that patient. This is particularly helpful for irregular or odd-shaped burns. The extent of a burn is often revised later, after the edema has subsided and demarcation of injury zones has occurred.

16. How do I determine the depth of the burn?

Burns are dynamic in their presentation. On first evaluation all but the most severe can be easily underestimated.

Burn Thickness

Thickness	Tissue Involved	Appearance	Pain
Superficial	Epidermis	Red Dry Blanches	Painful to touch
Partial thickness	Epidermis and dermis	Red Blisters, intact Blisters, open Weeping wounds Blanches	Exquisitely painful
Full thickness	Epidermis, dermis, and subcutaneous tissue	Color varies: yellow to black Dry Charred Leathery No capillary refill	No pain to areas that are full thickness*

*It would be extremely unusual for a patient to have full thickness burns as the only burn injury.

17. Is there a rule of thumb for scalds?

Water Temperature in Fahrenheit	Water Temperature in centigrade	Contact Time	Injury to be Expected
140°	60°	3 seconds	Deep dermal to full thickness
156°	68.8°	1 second	Deep dermal to full thickness

- Coffee is brewed at 180°F/82.2°C
- Cooking oil is used at 400°F/204.7°C
- Tar is spread at 400°F to 500°F/204°C to 260°C

18. How do I determine the severity of a burn?

This determination is based on a combination of the extent, depth, and location of the burn. It also considers the patient's age, concurrent injuries, airway/inhalation involvement, associated injuries, preexisting health issues, and circumferential burns of the chest.

19. What locations or body regions compound severity?

The face, neck, the palms of the hand and soles of the feet, joint spaces, and the perineum are all locations that acutely affect severity.

20. Where do I try for IV insertion?

Try and find a peripheral site in a nonburned area, but placement through burned tissue is common. Secure the line as well as possible. Crisis IV sites include antecubital and external jugular or a physician-inserted subclavian central line. Secure peripheral lines with dressings, and central lines with suturing.

21. How do I get the electrocardiogram leads to stay in place?

First look hard for nonburned sites. If you must work on the burned tissue, try wire/needle electrodes. You can use skin staples, and then attach the leads with alligator clips.

22. Why is fluid management so important?

Because of fluid shifts and their resultant hypovolemia, all major burn patients will require fluid resuscitation to maintain vital organ perfusion.

- 2 to 4 mL × % of the body surface area burned × the weight of the patient in kilograms, divided in half. This amount is infused over the first 8 hours postinjury.
- The second half is infused over the next 16 hours. Remember when estimating the percentage of the burn for fluid resuscitation—only calculate the areas that are partial and full thickness.

23. How will I know if fluid resuscitation is adequate?

"The kidneys are the windows to the perfusion of the viscera." Watch the urine output.

24. How can I help manage the patient's pain?

Medication is most effective when given early or even prior to onset. Once pain medication is given it should be given on a scheduled basis. Do not administer the medications intramuscularly (IM) in severe burns because the medication becomes sequestered in the third-space. Narcotics are the first-line drugs for the emergent phase of burn injury. Antianxiety drugs may also be prescribed.

25. Are ice-cold sterile dressings useful?

Patients state that they are more comfortable with ice-cold dressings or if they submerge their burn in ice water. Both these practices are harmful. The peripheral circulation is already compromised from the injury and application of extreme cold causes further vasoconstriction with decreased oxygenation to the tissues. Additionally, hypothermia is a looming threat.

26. What else can I do to improve the patient's comfort?

Protecting the exposed nerve endings improves comfort. Cover the wound as soon as possible. Also, elevate burned extremities to the level of the heart as dependent wounds have increased pain.

27. Who needs a gastric tube?

Patients with burns over 20% TBSA or more. In their hypermetabolic state, the gut of these patients shut down, resulting in ileus. They are also most likely patients to develop Curling's stress ulcers.

28. What types of burns must be reported to legal authorities?

There is no national standard for the reporting of burn injuries. Types of burns that are fairly standard for reporting include child and elder abuse, assaults, arson related, and radiation injury.

29. List assessment questions to ask related to a chemical burns.

Obtain the name of the chemical that caused the injury. Although only 3% of burns are chemical in nature, approximately 30% of burn-related deaths result from chemical injury. Also ask:

- What is the substance?
- How long were you in contact with the substance?
- What was the concentration of the substance?

30. Which type of chemical burn is worse, acid or alkaline?

Acids tend to tan the skin and make it impenetrable. Alkaline substances combine with the skin's fatty tissue to create soap. The soap acts to dissolve the skin. Alkaline substances are worse.

31. Discuss care of a burn from hydrofluoric acid.

Hydrofluoric acid burns are most common in those who work in the computer chip industry, with cleaning solvents, and/or with paint removers. Evaluate the benefits of calcium subcutaneous or local arterial injection combined with careful decontamination. These burns may require removal of nails under anesthesia if the nail beds harbor residual hydrofluoric acid.

32. Why is cement a possible source of chemical burns?

It is alkaline in nature and workers often kneel in it or drop it into their gloves or boots.

33. What is the initial management of a patient with a chemical burn?

Wear full protective clothing. Remove the patient's clothing. If the chemical can be brushed off, do so. Initiate irrigation with copious amounts of water for approximately 60 minutes, shunting the irrigation away from uninjured areas, if possible.

34. How do I remove tar or asphalt, so I can see the injury?

First cool the tar/asphalt via irrigation. Then apply a petroleum-based product and cover the wound with dressings. In 2 to 4 hours remove the dressing and the petroleum-based product and assess the need to repeat the process.

35. What information do I need about my patient's mechanism of electrical burn?

- Voltage
- Type of current
- Location of the electrical source
- Duration of the contact

36. What should I look for in patients with electrical burns?

Burns are normally equated with visible tissue damage and this is not always the case in electrical burns. Observable skin injury can be just the tip of the iceberg.

37. How do you mean, tip of the iceberg?

The electrical current meets the body's resistance and is converted into heat. Areas of the body that are smaller, like the wrist or ankle, do not allow for heat dissipation. Consequently, areas with smaller size are most susceptible to injury and destruction. Arcing may also occur as the current can jump joint spaces that are in proximity at the time of the injury.

38. What signs and symptoms are associated with electrical burns?

- Entrance and exit wounds
- Altered level of consciousness
- Dysrhythmias from a disruption in the electrical system of the heart
- Possible myoglobinuria, from muscle damage
- Possible elevations in compartment pressures, related to edema from muscle damage

39. What kinds of burn patients receive escharotomies?

Patients with full-thickness circumferential burns to any body region, especially the extremity or chest. The severe burns cause intense swelling, leading to a decreased blood flow to the periphery of the involved extremity, or limited chest expansion.

40. What burn patients should be considered for transfer to a burn care center?

The United States and Canada combined have 156 self-designated burn centers. The American Burn Association criteria for a burn unit referral include:

- Partial thickness burns greater than 10% TBSA
- Burns that involve the face, hands, feet, genitalia, perineum, or major joints
- Third-degree burns in any age group
- Electrical burns, including lightning injury
- Chemical burns
- Inhalation injury
- Burn injury in patients with preexisting medical disorders that could complicate management, prolong recovery, or affect mortality
- Any patients with burns and concomitant trauma (such as fractures) in which the burn injury poses the greatest risk of morbidity or mortality. In such cases, if the trauma poses the greater immediate risk, the patient may be initially stabilized in a trauma center before being transferred to a burn unit. Physician judgment will be necessary in such situations and should be in concert with the regional medical control plan and triage protocols.
- Burned children in hospitals without qualified personnel or equipment for the care of children
- Burn injury in patients who will require special social, emotional, or long-term rehabilitative intervention

Key Points

- Always stop the burning process first. Remove all clothing and jewelry.
- Flame events in closed spaces cause inhalation injury that is attributed to up to 50% of burn deaths. It can take 12 to 36 hours for signs to appear.
- The palm of the patient's extended hand, including the fingers, is equal to 1% of body surface area for that patient.

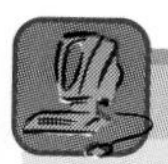

Internet Resources

American Burn Association
Prevention
http://www.ameriburn.org/Preven/Prevention.htm

Burn Unit Referral Criteria
http://www.ameriburn.org/BurnUnitReferral.pdf

America Association of Poison Control Centers
http://www.aapcc.org/

OSHA Construction e-tool: Burns and Other Injuries
http://www.osha.gov/SLTC/etools/construction/electrical_incidents/burns.html

Burn Survivor Resource Center Medical Care Guide: Types of Burns/Inhalation Injuries
http://www.burnsurvivor.com/burn_types_inhalation.html

FindLaw: Medical Demonstrative Evidence: Escharotomy and Harvest of Skin Grafts—Medical Illustration
http://findlaw.doereport.com/generateexhibit.php?ID=9620

Library of the National Medical Society: Burn Management
http://www.medical-library.org/journals2a/burn_management.htm

CDC Emergency Preparedness and Response: Hydrofluoric Acid
http://www.bt.cdc.gov/agent/hydrofluoricacid/index.asp

Bibliography

Eckle N, Haley K, Baker P: *ENPC provider manual,* ed 2, Chicago, 2000, Emergency Nurses Association, 207-222.

Herndon D: *Total burn care,* ed 2, London, 2002, WB Saunders.

Jacobs B, Hoyt K: *Trauma nursing core course instructor supplement,* ed 5, Chicago, 2000, Emergency Nurses Association, 117-131.

Jacobs B, Hoyt K: *Trauma nursing core course provider manual,* ed 5, Chicago, 2000, Emergency Nurses Association, 207-232.

Knipe CJ: Burns. In Lewis SM, Heitkemper MM, Dirksen SR, editors: *Dirksen's medical-surgical nursing,* ed 6, St Louis, 2004, Mosby.

McSwain N, Frame S, Paturas J: *PHTLS basic and advanced prehospital trauma life support,* ed 5, St Louis, 1999, Mosby, 248-263.

Newberry L, Sheehy S: *Budassi: Emergency nursing principles and practice,* Chicago, 1998, Emergency Nurses Association, 359-372.

Woods W, Young J, Just J: *Emergency medicine recall,* Philadelphia, 2000, Lippincott Williams & Wilkins, 484-491.

Chapter 44

Amputations

Mary E. Fecht Gramley

1. List some of the mechanisms of injury that may result in an amputation.

- Guillotine: clean cut that penetrates the full depth of tissue (e.g., knife)
- Crushing: intense internal pressure (e.g., finger in a drill press)
- Blast, traumatic: a body part is literally "blown away," shattered (e.g., firecracker)

2. What is the difference between a partial and a complete amputation?

In a partial amputation, the limb or part remains partially attached to the stump. This may involve skin only, muscle, or other connective tissues. In a complete amputation, the limb or part is completely severed from the stump.

3. Are all amputations categorized as emergent?

Those that meet the following criteria are emergent:

- Amputations associated with multiple traumatic injuries
- Patient is hemodynamically unstable
- Amputations proximal to the wrist or ankle

4. What are the nursing care priorities for the patient presenting with an amputation?

- Airway, breathing, circulation (ABCs).
- Start an intravenous (IV) line.
- One IV line if the amputation is an isolated injury.
- At least two large-bore (14G or 16G catheters) if the amputation is associated with multiple injuries.
- Assess neurologic status.
- Assess and relieve pain (by IV medications or nerve block).
- Wound care.
- Additional medications, usually an antibiotic and/or dT booster.

5. List examples that would signal a patient is hemodynamically unstable.

- Sustained hypotension in the field, or a blood pressure less than 90 systolic (80 systolic for pediatrics), on two consecutive measurements 5 minutes apart

- Blunt/penetrating trauma with hemodynamic compromise as evidenced by unstable vital signs
- Respiratory compromise as evidenced by respiratory rate less than 10 or greater than 29 in the adult
- Altered mentation with a Glasgow Coma Scale less than 10 or associated with focal neurologic signs
- Penetrating injury to the head/neck/torso/groin
- Limb paralysis and/or sensory deficit above wrist or ankle
- Two or more proximal long bone fractures
- Trauma victims with significant mechanism of injury: e.g., explosion, motor vehicle crash, fire exposure, or combined with greater than 20% total body surface area (TBSA) burn
- Two or more body regions with potential life or limb threat

6. How should I prioritize a patient who is hemodynamically unstable?

Then the principle is life before limb, and the amputation treatment is secondary.

7. What triage category is a patient with an amputation and hemodynamically unstable?

A hemodynamically unstable patient would be considered a category I in a three-level triage system or five-tier triage system, e.g., emergent, life-threatening, or red.

8. Is it appropriate to use a tourniquet on a stump after an amputation?

It is not recommended to use a tourniquet to control bleeding on an amputation because of the potential for damage to the tissue, which can compromise the possibility of replantation.

9. What should I use?

Pressure dressings and elevation. If bleeding is not controlled, use additional dressings without removing the original dressings. If this is not effective, an artery (arteries) may need clamping to prevent exsanguination.

10. Is there never a time to use a tourniquet?

The only time a tourniquet is recommended is if:

- Transport of the victim to a definitive treatment center is delayed.
- Bleeding to prevent exsanguination cannot be controlled by any other means.

11. Tell me the triage category if the patient with an amputation is hemodynamically stable.

The patient is considered urgent (as soon as possible). The goal is to preserve the limb/part and function of that limb/part. This is a patient who should not wait as a result of pain, anxiety, and potential for deterioration.

In a three-level triage system, this patient would be categorized as a Category II patient (yellow) or urgent. In a five-tier system, this patient would be categorized as a Category II also.

12. Name some treatment differences for an isolated amputation injury, compared to one with multiple injuries.

- The focus is on the attempt at replantation or repair of the stump.
- X-rays of both the amputated part and the stump are taken to determine the degree of injury.
- Referral(s) are made.

13. What solution should I use to cleanse the wound?

Normal saline (NS), 0.9% saline. Some texts also suggest using Lactated Ringer's solution. Do not use tap water or distilled water, as they may damage or macerate the skin and compromise the attempt at replantation.

14. How do I care for the stump?

Rinse the stump with 0.9% NS solution to remove gross contamination, apply a pressure dressing, splint, and elevate.

15. How do I care for the amputated part?

- Rinse the amputated part in 0.9% NS solution to remove gross contamination.
- Wrap the part in gauze sponges moistened with 0.9% NS solution.
- Store it in a plastic bag, keeping the part in a position of function if possible, and seal.
- Place the plastic bag in a container and label it.
- Put the container on top of crushed ice and water. This allows cooling of the tissue, but prevents the freezing and maceration that would occur if the part were placed directly in water or on ice.

16. Should I apply antibiotic ointment to prevent infection?

No, medications may damage the tissue and preclude the attempt at replantation.

17. How do I handle a tissue bridge?

Leave it in place and splint the entire extremity to help preserve tissue until evaluated by the physician.

18. Explain how it is decided which referral services are needed.

The principle is that anything proximal to the fingers and toes require orthopedic surgeon for bone stabilization. However, orthopedic services need vascular services to reattach vessels and perhaps plastic services to reattach nerves.

Therefore anything beyond fingers and toes needs a multidisciplinary approach.

19. Is the correct term replantation or reimplantation?

As one prominent orthopedic surgeon once said, "If you rip a plant out of the ground and wish to replace it, you replant it." An implant is something that is put into place that is not part of the original structure. Reimplant implies that you removed an implant and then replaced it. However, you will hear the two words used interchangeably by health care professionals.

20. List factors related to the patient that affect treatment outcomes.

- Age (>50 years)
- Current patient stability/instability
- Co-morbidity (diabetes mellitus, peripheral vascular disease, bleeding disorders, cardiorespiratory diseases)
- Smoker (vasoconstriction)
- Motivation and ability to participate in rehabilitation

21. The patient asked me if the body part would be the same after reimplantation.

The replanted part will not look exactly like the same, and function may not return.

22. Name wound/amputation characteristics that will affect the outcome.

- *Type of wound.* Guillotine is most amenable for reattachment and its vasospasm restricts blood loss.
- *Length of time that the part is ischemic.* Replantation can be considered up to 6 hours if the limb is not cooled (called warm ischemia time): 18 hours if cooled.
- *Location.* Upper extremities are more successful in replantation than lower extremities.
- *Avulsion.* In an avulsion wound, it is difficult to locate all tissues necessary to reconnect, control bleeding, and restore function.
- Wound contamination
- Previous injury to the affected part or limb
- Availability of an experienced replantation team

23. How can the frequency of amputation injury be decreased?

Injury prevention is the key! Organizations/programs involved with safety initiatives include (also see box, below):

- The American Trauma Society (Traumaroo).
- Pediatric Advanced Life Support Course, American Heart Association (PALS)
- Emergency Nursing Pediatric Course, Emergency Nurses Association (ENPC)
- Emergency Nurses Cancel Alcohol Related Emergencies, Emergency Nurses Association (ENCARE)

- Safe Kids
- Occupational Health and Safety Agency of the Federal Government (OSHA)

Related Organizations

American Academy of Pediatrics (AAP)
P.O. Box 927
Elk Grove Village, IL 60009-0927
www.aap.org
800-433-9016

American Association for the Surgery of Trauma
www.aast.org

American College of Surgeons (ACS)
Trauma Department
633 N. St. Clair St.
Chicago, IL 60611-3211
312-202-5005
www.facs.org

American Trauma Society
8903 Presidential Parkway
Suite 512
Upper Marlboro, MD 20772
800-556-7890
www.amtrauma.org

Center for Injury Prevention and Control (CIPC)
CDC
4770 Buford Highway NE, MS K-65
Atlanta, GA 30341-3724
www.cdc.gov/ncipchm.htm

Children's Safety Network
National Injury and Violence Prevention Resource Center
Education Development Center
55 Chapel Street
Newton, MA 02158-1060
617-969-7100
www.edc.org

Consumer Product Safety Commission
Washington, DC 20207
800-638-2772
www.cpsc.gov

Emergency Medical Services for Children (EMSC-C)
National Resource Center
Children's Hospital
111 Michigan Avenue NW
Washington, DC 20010-2970
202-884-4927
info@emscnrc.com

Harborview Injury Prevention and Research Center
325 Ninth Avenue
Box 359960
Seattle, WA 98104-2499
206-521-1520
http://weber.u.washington.edu/~hiprc

Harvard Injury Control Center
Harvard School of Public Health
677 Huntington Ave.
Boston, MA 02115
617-432-1090

Injury Control and Research Center
University of Alabama at Birmingham
CH-19, Suite 403, UAB Station
Birmingham, AL 35294
205-934-1448
www.uab.edu/icrc/icrc/htm

Injury Control Research Centers (ICRC)
Colorado State University
Dept. of Environmental Health
Fort Collins, CO 80523-1676
970-491-6156
www.colstate.edu/orgs/cicrc

Injury Prevention and Research Center
University of North Carolina
204 Chase Hall, CB 7505
Chapel Hill, NC 27599-7505
919-966-2251
iprc@unc.edu

Insurance Institute for Highway Safety
1005 North Glebe Rd.
Arlington, VA 22201
703-247-1678
www.hwysafety.org

Iowa Prevention and Research Center
University of Iowa
100 Oakdale Campus, IREH
Iowa City, IA 52242-5000
319-335-4458
www.info.pmeh.uiowa.edu/iprc/iprc.htm

The Johns Hopkins Center for Injury Research & Policy
624 N. Broadway, 5th floor
Baltimore, MD 21205
410-614-4025
www.sph.jhu.edu/Research/Centers/CIRP/

(NHTSA) National Highway Transportation Safety Administration
400 7th St. SW
Washington, DC 20004
www.nhtsa.dot.org

National Safe Kids Campaign
1301 Pennsylvania Ave.
Washington, DC 20004
202-662-0600
www.safekids.org

Rural Injury Resource Center
National Farm Medicine Center
1000 North Oak Ave.
Marshfield, WI 54449
800-662-6900
www.marshmed.org/nfmc/

The San Francisco Injury Center
San Francisco General Hospital
Ward 3A
1001 Potrero Ave.
San Francisco, CA 94110
415-206-4623
itsa.ucsf.edu/~sfic/INDEX.html

Southern California Injury Prevention Research Center
UCLA School of Public Health
10833 Le Conte Ave.
Los Angeles, CA 90095-1772
310-206-4115
http://www.ph.ucla.edu/sciprc/

Think First Foundation
22 S. Washington St.
Park Ridge, IL 60068
847-692-2740
www.thinkfirst.org

Trauma Foundation
San Francisco General Hospital
Bldg. 1, Rm. 300
San Francisco, CA 94110
www.trmafdn.org

University of Pittsburgh
230 McKee Pl, Suite 400
Pittsburgh, PA 15213
412-647-1110
www.pitt.edu/~icrin/

Key Points

- Use 0.9% NS to irrigate the wound, stump, and amputated part.
- Guillotine-type lacerations through a severed part or limb are more likely to be successfully replanted than are jagged lacerations or crush injuries.
- Upper extremity amputations are more successfully replanted than those of the lower extremities.
- The replanted part will not appear exactly as it was before the amputation and may not have normal function.

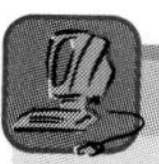

Internet Resources

National Injury and Violence Prevention Resource Center
www.edc.org

Emergency Medical Services for Children
info@emscnrc.com

Injury Prevention and Research Center
iprc@unc.edu

Think First Foundation
www.thinkfirst.org

Bibliography

American College of Surgeons, Committee on Trauma: *Resources for optimal care of the injured patient,* Chicago, 1999, American College of Surgeons, Committee on Trauma; available: www.facs.org/dept/trauma.

Gilboy N, et al: *Emergency severity index (ESI),* Des Plaines, Ill, 2003, Emergency Nurses Association, 12-19, 23, 29-33.

Jacobs BB, Hoyt KS, editors: *Trauma nursing core course,* ed 5, Des Plaines, Ill, 2000, Emergency Nurses Association, 195-196, 204.

Jordan KS, editor: *Emergency nursing core curriculum,* ed 5, Philadelphia, 2000, WB Saunders, 525-528.

Killian M, editor: *Standards of emergency nursing practice,* ed 4, Des Plaines, Ill, 1999, Emergency Nurses Association, 10-11, 23-29, 43-45.

Newberry L: *Sheehy's emergency nursing principles and practice,* St Louis, 2003, Mosby, 322-323.

Selfridge-Thomas J: *Emergency nursing: An essential guide for patient care,* Philadelphia, 1997, WB Saunders, 152.

Chapter 45

Minor Motor Vehicle Crashes

Robert D. Herr

1. Why are they called crashes instead of accidents?

Motor vehicle crashes are no longer considered accidents based on the premise that they are avoidable. Nonetheless, crashes are the leading cause of major trauma in the U.S., causing over 40,000 deaths and up to 1 million injuries each year.

Death and injury have decreased markedly over the past decade as a result of mandatory seatbelt and helmet laws in many states, better attention to rollover accidents, and use of airbags.

I'll never forget my first patient who'd survived a crash as a result of an airbag. In 1988, a young man walked in after driving his sports car at 50 miles per hour into a bridge abutment in a fit of rage. The airbag deployed and he was able to walk away. I could not believe he survived; the police confirmed the car had been totaled.

2. Does the information in this chapter apply to all vehicles?

No, it applies mainly to cars. Accidents in buses, trucks, farm vehicles, and others are beyond the scope of this chapter.

3. What do I consider at triage for the patient who's been in a motor vehicle crash?

The airway, breathing, circulation (ABCs) apply just as much at the triage desk as for the patient brought by emergency medical service (EMS) on a backboard with cervical collar. One recent "walk-in" was an older adult woman complaining of rib pain from a fall inside a motor home when her impatient husband stepped on the gas. She fell against a table in the motor home. At triage she became short of breath and had subcutaneous emphysema from a tension pneumothorax. By the time her husband had parked the motor home and found her in the emergency department (ED), she'd had chest tube placement and was being admitted.

4. How can I get "burned" or embarrassed by mistriage?

Not all crashes cause blunt trauma. The patient who cannot recall the crash most likely has mild retrograde amnesia. However, suspect syncope prior to the crash from hypoglycemia, seizure, or another cause.

5. What about the crash do I need to note and how is it important?

The following are associated with severe trauma—these are the same criteria EMS uses for immediate transport to a trauma center. Such patients are highest level triage:

- Death of an occupant
- Prolonged extrication
- Thrown from vehicle
- Auto-pedestrian accident
- Fall more than 30 feet

Additional factors to consider:

- Lap belts can still be associated with severe injury if they are loose, worn incorrectly, or the occupant is undersized for the lap belt.
- Airbag deployment in crashes involving undersized individuals including children can cause closed head injury and c-spine injury from sudden impact to head or neck.
- Starred windshield: suggests closed head injury, cervical spine trauma.
- Driver of a vehicle with a bent steering wheel: suggests chest injury with possible cardiac contusion.
- Lap belt without other restraints: evaluate for tears to large bowel w/signs of peritonitis
- Airbag deployed without seatbelt use: occupant can be thrown from vehicle or moved away from deployed airbag, resulting in a loss of airbag effectiveness.

Position of injured occupant with respect to impact:

- Driver injured in driver side impact: consider injury to spleen and closed head injury.
- Passenger injured with passenger side impact: consider injury to liver and closed head injury.
- Rear impact: injury to lumbar spine, more likely if seat collapsed backward or extensive damage to rear compartment or trunk.
- Frontal impact: injury to cervical spine.
- Rollover: suspect head or neck injury from downward impact to head.

6. If the crash happened a day or two ago, doesn't it change the triage to a minor?

The patient survived the crash but could, nevertheless, have injury threatening to life and limb. There are commonly cases of unstable cervical spine fractures and splenic ruptures among walk-ins. The prudent course is to consider all trauma to be potentially life-threatening and triage accordingly.

7. Why apply a cervical collar when the patient's been walking around for days post-trauma without one?

The reasons are medical, legal, and functional. From a medical standpoint the patient is about to undergo a neurologic and orthopedic examination that could apply stress to the c-spine unless it is immobilized. The collar also signals to the radiology tech that a complete cervical series is needed.

Legally any decline in neurologic function is your responsibility from the point of triage onward. Functionally a collar tells the patient not to stress the neck further.

8. Which type of motor vehicle crash (MVC) is the highest risk for neck trauma?

The highest risk accidents are rollovers. In a rollover, the head can impact the car roof with compressive forces shattering the upper c-spine. However, front- or side-impact collisions can create forces that cause flexion, rotation, bending, or any combination that can sprain neck ligaments.

9. How do I approach stiff or sore neck from trauma?

Stiff or sore neck is discussed in Chapter 23. The standard of care is to immobilize the patient's neck until the physician can evaluate the c-spine. Proper immobilization takes three elements:

- Backboard
- Properly fitted cervical collar
- Sandbags or intravenous (IV) fluid bags placed with tape to prevent head and neck movement.

10. But isn't the physician just going to clear the c-spine without radiographs?

Outcomes of studies suggest that certain patients with isolated head or neck trauma and normal exam are candidates for clinical clearance without radiographs. These patients are less than half of all victims of trauma.

11. Can a triage nurse clinically clear a c-spine?

This would be established with the ED physicians and hospital policy. However, the procedure is now an acceptable, widely used method by both nursing and prehospital paramedics, to safely reduce unneeded c-spine radiographs and get patients up off backboards faster, especially in low-risk situations. Departments with this procedure indicate it is also useful in determining when not to put on a c-collar for an ambulatory patient with neck complaints.

12. What are the components of the procedure for nursing to clear a c-spine?

The adult patient, must be English-speaking, alert and oriented, have no history of loss of consciousness, not be impaired (e.g., drunk, drugs), and deny any cervical or other severe painful injuries. The patient is physically and systematically assessed for cervical tenderness or deformity, neurologic intactness, and active range of motion.

The department must implement adequate staff instruction, with an emphasis on consistency and thoroughness, and competency documentation. Many departments that have had a nurse clearing protocol for years report no negative outcomes.

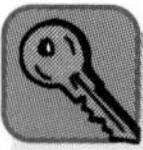

Key Points

- Minor MVC is not one injury but a spectrum of injury.
- Question witnesses and the victim for circumstances of the crash immediately.
- Look for key crash factors suggesting severe injury and communicate to the treating physician immediately.
- Identify mechanism of injury from victim's position and direction of vehicle impact.

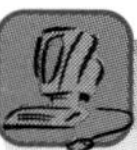

Internet Resources

National Highway Travel Safety Association
United States Department of Transportation
http://www.nhtsa.dot.gov

Bibliography

Bazarian JJ, Fisher SG, Flesher W, et al: Lateral automobile impacts and the risk of traumatic brain injury, *Ann Emerg Med* 44:2:142-152, 2004.

Cornwell EE: Initial approach to trauma. In Tintinalli JE, Kelen GD, Stapczynski JS, editors: *Emergency medicine,* ed 5, New York, 2000, McGraw-Hill, 1609.

Runge JW, Kanianthra JN: Risk analysis in road traffic injury research, *Ann Emerg Med* 44(2):153-154, 2004.

Section VII

Balance Alterations

Chapter 46

Falls in the Older Adult Population

Robert D. Herr

1. Why is there a chapter on this subject?

In the older adult, falls are the most common form of accidental injury and cause of death. It is the most frequent emergency department (ED) complaint for the older adult (although chest pain is the most common diagnosis). In the U.S. alone there are over a half million hospital admits each year from falls in the older adult.

2. What are the major causes of falls in the older adult?

Major causes are age-related changes in balance senses, chronic illness, medication, and environmental factors. Balance senses include changes in vision, hearing, and sensation in upper and lower extremities.

3. Discuss aging factors.

Normal aging includes reduced visual acuity, contrast sensitivity, dark adaptation, and peripheral vision. Cataracts, diabetic retinopathy, and not using prescribed corrective lenses may contribute. Hearing diminishes too, as do the warning signs of impending collision.

Other balance senses that diminish with age are proprioception, vestibular system, and hearing. Proprioception may further decrease with peripheral neuropathy from diabetes or degenerative central nervous system (CNS) disease. Vestibular dysfunction contributes to unsteadiness, disequilibrium, and vertigo. See Chapter 47 for further discussion.

4. Talk about causes from chronic illness.

Chronic illness leads to falls when it causes neuropathy (diabetes, renal failure, degenerative CNS conditions), visual impairment (diabetes, hypertensive retinopathy, macular degeneration), or muscle weakness. Muscle weakness accompanies many conditions and combined with reduced reflexes makes it hard for the patient to right himself or herself quickly. Even chronic foot disorders such as bunion or blister makes proper shoes tough to wear and prone to tip.

Acute illness can also be a cause if it results in dehydration from vomiting, diarrhea, or poor oral intake. The last fall patient I treated had a fever with delirium from urosepsis.

5. Explain medications as a cause for falls.

Medication-induced falls occur from direct sedative effects of benzodiazepines and other anxiolytics and muscle relaxants. Drug metabolism slows with age so low doses of these meds, especially when taken daily, can result in sustained high brain levels and impair balance.

6. Elaborate on home hazards.

Home hazards include uneven surfaces especially throw rugs, raised thresholds, small pets, and young children. Normal lighting may be inadequate to overcome age-related decrease in contrast (three times more light is needed with aging).

Stairs and transfers are major challenges. Most falls result while using stairs (descending mostly) and performing daily activities with standing, walking, and changing position.

7. How do I recognize patients who have had a fall?

Many older adult patients with history of a fall come in by ambulance. Of course, the nonverbal patient may not provide such a history. Even the verbal patient may not recall a fall as a result of syncope, dementia, or amnesia.

Key signs of a fall occurring are any patients "found down" or who were on the floor at any time. Anyone found at the bottom of stairs should be considered to have fallen down the entire staircase until proved otherwise. C-spine immobilization and backboard should be considered.

8. Are there any special concerns regarding the use of backboards with the older adult?

Merely 80 minutes on a backboard can cause a pressure ulcer in the older adult. One study found that the average time patients were left immobilized on a backboard was 54 minutes if there were no x-rays taken and 181 minutes if x-rays were taken. Early c-spine clearance should be a priority.

9. What is one of the most important aspects in the triage of a patient with a fall?

A key determination is whether the fall involved a systemic illness or is associated with an environmental factor alone. If the patient gives a history of tripping or falling he/she can be triaged without special concern for underlying illness. The patient who "fainted," became weak, dizzy, or lightheaded, or can't remember falling needs evaluation for underlying medical condition.

Such patients can benefit from cardiac monitoring, orthostatic pulse and blood pressure, blood draw (complete blood cell count [CBC], electrolytes, and medication levels, if appropriate) and an IV for medication access and potential intravenous (IV) fluid infusion. Refer to Chapters 47 and 48 for further discussion.

10. Discuss the assessment related to a patient who had a fall.

The skin and face exam should look for any signs of edema or bruising and an extremity exam should look for angulation and deformity. Bones break more easily because the bone mass diminishes with age.

Pain also diminishes with age, and even the alert patient may say it's only a bruise when in fact there is significant internal injury. Therefore in the older adult fall patient it's better to use radiography more generously than in younger fall patients.

11. Talk about the triage for a fall on a patient who has a coagulopathy.

Occasionally the patient with hemophilia will come in after a fall. More often the older adult patients who have a coagulopathy are taking anticoagulants, such as warfarin (Coumadin) or enoxaparin (Lovenox). Aspirin alone will not result in coagulopathy.

They might also have a medical condition that impairs liver-produced coagulation proteins. These conditions include liver cirrhosis, cancer metastatic to the liver, toxic liver insult, or alcoholism.

Consider the following actions for all of these patients:

- Maintain a high suspicion for bleeding throughout. The older adult brain (especially if there is a history of alcoholism) has some atrophy and may show delayed signs.
- Draw blood and send for prothrombin time/international normalized ratio (PT/INR) and/or partial thromboplastin time (PTT).
- Obtain a urine specimen as occult blood in the urinalysis implicates kidney injury.
- Any anticoagulated patient who had a head injury should have a head computed tomography (CT) to look for intracranial bleed.
- Any major fall should have CT abdomen and pelvis looking for intraabdominal bleeding.
- Any fall against the flank or side or back should have exam and CT to look for retroperitoneal bleeding.

12. Explain how to handle a patient who presents with an unsteady gait.

A patient with an unsteady gait might be evident as the person walks in. However, sometimes this type of patient presents in a wheelchair. Watch a patient in a wheelchair walk before he or she leaves if the individual indicates that walking is the normal capability.

The key question is establishing if the gait imbalance is chronic or acute. Usually the chronically gait impaired person has a cane, walker, or wheelchair. Ask to see it and look to see if it shows signs of heavy use and personalization by the patient.

13. What if the unsteady gait is new for this patient?

If the unsteadiness is new, then it's important to establish the cause. Anybody suspected of a new stroke, or anyone with signs of systemic illness, are placed in a medical bed on a monitor. The reason for this is that stroke and myocardial infarction (MI) occur together one fifth of the time.

Further questions to ask include if the patient has any new medications, medical conditions, weakness, speech difficulty, or change in responsiveness or orientation.

14. Can you ever place a patient with a new unsteady gait in a low-acuity room?

The only individual who can safely go to a low-acuity setting is someone with an identifiable low-acuity problem causing gait trouble. Many of these problems concern the feet such as new ulcers, corns, bunions, or foreign body in the shoe. Therefore make sure you remove the shoes and socks at triage to look for the obvious.

A more memorable patient with gait trouble that I treated had arrived in police custody. He was limping after he ran from police and hid behind a dumpster for a half hour in stocking feet before giving himself up. Unfortunately for him, the temperature was 14°F (−10°C) outside. When we removed the socks we saw that the gait problem came from frostbitten soles of the feet.

15. How do I handle a patient with a complaint of numbness in an extremity?

New numbness can result from vascular, neurologic, or even a psychogenic cause.

16. How would I know if it was a vascular or neurologic cause?

Vascular causes usually involve ischemic extremity. Look for a limb that is pale, pulseless, and painful compared to the other limb.

Neurologic causes are most commonly a pinched nerve in the lumbar spine and peripheral neuropathy. Look for pinched nerve—so called *sciatica*—as numbness of any side or top of a foot. The lateral foot is the S1 nerve root, the medial is L4, and the dorsal foot is L5. Numbness is typically experienced as dullness to pinprick (I used a broken tongue blade to test sensation discrimination between dull/sharp).

Peripheral neuropathy usually comes on slowly in someone with diabetes or renal failure. However, there are rare demyelinating neuropathies, such as Guillain-Barré Syndrome, that begin as numbness in both feet with weakness of calves that progresses upward.

17. When do I consider abuse or neglect?

Key signs of abuse are a history of unexplained "fall" in the presence of a caregiver, bad interaction among the patient and a caregiver, repeated "accidents," or suspicious bruising in the shape of a fist or object of assault. Because abuse is embarrassing and threatening to both abuser and victim, the skillful triage nurse tactfully and quickly considers whether the history of the fall sounds plausible and whether the injuries match the story. Sometimes the first response to the question "What happened?" is the best time to determine how valid the explanation sounds.

Some key tips to elder abuse:

- Signs of restraints such as wrist or ankle welts or bruising
- Circular burns from cigarettes
- Recent hair loss
- Scratches or bite marks
- Nail or hand contusions from defensive posture
- Black eye
- The patient may be teary-eyed and withdrawn especially around abuser.
- The abuser may decline to leave the bedside of the victim or to allow the patient to speak to the nurse privately, decline to call EMS or take the patient to the ED, or sustain bite marks or scratches because of the older adult fighting back.

Key signs of neglect are delayed presentation after a fall when a caregiver was present and able to respond. Such patients can sustain pressure sores, dehydration, hypothermia, and rhabdomyolysis from even a few hours on a floor.

Key Points

- Falls are common in the older adult.
- Look for drug related and other medical causes by careful attention to whether the patient may have fainted or felt dizzy before falling.
- The anticoagulated patient could have internal bleeding from a fall.
- Check tetanus and give a dT if its been ten years since the last one.
- Consider abuse if the story seems suspicious or injuries don't seem to match the story.

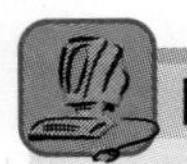

Internet Resources

MedlinePlus Health Topics: Elder Abuse
http://www.nlm.nih.gov/medlineplus/elderabuse.html

The Older Adult Place: Elder Abuse
www.older adultplace.com/abuse/index.shtml

Bibliography

Woolard RH, Becker B, Haronian TJ: Geriatric considerations. In Harwood-Nuss A, editor. *Clinical practice of emergency medicine,* ed 3, Philadelphia, 2001, Lippincott, Williams & Wilkins, 1769-1775.

Chapter 47

Dizziness, Vertigo, and Weakness

Robert D. Herr

1. What is dizziness?

Dizziness is a general term that has many meanings to the individual. Most people use it to describe the inability to orient themselves in their environment. They will feel "faint," as if they are about to pass out, especially when standing or walking. Other descriptions for dizziness are lightheadedness, giddiness, floating, swimming, unsteadiness, or ill-defined disequilibrium.

Some people ascribe the term dizziness to falling, unsteadiness, or limb weakness in an individual who has no head sensation. Such a person is not truly dizzy, but they may have a new sensory loss such as vision or proprioception. Their evaluation requires a separate approach.

2. Compare dizziness to vertigo.

True vertigo is a term used to describe the sensation of movement. Patients with vertigo feel as if either they, or the room they are in, is spinning. Other common terms include whirling, rocking, or tilting.

This symptom is often made worse by position changes, particularly moving or turning the head. Nausea, vomiting, diaphoresis, and abdominal cramping are common associated symptoms.

3. What are the causes of vertigo?

A key distinction is if the vertigo has central causes (cerebellar, hemorrhage, infarction) compared to a peripheral cause (such as otitis media). Assess the patient for nystagmus. If nystagmus is not observed at rest, perform the Nylen-Barany test.

Central causes are more likely to result in continuous nystagmus. There will be no latency period with a lateral gaze; it will be multidirectional or only present in one eye. Peripheral causes are accompanied by a nystagmus that is typically horizontal or rotary, never vertical, and in both eyes. When asked to look laterally, there is a generally a brief period before the nystagmus occurs and the nystagmus is suppressed by visual fixation.

4. Describe the Nylen-Barany test.

The patient is brought from sitting to lying with the head slightly off the top of the gurney and turned to one side. Then look at the patient's eyes for nystagmus, or quick saccades to one side and slow movement back. The patient with central nervous system (CNS) dizziness has immediate onset of dizziness, and vertical nystagmus. Repeat the maneuver, and turn the head the opposite way. When you repeat the maneuver, the patient feels no better and nystagmus recurs.

A reassuring result is when the patient feels better on repeat of the test or has horizontal or rotary nystagmus. These patients have a so-called vestibular dizziness that is, fortunately, the most common cause.

5. How do these differ from syncope?

Syncope is an abrupt onset of a true loss of consciousness in which period of time cannot be recalled. Recovery is usually rapid, compared with recovery from a seizure.

For this, the single most important historical clue is the patient's recollection of what happened just prior to the event. Cardiac will happen without warning or effort; vasovagal has premonitory symptoms of dizziness, yawning, nausea, and diaphoresis. See Chapter 48 for further discussion.

6. What are specific questions I should ask any patient presenting with "dizziness"?

Besides the routine triage history questions, additional helpful information may be elicited from asking about:

- Onset (new, with position change)
- Ear complaints
- Last time the person ate/what they ate
- Any history or signs/symptoms to indicate dehydration
- New medications (including over-the-counter [OTC])
- Alcohol intake
- Any signs/symptoms to indicate anemia

7. How do I detect the acutely life-threatening causes of dizziness or vertigo?

Dizziness is uncommonly life threatening, but key causes that are serious are cardiovascular, CNS, and metabolic causes. More concern is warranted with older adult patients, because they more frequently have a serious cause for their dizziness.

8. Talk about cardiovascular causes and the triage response.

With a presenting complaint of lightheadedness, the triage nurse should ask about palpitations and assess blood pressure and pulse with orthostatic changes. Ask the patient what they were doing when they noted the onset. The vertebral artery can be narrowed and cause dizziness when the head is extended, typically when the patient looks up into a cabinet over the refrigerator.

A "dizzy" patient with palpitations, arrhythmias, or a cardiac history should have electrocardiogram (ECG). Older adult patients, particularly if they have diabetes, can have a "silent" myocardial infarction (MI) as a result of neuropathy.

9. Discuss CNS causes and the related triage assessment.

CNS causes include stroke, brain tumor, and hydrocephalus. The triage nurse should look for level of alertness and any neurologic deficits. Lesions of cranial nerves are called neighborhood signs because they are close to the balance and dizziness centers (CN VIII). Such patients may have double vision or be unable to track a finger moved in front of their face (CN III, IV, and VI).

10. Discuss medications that might cause dizziness.

Medications more likely to cause a problem are antihypertensives (beta-blockers, calcium channel blockers), aminoglycosides, anticonvulsants, tranquilizers, and vasodilators.

11. Elaborate on metabolic causes and the triage actions.

Metabolic causes are mostly drug-induced, but can be blood sugar or electrolyte abnormalities. Check for blood sugar in diabetics and new medications and OTC drugs that can cause sedation.

12. What orders should I anticipate for suspected central causes?

These patients usually need immediate head computed tomography (CT) and referral to neurology or neurosurgery depending on what is found. Make them at least an urgent category in triage.

13. How are peripheral or vestibular causes of dizziness treated?

These patients need symptomatic therapy with antinausea agents and a vestibular suppressant such as meclizine (Antivert) or diazepam (Valium). Intravenous (IV) diazepam 1 to 2 mg can quickly reduce disturbing vertigo while evaluation continues. The dose can be repeated every 30 minutes until dizziness improves or the patient becomes sedated. These patients usually improve with time and are safely discharged with meclizine and ear, nose, and throat specialist (ENT) follow-up if not better.

14. Should I anticipate admission for all older adult patients who fell at home?

Simply falling is not a reason to admit a patient, but a period of observation is warranted if the patient has no caregiver until the patient can walk with a walker and safely transfer. In some cases an evaluation for a long-term care setting is needed.

15. How should I treat other types of dizziness such as ill-defined lightheadedness or loss of balance?

These are the toughest conditions because the cause is unknown, so treatment is symptomatic although leaving open the chance that a specific cause will declare itself. As above, the patient who is unable to safely walk or sit should have a home caregiver. If not, a period of observation is appropriate with repeat neurologic examination. Long-term care may be needed.

16. What causes weakness?

Weakness has many causes, but the serious ones are those that progress unless treated. They include:

- Cardiovascular causes, such as MI or volume depletion
- Infectious causes, such as sepsis
- Renal causes, such as acute or chronic renal failure
- Liver failure, as a result of overwhelming hepatic necrosis
- Neurologic causes, such as stroke, demyelinating neuropathy, or simple deconditioning

17. So what is the most prevailing cause of weakness in the older adult?

Deconditioning: the "use it or lose it" aspect to strength that the geriatrician is well aware of. Older adult patients who do not walk for even just a few days become weak. This weakness is self-perpetuating. Bed-ridden older adults have a high mortality rate.

18. How do I detect the acutely life-threatening causes of weakness?

Generally a history of chronic disease, acute insult, deconditioning, or new medication can detect serious causes. A complete blood cell count (CBC), urinalysis (UA), and basic chemistry screen may augment the evaluation, with ECG in the patient over 50 years.

Key Points

- When a patient complains of lightheadedness or dizziness, check level of consciousness (LOC), orthostatic vital signs, presence of palpitations/arrhythmia, blood glucose, and an electrocardiogram (ECG) if older than 50 years of age.
- Vertigo is differentiated from dizziness by the presence of the sensation of movement.

Internet Resource

Treatment for Positional Vertigo:
http://www.emedhome.com/resources/pdfdatabase/63.pdf

Bibliography

Eggers SD, Zee DS: Evaluating the dizzy patient: Bedside examination and laboratory assessment of the vestibular system, *Semin Neurol* 23(1):47-58, 2003.

Hotson JR, Baloh RW: Current concepts: Acute vestibular syndrome, *N Engl J Med* 339:680-685, 1998.

Chapter 48

Syncope

Robert D. Herr

1. What is syncope?

Syncope is a faint or loss of consciousness (LOC) with loss of postural control without an obvious head trauma or seizure. People may use the term fainting spell, drop attack, falling out, and other vernacular expressions. A key distinction is that syncope requires LOC whereas suddenly feeling faint without LOC is called near-syncope.

Other complaints may describe dizziness such as lightheadedness, giddiness, floating, swimming, unsteadiness, or ill-defined disequilibrium. These sensations are described in Chapter 47.

2. Is all LOC syncope?

No. Consider sleep, which is LOC without syncope. Consider partial complex seizures or temporal lobe epilepsy in which the patient loses consciousness but maintains upright posture. Likewise cataplexy is an uncontrolled fall with full consciousness.

3. What do I ask about?

- First grab any witnesses before they leave. Because the syncopal patient lost track of the event any witness can be a gold-plated gem of information.
- What did the faint look like? Was there a respiratory arrest? Did the patient lose a pulse? Studies show laypeople are poor at finding pulses, so lack of pulse must be interpreted in light of the skill of the examiner. How long was the patient unconscious? Did the patient exhibit seizure-like activity? Was the return of awareness slow with a period of grogginess or confusion? Or was return sudden like the lights coming on in a room? Slow return can mean there was seizure or hypoglycemia. Quick return of awareness is more common in vasovagal syncope unless the patient was kept sitting instead of laid down.
- How many syncopal episodes? Is this one episode or a pattern of several? Any known diagnoses related to past episodes? (The best predictor of current problem is past problems.)
- What symptoms occurred prior to syncope? Ask about nausea, sweating, lightheadedness, racing heart, chest pain, headache, abdominal pain. The first

three are warning or premonitory symptoms of vasovagal syncope (see below) and the duration of symptoms is a predictor of this.
- What position did the patient faint from? Did they arise suddenly to standing? Did they experience emotional upset? Did the patient have a glucose reading performed?

4. What do I ask the patient about current symptoms?

Ask if they feel palpitations, chest pain, nausea, headache, dizziness, or abdominal pain at the present time.

5. What are the key causes of syncope?

The rate of cardiovascular causes increases with age. Studies show cardiac syncope is a better overall predictor of mortality than is noncardiac syncope. The two broad classes are electrical dysfunction—arrhythmia—and mechanical dysfunction from hypertrophic cardiomyopathy or pulmonary hypertension. Electrical dysfunction is mainly arrhythmia in which the heart activity is either too slow such as bradycardia or heart block or not coordinated such as rapid ventricular tachycardia or fibrillation. A fall causes self-cardiovert tachyarrhythmia and the patient may present in sinus rhythm—until the next episode. Mechanical dysfunction includes sudden loss of pump during acute myocardial infarction (MI), cardiac outflow obstruction from asymmetric septal hypertrophy (formerly called IHSS), or valve dysfunction from aortic valve stenosis.

The so-called vasovagal syncope is common in adolescents to older adults. Studies show this may be due to inadequate cardiac response to a fall in blood pressure due to high vagal tone or other causes. Clinicians may use a tilt-table test to identify patients are at risk for repeated vasovagal syncope. The other term is vasodepressor syncope.

Seizure can cause syncope in all ages. One review cites 6% of children under age 15 years have a nonfebrile seizure, many of whom have syncope with them. Seizure in adolescents to adult can be associated with recurrent pattern of epilepsy to single seizure from use of neurostimulant drugs like cocaine to withdrawal of neurodepressor drugs like ethanol or benzodiazepines.

The "other" category of syncope is sudden abdominal bleeding of ectopic pregnancy, subarachnoid hemorrhage with sudden increase in intracranial pressure, and vertebrobasilar (brainstem) ischemia. Transient ischemic attacks (TIAs) and stroke of cerebral hemispheres does not cause syncope but rather focal neurologic deficits.

6. How do I triage the patient with syncope?

Postural hypotension can be detected at triage through examination of symptoms and blood pressure (BP). Recall that the patient with history of hypertension or carotid artery arteriosclerosis can get postural syncope even with a normal blood pressure. The reason is that these patients have carotid arteries that resist blood flow, so higher pressure is needed to perfuse the brain. The key to evaluating is taking the BP supine and upright. If the BP drops 10 points or more with symptoms, you have evaluated the patient as "postural." The postural patient may be unable to stand for long, so just record a BP at whatever upright position the symptoms allow even if it is just sitting up with legs dangling. Normally the pulse increases with postural drop in BP, but this sign is unreliable in those patients taking cardiac medication such as beta blockers or calcium channel blockers.

When orthostasis is new and contributing to syncope, it is normally treated by beginning an intravenous (IV) line and infusing normal saline (NS) or lactated Ringer's solution. In adults the IV should be at least 18-gauge to permit restoration of body fluid deficit within minutes to hours. I have seen adults rehydrated through a 22- or 24-gauge IV but it takes a long time and usually a pressure bag around the IV bag. Whatever pain you save the patient from the smaller stick of a 24-gauge will be inflicted many times over from lying on the hard gurney. If there are ongoing fluid losses from vomiting or bleeding it's even more important to start at least an 18-gauge IV.

The impossible IV stick often has an external jugular vein that the physician can cannulate, perhaps quicker than waiting for "IV therapy" nurse to come to the emergency room (ER) and try a conventional IV. Ask the doctor! Other sites are femoral vein catheters and in children intraosseous infusion.

Because the patient with cardiovascular syncope has early mortality without intervention, the bias is to evaluate for cardiac causes early and often. Consequently the adult patient could be placed on telemetry immediately to assess for arrhythmia. An electrocardiogram (ECG) can yield critical information to the physician so you may want to anticipate what she is looking for:

- Second or third degree heart block
- Bradycardia with pauses
- Normal sinus rhythm with long QT syndrome risks fatal ventricular arrhythmia.
- Normal sinus rhythm with delta wave and shortened PR interval have Wolf-Parkinson-White with recurrent tachycardia.
- Normal sinus rhythm with right bundle branch block and ST elevation in V1-V3 have Brugada syndrome, a dominant genetic condition accountable for one in five deaths in those with structurally normal hearts.

The patient without these ECG symptoms and normal vital signs may still have cardiovascular syncope. For this, the single most important historical clue is the patient's recollection of what happened just prior to the event. Cardiac syncope will happen without warning or effort; vasovagal syncope has premonitory or warning symptoms of dizziness, yawning, nausea, and diaphoresis.

Triage labs are complete blood cell count (CBC), glucose and electrolytes, beta human chorionic gonadotropin (HCG) and drug levels if appropriate.

7. What if no monitored beds are available?

Sudden syncope with no warning needs a monitored bed and telemetry. The only exception who could go to a non-monitored bed is younger (below 50 years) without history of either cardiac problems or seizures whose warning period was at least 20 seconds.

8. Describe how to prevent syncope.

Syncope happens to ER patients and visitors from painful or emotional situations. I've seen patients faint when I injected anesthetic to number a laceration—until I learned to always lie the patient flat before injecting—even before showing them the needle. Likewise the visitor who wants to hold the patients hand during suturing risks fainting, especially if they act tough and really want to see it. "The bigger they are, the harder they fall." Simply having the visitor sit and preferably look away during suturing will save you from having to check in another patient.

The patient who gets lightheaded can prevent syncope from by placing the head between the knees or from lying down with legs elevated.

9. How do I evaluate the patient with seizure?

Besides the routine triage history questions, additional helpful information may be elicited from asking the patient or witnesses about the following:
- Onset (what activity patient was engaged in)
- Preseizure sensations (called aura)
- New medications (including over-the-counter)
- Any stopped medications
- Recreational drugs especially cocaine, methamphetamine
- Alcohol intake

On examination evaluate for head injury, tongue biting, and urinary incontinence that go with seizure. Seizure can also cause shoulder dislocation from strong contraction of muscles or from direct trauma of falling onto the arms.

On laboratory the generalized seizure releases lactic acid. This depresses the serum bicarbonate level for up to a half hour. That is why serum electrolytes (that include bicarbonate) are important to draw at triage if generalized seizure is suspected but not known for sure. The clinician can evaluate bicarbonate level and measure the anion gap. This anion gap is the sodium level minus the sum of bicarbonate plus chloride. A level over 14 is suspicious for acidosis and lactic acid is the most likely culprit.

Key Points

- Syncope is often vasovagal and benign. However, evaluate for cardiovascular causes because these are more serious.
- Warning or premonitory symptoms are nausea, dizziness, lightheadedness, and sweating.
- Sudden syncope without warning is usually cardiovascular or seizure, until proven otherwise. These patients need a monitored bed in the emergency department (ED).
- When a patient complains of syncope, evaluate orthostatic blood pressure and anticipate an order for rehydration if needed. Triage labs include CBC, electrolytes, blood glucose, and an ECG.
- Prevent vasovagal syncope in patients and visitors by shielding them from sudden emotional stimuli or requiring that they lie down or sit down.

Internet Resources

Emedicine.com: Syncope
www.emedicine.com/emerg/topic876.htm

National Institute of Neurological Disorders and Stroke: Syncope Information Page
www.ninds.nih.gov/disorders/syncope/syncope.htm

American Heart Association: Syncope
www.americanheart.org/presenter.jhtml?identifier=4749

Virtual Hospital: Cardiology—Syncope
http://www.vh.org/adult/provider/familymedicine/FPHandbook/Chapter03/06-3.html

Merck Manual of Diagnosis and Therapy: Syncope (Fainting)
http://www.merck.com/mrkshared/mmanual/section16/chapter200/200b.jsp

Bibliography

Goldman JM, Martin TP: Syncope. In Harwood-Nuss A, Wolfson AG, Linden CH, Shepherd SM, Stenklyft PH, editors. *The clinical practice of emergency medicine,* ed 3, Philadelphia, 2001, Lippincott, Williams & Wilkins, 717-720.

Juang JM, Huang SK: Brugada syndrome—an under-recognized electrical disease in patients with sudden cardiac death, *Cardiology* 101(4):157-169, 2004.

Kenney RA: Syncope in the elderly: Diagnosis, evaluation, and treatment, *J Cardiovasc Electrophysiol* 14(9 suppl):S47, 2003.

Section VIII

Environmental

Chapter 49

Bites and Stings

Robert D. Herr

1. Is it typical for patients to not know what bit them?

Yes. The "bright side" is they don't bring any biting animal with them into the emergency department (ED). Some might prefer the patient who captures and kills it, maybe seals it in a clear smell-proof container and presents it in triumph to triage. I prefer the mystery and speculation about whether that red or painful area is a bite and what horrible ugly venomous creature might have done it.

2. Are most unknown bites from spiders?

Spiders get blamed for 80% of unknown bites as a result of their ubiquity, reputation, and the popular press. Studies show spiders actually cause less than 20% of bites, with the rest as a result of mosquitos, midges, ants, and other insects. Sometimes just scratches or other skin irritation mistakenly attributed to a bite. With due respect to shows like "CSI" unless somebody dies or there is an outbreak of similar bites I just don't see the authorities taking the time to investigate what bit them.

3. How should I handle an unknown bite?

Why argue with the patient? Sure, it's a bite. Could happen again; next time catch the critter if you see it. Yes, you might need an exterminator once you find out what to exterminate. Assure them more people die annually in the U.S. from lightning strikes than from spider and snake bite put together. The therapy for the unknown bite is symptomatic.

- Update tetanus status, if needed.
- Look for a stinger (if any) and remove it.
- Cleanse the wound with tap water and soap or antiseptic.
- Dress the wound with antibiotic ointment and a sterile dressing.
- Give instructions to return for signs of infection such as enlarging area of redness, pus, red streak, and more sore instead of less sore.

4. Is spreading redness always a sign of infection?

Spreading red area could represent growing cellulitis. A tick bite from the *Erythema chronicum migrans* of Lyme disease, however, could also cause it. This rash has a central clearing area as the redness spreads outward.

5. How do I handle a bee sting?

Bee and red ant stings cause pain, redness, and swelling that can resemble a cellulitis but is not, so antibiotics are not indicated. However, the patient feels better with an ice pack, elevation, and antihistamine such as diphenhydramine (Benadryl).

6. When is a bite serious?

The U.S. has a temperate climate in which bites by insects—six-legged creatures—are rarely serious. In contrast, bites can be serious when the animal has more than six legs (some arachnids such as the black widow, brown recluse, hobo), four legs (dogs, cats, raccoons, and other wild animals), two legs (human bites), no legs (some snakes), or scorpions. Marine bites are beyond the scope of this discussion, but lionfish are commonly kept in aquariums, and their bite is sometimes fatal.

7. Discuss black widow spider bites.

Black widow bites usually produce a brief pain like a needle stick. The bite may be two small puncture wounds, with a halo of pale skin surrounding the bite. Frequently no bite is visible. Over the next 30 minutes, an aching, burning, and deep pain begins near the bite. Within an hour there may be muscle spasms or cramps. The patient's abdomen or trunk may be rigid with muscle spasm. The key is there is no local tenderness on examination—just diffuse pain and spasm of the abdomen. The patient may writhe to find a comfortable position. He may develop headache, vomiting, and paresthesias. There are no confirmatory lab tests. Symptoms may not peak for 12 to 18 hours and last for days.

Triage treatment should be to get an order for 5 to 10 mL of calcium gluconate. Supplement with pain relievers up to morphine intravenously (IV) and lorazepam for muscle relaxation. The antivenin is made from horse serum. Because horse serum causes serum sickness in some patients the antivenin is reserved for severe pain or dangerous hypertension.

8. Talk about brown recluse spider bites.

The brown recluse has a violin-shaped mark on the dorsum of its cephalothorax. Brown recluse spiders are most common in the Midwest from April to October. As its name implies, this spider is reclusive. Most patients with brown recluse bites contact the spider in a hot dry private place such as in wood piles, closets, attics, and woodsheds. However, the spider is nocturnal when it hunts. Nighttime bites occur when the spider gets trapped in the bedding and bites the sleeper. Many are not aware of the bite when it occurs. Others might feel a pinprick.

The bite mark of the brown recluse shows a purplish center and irregular borders. Over the next 1 to 2 days the center becomes black with necrotic tissue. This necrotic eschar may slough off in 2 to 5 weeks and rarely involves underlying muscle.

At triage it is important to look for systemic effects of the brown recluse toxin. These effects are called loxoscelism after the genus for the brown recluse spider Loxosceles. Such symptoms are fever, nausea, vomiting, myalgias, and weakness.

All patients with systemic symptoms need medical attention urgently. Send a complete blood cell count (CBC) because hemolytic anemia can occur, coagulation measures prothrombin time/partial thromboplastin time (PT/PTT) as a result of blood clotting abnormality, and measure of renal function (blood urea nitrogen [BUN], Creatinine) as a result of renal compromise. The necrotic bite itself may need debridement and frequent outpatient follow-up.

Fortunately most *Loxosceles* species cause local necrotic bites without systemic symptoms, and some species are specific to regions of the U.S. and the world. Examples are the desert recluse of the intermountain region, Arizona recluse, and others.

9. How do I triage snake bite?

Any snake can be provoked to bite, but fortunately most have no venom. Venomous snakes native to the U.S. are the rattlesnake, copperhead, water moccasin, and the coral snake. Overall the chances of getting envenomated from a venomous snake are about 50%. These "dry bites" can be evaluated after an observation period of a few hours with no tissue or systemic injury. Snakes that are pets or kept in zoos are more likely to be exotic species. The victim of these bites requires special antivenin.

The victim of snakebite might feel sudden severe pain at the bite site, with two puncture wounds. The assessment of the affected extremity might also show signs that antivenin is needed. Even the patient who has no swelling or pain should be watched for 6 hours before being released from care.

Any effected extremity local redness or swelling should be immediately marked with a pen and the patient brought back for medical monitoring. Generally the presence of any progressive pain, swelling, or ecchymosis means antivenin is indicated. Triage labs should include CBC, basic chemistries, and coagulation studies (PT, PTT).

10. How do I triage the scorpion sting?

The sting is a small puncture surrounded by redness. There is immediate tingling or burning pain that many generalize into paresthesias. Triage treatment is with wound cleansing, cool compresses, and an order for analgesics. Most stings require no specific therapy beyond that.

It is helpful to identify those stings that cause systemic symptoms that occur only in the *Centruroides* species because these species inject a range of neurotoxins. *Centruroides* scorpions live in Arizona and other states in which it is hot and dry. Look for tachycardia, vomiting, wheezing, and jerking of arms or legs.

Muscle spasm may progress to convulsions, opisthotonic posturing, vision change, nystagmus, and in those under age 3 years, hyperactivity "like a child break-dancing in bed."

There is an antivenin for bites from Centruroides species whose bites cause neurotoxic symptoms or severe prolonged pain.

11. How do I triage the dog and cat bite?

The bite victim should have the wound assessed for any damage to underlying blood vessel, bone, muscle, tendon, and nerve. Bleeding should be controlled with direct pressure and elevation. Radiographs are helpful to rule out a broken tooth in the wound, and tetanus and rabies considered. Specific wound care is addressed in this chapter.

12. How important is the role of cleansing with these bites?

Bites introduce bacterial contamination, so they will all need cleansing. The biggest pitfall in bites is lack of adequate cleansing, which then promotes infection with organisms such as *Staphylococcus*, *Streptococcus*, and *Pasteurella*. Up to 15% of wounds get infected even with great wound care.

13. How should this cleansing be accomplished?

Adequate cleansing critically depends on good irrigation and debridement. Good wound care usually hurts so the skin should be anesthetized prior to cleansing the wound.

First any devitalized or dead tissue will need to be debrided with forceps. The only type of cleansing shown to reduce infection is irrigation with a jet of fluid directly into the wound. This washes away contamination by mechanical action. Wound scrubbing with a soft brush does the same thing on larger wounds.

14. What amount of irrigation solution is recommended?

There are published formulas for how much irrigant to use, and the word "copious" is found everywhere. I use 100 to 1,000 mL for wounds up to 2.5 centimeters. The worse the blood supply, the more irrigant is needed. Moreover, remember it is force used rather than the amount of irrigant that determines how effectively bacteria are washed away.

15. When are stitches required for bites?

The most common question of "Will I need stitches?" for a bite can be answered with "No," unless the bite is on the face. Animal bites are usually left open to heal because sutured closure is associated with higher infection rate. Open closure leads to a bigger scar, so on cosmetic areas like the face the wound is often closed with sutures, especially if debridement is good.

16. Talk about the risk of rabies. So many patients are worried about that aspect.

Rabies cannot be effectively treated, only prevented. Rabies prevention shots are expensive and bothersome, rather than painful. Preventive shots are widely overused for bites of dogs and cats because they rarely carry rabies. At the other extreme are the bat and skunk; rabies is endemic to both species. Bat or skunk bites or scratches always need rabies prophylaxis unless the animal can be killed and examined for rabies immediately. Rodents such as squirrels, chipmunks, hamsters, or gerbils are low risk because they don't eat animals that might be rabid (they're herbivores). There is a small risk a rodent could have contracted rabies from a bite from a rabid carnivore.

17. What helps determine the need for preventive shots?

Common questions that help guide the decision for rabies prevention include:

- Has the animal been vaccinated against rabies?
- Was the animal acting strangely or normally?
- Was the attack provoked or unprovoked? An unprovoked attack is when the animal runs up and bites the victim who is otherwise minding his or her own business. Rabies in cats and dogs can cause this aggressive behavior.

Consider calling the county animal control office. Most states have mandatory reporting of bites and can tell you if there are recent rabid dogs or cats in your area.

If you still suspect rabies and the animal can be captured, the animal can be observed for 2 weeks for signs of rabies or sacrificed on the spot with its brain autopsied for classic signs of rabies. Most families with pets opt for the observation, but should the pet die during the 2 weeks its brain should be immediately examined and shots begun presumptively.

18. How do I triage the human bite?

Wound assessment and debridement needs are identical to dog and cat bites. Children may bite when they are upset or angry. In adults a bite usually shows the bite victim was an aggressor who placed someone into a desperate situation that evoked biting as a primitive response. Assessing the circumstances of the injury is essential.

19. Discuss how a human bite on the knuckles is a special circumstance.

A common missed bite wound is the puncture wound over the knuckle. Consider these as bites incurred by the common practice of the punch to the jaw gone awry. When the closed fist contacts the tooth, the knuckle or metacarpophalangeal (MCP) joint is in a vulnerable position. The metacarpal joint cartilage is exposed and can be easily nicked by a tooth. This introduces infectious organisms in saliva to the cartilage and joint space. Without cleansing in surgery, the joint gets infected and can be lost quickly, leading to a crippling arthritis at that knuckle.

A radiograph of the MCP joint should be ordered to look specifically for a tooth mark indenting a bone cortex. A positive finding will change therapy and perhaps save the joint.

20. Any infections, besides bacterial, that I should be concerned about in a human bite?

Humans are not rabies carriers, so that is not a risk in human bites. Human bite victims can contract Hepatitis B from the donor, even in children. In children assess if vaccinations are up to date, including Hepatitis B immunization. Some adults may also be Hepatitis B immune. If the victim is susceptible to Hepatitis B and the donor either cannot be identified or has high risk for Hepatitis B, the options are the same as in the needlestick injury.

The Centers for Disease Control and Prevention (CDC) considers saliva alone to not be an agent for human immunodeficiency virus (HIV) transmission. However there are cases of HIV seroconversion in bite victims from assailants with HIV infection. It is thought the transmission occurred from blood in the assailant's mouth transmitted HIV to the human bite victim. Because it is impossible to completely be sure the assailant did not have blood in his or her mouth, the prudent course is to treat the human bite as a potential transmitter of blood-borne pathogens including HIV. Therefore post exposure HIV prophylaxis should be considered in anyone bitten by an assailant with known HIV or suspected HIV infection. Please consult your hospital's postexposure prophylaxis (PEP) protocol. In addition there is forensic value in documenting or photographing the bite mark because there is successful prosecution for assault, even murder, from intentional HIV transmission through a human bite.

21. Do human bites need to be reported to the authorities?

Most states have mandatory reporting of assaults, and human bites usually qualify. I am a skeptic that anyone could stretch their arm and accidentally hit someone on the tooth, or that someone's mouth happens to fall on someone else's knuckle, or that anyone other than a kid would play "cannibal." Why not document what you see and let the authorities take it from there?

Key Points

- Most insect bites are harmless and treated with cleansing and warning about infection.
- Dangerous spider bites either have central necrotic ulcers or systemic symptoms.
- Snake bites should be observed for at least 6 hours with frequent exams to look for local swelling or neurologic symptoms. Triage labs include coagulation studies.
- Rabies and tetanus risk should be considered in all bites.

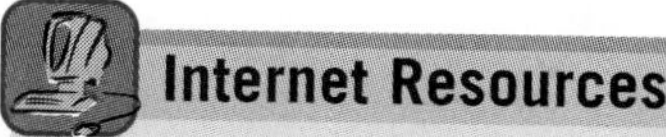

Internet Resources

Pictorial Atlas of Snakes
http://www.pitt.edu/~mcs2/herp/SoNA.html

Bibliography

Banner W: Scorpion envenomation. In Auerbach PS, Geehr EC, editors: *Management of wilderness and environmental emergencies,* ed 2, St Louis, 1989, Mosby, 603-616.

Herr RD, Zimmermann PG: Wound management. In Sheehy S, Lenehan G, editors: *Manual of emergency care,* ed 5, St Louis, 1999, Mosby, 361-381.

Playe SJ, Aghababian RV: Mammal bites and associated infections. In Harwood-Nuss A, Wolfson AB, editors: *The clinical practice of emergency medicine,* ed 3, Philadelphia, 2001, Lippincott, 1644-1647.

Pretty IA, Anderson GS, Sweet DJ: Human bites and the risk of human immunodeficiency virus transmission, *Am J Forensic Med Pathol* 20(3):232-239, 1999.

Rees RS, Campbell DS: Spider bites. In Auerbach PS, Geehr EC, editors: *Management of wilderness and environmental emergencies,* ed 2, St Louis, 1989, Mosby, 543-561.

Chapter 50

Near-Drowning

Barbara A. Weintraub

1. What is the difference between drowning and near-drowning?

Drowning refers to death from asphyxia within the first 24 hours after a submersion injury. Near-drowning refers to situations in which the patient survives at least 24 hours after the submersion injury, regardless of the eventual outcome.

2. What specific aspects of a history should the triage nurse obtain from a victim of a near-drowning?

In addition to the usual aspects of history that a triage nurse obtains, in near-drowning incidents there are other specific areas to ask about. I think of these factors as the 5 Ts. They are:

- Trauma preceding incident
- Temperature of water
- Time underwater
- Time until cardiopulmonary resuscitation (CPR) begun
- Tranquilizers/Tequila/Trembles: contributing factors such as alcohol or drug ingestion, or history a of seizure disorder

3. Why are these important? Shouldn't I just listen to the patient's lungs and get them a bed?

As a matter of fact, no. Submersion incidents can occur via a variety of mechanisms. For instance, people with seizure disorders are four to five times more likely to suffer a submersion incident than those without. Some submersion incidents occur after suffering an acute medical episode while in the water, such as having a myocardial infarction (MI) or a hypoglycemic episode. Still other episodes occur after diving accidents. Therefore, failure to get an adequate history can cause you to not only neglect some very important medical conditions, but to miscategorize their triage acuity as well.

4. What are the most important assessments in the situation in which someone was unresponsive after surfing in cold water, but responds after CPR?

The most important vital signs to check are respiratory rate, a very accurate temperature, and pulse oximetry. These are important because tachypnea can precede other clinical signs of either aspiration pneumonia or pulmonary edema, the elevated respiratory rate may be your only clue of impending respiratory failure.

The pulse oximetry is kind of a trick answer. Although clearly an oxygen saturation above 96% would be reassuring in this patient, because of the probable existence of some degree of hypothermia, accurate measurement may be difficult if not impossible. This said, an attempt at obtaining an SpO_2 should be undertaken on the extremity demonstrating the capillary refill time closest to normal (2 to 3 seconds).

Hypothermia frequently accompanies near-drowning episodes, even in water up to 80°F. Ideally this patient should have a rectal temperature done. If this can not be done at triage as a result of lack of privacy, an initial oral temperature should be done, with a follow-up rectal temperature done if abnormal.

5. Is it safe to discharge a patient such as this if there are normal vital signs, pulse oximeter, and a clear radiograph?

Because respiratory distress can develop up to 4 to 6 hours after an immersion incident, the patient should either be admitted for observation or kept 6 hours or so for observation. Studies have found that, in general, discharge from the emergency department is safe with reliable adults who are asymptomatic after 8 hours of observation, a normal chest radiograph, and normal pulse oximetry readings.

6. Which patient should I worry more about: the one who was submersed in freshwater or the one submersed in saltwater?

Although the pathways they take are different, both patients are at risk for pulmonary edema. In freshwater drownings, there is a washout of surfactant, and the alveolar basement membrane is damaged. This results in movement of proteinaceous material into the lung, leading to pulmonary edema. In contrast, aspiration of hypertonic seawater results in the movement of water from the intravascular space into the alveolar space. This then results in the same washout of surfactant, damage of the alveolar basement membrane, and eventual pulmonary edema.

7. Does that mean that regardless of what kind of water a patient is submersed in, the prognosis is the same?

No, it means no such thing. Aspiration of vomit, sand, mud, or pathogens found in sewage or seawater can cause pneumonitis, worsening the patient's condition and their prognosis.

8. Should antibiotics, and possibly steroids, be given to patients who are submersed in "dirty water"?

Although that would seem to make sense intuitively, research has not demonstrated this intervention. Although there is still controversy about the prophylactic use of antibiotics for victims who have aspirated grossly contaminated water, most experts recommend that antibiotics be restricted only to those patients demonstrating signs of bacterial infection or sepsis, and steroids have not shown to be of any use at all in aspiration pneumonitis.

9. What medications should I be prepared to give?

First of all, all symptomatic near-drowning patients should receive oxygen. As bronchospasm may be found in near-drowning victims, albuterol may be of some benefit. One study identified the use of artificial surfactant as beneficial in a small study of near-drowning victims. Otherwise, treatments are aimed at either underlying or resultant medical conditions. Seizures can be treated with anticonvulsants, spinal injury with corticosteroids, hypotension with fluids, hypoglycemia with dextrose, and elevated intracranial pressure (ICP) (as a result of anoxic injury) with Mannitol or furosemide.

10. A mother claims her 14-month-old daughter was found head-first in the bucket of water she was using to wash the floor. Although the child is in no distress now, should I be suspicious of child abuse?

No, you should not be suspicious as this could have happened in the manner the mother described. Each year, approximately 27 children drown in 3- to 5-gallon buckets filled with liquid. These buckets are very stable, and do not tip over easily. As toddlers are proportionately head-heavy, they fall in head first, but do not have the muscle strength to pull themselves out.

11. Are there any types of submersion incidents in which I should be suspicious for child abuse?

About 10% to 25% of residential drownings occur in the bathtub, usually when an infant is left alone or with inadequate supervision. In one study of 21 patients with a bathtub near-drowning incident, 67% had evidence of abuse or neglect. Of course, any time the injury doesn't match the history or the developmental level of the child, the triage nurse should have a heightened index of suspicion for child abuse.

12. A 3-year-old child is rushed in from falling through the ice and was submerged for 35 minutes. Your rapid assessment reveals an unresponsive, pulseless, apneic, very cold, blue child. All of the beds in the treatment area are full. What triage level (on a five-tier triage scale) should you assign this child?

Patients in full arrest are assigned a level 1, as they require immediate care. However, patients without vital signs for 35 minutes are generally nonresuscitatable, and thus do not require immediate treatment, as they are considered dead on arrival (DOA). Is the patient a "1" or a "5"?

There are multiple published reports documenting survival after prolonged cold-water submersion of up to 66 minutes, with no neurologic deficit. Thus, assign this patient a triage level 1. In general, patients aren't dead until they're warm and dead.

13. Let's take the same situation as above, but the waiting room is full of people waiting to be triaged, and waiting for a bed after triage. Now to what triage category would you assign this patient?

The triage level to which you assign a patient is based only on that patient's condition. You would never change your triage acuity rating because of conditions in the department. The patient is still a level 1.

Key Points

- Obtain the 5T history pertinent for near-drowning.
- Although the pathways are different, patients drowning in both fresh water and saltwater are at risk for development of pulmonary edema.
- Near-drowning is differentiated from drowning by survival of at least 24 hours after the event.

Internet Resources

What Immediate Care Should You Give a Near-Drowning Victim?
http://nursing.about.com/library/1999/bldyk062501.htm

Near-Drowning
http://www.findarticles.com/p/articles/mi_gGENH/is_/ai_2699003532

Submersion Injury, Near-Drowning
http://www.emedicine.com/emerg/topic744.htm

Near-Drowning
http://www.chclibrary.org/micromed/00057890.html

Cold Injuries and Cold Water Near-Drowning Guidelines
http://www.sarbc.org/sarbc/hypo2.html

Bibliography

Harley JR, Ochesenschlager DW: Near drowning. In Barkin RM, editor: *Pediatric emergency medicine: Concepts and clinical practice,* ed 2, St Louis, 1997, Mosby, 474-481.

Knopp R: Near-drowning. In Rund, DA, editor: *Essentials of emergency medicine,* ed 2, St Louis, 1996, Mosby, 345-347.

Manton AP: Pulmonary emergencies. In Sheehy SB, Lenehan GB, editors: *Manual of emergency care,* ed 5, St Louis, 1999, Mosby, 214-216.

Chapter 51

Environmental Thermo-Emergencies

Vicki Sweet

1. What are the contributing factors for a hypothermic/hyperthermic condition?

Pre-existing illness, prescription drugs, street drugs, alcohol use, and age can all be risk factors associated with both heat and cold emergencies.

2. I've heard that every triage area needs a "hypothermia thermometer." What is it and how is it different?

Every emergency department (ED) needs a thermometer that will read very low body temperatures. Many of the newer electronic temperatures will read as low as 80°F (36.6°C). It would be unusual, but not impossible, for a patient with a body temperature of <90°F (32°C) to walk in with a chief complaint of hypothermia, but just when you say it will never happen, you know that it will.

3. What is "hypothermia"? Some patients say, "My temperature always runs lower than normal."

Definitions vary, but most consider mild hypothermia is present when the body temperature is between 93°F and 95°F (33.8°C and 35°C). Therefore, a patient whose oral temperature is 97°F (36°C) is not necessarily hypothermic. The mildly hypothermic patient walking into the triage area would most likely have vague complaints, such as confusion, shivering, or lack of fine motor coordination. Confusion usually begins at 93°F (33.8°C).

The patient is considered to be moderately hypothermic when the temperature drops to between 90°F and 92°F (29°C to 32°C). These patients lose the ability to shiver and move by 90°F (32.2°C).

Patients who are severely hypothermic will probably always arrive via emergency medical service (EMS) with body temperatures of below 90°F (32°C). They will most likely be unconscious.

4. How would I recognize a hypothermic patient, other than taking their temperature?

There are the obvious signs of shivering and "goose flesh." Other signs and symptoms include complaints of fatigue, impaired fine motor coordination, confusion, or slurred speech. If the temperature is not taken, the true etiology for the neurologic deficits might be missed.

5. What are "chilblains"?

Chilblains is most likely a mild form of frostbite. The patient may present with a complaint of itchy, red, swollen areas on the ears, fingers, or toes after prolonged exposure in cold, damp weather. The ambient temperature does not need to be below freezing to produce this condition.

Do not have the patient rub the affected area. The condition usually does not result in any permanent tissue damage and patient teaching should focus on prevention.

6. If I think my patient has frostbite, what immediate steps can I take in the triage area?

- Frostbite occurs when the tissue temperature decreases to less than 32°F (0°C) and ice crystal formation damages the cellular architecture.
- Handle possible frostbitten areas very carefully. The tissues are quite fragile and subject to further injury. Never rub the affected area.
- Place in a warm environment.
- Prevent further heat loss.

7. How is complete "thawing" accomplished?

Rapid, complete thawing is done by immersion in 104°F to 105°F (40°C to 41°C) water; circulating water is the ideal recommendation for thawing. (Never use dry heat.) Reestablishing perfusion is intensely painful and analgesics will be needed so this step is done within the ED treatment area.

8. I work in southern California. How can someone in a warm climate become hypothermic?

The body loses heat by several mechanisms, including evaporation, convection, conduction, and respiration. Consider these possible scenarios.

- The older adult woman who goes to the kitchen at 1 AM for a glass of milk. She slips, falls, breaks her hip, and lies on the cold tile floor all night in her thin cotton nightgown.
- Prolonged exposure to cool lakes and oceans, in which temperatures might be in the 60s (compared to body temperature of 98.6°F [37°C]). Even heated pools (in the 70s) can be chilling, especially to children's increased body surface area.
- Homeless persons who spend cold, damp nights outside are also at risk for hypothermia, even in the warmest of climates.

9. How should I handle a severely hypothermic patient who is experiencing an arrhythmia?

Patients are not considered dead until they are "warm and dead." Arrhythmias don't respond well to standard cardiac treatment until the patient is "warmed." Both active and passive rewarming is necessary.

10. Aside from fever, what are some of the ways that a hyperthermic patient presents?

Patients with heat exhaustion will have cool, moist skin with muscle cramping. The core temperature might be slightly elevated or even normal, yet their symptoms result from salt depletion from excessive perspiration and the resulting hyponatremia and dehydration. Headache, nausea, and tachycardia can be present. This is an "urgent" triage category.

The patient with heat exhaustion might present with a history of syncope. The syncope resulted from the blood being diverted to peripheral tissues for cooling. It occurs frequently with coexisting cardiovascular disease and/or with patients receiving diuretics.

11. Compare that with heat stroke.

Heat stroke is an "emergent" condition that may have all the symptoms of heat exhaustion. However, the hallmark signs are:

- Central nervous system (CNS) dysfunction, usually of sudden onset, such as agitation, confusion (95% to 100%)
- High temperature >41°C or 106°F (95% to 100%)
- Aggressive, immediate definitive treatment is needed to help prevent permanent disability or death.

12. Who is most likely to experience a heat stroke?

The very young and the debilitated older adult during a sustained, sudden heat wave because they are unable to compensate for a change in the environment. It also can be exertion-induced in the physically fit population, such as the marathon runner. It is life-threatening and cooling treatment must begin immediately.

13. Is it true that heat stroke doesn't always present with hot, dry skin?

It is definitely possible to still perspire although having a heat stroke. Perspiration cools only 1 kcal for each 1.7 mL of perspiration and in the heat stroke, the cooling mechanism is no longer effective. The key distinguishers of a heat stroke are altered level of consciousness (LOC) and a high temperature (41°C or 106°F).

14. My patient had a fever after working out in the hot sun. Why was his urine sample so dark brown?

Strenuous exercise in a hot environment can cause muscle breakdown. Dark brown urine may be from myoglobin as a result of rhabdomyolysis. This is a serious condition that must be treated rapidly with copious intravenous (IV) fluids to prevent renal injury.

15. How should I prioritize the different temperatures?

The degree of temperature does not necessarily reflect the seriousness of the environmental emergency. In the case of heat stroke, in which there is up to 70% mortality, the core temperature will almost always exceed 105°F (40.6°C). However, in heat exhaustion, the temperature may be normal yet the patient might have a serious electrolyte imbalance as a result of excessive perspiration.

Perform a careful assessment of objective and subjective data and use sound clinical reasoning. Overall, frostbite/mild hypothermia, and heat exhaustion are "urgent," with the goal toward definitive care within 15 to 30 minutes.

16. Give an example of a triage category.

The Manchester Triage Group place any patient whose skin to touch feels "cold," a "hot child," or a "very hot adult" in the Level 2 (very urgent, 10 minutes). See Chapter 18 for further discussion. Objectively, cold is considered <89.6°F (<32°C), hot is >101.3°F (>38.5°C), and very hot is >105.8°F (>41°C).

17. My patient says he has recently used cocaine and has a fever. Does this increase his acuity?

Cocaine can cause the body's temperature regulating systems to go awry, resulting in an increased body temperature. In addition, agitation from cocaine use may result in increased motor activity. This, in turn, may cause increased heat production. A cocaine user with hyperthermia is at risk for complications and should receive a higher acuity rating. This is why it is always important to get a full set of vital signs in the triage area.

18. I've heard that I should always take a temperature if I suspect "rave drug" use. Why is this important?

One of the popular "rave drugs" is MDMA, or Ecstasy. There have been documented deaths from this drug and most of the fatalities probably have been as a result of hyperthermia and heat stroke. The combination of the drug's heat-producing effects, energetic dancing, inadequate hydration, and a crowded environment puts users at risk for serious complications, including brain damage if they survive.

Key Points

- All patients with systemic complaints should have a temperature taken, because presentations aren't always obvious.
- Never rub chilblains or frostbite.
- Be alert for "brownish" urine from rhabdomyolysis if there is a history of fever after strenuous exercise.
- Cocaine and "rave drug" use can cause elevated temperatures.

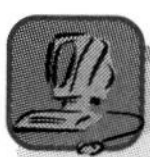

Internet Resources

California Emergency Nurses Association: Rave Drugs
http://www.enw.org/calena/Education/RaveDrugs.htm

Emedicine.com—Hypothermia
http://www.emedicine.com/emerg/topic279.htm

Emedicine.com—Heat Exhaustion and Heatstroke
http://www.emedicine.com/emerg/topic236.htm

Emedicine.com—Toxicity, MDMA
http://www.emedicine.com/emerg/topic927.htm

Bibliography

Danzl DF: Hypothermia and frostbite. In Markovchick VJ, Pons PT, editors: *Emergency medicine secrets,* ed 3, Philadelphia, 2003, Hanley & Belfus.

Mackway-Jones K: *Emergency triage,* London, 1997, Manchester Triage Group.

Metheny NM: *Fluid and electrolyte balance: Nursing considerations,* Philadelphia, 2000, Lippincott, Williams & Wilkins.

Perry SJ, Vukich DJ: Heat illness. In Markovchick VJ, Pons PT, editors: *Emergency medicine secrets,* ed 3, Philadelphia, 2003, Hanley & Belfus.

Ribiero VM: Fever (elevated temperature). In Dais MA, Votey SR, Greenough PG, editors: *Signs and symptoms in emergency medicine: Literature-based approach to emergency conditions,* St Louis, 1999, Mosby.

Section IX

Psychiatric

Chapter 52

Triage of the Psychiatric Patient

Gail Lenehan

1. What do I need to determine at triage for the psychiatric patient?

Your first priority is to decide what will be needed to keep the patient and the staff safe, both at triage, and then when they go back into the emergency department (ED). If there is any question about safety, have emergency medical service (EMS) personnel wait until hospital security arrives and you decide whether a "sitter," a security guard, or restraints, etc., will be needed. It is helpful to ask EMS, friends, or family about the most dangerous thing the patient has done.

Next, decide whether the patient needs someone to evaluate them medically (e.g., an ED physician or nurse practitioner), or someone to evaluate them for psychologic or psychiatric problems (e.g., a psychiatrist/psychiatric nurse clinician).

2. How do you know whether the patient will be safe?

When you ask the family, EMS, or whoever accompanies the patient, what the most worrisome thing the patient has done prior to coming in, listen carefully, and trust that they are not exaggerating or "hysterical." It is likely that what the patient was doing outside the ED is just what he will do once he is inside the ED, only worse. If the police say that the patient was reported to have assaulted people passing by in the subway, without provocation, then it is perhaps more likely that he will assault hospital staff who will be more intrusive and possibly more threatening, in the patient's mind, than any passerby could be.

If the patient is suicidal, ask the patient directly whether he or she can control an urge to hurt himself or herself while in the ED. Contracts are often used in psychiatry, but whether the triage nurse has the time and expertise to assume this responsibility is arguable.

3. How much of a role should my intuition play at triage?

Although nothing is as important as history, do listen to your intuition. It is often a good diagnostic and prognostic indicator. Are you annoyed and angry with a patient? Are you feeling manipulated? The patient may have characterologic qualities and may even be a sociopath. On the other hand, do you feel sympathetic? In my experience, psychotic patients elicit more sympathy than patients with characterologic problems. Do you feel afraid, uncomfortable? Trust your instincts. The patient may be potentially violent. Err on the side of protecting the patient and others.

4. What questions are most helpful to ask?

A question like, "What did you hope that we could do for you here today?" It can cut to the chase and let you know what the patient expects. The patient may say that he wants to go to the hospital, or wants to see a doctor for medicine, etc. Asking directly encourages the patient to tell you, rather than forcing them to show you, acting out how sick and in need they are.

Consider asking all psychiatric patients if they have hurt themselves or if they are having any pain. Homeless psychotic patients are vulnerable to physical assaults on the street. They may respond that their head hurts and reveal an otherwise less than obvious head trauma, or they may have a fractured extremity that isn't obvious.

5. What, if anything, should I avoid asking in an initial encounter?

It is not usually helpful to say, "What's wrong?" So many things are wrong in the eyes and experience of someone with psychiatric illness, particularly chronic psychiatric illness, that they may not even know where to begin and they may ramble or, at the least, become more anxious.

6. If I can't get any information from the patient at triage, what can I do?

Look for a wallet and see if there are any numbers with which to reach key people. Parents can be especially helpful, even when the patient is an adult. Patients with a psychiatric history may have parents who are concerned and knowledgeable and who try and monitor their children's welfare, even when they are only able to do so from a distance.

Ask to see their medication container. It's a way of finding out the name of their primary psychiatrist when they are too confused to tell you. If you can find out the name of their primary psychiatric clinician, if not to call yourself, then to pass on to the ED psychiatric clinicians, it will save a world of time.

Ask patients if they have been started on drugs recently. They may be reacting to a single new psychiatric medication, or could be reacting to a drug interaction, as occurs with patients with medical illnesses.

7. What should I be aware of when asking about the patient's medications?

Just because patients have been prescribed a medication, and just because they say they are on a medication doesn't mean that they are actually taking the medication, or taking it regularly. It may be that the side effects are too frightening or unpleasant, and they have stopped the medication and they have deteriorated.

8. Is it better to ask general or specific questions?

It is better to be fairly concrete at triage. Try to ask specific questions, such as, "What medicines have you taken? If the patient says, "lithium," then you know that at least one clinician, at one point in time, thought that this patient suffered from mania. Ask patients what hospital/s they've been to, or who their clinician is as a way of discerning the extent of their mental illness. If they say they've had twenty admissions to a chronic psychiatric hospital, then you will have a better sense of the problem. Although this doesn't always work, when it does, a quick call to that clinician can provide a goldmine of information. Ask specifically about the last time the patient took their medications. It may be that the patient has simply run out of medication, and, in their resulting confusion, has not been organized enough to get back to their normal clinician.

9. Any hints about particular questions?

It's important to know whether the patient's behavior is chronic or has come on suddenly, for the very first time. When you ask the patient's friends and relatives whether the patient has ever "been like this" before, they will often, and emphatically say "No!" After much research, it is not uncommon to find out that the patient has, in fact, exhibited similar behavior, but not as severe. When this information is presented to friends and family, the response is usually, "Well yes [acknowledging similar behavior], but never THIS bad". This has happened so often in my experience that I have labeled it the "yes, but never this bad" syndrome. Families are so frightened by the worse behavior, that they see it as qualitatively, not just quantitatively, different from the patient's past history.

10. Do I have to take a full set of vital signs on a psychiatric patient?

Yes, definitely. The reason for a patient's bizarre behavior might be "organic" and vital signs can offer important clues. Not only that, but psychiatric patients, like other patients, do become physically sick. In fact, when patients become psychotic, they also become disorganized and may not eat, drink, or rest, making them more vulnerable to dehydration and illness. By the same token, physical symptoms can frighten someone with psychiatric disease so much so that they "decompensate" and become, or at least seem, psychotic, or in panic.

11. What might vital signs reveal?

A temperature might mean that there is an infection, possibly a serious one, and possibly one that is causing neurologic signs and symptoms. Elevated temperature, blood pressure, and pulse could all be as a result of dehydration, and it would be important to hydrate the patient before sending them to another facility with less acute care resources. A rapid pulse or elevated blood pressure could reflect the ingestion of illicit drugs. No amount of nervousness causes a patient's pulse to go to 160 beats per minute. In my experience, if a patient's pulse is above 120, even above 112, then a careful look at ingestion of drugs, an allergic reaction, or other causes is in order.

12. How do I separate out what are "physical" (organic) from what is "psychiatric"?

Look at key organic causes of bizarre behavior such as medications. Just as everything is as a result of medications until proven otherwise for the older adult, similarly, medication side effects are a good place to start with psychiatric patients. The dystonia that a patient can get from an antipsychotic medication is so frightening that the patient will understandably become fearful and may possibly decompensate emotionally and posturing in what looks like a bizarre fashion. Everything that looks crazy isn't necessarily.

13. Are there any quick checks for clues that a psychiatric patient's behavior has an organic (medical) cause besides abnormal vital signs?

Check pupil size. A patient's pupils can be very telling. Very small, even "pinpoint" and very large pupils must be taken to mean drug toxicity until proven otherwise. Functional ("psychiatric") illness does not cause someone's pupils to be huge or very small. Illicit drugs and prescription medications can.

Check for a nystagmus. Have the patient follow your finger with their eyes both up and down and side to side. If the eye "bounces," it is often indicative of drug or toxin ingestion.

Don't dismiss incontinence as insignificant. The fact that a patient is incontinent raises some serious concerns about organic illness. The patient may have had a seizure, for example, and lost control of their bladder, or they may have lost control of their musculature because of temporary anoxia or other reasons.

14. If someone is psychotic, they don't need to be triaged as urgent because they are "out of it"; it doesn't matter how quickly they are assessed, right?

Wrong. First, it may be that the patient has a rapidly progressing neurologic problem. But even if the problem is that a schizophrenic is in a "functional" psychotic state, this can be terrifying for the patient. It would be just as inhumane to make a patient wait with acute paranoid delusions who is struggling to escape his restraints as it would be to subject patients in excruciating physical pain to extended waits. Moreover, there is always the possibility that, even when restrained, psychotic patients can cause harm to themselves or others. There are instances, for example, in which a patient on phencyclidine (PCP) has managed to pull their own teeth out in the course of biting on sheeting and restraints. Patients have also set fires and hit their head against stretcher rails or walls.

15. What if the patient is wearing or doing something bizarre and it is too awkward to ask about it?

Become used to asking about awkward things in a way that isn't awkward. Usually, the patient is much more aware of that upside down cooking pot on his head than you are. Such behavior is only the tip of an iceberg that the patient knows much more about than you. Ask the patient directly, but respectfully, if he or she minds if you ask about the pot to better understand why it is there. Patients are sometimes relieved to be able to tell someone that the pot is warding off radiation from the Federal Bureau of Investigation (FBI), to let others know why it's important to keep it on. Guard against sounding too patronizing. It may make patients with paranoia all the more suspicious.

16. What should I document at triage?

One thing that is becoming more important is the documentation of a reason for your decision to have the patient restrained, medicated, or put in a seclusion room. Even if it's a small threatening utterance, or darting paranoid-like eye glancing, jot down a few words that will make anyone reviewing the chart understand the rationale. Similarly, if you decide not to restrain, put a few words down to suggest why you felt comfortable with the less restrictive means of protection for the patient.

Also document any breaches of confidence. New Health Insurance Portability and Accountability Act of 1996 (HIPAA) regulations have made it necessary to document what information was obtained and how; it is also helpful to document the reason for the urgency in obtaining information. Include a few words to underscore what imminent danger to the patient or others existed and why information was obtained. Document that patients were not able to communicate permission or sign waivers for health information because the patient appeared to be psychotic, or that they refused but that their history or current behavior indicates a danger of suicidal or homicidal behavior, for example.

17. Any overarching principles with psychiatric patients at triage?

Treat psychiatric patients with the same concern, and be as suspicious of hidden disease or injury, as you would employ with any "medical" patients at triage. And remember to be kind and respectful. Psychiatric patients, like all of the other patients you'll triage, are simply trying to survive. See also Chapter 69.

Key Points

- Trust your intuition. If you are feeling angry, the patient may have characterologic problems. If you are feeling sympathetic, the patient may be psychotic. If you are feeling afraid, there is probably a good reason to be.
- Ask specific questions, such as "What did you hope that we could do for you here today? rather than a vague "What's wrong?" Someone with psychiatric illness has so many things wrong, a general question won't elicit what you need and, as the patient rambles, you both become more anxious.
- Be alert to the "yes, but never this bad" syndrome. The family may initially say that the patient never did this before. But often, they really mean that it is only quantitatively, not qualitatively different. The patient has done it, just never to this degree.

Internet Resources

Emergency Nurses Association Position Statement: Medical Evaluation of Suspected Intoxicated and Psychiatric Patients
http://www.ena.org/publications/statements/PositionPDF/MedEval-of-Intoxicated.PDF

FERNE: Foundation for Education and Research in Neurological Emergencies
Evidence Based Evaluation of Psychiatric Patients
http://www.ferne.org/Lectures/evaluation_of_psychiatric_patients_zun_saem0503.htm

Psychiatric News: Resident's Forum

New Solutions to Old Problems
http://www.psych.org/pnews/97-10-03/res.html

Bibliography

Allen MH: Emergency psychiatry. In *Review of psychiatry,* Arlington, Va, 2002, American Psychiatric Press.

Holdsworth NE: Effective approach to psychiatric patients (Clinical Nurses Forum), *J Emerg Nurs* 30(2):155-156, 2004.

Petit J: *Handbook of emergency psychiatry,* Philadelphia, 2003, Lippincott.

Chapter 53

Depression and Suicide

Nina M. Fielden

1. Define depression.

The diagnosis of depression is a depressed mood that is present at least half of the time over a 2-week period. (The average adult American feels "sad, blue, or depressed" an average of 3 days a month.) In addition, there must be at least four of the following symptoms during the same period: sleep disturbance, loss of interest or pleasure in usual activities, feelings of guilt or worthlessness, lack of energy, decreased concentration or ability to make decisions, appetite disturbance (usually diminished), psychomotor changes (agitated or slowed), and suicidal thinking. Depression is the most common psychiatric disorder in older adults.

2. What might make the triage nurse suspect a patient is depressed?

The person may have a sad affect, but often the person's depression is to be expressed in physical rather than emotional terms. They may report nonspecific complaints, such as fatigue, headache, nonspecific pain, gastrointestinal complaints, or vague "just feeling bad." Anxiety may also be present and manifested as shortness of breath, nervousness, irritability, or difficulty swallowing. Another signal can be answering questions with "I don't know."

3. Explain why frequent answers of "I don't know" could signal depression.

This type of response is more common in the older adult person who is depressed, but it can be wrongly attributed to confusion or ignorance. It can mean "I don't care." People with true cognitive loss are usually unaware of it (or its extent). They will tell you "no one tells me anything" or will think it is 1932, but the person "cares" enough to try to answer your question.

4. Provide something to help you remember what to ask about when screening for depression.

Rund and Nockowitz (2003) suggest using the mnemonic SIG E CAPS. Remember it by thinking of what you want to do for depressed people: in a figurative sense you want to "prescribe energy capsules" that help with the following:
Sleep disturbance
Interests
Guilt

Energy
Concentration
Appetite disturbance
Psychomotor changes
Suicidal thinking

5. Are generalized unexplained persistent musculoskeletal pains always indicative of depression?

In one study, 93% of patients with these complaints had low serum vitamin D levels, with 28% being severely low. The severest deficiency was in African-American patients. However, this nutritional deficiency could also be a result or symptom of depression.

6. What is the incidence and recommendation for screening for depression?

Depression is associated with being female, being divorced or separated, low socioeconomic status, poor social support, and a recent adverse and unexpected event. Women have a 1.7 to 2.7 lifetime incidence of depression that is greater than men. Approximately 15% of the community-dwelling older population has symptoms of depression: it is the most common mood disorder in older adults. The U.S. Preventive Services Task Force recommends screening for depression, although there is no current agreement on a specific screening tool to use.

7. Provide a simple way to screen for depression.

Arroll (2003) tested whether two questions about depressed mood were sensitive enough to suffice as a depression-screening tool for adults. The questions were:

- "During the past month, have you often been bothered by feeling down, depressed, or hopeless?"
- "During the past month have you often been bothered by little interest or pleasure in doing things?"

They found the questions had 97% sensitivity and 67% specificity for depression if the person answered "yes" to either one of the questions. It also had a 99.6% negative predictive value; e.g., those who answered "no" to both questions were not depressed.

8. Describe the short form of the Beck Depression Inventory.

The Beck Depression Inventory is a questionnaire of 13 items with four options for each item. The questions' responses measure varying degrees of sadness, pessimism, sense of failure, dissatisfaction, guilt, self-dislike, self-harm, social withdrawal, indecisiveness, self-image change, work difficulty, fatigability, and anorexia. For instance, with self-dislike, the respondent scores zero points for "I don't feel disappointed in myself," one point for "I am disappointed in myself," two points for "I am disgusted with myself," and three points if they choose "I hate myself." The total score indicates no, mild, moderate, or severe depression. One advantage is that the patient can complete the questionnaire independently while waiting.

9. What is suicidal behavior?

1. Suicidal behavior includes suicidal gestures, suicidal ideation, attempted suicide, and completed suicide.
2. Suicide gestures are plans and actions that appear unlikely to succeed.
3. Suicidal ideation is primarily a communicative act and should be regarded as a plea for help.
4. Attempted suicide is a suicidal act that is not fatal. This could be because the intention was ambiguous, the person was discovered early, or the action had a low lethal potential. Most persons who attempt suicide are ambivalent about dying; however, patients who attempt suicide are five to six times more likely to attempt suicide again.
5. Completed suicide results in death.

10. What is the prevalence of suicide?

According to the Centers for Disease Control and Prevention (2004), suicide is the thirteenth leading cause of death worldwide (the eleventh in the United States). The World Health Organization estimates that 1 million people died from suicide in 2000, with ten to twenty times more people attempting suicide worldwide.

11. What ages are at increased risk of suicide?

It is now the third leading cause of death among U.S. residents aged 10 years up to 24 years and accounts for 11.7% of all deaths in this age group. However, suicide increases in the older adult; 20% of all suicides are over the age of 65. Suicides in women peak between ages 55 and 65, and the suicide rate for men age 85 years and older is 5.5 times the rate of the general population.

12. List factors that increase the risk of suicide.

People with:

- Mental disorders (schizophrenia, personality disorders, mood disorders, anxiety disorders, disruptive disorders)
- History of depression. The lifetime suicide rate is 15% in patients with recurrent depression. The highest risk is early in the treatment of depression when the depressed mood is starting to lift but still present (the person has the "energy" to carry out the plan now).
- Social factors (abuse, unemployed, living alone, sudden, dramatic change in life, anniversary of significant loss). Up to 50% of women who are battered attempt suicide.
- Physical disorders, chronic illnesses (cancer, chronic obstructive pulmonary disease [COPD], chronic pain, on renal dialysis, human immunodeficiency virus positive [HIV+])
- History of self-destructive behavior (reckless driving, self-mutilation, and violent antisocial acts)
- History of previous suicide, family history of suicide. Twenty percent of persons who attempt suicide will try again within a year with 10% succeeding.
- Alcoholism/substance abuse. Alcohol use is involved in 33% of suicides.

13. Compare men and women in suicide risk.

Men are more likely to complete suicide than women but women are more likely to attempt suicide. Men tend to use more violent means such as guns, hanging, or jumping, although women are more likely to use drug overdose in a suicide attempt.

14. How is suicide most commonly attempted?

The most common method in suicide attempts is drug ingestion (psychoactive and acetaminophen drugs). In 20% of the cases, two or more methods or a combination of methods is used in attempted suicides that increase the risk of death.

15. Should I take a suicide gesture serious if the used method wasn't lethal?

Any suicidal act or threat must be taken very seriously. If a person threatens suicide, s/he is in immediate crisis and should be cared for immediately. Friends or family may have missed previous warning signs and the person is "crying for help."

16. Provide a tool that can help identify the risk of suicide in a patient.

SAD PERSONS is an acronym that may assist the triage nurse in identifying the risk of suicide in the patient.

Sex	Male	1 point
Age	<19, >45	1 point
Depression	Mood disturbance Somatic symptoms	2 points
Psychiatric care Previous attempts	Formal psychiatric history	1 point
Ethanol Excessive drug use	History of excessive alcohol or drug use	1 point
Rational thinking	Loss, psychosis Severe depression	2 points
Social supports Single	Single, separated Widowed, divorced	1 point
Organized plan	Serious, well-planned attempt/ideation	2 points
No social support	Interpersonal isolation No significant other	1 point
Sickness States future intent	History of debilitating illness Determined to repeat	2 points

Total >8 = very high risk of suicide

17. Should I avoid asking a patient if they have any thoughts about suicide? I don't want to give the person any ideas.

You will not initiate suicidal thoughts or actions by asking questions about it. The person many require prompting to verbalize their suicidal thoughts, but many will appreciate or be relieved at the opportunity to talk about them. They often have ambivalent feelings about the suicide.

18. What should I evaluate when the person admits to having suicidal thoughts?

A patient with threats of suicide should be evaluated for a plan and intent. Ask about:
- Content and duration of the suicidal thoughts
- Changes in the suicide thoughts and how the patient is controlling them
- Hopelessness
- Impulsivity
- Alcohol and other substance abuse

19. Provide more specifics about what I should determine regarding these areas.

- Has a plan been formulated or implemented?
- Are the means to carry out this plan available or readily accessible and does the patient know how to use these means?
- Have preparations been made such as hoarding pills, writing or changing a will, writing a suicide note? Has the patient practiced the suicidal act or already tried to commit suicide?
- Is there a specific method (place and time)?
- What is the expected outcome of the suicide plan? Do they think about dying and how often?
- Do they think they would be better off dead?
- Are there support systems to the patient? Is there anyone among their family or friends that would make them less likely to kill themselves?
- Are there recent stressors that make it difficult for the patient to cope?
- Has the patient attempted suicide in the past and is there a history of suicide in the family?

Health care personnel would internally also consider:
- How lethal is the plan?
- Is there a chance of a rescue?

20. List some significant historical factors that a family member or friend might relate.

- Vague but good-bye or leaving theme (giving away possessions)
- Sudden change in behavior, especially calmness, after a history of anxiety or agitation
- Specific statements about suicide or self-harm
- Preoccupation with death

- Overwhelming sense of shame, guilt, or self-doubt
- Significant life event

21. Who is at the highest risk to attempt suicide?

Patients who have:

- A specific plan
- Lethal means to commit suicide
- Psychosis and are hearing voices telling the person to commit suicide
- Cognitively impairment or lack judgment
- A high risk in those who have attempted suicide and still want to die

22. How do I evaluate the suicide risk in a patient who is intoxicated?

Patients who are intoxicated must be treated for the intoxication before the evaluation for suicide risk can be made.

Suicidal precautions should be maintained until the patient is evaluated and suicidal risk is ruled out.

23. Can I put the patient who presents to triage with suicidal ideation in the waiting room if a parent or friend says he or she will stay with the patient?

This is not recommended, no matter how busy the emergency department (ED) is. It is better to place the patient in a room in the main ED to isolate the patient. The patient should be placed in a room with all clothing and belongings removed and searched for potential weapons to cause self-injury. If it is not a security room, remove any items from the room that can be used as a weapon, including sheets to create a noose. In addition, the patient may need a sitter in the room with them.

24. What is the incidence of suicide in children?

Suicidal thoughts are common in children and adolescents and may not be associated with psychopathology. However, the risk of suicide increases when the thoughts become threats. Suicide attempts are much less common than suicidal ideation.

Approximately 2 million U.S. adolescents attempt suicide each year and are usually associated with psychopathology, especially mood disorder. Suicide is now the third leading cause of death in children age 10 to 14 and ages 15 to 34. Adolescent girls attempt suicide more than boys, but boys are more successful at completing suicide, primarily with firearms.

25. Which children are most at risk of suicide?

Older male children, age 16 to 19 or adolescents of either gender.

26. Provide a tool that can help evaluate a suicidal child.

Press and Khan (2003) suggest the MALPRACTICE acronym can be used to evaluate the suicidal child or adolescent:

Mental Health	Psychiatric diagnosis, taking psychotropic medications, family history of mental health illness
Attempts	When did patient first consider suicide? Has patient tried to harm him/herself before? Did he/she receive medical attention for that attempt?
Lethality	Did the patient want to die, does he/she still want to? Does he/she have access to lethal means?
Plans	Is the patient able to make plans for the future? Will he/she graduate from school? What kind of job will he/she do?
Risk-taking	Engaging in activities that may be disguised attempts at self-harm, engaging in unprotected sexual activity
Alcohol and drugs	Were substances involved in current attempt? How long have substances been used, what substances, when was last use?
Conflict	Is there an interpersonal conflict that precipitated the event?
Trauma	Physical or sexual abuse, witness to violence, recently lost a loved one
Impulsivity	Was the act premeditated? How much planning went into the suicide attempt? Was a suicide note written? Did he/she tell anyone about his/her plans?
Community	Does the patient have a social support system? Resources?
Exposure	Have other family members or friends attempted/completed suicide? Exposure to suicide in the media, attempt part of a suicide epidemic?

27. What should I ask when a patient admits to ingesting a substance?

Ask what the substance was, how much was ingested (have family and friends try to find all the containers or pill bottles and try to determine how many pills or liquid were in the bottles), how long before arrival, and any prehospital treatment.

28. Anything to consider for the toxicology lab value besides the known ingested substances?

Many recommend routinely adding acetaminophen levels on all suicidal patients as a result of its availability and common use in suicide attempts.

29. What does the Canadian Triage and Acuity Scale (CTAS) recommend for patients at risk for suicide?

Level II (emergent, ≤15 minutes): Attempted suicide, history of attempted suicide, and aggressive and/or violent behavior

Level III (urgent ≤30 minutes): Acute psychosis with or without suicidal ideation. These patients are described as not really agitated or violent and reasonably cooperative. They may be emotional but there is some uncertainty regarding whether they are threat to themselves or others. They have normal vital signs.

Level IV (less urgent ≤1 hour): Patients who are complaining of suicidal thoughts or have made gestures but do not seem agitated. These patients should have a responsible person staying with them and periodic reassessments should occur.

The CTAS also indicates patients with depression should also be evaluated for their potential for suicide. All clinicians should show empathy and try to have the patients placed in a quiet and secure area.

30. How about the Australian Triage Scale (ATS)?

Patients with an immediate threat to self or others fall in the ATS II category. Patients who are very distressed with risk of self-harm or deliberate self-harm are categorized as ATS III. The ATS recommends that patients presenting with mental health or behavioral problems should be triaged according to their clinical and situational urgency, as with other ED patients. Where physical and behavioral problems co-exist, the highest appropriate triage category should be applied based on the combined presentation. Evidence of acute deliberate self-harm should be triaged to ATS III or higher.

31. Give the Manchester Triage Scale rating.

Manchester Triage Scale places patients at high risk of harm to others and self as Level 3 (urgent, 60 minutes) and moderate risk to harm others or self as Level 4 (standard, 120 minutes).

Risk of self-harm is defined as whether the patient is actively trying to harm himself or herself or trying to leave with the intent of harming himself or herself. Risk of harm to others is defined by evaluating the patient's posture (tense and clenched), speech patterns (loud and using threatening words), and motor behavior (restless, pacing). High risk should also be assumed if weapons and potential victims are available or if self-control is lost.

32. Provide the Emergency Severity Index (ESI) rating.

Emergency Severity Index (ESI) place suicide attempt/complaint as a High Risk Situation, Level 2.

33. How can we prevent suicide?

- Screening for depression and asking about suicidal thoughts if signs of depression are present.
- Do not ignore any threats or gestures of suicide because the person is asking for help.
- Assess the lethality and potentiality of any suicidal threat or plan.

Key Points

- The U.S. Preventive Services Task Force recommends screening for depression.
- One study found a simple screen for depression in adults was asking "During the past month, have you often been bothered by feeling down, depressed, or hopeless?" and "During the past month have you often been bothered by little interest or pleasure in doing things?"
- Any suicidal act or threat must be taken seriously. Evaluate for plan and intent.
- Patients who are at most risk are those who have a specific plan, lethal means, hearing voices telling them to commit suicide, or cognitively impaired or lack judgment.
- Patients who are suicidal should have personal clothing and belongings (searched for weapons) removed and placed in a safe environment.

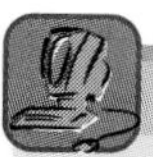

Internet Resources

Canadian Association of Emergency Physicians (CAEP): Implementation Guidelines for the Canadian ED Triage and Acuity Scale (CTAS)
http://www.caep.ca/002.policies/002-02.CTAS/CTAS-guidelines.htm

National Guideline Clearinghouse: The Assessment and Management of People at Risk of Suicide
http://www.guideline.gov/summary/summary.aspx?ss=15&doc_id=4340&nbr=3273

Emergency Nurses Association: Psychiatric Patients in the Emergency Department: How Can the System Respond?
http://www.ena.org/publications/OnlineConnection/2004/Apr/PsychiatricPatientsInED.asp

Bibliography

Alexopoulos G: Mood disorders. In Kaplan H, Sadock B, editors: *Kaplan and Sadock's comprehensive textbook of psychiatry,* Philadelphia, 2000, Lippincott, Williams & Wilkins.

American Academy of Child and Adolescent Psychiatry: Practice parameter for the assessment and treatment of children and adolescents with suicidal behavior: *J Am Acad Child Adolesc Psych* 40 (7 suppl):24S-51S, 2001.

American Psychiatric Association: Practice guideline for the assessment and treatment of patients with suicidal behaviors, 117, 2003.

Arroll B, et al: Screening for depression in primary care with two verbally asked questions: Cross sectional study, *Br Med J* 327:1144-1146, 2003.

Australasian College for Emergency Medicine (ACEM): Policy Document—The Australasian Triage Scale, ACEM [serial online], 2000, available: http://acem.org/au./open/documents/triage, accessed March 4, 2004.

Australasian College for Emergency Medicine (ACEM): Guidelines for Implementation of the Australasian Triage Scale in emergency departments, ACEM [serial online], 2000, available: http://www.acem.org.au/open/documentas/triageguide, accessed Nov 4, 2004.

Canadian Association of Emergency Physicians: Canadian Emergency Department Triage and Acuity Scale implementation guidelines, 1(3 suppl), 1999.

Centers for Disease Control and Prevention: Suicide and attempted suicide, *MMWR* 53(22):471, 2004.

Gilboy N, et al: Emergency severity index, Des Plaines, Ill, 2003, Emergency Nurses Association.

Kennebeck S: Suicidal behavior in children and adolescents, *UpToDate Online* 11:3, 2003.

Mackway-Jones K: *Emergency triage,* Manchester Triage Group, London, 1997, BMJ Publishing.

Press BR, Khan SA: (From Kennebeck S: *UpToDate* reprint, *Curr Opin Pediatr* 9:237, 1997), 2003.

Rund DA, Nockowitz RA: Depression and suicide. In Markovchick VJ, Pons PT, editors: *Pons' emergency medicine secrets,* ed 3, Philadelphia, 2003, Hanley & Belfus.

US Preventive Services Task Force: Recommendations. *Ann Intern Med* 163(2):760, 2003.

Zimmermann, PG: Tricks for the ED trade, *J Emerg Nurs* 29(5):453-458, 2003.

Chapter 54

Toxicologic Emergencies

Susan Bednar and Jerrold Blair Leikin

Poisonings are responsible for more than 1 million emergency department (ED) visits annually in the United States, with more than two thirds of them involving children. The fact is, *all* chemicals have the potential to be poisonous, if given in large enough doses. For confirmation of this fact, one can open any clinical pharmacology textbook and note therapeutic agents that can lead to specific toxic syndromes. Despite the potential for the wide range of clinical presentations as a result of a virtually unlimited amount of toxins, <0.05% of all poison exposures called to a poison control center result in death. It is evident that if one follows a consistent treatment algorithm of the poisoned patient, the outcome will be favorable in the vast majority of cases.

The intent of this chapter is to review what questions the RN should consider when triaging the patient with a suspected ingestion/overdose, and practical advice (in the form of "commonly asked questions") on what to do with that information. We will also review "red flags" or symptoms/complaints that require immediate action. Finally we will provide some resources to help guide your care of the patient with a suspected or known overdose/ingestion.

1. What information is most important when triaging a patient with suspected overdose/ingestion?

It's important to get as much detailed information that you can about the incident. What they took, the amount they took, when they took it, and the route of exposure are all salient questions. If an overdose attempt is suspected, family and the patient's physician may be able to give more detailed information regarding the patients' motives. The old chart may be invaluable for this information as are any pharmacy records. If accidental ingestion/exposure, witnesses to the event or emergency medical technicians (EMTs) on the scene might be able to provide more information.

Although attempting to obtain the history of a suspected overdose/ingestion (accidental or intentional) is important, it is often unreliable and/or inaccurate. Take home message here—don't spend a lot of time at triage trying to figure out the specifics. A physical examination (including vital signs) is more helpful in that it allows the examiner to objectively identify any physical abnormalities present.

2. We are big on "less is more" in the ED. Is there a "toxicology algorithm" that we can use in the ED for quick reference?

The recommended treatment plan for the poisoned patient is not unlike general treatment plans taught in advanced cardiac life support (ACLS) or advanced trauma life support (ATLS) courses. In this manner, the initial approach to the poisoned patient should essentially be the same in every case, irrespective of the toxin ingested, just as the initial approach to the trauma patient is the same irrespective of the mechanism of injury. This approach, which can be termed as routine poison management, essentially includes the following aspects, the first three of which are especially applicable for the triage nurse.

- Stabilization: "ABCs" (airway, breathing, circulation): administration of glucose, thiamine, oxygen, and naloxone
- History, physical examination leading toward the identification of class toxin (toxidrome recognition)
- Prevention of absorption (decontamination)
- Specific antidote, if available
- Removal of absorbed toxin (enhancing excretion)
- Support and monitoring for adverse effects
- If discharged, preventative education and environmental detoxification

3. Are there common groups of physical findings that lead the clinician to suspect a specific category of toxins?

With so many things that can be "ingested" or "overdosed on" where do you start in trying to figure out what the patient might have taken/ingested? Clues that clinicians discover on the physical examination have been grouped into specific symptom complexes called "toxidromes." Toxidromes are grouped, physiologically based abnormalities of vital signs, general appearance, skin, eyes, mucous membranes, lungs, heart, abdomen, and neurologic examination that are known to occur with specific classes of substances and typically are helpful in establishing a diagnosis when the exposure is not well defined (Tintanelli, p. 1016).

Examples of toxidromes can be seen in the following table:

CLASSIFICATION OF TOXINS (TOXIDROMES)
Examples of Toxidromes

Toxidromes	Pattern	Example of Drugs	Treatment Approach
Anticholinergic	Fever, ileus, flushing, tachycardia, urinary retention, inability to sweat, visual blurring, and mydriasis. Central manifestations include myoclonus, choreoathetosis, toxic psychosis with lilliputian hallucinations, seizures, and coma.	Antihistamines Atropine Baclofen Benztropine Jimson weed Methylpyroline Phenothiazines Propantheline Tricyclic antidepressants	Physostigmine for life-threatening symptoms*
Carbolic marasmus	Headache, dizziness, salivation, anorexia, and skin pigmentation changes	Phenol	Lavage/activated charcoal (AC) with cathartic Possible endoscopy
Cholinergic	Characterized by salivation, lacrimation, urination, defecation, gastrointestinal (GI) cramps, and emesis ("sludge"). Bradycardia and bronchoconstriction may also be seen.	Carbamate Organophosphates Pilocarpine	Atropine* Pralidoxime for organophosphate insecticides
Extrapyramidal	Choreoathetosis, hyperreflexia, trismus, opisthotonos, rigidity, and tremor	Haloperidol Phenothiazines	Diphenhydramine Benztropine
Hallucinogenic	Perceptual distortions, synesthesia, depersonalization, and derealization	Amphetamines Cannabinoids Cocaine Indole alkaloids Phencyclidine	Benzodiazepine
Metal fume fever	Pleuritic chest pain, cough, dyspnea, thirst, metallic taste, fever (temperature ranges from 102°F to 104°F), tachycardia, chills, nausea, myalgia	Most common: Zinc and copper Also: Cadmium, mercury	Supportive (usually resolves within 2 days) Avoidance of further exposure

Continued

CLASSIFICATION OF TOXINS (TOXIDROMES)—*cont'd*
Examples of Toxidromes

Toxidromes	Pattern	Example of Drugs	Treatment Approach
Monosodium glutamate symptom complex	Burning sensation of back of neck, forearm, and chest; numbness in back of neck radiating to arms and back; tingling, warmth, and weakness in facial area, temples, upper back, neck, and arms; facial pressure or tightness, chest pain, headache, nausea, tachycardia, bronchospasm, drowsiness, weakness	Monosodium glutamate	Usually self-limited; diphenhydramine may be useful
Narcotic	Altered mental status, unresponsiveness, shallow respirations, slow respiratory rate or periodic breathing, miosis, bradycardia, hypothermia	Opiates Dextromethorphan Pentazocine Propoxyphene	Naloxone*
Retinoic acid syndrome	Fever, dyspnea (60%), arrhythmias (23%), tachycardia, hypotension, cardiac failure (6%), respiratory distress, nausea, vomiting (57%), renal failure (seen in patients with acute promyelocytic leukemia treated with >45 mg/m^2 per day of tretinoin)	Tretinoin	Dexamethasone (10 mg intramuscularly [IM] every 12 hours for 3 or more days)
Sedative/ Hypnotic	Manifested by sedation with progressive deterioration of central nervous system (CNS) function. Coma, stupor, confusion apnea, delirium, or	Anticonvulsants Antipsychotics Barbiturates Benzodiazepines Ethanol Ethchlorvynol Fentanyl	Naloxone* (opiates) Flumazenil* (benzodiazepines) Urinary alkalinization (barbiturates)

CLASSIFICATION OF TOXINS (TOXIDROMES)—*cont'd*
Examples of Toxidromes

Toxidromes	Pattern	Example of Drugs	Treatment Approach
	hallucinations may accompany this pattern.	Glutethimide Meprobamate Methadone Methocarbamol Opiates Quinazolines Propoxyphene	
Epileptogenic†	May mimic stimulant pattern with hyperthermia, hyperreflexia, and tremors being prominent signs	Anticholinergics Camphor Chlorinated hydrocarbons Cocaine Isoniazid Lidocaine Lindane Nicotine Phencyclidine Strychnine Xanthines	Anticonvulsants (although generally not phenytoin) Pyridoxine for isoniazid* Extracorporeal removal of drug (i.e., lindane, camphor, xanthines) Physostigmine for anticholinergic agents* Avoid phenytoin
Serotonin†	Confusion, myoclonus, hyperreflexia, diaphoresis tremor, facial flushing, diarrhea, fever, trismus	Clomipramine Fluoxetine Isoniazid L-tryptophan Paroxetine Phenelzine Sertraline Tranylcypromine Drug combinations include: monoamine oxidase (MAO) inhibitors with L-tryptophan Fluoxetine or meperidine Fluoxetine with carbamazepine or sertraline	Withdrawal of drug/ benzodiazepine Beta-blocker (?) Cyproheptadine (?)

Continued

CLASSIFICATION OF TOXINS (TOXIDROMES)—*cont'd*
Examples of Toxidromes

Toxidromes	Pattern	Example of Drugs	Treatment Approach
		Clomipramine and meclobemide Tramadol and buspirone Paroxetine and dextromethorphan	
Solvent	Lethargy, confusion, dizziness, headache, restlessness, incoordination, derealization, depersonalization	Acetone Chlorinated hydrocarbons Hydrocarbons Naphthalene Trichloroethane Toluene	Avoid catecholamines
Stimulant	Restlessness, excessive speech and motor activity, tachycardia, tremor, and insomnia—may progress to seizure. Other effects noted include euphoria, mydriasis, anorexia, and paranoia.	Amphetamine Caffeine (xanthines) Cocaine Ephedrine/ pseudoephedrine Methylphenidate Nicotine Phencyclidine	Benzodiazepines
Uncoupling of oxidative phosphory- lation	Hyperthermia, tachypnea, diaphoresis, metabolic acidosis (usually)	Aluminum phosphide Aspirin/salicylates 2.4-Dichlorophenol Dinitrophenols Dintrocresols Glyphosate (?) Hexachlorobutadiene Phosphorus Pentachlorophenol Tin (?) Zinc phosphide	Sodium bicarbonate to treat metabolic acidosis Patient cooling techniques Avoidance of atropine or salicylate agents Hemodialysis may be required for acidosis treatment.

*From Nice A, Leikin JB, Maturen A, et al: Toxidrome recognition to improve efficiency of emergency urine drug screens, *Ann Emerg Med* 17:676-680, 1988.
†Poisoning toxicology handbook, 1978-2003 by Lexi-Comp, Inc.

Within the toxidromes are common physical findings along with examples of drugs that can cause that particular pattern of physical findings.

4. **Can you talk about abnormal vital signs at triage and common physical findings with the suspected overdose/exposure/ingestion patient and specific drugs/toxins?**

   Instead of trying to commit this information to memory, what might help here is a quick reference for the triage nurse. The following boxes list drugs that commonly increase vital signs and those that commonly decrease vital signs.

Agents That Increase Vital Signs

Antihistamines
Anticholinergic agents
Sympathomimetic agents
Theophylline/caffeine
Cocaine
Lysergic acid diethylamide
Narcotic/drug withdrawal
Nicotine
Amphetamines
Mushrooms (amarita, muscaria)
Antidepressants (MAO inhibitors and tricyclic antidepressants)
Methylphenidate
Atropine
Salicylates
Pentachlorophenol
Dinitrophenol

Agents That Decrease Vital Signs

Carbamazepine
Choral hydrate
Clonidine
Colchicine
Ethchlorvynol
Glutethimide
Guanabenz
Guanfacine
Maprotiline
Opioid agents
Naphazoline
Barbiturates
Phenytoin
Prazosin
Rivastigmine
Benzodiazepine
Baclofen

A bit of discussion on the effects of different categories of drugs and their effects is warranted. Sympathomimetics (i.e., cocaine, amphetamines) and anticholinergics (i.e., atropine, most antihistamines, Scopolamine) essentially cause an increase in all of the vital signs parameters. This is particularly true for cocaine intoxication, in which it has been noted that hyperthermia may be a particularly ominous sign for mortality. Conversely, organophosphates, opiates (i.e., heroin, morphine), barbiturates, beta blockers, benzodiazepines, alcohol, and clonidine toxicities result in hypothermia, respiratory depression, and bradycardia.

Tremors, reflexes, pupillary findings, nystagmus, and even the nature of seizures can be useful diagnostic tools. Like hallucinations, seizures caused by specific toxins can exhibit certain specific properties. For example strychnine is unique in that it can cause generalized seizures while the patient is alert. This can be referred to as a "spinal seizure." Other drug-induced seizures will respond only to specific antidotal therapies and not to conventional antiseizure medication. Examples of this property include anticholinergic-induced seizures, which may respond to physostigmine, and isoniazid-induced seizures, which respond to pyridoxine. Additionally, theophylline-induced seizures rarely respond to phenytoin alone and often only to multidrug therapy.

In addition to these physical signs, *odors* emanating from the patient may also provide important directions in management. For example, a garlic odor is often caused by arsenicals, phosphorus compounds, or organophosphates. A rotten egg odor can be associated with decomposition of organic materials (hydrogen sulfide) or disulfiram.

5. What are the most common drug interactions that lead to toxicities?

The following is a list of commonly used agents that can lead to drug toxicity.

- **Anticoagulants:** Coumadin administered with alcohol, macrolides, sulfonamides, azole antifungals, and amiodarone can increase the effects of the coumadin
- **Antimicrobials:** Rifampin, erythromycin, isoniazid, and azole antifungals can cause problems by either inducing or inhibiting hepatic and renal metabolism of other drugs
- **Serotonin syndrome** (see following box)

Serotonin Syndrome

Diagnostic Criteria for Serotonin Syndrome

* Recent addition or dosage increase of any agent increasing serotonin activity or availability (usually within 1 day)
* Absence of abused substances, metabolic infectious etiology, or withdrawal
* No recent addition or dosage increase of a neuroleptic agent prior to onset of signs and symptoms
* Presence of three or more of the following: (% incidence)

Agitation (34%)
Abdominal pain (4%)
Ataxia/incoordination (40%)
Diaphoresis (45%)
Diarrhea (80%)
Hyperpyrexia (45%)
Hypertension/hypotension (35%)
Hyperthermia
Hyperreflexia (52%)
Mental status change-cognitive behavioral changes
Anxiety (15%)
Euphoria/hypomania (21%)
Confusion (51%)
Agitation (34%)
Disorientation
Coma/unresponsiveness (29%)
Muscle rigidity (51%)
Mydriasis
Myoclonus (58%)
Nausea (23%)
Nystagmus (15%)
Restlessness/hyperactivity (48%)
Salivation (2%)
Seizures (12%)
Shivering (26%)
Sinus tachycardia (36%)
Tachypnea (26%)
Tremor (43%)
Unreactive pupils (20%)

Drugs (as Single Causative Agent) That Can Induce Serotonin Syndrome

Specific serotonin reuptake inhibitors (SSRIs)
Clomipramine
MDMA (Ecstasy)
Mirtazapine

Drug Combinations That Can Induce Serotonin Syndrome*

Alprazolam—Clomipramine
Bromocriptine—Levodopa/carbidopa
Buspirone—Fluoxetine
Buspirone—Trazodone
Citalopram—Moclobemide
Clomipramine—Clorgiline
Clomipramine—Lithium

6. More people are taking herbal supplements than ever before. Are there any herbal medicines that interact adversely with prescribed drugs? Which are the interactions that the clinician should be concerned about?

Because herbal supplements are not strictly regulated by the Food and Drug Administration, information regarding interactions is limited. See the Internet Resources Box at the end of this chapter for some websites that provide information on specific substances.

7. What are the most common drugs on which people intentionally overdose?

The most common drugs that people overdose on intentionally are analgesic agents. In fact, according to the 2002 annual report of the American Association of Poison Control Centers Toxic Exposure Surveillance System, analgesics, sedatives, and tricyclic antidepressants are associated with the largest number of drug-related deaths than any other classes of medication. It should be noted that only 2% of poisoning deaths involve children who are under 6 years old.

Tricyclics (TCAs) are well-absorbed from the GI tract and difficult to remove once absorbed. So limiting the amount of time these patients spend at triage is paramount.

The symptoms of TCA toxicity fall into three distinct categories, neurotoxicity, cardiotoxicity, and anticholinergic effects. Common findings with neurotoxicity are lethargy, hallucinations, and seizure activity. Cardiac symptoms include hypotension, electrocardiogram (ECG) changes (ST and T wave abnormalities, prolonged QT intervals, bradycardia). Anticholinergic effects include flushed skin, dry mucous membranes, anxiety, tachycardia, hyperthermia, and urinary retention. Key points for nursing care are the following:

- Because CNS depression can develop quickly, do not induce vomiting.
- AC binds TCAs well: give it promptly! (if airway patency is a concern, endotracheal intubation prior to charcoal administration is needed).
- All patients with TCA overdose must have continuous cardiac monitoring.
- Consider sodium bicarbonate administration as needed.

Point to consider: Many times you will not know "what" the patient ingested. Because of the gravity of a tricyclic overdose/ingestion, if the patient has any symptoms of a tricyclic overdose (i.e., lethargy, electrocardiogram [ECG] changes, hyperthermia, hypotension) they should be treated as if they did overdose on/ingest tricyclics, until proven otherwise.

8. What are the most common drugs that people overdose on accidentally?

The most common drugs that people overdose on accidentally are iron, acetaminophen, and salicylates.

9. In and around the household, what do children most commonly ingest?

Common things that are nontoxic:

- Crayons

- Common household plants
- Chalk
- Coins
- Small plastic toys
- Foil, cellophane, paper, and other candy wrappers
- Small amounts of soap or detergent

Common things that are toxic:

- Pesticides, gardening stuff, diazinon, plants (lily of the valley)
- Foxglove plants (contain digitalis)
- Bleach
- Iron-containing vitamins
- Folk remedies such as Oil of Wintergreen, Iodine, Mercury or other heavy metals, assorted over-the-counter (OTC) vitamin preparations, and aphrodisiacs
- Adult medications such as discarded patches of nicotine, nitroglycerin, Cardizem, or estrogen/testosterone
- Adult medications such as tablets of aspirin, acetaminophen, opioid analgesics, just about anything in Grandma's medicine cabinet

10. How is absorption of the ingested substance averted?

There are essentially four modes of gastric decontamination that work to prevent absorption of the substance:

- Emesis (which is no longer utilized)
- Gastric lavage (rarely utilized)
- Whole-bowel irrigation (used for iron, lithium, sustained-release medications, and body packers/stuffers)
- AC (most commonly used decontamination method. It can be used usually up to 2 hours post-ingestion)

11. When should ipecac be used? When should charcoal be used?

The use of syrup of ipecac has become increasingly unpopular in the management of acute ingestions for several reasons:

- It is seldom used in the emergency room (ER) because it is ineffective if time since ingestion is greater than 30 to 60 minutes.
- One hundred percent rate of emesis does not equal 100% rate of removal of toxin.
- Not effective for drugs that are rapidly absorbed.
- Syrup of ipecac has an unpredictable onset of action and intensity of effect.
- No longer the agent of choice for GI decontamination and should not be utilized.

AC, on the other hand, is one of the most important therapeutic interventions for the management of most toxic ingestions. AC works by allowing the toxin to be adsorbed to the charcoal within the lumen of the gut, and not into the tissues. The dose of AC commonly used is 1 g/kg. It is either administered via a nasogastric or Ewald tube, or given orally (mixed with juice). Charcoal can be used with any ingestion of a drug known to absorb it, and you can give it to patients with "unknown ingestions," as long as the patient's airway is protected.

12. What kinds of measures are taken to promote elimination?

- Urinary alkalinization (used for salicylate and Phenobarbital overdoses)
- Multiple dosing of charcoal
- Forced diuresis (rarely used)
- Hemodialysis (used for toxic alcohols and lithium)
- Hemoperfusion (only used 30 times in 2002)

13. What resources are available to help me in the ED?

The following phone number is the most valuable piece of information that the triage nurse can have at her fingertips in the ED. I encourage you to post it in several places in the ED (at triage, on the phones, at the charge desk). A triage nurse in any state can pick up the phone and dial **1-800-222-1222** and be directly connected to a poison control center to assist with information and patient management. These are the people that can help you ask the right questions and will review for you and the physician the treatment plan. Most hospitals also have access to Micromedex.

14. List some types of hazardous materials exposure.

- Accidental
- Intentional
- Chemical
- Biologic
- Nuclear

15. What agents have been used intentionally to create a hazardous exposure (terrorist activity)?

Ricin and sarin. Ricin is made from the castor bean. It is hazardous only if injected. However, its deadly nature promotes fear from the powder form even though it is nontoxic. Sarin or nerve gas has been used on the Tokyo subway with lethal effect. Fortunately those are the only two at the time of this writing. Anthrax is a microbe rather than a poison, so it is discussed elsewhere.

16. What should I do if someone walks into triage and I think that they have been exposed to an aerosolized chemical?

Take them to a decontamination room and have them shower immediately. If a decontamination room is not available, then keep them outside (in a protected area if possible), but out of the main ED in which the fumes can spread and possibly contaminate other patients and staff.

17. What substances are most dangerous with an "ocular exposure"?

Both acid and alkali exposures to the eye can be blinding. However, alkalis can penetrate the cornea quickly and thus can cause extensive damage. Treatment includes immediate flushing affected eye(s) with normal saline (NS) wash using a Morgan lens for 30 to 40 minutes. The pH should be checked until the runoff solution is either neutral or slightly acidic.

18. Can you talk a bit about common mistakes that you—as a toxicologist—see with emergent care of the overdose/exposed patient?

Top mistakes:

- Use of excessive sorbitol (it can promote vomiting)
- Use of ipecac
- Not recognizing medicines, which can cause delayed toxicity (i.e., iron, acetaminophen, lithium)
- Underestimating the effects of chronic supratherapeutic toxicity
- Missing carbon monoxide poisoning

Key Points

- History of ingestion is unreliable, so get patient to treatment area quickly.
- Clinical examination focuses on toxidrome.
- Common intentional drug ingestants are analgesics, sedatives, and antidepressants.
- Chemical splash to eye should have immediate eye irrigation.
- Oral ingestion should involve some gastric decontamination.
- Ipecac is rarely used in acute ingestion in the ER.
- Suspect poisoning any time there is unusual metabolic state/abnormal vital signs at triage.
- AC can be useful if given early.
- Ask about all medication and hazardous materials exposure.
- For a child, remember access can equal exposure.
- The confused patient is not competent to leave against medical advice (AMA) and should be kept until they have regained mental capacity to leave knowing the risks.

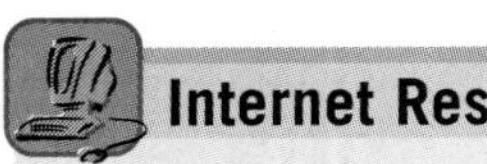

Internet Resources

The Natural Medicines Comprehensive Database
http://www.naturaldatabase.com

The NIH Office of Dietary Supplements
http://dietary-supplements.info.nih.gov/

IBIDS Consumer Database
http://ods.od.nih.gov/Health_Information/IBIDS_Overview.aspx

CBRNE—Ricin
http://www.emedicine.com/emerg/topic889.htm

Ricin Emergency Response Card
http://www.bt.cdc.gov/agent/ricin/erc9009-86-3pr.asp

Ricin Fact Sheet
http://www.bt.cdc.gov/agent/ricin/facts.asp

Sarin Emergency Response Card
http://www.bt.cdc.gov/agent/sarin/erc107-44-8.asp

Sarin Fact Sheet
http://www.bt.cdc.gov/agent/sarin/basics/facts.asp

The Poisoned Patient: The Overdosed and the Underdosed
http://www.enw.org/TOX.htm

Management of the Poisoned/Overdosed Patient
http://www.uspharmacist.com/ce/poisoning/default.htm

Bibliography

Delgado G, Pilarowski J: Principles of drug interactions. In Tintanelli, editor: *Emergency medicine: A comprehensive study guide,* New York, 2004, McGraw Hill.

Delgado G, Pilarowski J: Principles of drug interactions. In Criddle L, editor: *Toxicologic emergencies: Emergency nursing,* St Louis, 1999, Mosby.

Hack J, Hoffman R: Toxicology and pharmacology. In Tintanelli J, editor: *Emergency medicine: A comprehensive study guide,* New York, 2004, McGraw Hill.

Keyes DC, Dart RC: Initial diagnosis and treatment of the poisoned patient. In Dart RC, editor: *Medical toxicology,* ed 3, Philadelphia, 2004, Lippincott, Williams & Wilkins.

McCaig L, Burt C: Poisoning-related visits to emergency departments in the United States 1993-1996, *J Toxicol Clin Toxicol* 37(7):817, 1999.

Nice A, Leikin, JB, Mauturen A, et al: Toxidrome recognition to improve efficiency of emergency urine drug screens, *Ann Emerg Med* 17(7):676-680, 1998.

Watson WA, Litovitz TL, Rodgers GC, et al: 2002 Annual report of the American Association of Poison Control Centers Toxic Exposure Surveillance System, *Am J Emerg Med* 21(5):353-421, 2003.

Chapter 55

Differentiating Dementia from Delirium

Karen L. Rice and Joseph E. Williams

1. Define delirium.

Delirium is an acute, reversible state of agitated confusion. Common causes include drug and alcohol withdrawal, medication side effects, infections, hypoxia, electrolyte imbalance, and surgery/trauma.

2. Define dementia.

Dementia is a memory disorder, which generally occurs gradually over a period of time. There are exceptions, such as the result of stroke or brain injury (e.g., trauma, neurosurgical procedure).

In addition to problems with memory, the individual must have at least one other capability affected: judgment, thinking, language, visual-spatial perception (coordination), emotional behavior or personality, or cognitive skills. The symptoms associated with dementia are related to the type (e.g., Alzheimer's, multi-infarct, Lewy Body, Pick's disease), and the area of the affected brain.

Generally, early stages of dementia may be limited to poor short-term memory recall and may not be obvious to the casual observer. However, as the disease progresses, functional independence becomes compromised because of a decline in both cognitive and physical abilities to function.

3. How prevalent is Alzheimer's disease?

It is estimated that 10% of people over age 65 and 50% of those over age 85 have Alzheimer's disease. It is often not officially diagnosed. The Alzheimer's Association estimates that up to 12% of patients seen in primary care fail to be diagnosed at an early stage.

4. Compare the differences between age-appropriate changes in memory loss and dementia.

Dementia differs from expected age-related changes in cognition by the severity and progressive nature of cognitive decline. Anyone can become distracted and lose track of the house key. The person with dementia will not remember what the keys are for.

- Normal age-related memory impairment may entail forgetting parts of an experience, but remembering it happened. Patients with dementia forget the entire experience and are rarely able to recall it.
- Normal age-related memory impairment is associated with the ability to follow directions and keep helpful notes. Patients with dementia are gradually unable to follow any direction or to use notes as an aid.
- Those with normal age-related memory impairment are aware, and usually bothered by, the effects of age-related memory difficulties. In comparison, the patient with dementia is usually unaware of memory dysfunction and the family is often the first to notice.

5. Are there clues to early mild dementia?

An early clue is the patient's inability to perform a new task or retain new information. Although the diagnosis of dementia should occur in the primary care setting, it's not uncommon for the emergency department (ED) to be the first to suspect the diagnosis. Studies report that approximately 30 months prior to the establishment of a dementia diagnosis, certain clues are manifested. These may include:

- New onset of anxiety
- Forgetfulness
- Depression
- Insomnia
- Paranoid ideation

The early manifestations may underlie frequent presentation for emergency treatment for unexplained chest pain, dyspnea, the same complaint or conditions related to nonadherence with medication regimens. In addition, instances of poor hygiene and malnutrition may also be related to cognitive dysfunction.

6. Why is it important to selectively screen for dementia in the ED?

Although the ED is not the most suitable environment to screen for dementia, screening of certain patients may be appropriate. Older patients seen frequently in the ED for accident-related injuries, unsubstantiated complaints, and events related to medication noncompliance should be screened because of the likelihood that these are symptoms of an underlying dementia.

Although Folstein's Mini Mental State Exam is an accepted method to screen for cognitive dysfunction, its length and dependence on patient cooperation makes it frequently difficult to administer. Screening tests of executive function are likely to be more useful in the ED. These include Royall's Clox clock drawing, the Controlled Oral Word Association Test, and the Trailmaking Test (www.hartfordign.org).

7. Describe the clock test.

The nurse draws a circle on a piece of paper and asks the patient to put in the numbers as they appear on the face of the clock, then asks the patient to draw the hands to read a specific time, such as 10:40.

To score the test, the nurse divides the clock drawing into eighths, assigning a point for each number that is in the right octant of the circle and a point for each proper hand position. The numbers 12, 3, 6, and 9 are not counted. A perfect score is 10 points; less than 8 is a mild impairment. Less than 5 points is considered a severe impairment.

8. It seems so basic. I can't believe it works.

In one true illustrative example, the family brought in their mother for symptoms that were a result of subtherapeutic medication levels, although the woman denied any nonadherence. Was this an issue of needing more drugs? We knew the answer when she made the clock drawing with the number running horizontally, like a calendar, and insisted it was like a clock. Older adults sometimes hide their increasing disability, even from themselves.

9. Discuss the effects of dementia on a patient's ability to communicate.

As the disease progresses, the person with dementia has a decreased ability to communicate.

- New stimuli cannot be properly processed or retained. Reorienting will not work because it must be continuous to be effective.
- All environmental events can be perceived as vague threats because the person cannot understand.
- The person is incapable of behaving differently; the nurse must modify his or her approach to be effective.

10. List approaches that can help in communicating with patients with dementia.

- *Always identify yourself and call the patient by his or her name during every interaction.* The person will not remember you. Include gentle physical contact, unless the person withdraws (stand a handshake's distance away)
- *Always face the patient, approaching slowly, with eye contact.* Place a light behind the patient (not the nurse) to illuminate the nurse's face. As we age, up to 50% more light is required for the same sight ability.
- *Try to place the person in an environment with limited extraneous stimuli.* When they are right next to the nursing station, they cannot separate out important information from the commotion.
- *Speak slow, short, simple phrases, with one thought at a time.* For example, avoid "When did the pain start and what does it feel like?"
- *Initiate asking about complaints.* In patients with dementia, up to 80% to 90% of the interaction is provided by the staff. Rather than say, "Any pain anywhere?" or wait for the patient to ask for pain medication, ask specifically, "Does it hurt here? Here?"
- *Avoid jargon.* Keep the content concrete. The person will literally interpret statements, such as "hop into bed" or "going to the floor."
- *Avoid varying the terms used if a question is repeated.* Many nurses are used to trying another word if the patient has problems processing a question.

For instance, with someone who has limited English, the nurse might ask, "Does this hurt? Pain? Ouch?" With dementia, it takes the person longer to process the inquiry. Changing the word starts the intellectual process all over again from the beginning—keep it the same each time.

- *Phrase communications positively.* Research shows that excessive use of "no" or demanding commands ("Hold still!") actually increases resistance. Say, "You can rest here," versus "Don't get up!"
- *Reinforce safety and comfort.* The patient is able to feel emotions even as language difficulties set it. A frequent reference to "home" is often actually a cry for security and reassurance. Remind the patient often that you are here and will take care of them, not that they can't go home.
- *Consider a different nurse if the patient responds negatively.* We tend to assume that the patient must adjust to whomever they have as the nurse but try a total different individual (e.g., young male instead of older woman; black instead of white nurse). The patient cannot distinguish the nurse and that role from the person's characteristics that may be similar to a past negative person or experience.
- *Consider a "therapeutic fib."*

11. Explain the "therapeutic fib" concept.

Championed by Alzheimer care expert Carly Hellen, the approach focuses on providing emotional comfort. The physical changes in the person's brain make it impossible for the patient to comprehend and assimilate the new information for them.

For instance, if a woman with advanced dementia says "I have to go home to feed the baby." That is her reality: imagine how concerning that is to her to believe she has a hungry baby at home. It does not help to remind her she is too old to have a baby. Instead, reassure her that someone is already feeding the baby for her.

12. Talk about safety.

Falls are always a risk and concern. Try diversional activity, such as music, TV, activity, or even toys. One ED had great success with a water-filled infant's "pillow" that contained floating objects.

13. Describe and compare delirium to dementia.

In contrast to dementia, delirium reflects a clinical state rather than a disease. An acute, sudden onset, fluctuation of mental status, and disturbances of the sleep/wake cycle characterize delirium. Generally, visual and/or auditory hallucinations in the older adult population suggest delirium rather than dementia. Symptoms can fluctuate throughout the day, but tend to be worse at night. Delirium accounts for 10% to 15% of admissions to acute care hospitals.

14. List some causes of delirium.

- Medical conditions (liver, heart, or renal failure)
- Withdrawal from medications/new medication
- Alcohol withdrawal
- Fluid and electrolyte imbalance
- Acute infection (cellulitis or a urinary tract infection [UTI])

15. Name one of the most obvious differences between dementia and delirium.

Awareness. Although the demented patient is usually alert, the delirious patient exhibits a reduced awareness along with a decreased ability to focus, maintain, or shift attention. The person is often oriented to person, but not time or place. However, because of the fluctuation of symptoms, delirium can be present in an oriented patient.

16. Recommend a tool to use for evaluation of delirium.

Although there are many useful tools for the evaluation of delirium, the Confusion Assessment Measurement (CAM) has been reported to be useful in the ED setting.

17. Can a patient have both dementia and delirium?

Although dementia and delirium are different, the demented patient may present with delirium. Similarly a presentation of delirium may be the first clue of an underlying dementia that has not been diagnosed. In fact, one third to one half of delirious patients have an underlying dementia.

18. Who is at risk for delirium?

Patients with dementia are at a two-to-five increased risk for developing delirium. Other predisposing factors include:

- Preexisting cognitive dysfunction or dementia
- History of stroke
- Chronic renal insufficiency
- Parkinson's disease
- Cancer
- Multiple comorbidity or any severe underlying illness
- Advanced age (>75 years)
- Dehydration
- Malnutrition
- Visual or hearing impairment

19. What medications commonly affect mental status?

All medications pose a potential risk for inducing a mental status change, particularly in cases of polypharmacy (>8 medications). However, commonly used medications that exert a mood altering effect (e.g., opioids, benzodiazepines, ethyl alcohol, tricyclic antidepressants), nonsteroidal anti-inflammatory agents, steroids, lithium, anti-Parkinson drugs, and those that negatively impact acetylcholine levels (e.g., histamine blockers, anticholinergics, antiemetics) likely pose the greatest risk of confusion or impaired judgment. Similarly, withdrawal syndromes related to abrupt cessation of ethyl alcohol, opioids, or benzodiazepines may present as an acute confusion.

20. What is meant by the term "a change in mental status"?

A mental status change in the general population is defined as a change in the ability to appropriately respond to mental stimuli, such as specific questions. The definition of a mental status change in the older adult includes any change in daily activities, such as new-onset or sudden anorexia, incontinence, or apathy/depression. Another important change may be associated with the new onset of frequent falls. Although all of these symptoms are very nonspecific, they may represent illness in the older adult.

21. How prevalent are mental status changes in the older adult ED patient?

Hustey and Meldon (2002) concluded that impaired mental status is common in older adult ED patients. In a prospective, observational study they identified mental status impairment in 78/297 (26%) of patients ≥70 years seen in the ED for varied complaints. Thirty of the 297 (10%) patients exhibited symptoms consistent with delirium and 48 (16%) had cognitive impairment without delirium. In a prospective cross-sectional study, Hustey and coworkers (2003), again reported a high prevalence of mental status changes in older ED patients.

22. What are the most frequent causes of lethargy or confusion in the older adult?

A change in mental status in an older adult may be from a great variety of causes that do not cause confusion in a younger person, including:

- Recent stressful events or changes in the environment
- Infections, such as a UTI, pneumonia, or bacteremia
- Gastrointestinal (GI) bleeding, including nonsteroidal anti-inflammatory drugs (NSAID)-induced blood loss
- Dehydration
- Medications (both new and old)
- Alcoholism

23. Why should you perform a mental status exam on all older adults?

Studies of older adults treated in the ED have shown that mental status impairment is often overlooked. To some extent, this is probably from the myth that all older adults will experience cognitive impairment. During the mental status examination note:

- The ability to answer questions
- The ability to place occurrences in their proper order
- Orientation to person, place, time, and situation

- Physical appearance (poor hygiene?)
- General emotional tone (calm? nervous?)

24. Outside of wrong answers, what else might be a clue that the patient is experiencing confusion?

Avoidance of answering a question is often a clue. They may also explain their wrong or inappropriate responses with "No one ever tells me anything." Some are skilled in "covering up" with charm or humor, such as "At my age, it doesn't matter because every day is a good day." However, despite the clever response, the reality is a fully functional person should be able to tell you the day.

25. What are the key historical questions to ask the patient and/or the patient's family?

In assessing mental status changes the most important questions should deal with the timing of, or length of time from, onset of symptoms. Establish:

- The patient's baseline mental status and activity before the change occurred
- Recent changes in the patient's life or environment
- If the change was sudden or there were subtle changes over a period of time
- What changes made the caregiver or patient seek emergency treatment today

26. Why is it important to know how long the patient has experienced mental status changes?

Generally, an acute mental status change in the older adult is more serious than that which occurs over a longer period of time. However, acute changes are more likely to respond to treatment.

27. What may be the most helpful when obtaining the history?

The elderly are more likely to have a number of processes going on that may be contributing to the mental status change. Obtaining the point in time when the subtle changes began can help pinpoint the cause(s).

28. Is there anything I should be aware of?

Casual contact may have precluded the family from noticing a progressive decline in cognition. For example, a visit from out-of-town family may lead to the perception of an acute mental status change when in fact the chronic cognitive dysfunction had not been recognized in brief telephone conversations.

29. How extensive must the history and physical be for the older adult with mental status changes?

The examination should include:

- Neurologic examination
- Level of consciousness (LOC)

- Level of attention
- Nutritional status
- Evidence of pyrexia
- Cognitive function using a standardized instrument (e.g., Orientation Memory, Concentration examination, Folstein MMSE, Neecham Confusion Scale)
- Evidence of alcohol or signs of withdrawal syndrome

For further discussion, see Chapter 4.

30. Why is it important to identify possible alcohol abuse when treating the older adult?

Alcohol abuse is a common, but often unrecognized, problem in the older adult, particularly for individuals who drank alcohol throughout their life. They may now increase use to deal with aging effects (e.g., "empty nest"), but are less physiologically able to metabolize it.

Benzodiazepines should not be used if the older adult person has agitation without alcohol abuse. However, benzodiazepines are used in the older adult if the agitation is from a withdrawal syndrome. For further discussion, see Chapter 61.

31. Discuss caregiver assessment.

It's important to remember that the caregiver usually has no training to do what they are asked to do. Caregivers (sometimes older adults themselves) often are under a great deal of stress. They have to deal with aggression, disturbed nights, or incontinence. Although they may be holding down a job at the same time, financial issues may further strain relationships.

Stress of the caregiver has been shown to be a direct result of how the caregiver perceives their responsibilities. Those that feel "out of control," or feel that they get very little support have higher levels of stress. Higher stress levels have been associated not only with elder abuse but also with increased illness of the caregiver. For further discussion, see Chapter 59.

32. Is the confused patient competent to make decisions?

Confusion of itself does not preclude competence to make decisions regarding treatment options. Although most institutional policies dictate that a legally authorized party makes consent for treatment of the confused patient, the patient's input should not be discounted. Studies report that long-standing values and beliefs, such as those associated with end-of-life decision making do not change with cognitive impairment.

33. Which diagnostic and laboratory studies provide useful information?

Because of the multiple factors that frequently contribute to delirium, the workup of the patient with a mental status change cannot always be predicted.

However, several standard diagnostic and laboratory studies have been identified as being useful to rule out sepsis, metabolic imbalance, and cerebral pathology.

Laboratory studies, which should be considered for all patients include: pulse oximetry, a complete blood count with differential, glucose, electrolytes, calcium, blood urea nitrogen (BUN), liver function, thyroid function, and urinalysis. An electrocardiogram (ECG) and chest radiograph should also be included.

Other investigations indicated the findings from the history and physical examination may include: arterial blood gases, drug levels (e.g., digoxin, theophylline, phenytoin, drug panel), B_{12} and folate, specific cultures (e.g., urine, blood, sputum), electroencephalogram (EEG), computerized tomography of the head without contrast, and lumbar puncture. Remember that the older adult may manifest the clinical signs of drug toxicity without having a drug level that's consistent with toxicity.

34. When is pharmacologic intervention indicated?

Pharmacologic management of acute mental status changes in the older adult should be reserved for those patients whose behavior poses a risk to the safety of self and staff. Generally, a quiet environment with the support of individuals who are familiar to the patient is quite effective. Limiting contact to as few staff as possible will also minimize overstimulation and anxiety-provoking situations.

However, in the event a pharmacologic agent is required, a low dose antipsychotic, such as haloperidol 0.5 mg intravenously (IV), may be useful. Newer atypical parenteral agents such as ziprasidone (Geodon) may also provide a suitable option for those unable to take an oral agent. For urgent situations or withdrawal syndromes, short acting benzodiazepines such as lorazepam 0.25 to 0.5 mg IV should be considered.

35. Discuss important guidelines with pharmacologic management.

Pharmacologic management should be guided by the premise of "start low and go slow." Whether using haloperidol, a newer atypical antipsychotic, or benzodiazepine, dosing can be repeated every 30 minutes until reaching the desired effect. In addition, the desired effect should be "mellow" rather than sedated.

36. Tell me the current Food and Drug Administration-approved agents for the treatment of delirium.

Currently there are *no* Food and Drug Administration (FDA)-approved agents for the treatment of delirium. Guidelines for the management of delirium are available at www.guideline.gov and www.psych.org.

37. Discuss depression.

Depression effects on cognitive impairment may be similar to dementia, but it develops over short time and troubles the patient. It is specific, rather than global, language skills remain intact (although the person may withdraw), and the person can learn new information. It can sometimes manifest as vague, unexplained somatic complaints, such as headaches, stomachaches, and back pain. One woman kept saying she "just didn't feel right," but nothing specific was revealed in the specific follow-up assessment questions. I finally asked, "Do you think there is anything contributing to this feeling?" She answered, "You know, my husband died 1 year ago today in this hospital."

Depression is diagnosed by a distinct change in behavior marked by a depressed mood and at least five symptoms lasting over a 2-week period (psychomotor retardation, irritability, a negative outlook, sleep pattern changes, less energy, decreased appetite, weight loss, difficulty concentrating, memory loss, inappropriate feelings of guilt, suicidal ideation/preoccupation with death). For further discussion, see Chapter 53.

Key Points

- One of the most frequent causes of mental status changes in the older adult is UTI.
- Attempt to identify the point in time when subtle changes began.
- Patients with dementia are at the highest risk for developing delirium.
- Confusion of itself does not preclude competence to make decisions: long-standing values and belief do not change with cognitive impairment.

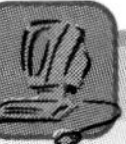

Internet Resources

University of California, San Diego. A practical guide to clinical medicine: The mental status exam
http://medicine.ucsd.edu/clmicalmed/mental.htm

The Alzheimer's Association
http://www.alz.org

American Psychiatric Association
http://www.psych.org

National Alliance for the Mentally Ill
http://www.nami.org

National Guideline Clearinghouse
http://www.guideline.gov

National Mental Health Association
http://www.nmha.org

Bibliography

Arnold E: Sorting out the 3 D's: Delirium, dementia, depression, *Nursing* 24(6):36-43, 2004.

Elie M, Rousseau F, Cole M, et al: Prevalence and detection of delirium in elderly emergency department patients, *Can Med Assoc J* 163:977-981, 2000.

Fick DM, Agostini JV, Inouye SK: Delirium superimposed on dementia: A systematic review, *J Am Geriatr Soc* 50:1723-1732, 2002.

Hustey FM, Meldon SW: The prevalence and documentation of impaired mental status in elderly emergency department patients, *Ann Emerg Med* 39:248-253, 2002.

Hustey FM, Meldon SW, Smith MD, Lex CK: The effect of mental status screening on the care of elderly emergency department patients, *Ann Emerg Med* 41:678-684, 2003.

Kakuma R, Galbaud du Fort G, Arsenalut L, et al: Delirium in older emergency department patients discharged home: Effect on survival, *J Am Geriatr Soc* 51:443-450, 2003.

Manos PJ: 10-point clock test screens for cognitive impairment in clinic and hospital settings, *Psychiatric Times* 15:10, 1998.

McCurren C, Cronin SN: Delirium: Elders tell their stories and guide nursing practice, *Med Surg Nurs* 12:318-323, 2003.

Monette J, Galbaud du Fort G, Fung SH, et al: Evaluation of the confusion assessment method (CAM) as a screening tool for delirium in the emergency room, *Gen Hosp Psychiatry* 23:20-25, 2001.

Nerenberg L: *Caregiver stress and elder abuse*, Washington DC, March 2002, National Center on Elder Abuse.

Nicholls PH: A simple test for evaluating cognitive impairment, *RN* 65:72, 2002.

Samuels SC, Evers MM: Delirium: Pragmatic management for managing a common, confounding, and sometimes lethal condition, *Geriatrics* 57:33-38, 2002.

Zimmermann PG: Effective communication with patients with dementia, *J Emerg Nurs* 24(5):412-415, 1998.

Chapter 56

Domestic Violence

Jill Cash

1. What is domestic violence?

Domestic violence is any act of physical, emotional, or sexual abuse that occurs to any person. The definition of physical abuse includes hitting, slapping, kicking, choking, or physically causing harm or injury to another person. Sexual abuse includes performing sexual contact with another person without mutual consent of contact.

2. Who needs to be screened for domestic violence?

All patients should be screened for the presence of violence or abuse over the past year. One emergency department (ED) screens even infants, asking the parents if they are aware of resources if someone was abusing their child.

3. I'm afraid of offending the patient by asking about abuse.

It is estimated that 25% to 30% of women who seek care in the ED are victims of domestic violence. What is concerning is that 92% of women who are abused did not discuss it with their clinicians. Many patients indicate they are glad EDs are doing screening.

4. Is it a regulatory requirement?

The Joint Commission on Accreditation of Healthcare Organizations (JCAHO) mandates all hospital EDs screen patients for domestic violence.

5. Why would we screen men as victims of domestic violence?

Police reports have a ratio up to 12 to 1 of battered women to battered men. However, one study found that 12% of husbands were violent to their wives, but 12% of wives were violent to their husbands. The method of battering differs. Men are more apt to push and shove; women are apt to throw things, kick, or hit with a fist. Men tend to inflict more damage because of their strength and size. It is believed that only men have the reputation as abusers because men tend to keep quiet, often out of embarrassment.

6. How often should a patient be screened for violence?

Each visit if time and resources permit. It establishes that the facility is a safe and appropriate place to talk about these things and circumstances could have changed since the last visit. It is recommended that pregnant women be screened each trimester of the pregnancy, as it is a risk factor for physical abuse to escalate.

7. How should the screening be done?

The assessment should be performed in a private and confidential environment, without anyone else present. It is acceptable to perform it either verbally or with a written questionnaire, but it should be done in the primary language (if at all possible).

8. What do I do if the partner is very controlling and won't leave the patient alone?

Be creative in separating them.
- Have a same-sex nurse take the patient into the bathroom for a specimen collection.
- Indicate this part of the exam is private and ask the partner to leave.
- One nurse put the patient in a wheelchair and took the patient to get an x-ray (even though none was ordered), indicating the spouse could not follow because of radiation exposure.

9. I'm not sure what to say. It seems so abrupt to ask.

It is recommended to do the screening in two parts. Start with a framing statement to put the actual question in context, and then ask a direct verbal question.

10. Give some examples of framing statements.

- "Because violence is so common in many people's lives we now ask all patients about it."
- "I'm concerned that your symptoms may have been caused by someone hurting you."
- "I don't know if this is a problem for you, but many of the women I see as patients are dealing with abusive relationships. Some are too afraid or uncomfortable to bring it up themselves, so I've started asking about it routinely."

11. Give me some examples I could use for direct questions.

- "Are you currently in a relationship in which you were physically hurt, threatened, or made to feel afraid?"
- "Have you ever been hit, kicked, slapped, pushed, or shoved by your ____________ (boyfriend/husband/partner) during this pregnancy?"
- "Have you ever been forced or pressured to have sex when you did not want to?"

12. What aspects do I need to include in my questions?

Using the mnemonic SAFE can assist you in remembering assessment components.

S: Do you feel SAFE at home and/or work?
A: Have you felt ABUSED in your current or past relationships? If so, how?
F: Do you have FRIENDS or FAMILY to turn to for support or help?
E: Do you have an ESCAPE plan or route for emergency if needed?

13. Give some more sample questions for asking about safety.

- Has anyone close to you ever threatened or hurt you?
- Have you ever been afraid of your partner?
- Does he blame you for things that are out of your control?

14. List some additional sample questions to ask about abuse.

- Have you ever been kicked, choked, hit, or physically hurt?
- Has anyone ever forced you to have sex?
- Do you feel that your partner controls you and/or isolates you from daily activities?
- Has he ever destroyed your personal things or things that are important to you (personal belongings, pets, etc.)?

15. Name other sample questions related to asking about family or friends.

- Does he restrict you from seeing your friends and family and control who you have contact with daily?
- Does he always stay by your side and never leave you alone to talk privately?

16. Tell me ways to ask about an escape plan.

- Do you have a planned destination?
- Do you know how you will get to your destination?
- Do you have money readily available?

17. Many victims are so stressed and terrified in times of trouble, how can I help the victim to remember the escape plan and find the phone numbers when it is needed?

Recommend the escape plan, money, phone numbers, or other information is put in a safe hidden place. One suggestion is keeping this information underneath the padding in the shoe (a place in which no one would look). Another is behind the refrigerator.

18. List some clues that violence may be a factor of the patient history.

- Presents to office or ED with trauma to head, neck, trunk, or unexplained injury
- Injury explanation inconsistent with type of injury

- Frequent office or ED visits
- Somatic complaints requiring treatment (headache, stomachache, pelvic pain, abdominal pain)
- Psychiatric illness such as anxiety and/or depression, posttraumatic stress syndrome, suicidal attempts
- Alcohol, tobacco, or drug abuse
- Threatened miscarriages or pregnancy with late entry or no prenatal care

19. Are there any inappropriate approaches that should not be used when screening for domestic violence?

Do not accuse or be judgmental when asking questions, even if you do not believe the answers. Accept her answers and go on with the visit. Chances are you will have a second opportunity to assess for domestic abuse at a later time. In addition, it takes some women repeated episodes or opportunities until she is willing to admit and/or deal with the problem.

20. Are there any comments that should be avoided?

The goal is to develop a trusting relationship and not appear judgmental. The nurse's role is to provide support and guidance. Do not ask questions that will lower self-esteem or self-confidence, imply failure, or insinuate that the victim is responsible for the abuse.

- "I would have left him/her long before now!"
- "What did you do to make him/her hit you?"
- "Why didn't you tell anyone that he/she was abusing you?"

21. What do I do if domestic violence is confirmed?

- Validate the feelings. Affirm the right to not be afraid or hurt.
- Investigate the immediate safety. Where is the perpetrator? Does he have a gun?
- Document.
- Connect the abuse to the patient's health issues. "How people get along with other people affects their health. Abuse contributes to chronic health problems including pain, depression, alcohol/drug abuse, and noncompliance in other disease management." Many have convinced themselves the abuse doesn't matter.
- Current access to advocacy and support resources. Provide brochures and phone numbers. Offer to let her read it there and call now.
- Discuss future safety and risk of significant injury. This includes acknowledging the potential for future harm, the classic escalation pattern, and a flight plan. The woman will be at most risk when leaving.

Law enforcement must be contacted if you suspect the patient or children are in immediate danger. Consider involving social services.

22. What other educational information would be appropriate?

Safety behaviors such as self-protection advice (remove all weapons, guns, knives from the house) and a safety escape plan for a future-threatening situation.

23. What should a safety plan include?

McFarlane recommends:

- Hide money.
- Hide an extra set of house and car keys.
- Establish a code with family and friends.
- Ask a neighbor to call the police if violence begins.
- Hide a bag of extra clothes.
- Have available social security numbers (his, yours, and the kids'), birth certificates, marriage license, driver's license, bank account numbers, insurance policies and numbers, rent and utility receipts, and important phone numbers.
- If you call the crisis shelter, after you finish the conversation call someone else immediately so the abuser won't know you called the shelter.
- Consider a protective order.

24. Why is a protective order important?

Judy McFarlane's research suggests it is the single most important thing because the order exposes the abuser and limits the abuser's control.

25. How do I document/record the abuse?

- Provide a picture of a body map and ask the patient to use a pen and draw an "x" on the sites of her body that she has been abused.
- If the abuse has been recent, view the sites and objectively describe your observations.
- Document.
- The difference between the time of the injury and now.
- Time missed from school or work as a result of the abuse.
- Frequency and severity of abuse.
- Treatment, referrals, and follow-up care.
- Take pictures after obtaining the patient's consent.
- Keep all documentation accurate without generalizations or opinions.

26. Do I have any legal responsibilities when abuse is identified?

Yes, some states mandate that domestic violence must be reported to the police.

27. The patient begs me not to report the battery because her husband has warned her that if she reports the abuse, he will kill her. What do I do?

Discuss the situation with the patient. If your state mandates reporting abuse, explain that you must report the abuse by law because domestic abuse is a crime. When you report the abuse, it takes the situation out of the patient's hands and she actually may be relieved. The law is there to protect her and to provide safety.

28. What if the patient reports previous episodes of abuse months or years ago and considers herself safe at the present time? Do I need to report the previous abuse?

If the patient is not presently threatened or injured, you do not need to file a police report of previous episodes of abuse. However, educate the patient about the cycle of violence (tension builds with isolation, blow-up/abuse, honeymoon period) and that violence tends to escalate with future episodes of abuse.

29. Why do women not report domestic abuse?

Reasons could include:

- Embarrassed and humiliated to admit it.
- Religious or cultural beliefs that abuse is acceptable in the family.
- Threatened by the abuser if she discloses the abuse.
- Believes abuser won't do it again.
- Thinks help is not available for her.
- Dependence (financial, etc.) on the abuser.

30. Why do victims stay in abusive relationships?

Victims do not like being abused but stay in abusive relationships for reasons including:

- *Fear of the unknown.* The victim may face financial burdens, concerns of where to stay, worries about the children, fear of future harm.
- *Believe the abuse is deserved.* The abuser often blames the victim.
- *Believe that abuse is the norm.* They grew up in an abusive environment and so are not aware of the dysfunction.
- *Abuse is intermittent.* Between the abuses, the times can actually be pleasant and they have affection for the person. The victim may believe it won't happen again.

31. Are there any characteristics common to those who perpetrate domestic violence?

Yes. It can become an intergenerational way of controlling or coping. They project blame, "You made me do it." Perpetrators of abuse often have one or more of the following characteristics:

- Frequent use or abuse of alcohol and/or drugs
- Previous exposure to family violence as a child or adolescent
- Inappropriate social skills, lacks communication skills, difficulty dealing with problematic situations
- Hostile and/or aggressive personality, low self-esteem
- Personality disorders such as schizophrenia, dependency/attachment problems, and narcissistic behaviors

32. Should I give the patient a card with abuse resource numbers on them?

Most do not want anything that will identify this phone number for fear the abuser will find it. Write the resource numbers on regular physician business card or even something feminine, such as an emery board. One hospital puts posters on the inside door of the women's bathroom stalls.

Key Points

- It is estimated 25% to 30% of women who seek care in the ED are victims of domestic violence.
- All women should be screened each visit.
- Use the mnemonic SAFE to cover components for screening.

Internet Resources

National Domestic Violence Hotline
http://www.ndvh.org

Family Violence Prevention Fund
http://endabuse.org

National Center for Injury Prevention and Control: National Health Resource Center on Domestic Violence (888 Rx-Abuse)
www.cdc.gov/ncipc/default.htm

Nursing Network on Violence Against Women International:
www.nnvawi.org

National Coalition Against Domestic Violence Hotline:
www.ncadv.org

Bibliography

American College of Nurse Midwives: *Violence against women (Position Statement),* Aug 1997, available: www.midwife.org.

American Nurses Association: *Physical violence against women,* 1991, available: www.nursingworld.org.

Beckmann C, Ling F, Laube D, et al: Caring for the adult sexual assault victim. In *Obstetrics and gynecology,* ed 4, Philadelphia, 2002, Lippincott, Williams & Wilkins, 619-623.

Dienemann J, Campbell J, Wiederhorn N, et al: A critical pathway for intimate partner violence across the continuum of care, *J Obstet Gynecol Neonatal Nurs* 32(5):594-603, 2002.

Emergency Nurses Association Position Statement: *Domestic violence, maltreatment, and neglect,* 2003; available: www.ena.org/about/position/.

McFarlane J, Gondolf E: Preventing abuse during pregnancy: A clinical protocol, *Am J Maternal Child Nurs* 23:22-27, 1998.

McFarlane J, Soeken K, Wiist W: An evaluation of interventions to decrease intimate partner violence to pregnant women, *Public Health Nurs* 17(6):443-451, 2000.

Rodriguez M, Bauer H, McLoughlin E, Grumbach K: Screening and intervention for intimate partner violence, *JAMA* 282(5):468-474, 1999.

US Preventive Services Task Force: *Guide to clinical preventive services,* Philadelphia, 1996, Lippincott, Williams & Wilkins.

Chapter 57

Bullying

Susan M. Hohenhaus

1. There's not enough time in triage to screen for everything. Why is bullying such a big deal?

Just like domestic violence, bullying is now viewed as inappropriate behavior and a serious health problem. When a child bullies another child, the abuse can cause lasting effects.

2. Bullying is just a right of passage for kids. I went through it; I suppose kids always will.

- Bullying is not a "normal" or socially acceptable behavior.
- Bullies receive power when adults do not protest the behavior and this has serious consequences for the child being bullied.
- It can lead to behavior problems. It is cited as why more than 160,000 children skip school every day. In more than two-thirds of school shootings, the attackers had been bullied.
- There are more subtle health risks also. Those who are bullied are two to three times more likely to have other illnesses. These include headache and depression.

3. How common is bullying?

Almost 30% of teens (grades 6 to 10) in the United States (over 5.7 million) are estimated to be involved in bullying as either a bully, a target of bullying, or both.

4. So what is "bullying" anyway?

Bullying is characterized as an imbalance of power, an intention to harm or disturb, with repeated occurrences. The focus should not remain on the action per se, but the attempt to have a certain effect or domination of the other person.

5. I've heard there are different types of bullying—what are they?

There are several categories of bullying:

- Verbal (such as name-calling, or threats of physical violence).
- Psychologic and emotional intimidation (such as spreading rumors and persistent teasing).

- Physical (kicking, hitting, biting, pinching, hair pulling).
- Relational (excluding the person from conversations and activities).
- Racist bullying may take these forms: making racial slurs, spray painting graffiti, mocking the victim's cultural traditions, and making offensive gestures.
- Sexual bullying is characterized by unwanted physical contact or abusive comments.
- Cyberbullying occurs when children are harassed in print via website or email campaign. It is difficult to stop as a result of a 1997 U.S. Supreme Court decision that defends a person's right to free speech.

In one survey, 61% of the respondents had comments made about their looks or speech; 60% had been the subject of vicious rumors; 56% had been hit, slapped, or pushed; 52% had been the subject of sexual comments or gestures; and 26% had been belittled about their religion or race.

6. Does bullying affect boys more than girls?

Bullying does occur more frequently among boys than girls. Teenage boys are much more likely to bully others and to be the targets of bullies. Although both boys and girls say others bully them by making fun of the way they look or talk, boys are more likely to report being hit, slapped, or pushed. Teenage girls are more often the targets of rumors and sexual comments.

7. What does a child who has been bullied "look like"?

There are many signs and symptoms to look for that indicate a child may be being bullied. Some of them may cause a caregiver to seek medical attention for the child:

- Avoidance of certain situations, people, or places, such as pretending to be sick so that he or she does not have to go to school.
- Changes in behavior, such as being withdrawn and passive or being overly active and aggressive.
- Self-destructive behaviors.
- Signs of injuries.
- Recurrent unexplained physical symptoms, such as stomach pains and fatigue.

8. How do I screen for bullying?

Don't make things complicated. Try adding a question to your triage assessment such as "Has anyone at school made you sad or afraid?" Other suggested terms include "mad" or "upset."

9. How do I get children to tell me what is troubling them in triage?

If the child answers yes to your screening question, ask him/her to tell you about it. You can also ask the parent if the child has had frequent school absences or signs of chronic illnesses, such as headaches or stomachaches while at school.

10. What information can I share with parents about keeping their child safe from bullying?

Schools have effectively changed the culture with institution-wide programs. In the meantime, if the school has nothing in place, encourage the child to respond verbally rather than physically fighting back or tolerating the bullying.

First statement:	"I don't like what you said to me."
Second statement:	"I'm asking you to stop."
Third statement:	"I'm going to get help." And then do.

Teach a child to report bullying to his or her teacher and to the parent. Teaching all children to implement this process at one school in Missouri decreased school fights from 55 to 6 a year, while raising standardized math and reading scores. Children deserve a safe environment.

11. Why isn't there more publicity about this issue?

To address these issues, the U.S. Department of Health and Human Services and the Maternal and Child Health Bureau have launched the National Bullying Prevention Campaign. They are using the slogan "Take a Stand. Lend a Hand. Stop Bullying Now!"

The campaign aims to inform health and safety professionals about the prevalence of bullying, early warning signs, consequences, and strategies for prevention, intervention, and advocacy.

Key Points

- Bullying is no longer regarded as "just a right of passage."
- Approximately 30% of children in grades 6 through 10 are involved in bullying.
- Screen for bullying by asking "Has anyone at school made you sad or afraid?"

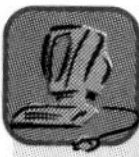

Internet Resources

Health Resources and Services Administration: Stop Bullying Now!
www.stopbullyingnow.hrsa.gov

Bibliography

Cavendish R, Salomone C: Bullying and sexual harassment in the school setting, *J Sch Nurse* 17(1):25-31, 2001.

Dake JA, Price JH, Telljohann SK: The nature and extent of bullying at school, *J Sch Health* 73(5):173-180, 2003.

Nansel TR, Overpeck M, Pilla RS, et al: Bullying behaviors among US youth: Prevalence and association with psychosocial adjustment, *JAMA* 285(16):2094-2100, 2001.

Olweus D: *Bullying at school: What we know and what we can do*, Cambridge, Mass, 1993, Blackwell Publishers.

Reeves K: More on children's bullying, *J Emerg Nurs* 27(3):232, 2001.

Sanborn PA: Stomachaches and other complaints in children: Is it really bullying? *J Emerg Nurs* 27(1):85-87, 2001.

Williams K, Chambers M, Logan S, Robinson D: Association of common health symptoms with bullying in primary school children, *Br Med J* 7048:9-17, 1996.

Chapter 58

Child Abuse

Shelley Cohen

1. How is child abuse defined, and who defines it?

State definitions vary but all have a common theme in that maltreatment of children is against the law. The categories of abuse with their frequency are:
Neglect 63%
Physical abuse 19%
Sexual abuse 10%
Emotional (including verbal) abuse 8%

2. Name some red flags that indicate a child could be a victim of neglect.

- Sudden change in behavior or ability to perform schoolwork
- Inappropriate growth and development for age
- Dehydration without presence of illness
- Stealing or hiding food
- Overt lack of dental or other medical care
- Not dressed appropriate for weather
- Left alone unsupervised at home

3. What age group is most commonly the victim of fatality related to abuse or neglect?

Children 5 years and younger. Their size and inability to independently provide self-care explain why they are the most vulnerable.

4. List some red flags that indicate a child could be a victim of physical abuse.

- Unexplained wounds or bruises
- Bruises in various stages of healing
- Wounds that appear to be the shape of objects such as a curling iron, a belt, or a cigarette butt
- The story from the caregiver of the injury does not match the capability of the child's age and growth and development
- The child appears frightened in the presence of adults who are their caregiver

5. Won't it be obvious if the physical abuse is really bad?

The majority of children with head injuries from abuse have no outward signs of the abuse. Many perpetrators inflict physical abuse in areas that they think a health care worker will not look, such as cigarette burns to the soles of the feet.

6. Tell me some red flags that could indicate a child could be a victim of sexual abuse.

- The child does not want to sit or walk or it appears painful to do so.
- Bedwetting as a new behavior
- Pregnancy at an inappropriate age
- Presence of sexually transmitted disease (especially in children younger than 12 years because they are usually not sexually active)
- History of running away
- Anorexia
- Overtly sexually aggressive toward adults or other children

7. Are some of the psychologic issues related to child victims of sexual abuse different than the other forms of abuse?

- They blame themselves.
- They have different levels of anger toward both parents. They are angry at the one abusing them and angry with the other parent for not stopping the abuse.
- They may believe this behavior between an adult and child is normal and expected in everyone's household.
- They feel trapped if they have tried to tell someone and were not believed.

8. Is there more specific data on child victims of sexual abuse?

The National Incident Base Reporting System gathers information from law enforcement agencies and their data from 1991 to 2002 reveals:

- Sixty-seven percent of sexual assault victims were under the age of 18.
- Thirty-four percent were under the age of 12.
- One out of every 7 victims were under the age of 6.
- Forty percent of the offenders who victimized children in this manner were juveniles (under 18). In the majority of the cases, the offender was known by the child.

9. What might be signs that indicate a child could be a victim of emotional abuse?

- Suicide attempts
- Developmentally delayed
- Cares for the other siblings as an adult would
- Flat affect
- Demonstrates extreme attempts to please caregiver
- Regressive child-like behaviors (rocking) in an older child

10. Anything else I should be alert for?

An estimated 3 to 10 million children witness domestic violence in their home and between 65% and 75% of those children are also abused. Often abused women do not leave their batterers until their children are endangered. Ask an adult victim of domestic violence about the children.

11. List some of the elements in the triage documentation that can assist in validating the concern.

- Document what you see, hear, smell
- Use the actual quotes of both the patient and caregiver
- Identify specific behaviors of child (e.g., makes no eye contact with father)
- Consider statements of other siblings present ("We didn't eat yet today.")

In one case I triaged, both the parent and child claimed he had fractured his femur when he fell off the swing in their back yard. The young sister at the bedside stated, "We ain't got no swing." The police photographed the backyard without the swing and we had a validated need for children's services.

12. Why is it not recommended that you document your assessment of the age of a wound?

A nurse cannot know a wound's age for a fact because the nurse was not there. Put anything stated by the caregiver or child in quotes. The goal is for documentation to be objective, accurate, and be able to support the victim, not the perpetrator. For instance: Mother states, "She fell a week ago at school." Purplish-blue circular bruise, 3-inch diameter noted in mid-lower abdomen.

13. What are some common errors made in triage documentation?

Documentation about the patient or caregiver that are either not within the nurse's expertise to document, imply something that may not be true, and/or would be difficult to defend in court. Examples of these could include:

- "Father is angry." (How do you know another person's emotion?) A better way to state this would be: Father states, "I'm angry that this child is such a brat."
- "Poor social interaction between mother and child." (What is your training and expertise to make this judgment?) Again, a better way to state this would be: "Mother does not reach out to comfort crying child."

14. What are some red flags related to the perpetrator?

Some commonly demonstrated behaviors by the parent who is mistreating the child are:

- Minimal physical contact (no hugging or hand holding)
- Unrealistic expectations for a child of that age
- Encourages others to use severe punishment in their absence
- Does not address the child by their given/legal name
- Speaks of the child in a negative way and does this in the presence of the child

- Blames and berates the child for issues out of the control of the victim
- Overtly treats the child in a way that suggests they prefer not to recognize them at all

15. Who are the common perpetrators of child maltreatment?

1999 statistics gathered from twenty-one state child protective service systems reveal the following:

- Women: 61.8% (almost half of them under the age of 30)
- Men: 38.2%
- Mother: 44.7 %
- Both parents: 17.7%
- Father: 15.9%

16. For specific types of maltreatment, the data collected reveals:

- The mother is the perpetrator and acted alone in 51% in cases of child neglect.
- The mother acted alone in 35.6% of cases involving physical abuse.
- The father acted alone in 20.8% of sexual abuse cases.

17. What are red flags that the person presenting with the child may be the perpetrator?

- They are overly protective of child or the extreme opposite and have no concern.
- They will not allow the child to speak to anyone unless they are present.
- Their story changes in detail as different members of the health care team interact with them.

18. How do you separate the parent from the child so you can screen them alone?

Triage may not be the most appropriate place to do the screening/assessment. You have to look for opportunities during their emergency department (ED) visit. Examples could include walking the child to the bathroom for a specimen collection, offering to sit with the child so the parent can smoke a cigarette outside, or staying with the child while the doctor reviews the radiology results with the parent.

19. What are some of the strong motivators for kids that prompts them not to tell us what is really happening to them?

These motivators vary with age, but include threats for separation from someone they trust or love (grandparent), loss of access to food or privileges, and physical beating.

20. Are there any particular questions that can help prompt a child to tell you their story?

The nature of the questions will vary with the developmental capability of each child. Some examples that help eliminate the sense that the child is "telling" on a parent include "We had spaghetti at our house last night, what did you have to eat at yours?" and "Does anyone wake you up at night and crawl into your bed?"

21. What motivates a person to want to harm or neglect a child?

- Substance abuse on the part of one or both parents plays a role in almost one-half of the cases of child neglect and abuse categories.
- Lack of tools or skills to cope and deal with life stressors appropriately. The child becomes the target of the person suffering the stress.
- Victims of unhappy or unsuccessful relationships or an unwanted pregnancy.
- Mental illness.
- A history of the perpetrator being abused as a child.

22. Isn't it the role of the physician to identify and report the suspicion?

In most states it is the role of all health care workers, teachers, clergy, police officers, and many others to report the suspicion. Assessment for any abuse begins at triage.

23. Sometimes I am not sure if there is an abuse issue or not. What should I do?

Always go with your gut. It is in the better interest of the child to file the reports than to not. Your phone call on file may be the one that gives the caseworker enough validation to remove a child from the home or to require that another person in the home move out.

24. What if the physician disagrees with the assessment of the triage nurse and feels there is no validation for concern? Should the nurse still file a report?

The nurse has a duty to follow state and facility requirements regardless of whether the physician agrees.

25. What if I am wrong and no abuse is found? Can I be sued by the family?

No, not if the report was made with legitimate intentions (vs. revenge, etc.).

26. How can I find out the statutes for the state in which I practice?

- You can access this information from several sources:
  - Facility policy/resource manual
  - Local Department of Children's Services

- Via the internet by searching with the name of your state and the words child abuse
- Police department

27. What is the role of the Department of Children/Human Services?

Some aspects of the role may vary by state, however the primary responsibility is to respond to reports of concerns related to child maltreatment, investigate complaints, and identify living situations that are unsafe for the child. The staff may present to the ED or request to take a telephone report only.

28. Is child abuse an issue that the media has exaggerated?

The National Child Abuse and Neglect System reported 1,300 children fatalities in 2001. The U.S. Department of Health and Human Services data from 2002 reveals that more than three children die each day as a result of child abuse in the home. Altogether, 14 million kids a year are suffering abuse or neglect, or sometimes both.

29. Discuss abandoned baby laws.

Since 1999, at least 35 states instituted some form of "abandoned baby" or "dumpster baby" laws after a government report revealed a 62% increase in the number of discarded newborns left to die in public places. These state laws permit an unwanted newborn infant (the range of allowed ages varies from 3 days to 1 month) to be "dropped off" at an ED without question or legal consequence.

Most EDs want any nursing staff that has contact with the individual dropping off the infant to ask about health information. However, the person should be allowed to leave immediately if the infant has no obvious signs of trauma or abuse. Organizations with literature and additional information include Project Cuddle (www.projectcuddle.org), Garden of Angels and Safe Arms (www.gardenofangels.org), and A Secret Safe Place for Newborns (http://secretsafeplace.org).

Key Points

- Never assume that because the caregiver has a professional occupation and is well known in the community that they cannot be the offender.
- Absence of wounds or bruises does not indicate absence of abuse.
- Use quotations to document comments made by both the patient and the adult.
- Listen to the child's story and believe them, it is someone else's job to disprove it.
- Become familiar with red flag alerts for neglect because this is the most common form of child abuse.

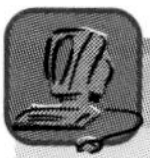

Internet Resources

Administration for Children and Families—Child Abuse and Neglect
http://nccanch.acf.hhs.gov/

Childhelp USA—National Child Abuse Statistics
www.childhelpusa.com.

For the Love of Our Children—Statistics
www.fortheloveofourchildren.org.

Faulkner, Nancy, PhD, Pandora's Box—Sexual Abuse Statistics
www.prevent-abuse-now.com.

Bibliography

Child Welfare League of America: *Making managed health care work for kids in foster care,* Washington, DC, 1996, CWLA Press.

Mulryna K, Cathers P, Fagin A: How to recognize and respond to child abuse, *Nursing* 34(10):52-56, 2004.

Rosen P: *The 5-minute emergency medicine consult,* Philadelphia, 1999, Lippincott, Williams & Wilkins.

Chapter 59

Elder Abuse

Shelley Cohen

1. What are the types and frequency of elder abuse?

The Physicians for a Violence Free Society indicates:
Neglect 55%
Physical abuse 14.6%
Financial exploitation 12.3%
Emotional abuse 7.7%
Sexual abuse 0.3%

2. Name red flags that may indicate neglect of the older adult.

Withholding food, shelter, appropriate clothing, or medical care in any form is neglect. Indications this is occurring include:

- Weight loss
- Unsanitary living conditions
- Caregiver is well dressed but the patient is not
- Decubiti
- Necessary medical care not provided in a timely manner

3. List some red flags that may indicate physical abuse of the older adult.

- Bruises of odd shapes that resemble an iron, belt, or teeth marks
- Bruises in various stages of healing
- Medication overdose

4. Are the bruises from elder physical abuse always obvious?

No. The perpetrator learns the places that health care workers tend not to check during an exam. For instance, socks cover restraint marks around ankles, undergarments hide trunk bruising or collars hide grip marks around the neck.

In addition, many caregivers have a story to explain how the older adult person was injured in the course of normal life events.

5. Talk about financial abuse.

Financial abuse involves misusing the senior's funds or forcing them to sign over checks. Signs can include:
- No control over their money ("I have to ask my son for the money to buy food.")
- Loss of personal valuable possessions
- Sudden changes in their will

6. Discuss sexual abuse.

Sexual abuse can range from rape to exploitation through photography. Signs can include vaginal/anal tears, abrasions, pain, or bleeding, and/or presence of sexually transmitted diseases (STDs).

7. Describe what is meant by emotional abuse.

The victim is subjected to constant remarks, public or private, that are intended to lower their self-worth and embarrass them. Signs a patient is experiencing this can include:
- Agitation
- Appears frightened in front of perpetrator
- Behavior that appears regressive such as rocking or sucking
- Verbally berated publicly such as, "Dad—you are so clumsy! That's why you fall all of the time!"

8. Discuss common wrong assumptions made at triage that can hinder perceiving that the patient is a victim of elder abuse.

Mistaken beliefs that influence nurses can include:
- The caregiver has the patient's interest in mind.
- A physical complaint is simply age-related rather than from an injury, such as a loss in hearing.
- Age stereotypes are true, such as the elderly do not have sex.

9. Give characteristics of those who are more likely to be a victim of elder abuse.

- The median age is 77.9. Those older than 80 years experience abuse and neglect two to three times to their proportion of the older adult population.
- Women (68.3%).
- White (66.4%).
- Developmentally disabled. They have a four to ten times higher rate for physical or sexual assault.

10. What is the type of environmental situation in which older adult abuse is more likely to occur?

Abuse/neglect can occur in any setting in which this vulnerable population resides. Don't be fooled by the fact that the older adult person lives with family members. Some scenarios can include:

- Disrupted family routines/lifestyles as a result of addition of older adult person to household
- Substance abuse on the part of the caregiver
- Mental illness on the part of the caregiver
- Lack of awareness and knowledge
- Financial constraints
- Overburdened caregiver who is doing the best they can
- Family members with a history of violence and/or control issues
- Social isolation
- Chronic illness/disease on the part of the caregiver

11. Who are the perpetrators of elder abuse?

Two thirds of perpetrators are family members of the patient, most often adult children (47.3% of the time). The likelihood is higher if the adult child is also the caregiver. Sometimes there is an attitude of a "pay back": revenge for real or perceived past parental mistreatment.

Spouses were the perpetrator 19.3% of the time for abuse, and spouses commit 24% of family murders of persons over the age of 60. Grandchildren played a role 8.6% of the time.

12. Why doesn't the older adult patient tell someone?

There is a large measure of control in place in an abuse situation that is quite powerful and overwhelming for the patient. The older adult victim can feel trapped by their situation even though they may realize they don't deserve to be treated that way. Reasons can include:

- Perpetrator threats to withhold medication.
- Perpetrator threats to place the patient in a nursing home.
- Misperception that family business is personal (just like domestic violence use to be regarded).
- Victim's feelings of being ashamed or embarrassed to tell on a family member.
- Victim lack of awareness of state laws and/or resources available for help.
- Cultural and/or generational beliefs that do not emphasize women's rights.

13. Am I legally required to report elder abuse?

According to the American Bar Association web site, at the time of this printing, there are still 17 states with no mandatory reporting requirements for elder abuse. Some states have laws that the adult child must support an indigent parent. However, regardless of the law, the nurse must also consider the state's Nurse Practice Act and the professional advocacy responsibilities, code of ethics, and moral expectations.

14. How do I report elder abuse?

States vary regarding the agency that oversees these cases, but in some it is adult protective services. Check with your local authorities and have the contact name and phone number at hand in the department.

15. Isn't the issue of elder abuse overexaggerated?

Definitely not. In 1996, there were more than 500,000 American victims aged 60 and over and 84% of these were not referred for help. The Senate Committee on Aging estimates that there are as many as 5 million older adult abuse victims each year. Because there is no uniform system to report these victims, gathering accurate statistics is a challenge. Clinician awareness is a start in the right direction.

Key Points

- The majority of elder abuse is not reported.
- Never assume the caregiver has the patient's best interest in mind.
- The most common perpetrator is a family member.
- Many older adult patients are too ashamed to tell you someone in their family is abusing them.
- Neglect is the most common form of abuse in the older adult population.
- The presence of an STD is a red flag for possible sexual abuse.

Internet Resources

Physicians for a Violence-Free Society—Get the Facts About Elder Abuse
www.pvs.org/elder.shtml.

American Psychological Association—Elder Abuse and Neglect: In Search of Solutions
www.apa.org/pi/aging/eldabuse.html

National Center on Elder Abuse—Abuse Statistics
www.elderabusecenter.org

Brayton Purcell Law Firm—Elder Abuse Information
www.elder-abuse-information.com.

American Bar Association
www.abanet.org/media/factbooks/eldt1.html.

National Elder Law Network—Adult Protective Services
www.keln.org

Kari and Associates—Elder Abuse
www.karisable.com/elderabuse.htm.

Bibliography

Emergency Nurses Association: *Care of older adults in the emergency setting (Position Statement),* Des Plaines, Ill, 2003, Emergency Nurses Association, available: www.ena.org.

Emergency Nurses Association: *Domestic violence—maltreatment and human neglect (Position Statement),* Des Plaines, Ill, 2003, Emergency Nurses Association, available: www.ena.org.

Forciea MA, Lavizzo-Mourey R, Schwab EP, Raziano DB: *Geriatric secrets,* Philadelphia, 1996, Hanley & Belfus.

Gray-Vickrey P: Combating elder abuse, *Nursing* 34(10):47-51, 2004.

Rosen P, Barkin RM, Hayden SR, et al: *The 5-minute emergency medicine consult,* Philadelphia, 1999, Lippincott, Williams & Wilkins.

Stabb AS, Hodges LC: *Essentials of gerontological nursing,* Philadelphia, 1996, Lippincott.

Chapter 60

Sexual Assault

Linda Ledray and Carol J. Schwartz

1. What is a sexual assault nurse examiner?

A sexual assault nurse examiner (SANE) is a registered nurse (RN) who has advanced education in forensic examination of sexual assault victims. A SANE is typically on call to the emergency department (ED) 24 hours a day, 7 days a week to provide medical forensic care for any sexual assault survivor (male or female).

2. List the functions of a SANE role.

The SANE is responsible for completing the entire sexual assault evidentiary examination. This includes:

- Crisis intervention
- Helping the survivor decide if she will report the crime
- Sexually transmitted infection (STI) prevention
- Pregnancy risk evaluation
- Emergency contraception (EC), if needed, following a pre-established medical protocol or with the approval of a consulting physician or advanced practice nurse
- Collection of forensic evidence
- Referral for additional follow-up support and care
- Reporting in states with mandatory reporting laws for felony crimes or child abuse

3. Does the SANE provide medical treatment?

The SANE conducts a limited medical examination to identify injuries, but does not complete a routine physical examination. The SANE may treat minor injuries, such as washing and bandaging minor cuts or abrasions, but further evaluation and care of any major physical trauma is referred to the ED or a designated medical facility.

4. How is a SANE-A different from a SANE?

SANE-A is the credential that a SANE receives when the nurse has passed the sexual assault nurse examiner certification examination offered through the International Association of Forensic Nurses. SANE is a nurse who has completed the SANE training.

5. What is a SART?

The sexual assault response team (SART) is the primary group of people who provide support and assistance to the rape survivor directly after the sexual assault. They include the SANE, rape crisis center advocate, law enforcement officer, prosecutor, and crime laboratory specialist.

6. Describe a rape crisis center advocate.

The rape advocate is usually a volunteer who has completed approximately 40 hours of special training to prepare her to provide support and advocacy to victims of sexual assault. The rape advocate will likely stay with the victim during the evidentiary examination and when the victim meets with the sex crimes detective and prosecutor at a later point in time.

7. Discuss the occurrence of rape/sexual assault.

For reported rape, the incidence for women (12 years and older) was 2.3 per 1,000 persons. One out of every four women will be sexually assaulted sometime during her lifetime; college campuses pose a particular greater risk for rape than the general population (350 rapes per year per student body of 10,000 females). For males (12 or older) the reported incidence was 0.4 per 1,000 persons.

8. What should I do if a patient comes to triage and says, "I have been raped"?

- Determine medical stability.
- Provide privacy. Even if there are no urgent physical injuries, a rape victim should be given a priority triage category.
- Notify an on-call SANE program, a SART, sometimes also referred to as a coordinated community response team, or a rape advocate program. Research shows it is best to call the SANE or advocate automatically (without asking the patient). You are calling a specialist, just like you would if the victim had a medical condition requiring a specialist's involvement.

9. How do I handle a patient who is upset and crying?

- Provide privacy.
- Allow any family or friends to stay with the patient (if the patient desires that).
- Make an initial assessment to determine if the victim is actively suicidal, currently oriented, or in need of mental health involvement.
- Reassure the victim that it is normal to be upset.
- Offer a warmed blanket to wrap around the victim.

10. Should we still page the SANE or advocate immediately if the rape victim is not medically stable?

Yes. Depending on the circumstances, the SANE could collect evidence during the medical treatment. It is also possible that the SANE may ask you to call back after the victim is stable.

11. Tell me what aspects are essential to cover with a sexual assault victim.

Time of the forced sexual contact. The guideline for a sexual assault evidentiary examination in most areas is within 72 hours. Some, however, use 96 hours, and epithelial cells have even been obtained from around the cervix up to a week later.

Decision about making a police report. Even if the victims do not want to make a report, and it is not mandated reporting, still give the option of having a sexual assault forensic examination to collect evidence in case they change their mind later.

Need for treatment to prevent STIs and/or pregnancy (EC). This should occur even if the victim refuses the sexual examination.

12. Talk about clues that might indicate that the victim had a drug-facilitated sexual assault.

Statements such as, "I don't remember what happened" or "I don't know how I got home." This is important as some date rape drugs, such as Xyrem (GHB), dissipate very quickly and specimen collection needs to be done as soon as possible.

13. Should I write "alleged rape" for the presenting complaint because I don't know for sure?

No! It implies that you do not believe the victim. Nurses do not write "alleged myocardial infarction" even though that diagnosis is not confirmed. Use "sexual assault," "reported sexual assault," "sexual assault forensic exam," or "chief complaint, sexual assault." The incidence of people falsely claiming rape is no greater, and probably less, than people falsely claiming that they have been victims of any other crime. It is much more likely that someone who has been raped will minimize or deny the fact.

Remember, it is not your responsibility to decide if the victim was really raped. That is what law enforcement will investigate and a jury will ultimately decide. It is your job to provide complete and comprehensive evidence collection and treatment.

14. Should the physician automatically see the victim before the SANE forensic examination if there is vaginal bleeding?

No, unless the bleeding is profuse. It is not uncommon for there to be some vaginal bleeding. The physician should be asked to examine the victim before the SANE arrives only when it is a medical necessity.

15. I paged the SANE. Now what?

The SANE typically responds within an hour. While waiting, the ED staff should:

- Verify the patient is medically stable.

- Consider a chaplain or social worker to wait with the victim.
- Call the police if the victim wants to make a report.
- Wait for treatment, if possible, until the SANE arrives for evidence collection.

16. Anything I should remember if treatment must be started?

If clothes or objects are removed from the victim, avoid cutting through tears or stains on the clothing. Each piece of clothing should be put in a separate paper bag with chain-of-custody documentation. When possible, take pictures of the victim's injuries before treatment is begun.

17. Should I offer something to eat or drink to a rape victim who is waiting?

No, unless you know for certain there was no oral involvement. It eliminates evidence.

18. What should I do if the victim asks to use the bathroom?

It is best if the rape victim does not use the bathroom until after the sexual assault forensic examination (whenever there has been genital contact). However, if it is necessary, ask the victim to catch the urine and not wipe ("drip dry"). Wiping destroys more evidence. Most crime laboratories do *not* want you to save toilet paper, or toilet water that might contain sperm. Maintain chain-of-custody for the specimen if a drug-facilitated sexual assault is suspected.

19. Is it possible a rape victim could come to the ED and not disclose that she was raped?

It is estimated that there are actually more than a million sexual assaults each year (male and female) and two-thirds go unreported. It is also estimated that only 30% of sexual assault victims report that they were sexually assaulted when seeking follow-up care after a sexual assault. Signs that the ED patient is a victim of sexual assault could include:

- Requests testing for STIs or EC, but is very vague about why there is a need.
- Appears upset or preoccupied.
- Is a domestic violence victim. Nearly one in three domestic violence victims are believed to also be a victim of sexual assault. The pervasive belief remains that a man always has a right to have sex with his wife or domestic partner. As a result, many of these women do not label forced sex as a sexual assault or rape.

20. Who is least likely to disclose a rape?

Classically it is male victims. They fear not being believed, considered gay, or blame themselves.

21. List some physical clues that might indicate a patient was a victim of sexual assault.

- Vaginal or rectal soreness
- Vaginal or rectal tearing or trauma, especially if it results in bleeding
- Bruising on the inner thighs
- Unexplained injury
- Unusual pain or sensitivity or the patient becomes tearful when a speculum is inserted

22. How can I help a victim recognize and/or disclose that he or she was a victim of rape?

Never hesitate to ask but initially avoid the term "rape." The victim might not label the forced sex as "rape." Instead ask, "Did anyone touch you sexually in a way that made you feel uncomfortable, that was against your will, or that hurt you?"

23. What do we do if the police bring in a patient for a rape examination, but the patient passes out from drugs or alcohol before giving consent?

Perform the examination if there is good reason to believe she was sexually assaulted or if law enforcement requests it under the law of exigent circumstances. The exam presents limited risk and valuable evidence will be lost if you wait. The only time the authors recommend to not proceed is if the victim actively refuses or physically resists the examination.

24. What if the parents or the police insist we do an exam on a teenager who is refusing?

Every patient has the right to refuse the examination, including an underaged, informed teenager. At what age you would sedate a child and complete an examination regardless becomes a matter of policy. Our program has agreed to decide on a case-by-case basis for children less than 11 years of age.

This type of situation is often an issue with a teenager who has admitted, or was witnessed, having sex with a "boyfriend." The parents can certainly report it to law enforcement if it fits the statutory rape guidelines, but the teenager can still refuse an evidentiary examination.

In this kind of case, explain to the parents that the evidentiary exam will really not provide any additional information. The evidence collected confirms recent sexual contact, which is not being denied. All that is really needed now is full and accurate documentation.

25. What if a teenager who has been raped wants EC and STI prevention medications, but the parent is not available to give consent?

Unless your state has passed a law requiring parental or court consent, federal statutes allow you to complete an evidentiary examination, treat to prevent sexually transmitted diseases (STDs), and provide emergency contraception (EC) without parental consent.

26. What if there was only digital vaginal penetration and no injuries are evident?

The victim still needs a forensic examination; so you should still page the SANE. With the advances in DNA recovery and identification, it may still be possible to recover the assailant's DNA. There may be internal (vaginal, cervical) injuries or additional information will emerge from the interview.

27. How should we triage a patient who has had multiple sexual assault examinations, but who has always failed to follow through with a police report?

Treat every sexual assault report individually, even though it may be frustrating. Someone who is being raped multiple times obviously needs help.

28. What STDs should be treated?

The Centers for Disease Control and Prevention recommends prophylactic treatment for chlamydia, gonorrhea, syphilis, hepatis B (if not immunized), and trichomonas (2002).

29. What if the victim is from a different culture?

It is always important to consider the language and cultural issues and their impact on sexual assault. Call an interpreter, as it is not appropriate to use a family member or friend, as the victim may be hesitant to provide detailed information in front of someone they know. For further discussion, see Chapter 71. Cultural issues may also play a role in not wanting to report the rape to law enforcement, or being concerned that others will find out what happened.

30. Are we violating the Emergency Medical Treatment and Active Labor Act if the physician does not do a complete medical screening examination before the SANE arrives?

The Emergency Medical Treatment and Active Labor Act (EMTALA) does *not* require that a physician complete the medical screening exam (MSE), but just that an appropriate MSE is completed. The requirement is that the same procedure should be used for all patients with similar symptoms. The SANE could be designated as the person to complete the MSE for all patients coming because of a reported sexual assault. Even when the injuries required a physician, they often can be treated after the SANE has completed the evidentiary examination.

31. Do we have a responsibility to provide forensic evaluation and care to victims?

The Joint Commission on Accreditation of Healthcare Organizations (JCAHO) requires health care facilities to develop protocols and train their staff to use criteria to identify possible victims of physical assault, rape, or other sexual molestation, domestic abuse, and abuse or neglect of older adults and children.

32. Do I have to report the rape to the police?

The mandated reporting statutes vary state to state. Check your local requirements.

- Mandated reporting of child sexual abuse: You must report when the victim of sexual assault is legally a minor and the perpetrator is a relative, lives in the household, or is in a position of authority over the child, such as a babysitter, troop leader, teacher, etc.
- Statutory rape: In most states this means the victim is legally a minor, and the perpetrator is legally an adult at least 4 years older than the minor. In most states you are not mandated to report statutory rape. Even though it is a crime, the victim still has the right to decide if she wants to report.
- Vulnerable adult laws: In most states you are mandated to report the rape of vulnerable adults, such as adults who are living in an institution or who are not competent to make their own decisions.
- Use of deadly weapons: If a deadly weapon, such as a knife or gun was used during the rape and it resulted in injury, you are mandated to report the use of the weapon and the injury.

33. How do I handle it when a victim does not want to make a report?

Clarify if the victim does not want to report because of a specific fear or concern and if the decision is informed. Common reasons a victim may be hesitant to report include:

- Not labeling the forced sex rape
- The assailant threatened to come back if she reported
- Blaming herself or himself because the victim was drinking with the assailant, willingly went to the assailant's apartment, or invited the person to the home
- Not wanting other people to find out because she is ashamed
- Fears people will blame her
- Bad past experience with the police
- Fear of arrest because the victim was drinking when under age or using illegal drugs prior to the rape
- Fear because of some minor past infraction (e.g., parking tickets)
- Fear the media will report the rape in the paper
- Belief it won't do any good to report anyway

Talk through the concerns. For instance, most law enforcement agencies will not check a victim's past record or will not charge the victim with alcohol or drug use when reporting a rape. Ledray found 38% of the 337 rape survivors were uncertain about reporting at first. After talking with a knowledgeable SANE, an additional 12% decided to report to the police in the ED. Only 3% of the 337 survivors in this study did not ever make a report.

34. How do I handle it if the victim still does not want to report after talking with the SANE, advocate, or me?

Offer to have evidence collected now (just in case). The victim can make a report years later. In Ledray's study (1999), an additional 23% agreed to have an examination because they might report later. However, the longer a person waits, the more likely credibility may be an issue and crime scene evidence will be lost. Always offer medical treatment, care for STI and EC, and referrals.

35. How long should we keep the evidentiary examination kit? The police won't take it unless there is a report filed.

Your facility should have a policy with a specified time period, but usually it is 1 month.

36. Will I have to testify in court?

In most cases the SANE will testify. The exceptions are if the victim tells you something she does not tell the SANE or if you helped treat significant injuries. Clear and accurate documentation is key. After a group of physicians at a Kansas City hospital began dictating their records, they were called to testify 70% less because the prosecutor could read the records.

37. Do emergency nurses' personal experiences of being a victim of violence affect the nurses' care of battered women?

Early et al (2002) found it did not affect the nurses' proposed nursing care of battered women using vignettes.

38. Where can I get help to start a SANE or SART program?

Go to www.sane-sart.com for a free guide that you can download or order.

Key Points

- Call a SANE or advocate automatically without asking the patient.
- The guideline for a sexual assault evidentiary examination in most areas is 72 hours.
- Never write the complaint as "alleged rape." Use "sexual assault" or "reported sexual assault."
- Ask, "Did anyone touch you sexually in a way that made you feel uncomfortable, that was against your will or that hurt you?" Some victims do not initially label the sexual assault as a "rape."
- Avoid cutting through tears or stains on the victim's clothing.
- It is estimated only 30% of sexual assault victims report the reason when seeking follow-up care.

Internet Resources

Emergency Nurses Association Position Statement: Care of Sexual Assault Victims
http://www.ena.org/publications/statements/positionpdf/care-sexual-assault-victims.pdf

Emergency Nurses Association Position Statement: Forensic Evidence Collection
http://www.ena.org/publications/statements/positionpdf/forensicevidence.pdf

American College of Emergency Physicians: Management of the Patient With the Complaint of Sexual Assault
http://www.acep.org/1,614,0.html

National Center for Victims of Crime (NCVC): Sexual Assault
http://www.ncvc.org/ncvc/main.aspx?dbName=DocumentViewer&DocumentID=32369

National Center for Victims of Crime (NCVC): Male Rape
http://www.ncvc.org/ncvc/main.aspx?dbName=DocumentViewer&DocumentAction=ViewProperties&DocumentID=32361&UrlToReturn=http%3a%2f%2fwww.ncvc.org%2fncvc%2fmain.aspx%3fdbName%3dSiteSearch

Sexual Assault Nurse Examiner—Sexual Assault Response Team
www.sane-sart.com

Bibliography

Bobak IM: Violence against women. In Bobak IM, Jensen MD, editors: *Maternity and gynecologic care,* St Louis, 1992, Mosby.

Chasson S, Russell A: Do SANE examinations satisfy the EMTALA requirement for "medical screening"? Sexual assault nurse examiners, Emergency Medical Treatment and Active Labor Act, *J Emerg Nurs* 28(6):593-595, 2002.

Chivers CJ: In sex crimes, evidence depends on game of chance in hospitals, *The New York Times,* August 6, 2000, 1-6.

Early MR, Williams RA: Emergency nurses' experience with violence: Does it affect nursing care of battered women? *J Emerg Nurs* 28(3):199-204, 2002.

Fisher BS, Cullen F, Turner M: *The sexual victimization of college women,* Washington, DC, 2000, US Department of Justice.

Joint Commission on Accreditation of Healthcare Organizations: *Comprehensive accreditation manual for hospitals: The official handbook,* Oakbrook Terrace, Ill, 1997, Joint Commission on Accreditation of Healthcare Organizations.

Ledray LE: *Sexual assault nurse examiner (SANE) development and operation guide,* Washington, DC, 1999, US Department of Justice, Office of Victims of Crime.

Ledray LE, Kraft JE: Sexual assault: Clinical issue—"Evidentiary examination without a police report: Should it be done? Are delayed reporters and nonreporters unique?" *J Emerg Nurs* 27(4):396-400, 2001.

Chapter 61

Alcohol Use and Abuse

Polly Gerber Zimmermann

1. Is alcohol misuse and abuse really that prevalent of an issue in emergency department patients?

Cherpitel (1999) found that patients presenting to an emergency department (ED) (compared to those presenting to a primary care setting in the same metropolitan area) were one and a half to three times more likely to report heavy drinking, consequences of drinking, alcohol dependence, or ever having treatment for an alcohol problem. Alcohol-related ED visits are estimated to be 7.6 million annually or 7.9% of all ED visits. This is three times higher than previously thought (an 18% increase over a 9-year period). Outside of obvious intoxication, alcohol can be a factor in many other presentations, including falls, domestic violence, or chronic conditions. We know:

- Three out of 10 American adults engage in risky drinking.
- Eighteen percent of the hospitalized drivers meet the criteria for alcohol dependence.
- Fifty percent of patients in all trauma beds were injured in an alcohol-related event.

2. What must a triage nurse never do?

Regard an intoxicated person as "just another drunk." This can lead to being less vigilant than a nurse would be with other patients who had a similar level of impairment.

3. What behaviors might make me suspect a person has a problem with excess alcohol?

- *Delay in seeking care for a significant injury.* One young man with a serious injury explained he laid on the floor for 12 hours because he was "tired."
- *Indicate a blackout period but do not seem concerned about it.* In my experience, people are worried if they have a blackout for the first time. A nonchalant attitude signals there has probably been a previous experience or awareness of the cause.
- *Frequent complaint of gastritis/heartburn.* The complaints are often after weekends and/or "big" events, such as the NBA finals.

4. Define "binge drinking."

Binge drinking is defined as consuming five or more alcoholic beverages (four or more for women) in a row at one "sitting."

5. How can I get an accurate response when I ask about alcohol consumption?

Make the patient quantify. Do not ask, "Do you drink?" Ask:
- "When did you last take a drink?"
- "What do you normally drink?"
- "How much do you normally drink?"

6. What can I do if I get an answer that I doubt?

- *Overestimate and let the individual correct you.* For instance, "Do you think you drank two cases of beer?" The person will then be more likely to respond "Oh no, just one case." It puts it in the realm of possible.
- *Feign surprise with a negative or low answer.* "Really? Is that all?" Then the person will sometimes sheepishly admit to a higher amount.
- *Ask unexpectedly.* Move on to another subject but then suddenly ask again, "How much did you say you drink?" Sometimes, caught off guard, a more truthful answer is given.

7. Do these ideas really work?

The key is to always remain matter of fact as if that is a "normal" answer. Alcohol abusers often become used to the excessive intake and probably have found others whose similar habits enable acceptance of their drinking patterns.

8. Discuss the times most likely for withdrawal symptoms.

The likelihood for onset for delirium tremors (DTs) is 8 hours (peak 24 hours) after the last drink. Alcohol-withdrawal seizures (AWDS) occur within 6 to 96 hours after the last drink. The AWDS occur in clusters of one to four seizures and tend to be self-limiting. They can be prevented with benzodiazepines.

9. Talk about the risk of alcohol-induced hypoglycemia.

Alcohol-induced hypoglycemia (AIH) results from insufficient glycogen stores and the alcohol-induced impairment of gluconeogenesis. It occurs during intoxication or up to 20 hours after the last drink. Patients vulnerable to AIH are chronic alcoholics, binge drinkers, and young children.

The classic signs and symptoms of the diabetic hypoglycemic response (tremulous, diaphoresis, anxiety) do *not* usually occur. Manifestations are related to the central nervous system's glucose deprivation (headache, depressed mental status, seizures). It can cause a stroke-like presentation in adults.

10. List some objective evidence that can help determine alcohol consumption.

The mean corpuscular volume (MCV) of the complete blood cell count (CBC). It is normally low in patients with chronic obstructive pulmonary disease, pernicious anemia, and B_{12} deficiency, but is also low in chronic alcohol abuse related to the poor nutrition.

The gamma-glutamyl transferase (GGT) liver enzyme. If it is high, although other liver enzymes are normal, there has been regular alcohol consumption in the last 2 months.

11. What age group has the most problems with alcohol excess?

Excessive alcohol consumption is an issue throughout all age groups, starting even in the grade schools.

- Twenty percent of eighth graders and 50% of high school seniors surveyed indicated they had had a drink in the past month, and 30% admitted to binging within the previous 2 weeks.
- Among U.S. college students, 22.8% did binge drinking three or more times in the previous 2 weeks and 21.6% did it one to two times in the previous 2 weeks.

12. Isn't this just a harmless phase in young people?

About 7.2 million said young people age 12 to 20 admitted they were binge drinkers and 2.3 million said they were heavy drinkers. Seventh grade drinking status was significantly associated with the number of problems in twelfth grade and at age 23.

13. What happens to the drinking habits as people grow up into adulthood?

In one survey, 17% of all adults were binge drinking, with an episode in the last 30 days. In moderate drinkers, the binge drinking was more than 50%.

14. Discuss drinking in the older adult.

Excessive drinking is more likely in the older adult if they had a pattern of drinking earlier in their life. There are more problems with alcohol abuse because of social isolation and they cannot physiologically handle alcohol as well.

15. Tell me the recommendations regarding moderate drinking for the older adult.

The current recommendation from the National Institute on Alcohol Abuse and Alcoholism (NIAAA) is that healthy adults > age 65 years should consume no more than one drink per day. One standard drink is defined as one 5-oz glass of wine, one 12-oz can of beer, or one mixed drink containing 1.5 oz of distilled spirits.

16. Are older adults aware of this?

Masters (2003) found that 52% of the older adults were aware of the health benefits of moderate drinking. Of those adults, 86% mistakenly believed these benefits applied to all individuals. And 40% defined moderate drinking as two or more drinks per day.

17. Why is it important to identify possible alcohol abuse when treating the older adult?

Benzodiazepines should not be used if the older adult person has agitation *without* alcohol abuse. Up to 25% of older adults have a paradoxical reaction to benzodiazepines and become agitated. This reaction is often not recognized and so *more* drugs are given. Benzodiazepines are used in the older adult *if* the agitation is from alcohol withdrawal.

18. Discuss the more recent emphasis on ED alcohol screening.

The focus is on identification and help of people who drink amounts that increase the risk for future consequences or drink amounts that cause harm, but not alcohol dependence. Alcoholism is a progressive disease that can respond to early intervention.

The third U.S. Preventive Services Task Force (USPSTF) guidelines recommend screening and counseling for alcohol misuse (category B). The Emergency Nurses Association (ENA) adopted a supportive position statement in 2004. The American College of Emergency Physicians (ACEP) also endorses and promotes screening.

19. What amounts are considered excessive?

The USPSTF indicates:
- Two standard drinks daily or >4 per occasion for men
- More than 1 daily or >3 per occasion for women.

The NIAAA indicates:

Men	>14 drinks/week or >4 drinks/occasion
Women	>7 drinks/week or >3 drinks/occasion
>65 years old	>7 drinks/week or >3 drinks/occasion

20. What approach should I use?

ED nurses are the first part of the **SBIRT** approach (**S**creening, **B**rief **I**ntervention of promoting education, provide **R**eferral, and formal evaluation and **T**reatment). Timing is important because an alcohol-related illness or injury can result in a "teachable moment." Studies have found up to 80% of those referred from an emergency room do follow-up.

The USPSTF recommends using validated questionnaires such as CAGE, AUDIT (Alcohol Use Disorders Identification Test), or TWEAK (for pregnant women). The NIAAA recommends the use of quantity and frequency (Q&F) questions and the CAGE questionnaire. Some emergency departments just ask the Q&F questions, moving on to CAGE only if the patient is above moderate levels.

21. List the quantity and frequency questions.

- On average, how many days per week do you drink alcohol?
- On a typical day when you drink, how many drinks do you have?
- What is the maximum number of drinks you had on any given occasion during the last month?

If the patient is in the excessive amounts, or you already know there is a problem, go to the CAGE questionnaire.

22. Describe CAGE.

CAGE screens for alcohol dependence in the last 12 months. Its rapid application makes it well suited for emergency department use. The acronym comes from:

- Have you ever felt you should **Cut down** on your drinking?
- Have people **Annoyed** you about your drinking?
- Have you ever felt bad or **Guilty** about your drinking?
- Have you ever had a drink first thing in the morning to steady your nerves or get rid of a hangover (**Eye-opener**)?

CAGE has a sensitivity ranging from 72% to 91% and specificity from 77% to 96% for recognition of alcohol dependence (positive predictive power of 87%). Its weaknesses are that it may fail to detect low, but risky, drinking and it does not perform as well among women and minorities.

23. What is different about enhanced CAGE or CAGEAID?

Enhanced CAGE adds quantity and frequency questions that result in better sensitivity, especially with minorities. CAGEAID is Adapted to Include Drugs. It adds the phrase "or drug use" to each question. Many believe the addition of drugs is warranted as more than one in ten Americans have a substance dependence or abuse.

24. How do I evaluate the answers?

A screen is positive if one or more questions from CAGE is answered "yes" and/or increased consumption. If the patient screens positive, move to a brief intervention.

25. Isn't the ED too busy to do screening for alcohol abuse?

One emergency department found it takes only a few seconds for about 40% of their adult patients because they do not drink alcohol (e.g., "no" to the first question). It then takes only about 10 additional seconds for moderate drinkers who are under the low-risk limits and 30 seconds total to complete all CAGE questions. Other alternatives include:

- Screen only "high-risk" patients, such as those with an injury, hypertension, gastrointestinal complaints, seizures, change in mental status, or 16- to 24-year-olds.
- Use questionnaires in the waiting room or computer-assisted entry.
- Involve outside resources. Project ASSERT in Connecticut has social workers and community outreach workers for substance abuse screening.

26. What is a brief intervention?

Brief interventions are short counseling sessions, often less than 5 minutes. They often incorporate the six elements summarized in the acronym **FRAMES**.

***F**eedback:* Review problems experienced because of alcohol
***R**esponsibility:* Changing alcohol use is the patient's responsibility
***A**dvice:* Advise to cut down or abstain
***M**enu:* Provide options for changing behavior
***E**mpathy:* Use an empathetic approach
***S**elf-Efficacy:* Encourage optimism that one is capable of changing behavior

27. Provide an example.

The acronym **ED DIRECT**, recommended by ACEP, incorporates these elements:
***E**mpathy.* Adapt a warm, understanding style
***D**irectness.* Maintain eye contact and state, "I would like to take a few minutes to discuss your alcohol use."
***D**ata.* Give feedback ("I'm concerned about your drinking because our screening indicates you are above what we consider the normal safe limits/at risk for alcohol-related injury, illness, or death.") Compare with national norms.
***I**dentify* willingness to change.
***R**ecommend* action/advice.
***E**licit* response.
***C**larify* and confirm action.
***T**elephone* referral.

28. Describe how to identify a willingness to change.

Ask the patient, "On a scale of 1 to 10, how ready are you to change your drinking patterns?"

- If the response is ≤6 or less, then ask "Why not more?"
- If the response is ≥7, then move on to recommendations.

Regardless of the answer, the clinician identifies discrepancies and assists the patient to move along from ambivalence to change.

29. How would I recommend action/advice?

- Use the **Five Rs** for individuals unwilling to change or abstain:
  Relevance: Ask the patient to indicate why a change is personally relevant (e.g., family, health).
  Risks: Ask the patient to identify negative consequences of current alcohol use (e.g., health, injury risk).
  Rewards: Ask the patient to identify potential benefits of changing (or stopping) alcohol use (e.g., feel better, save money).
  Roadblocks: Ask patient to identify barriers or impediments to changing/quitting (e.g., partner drinks, social events, lack of alternative coping skills).
  Repetition: Repeat process on a regular basis.
- Use the **Five As** for individuals who express a desire to change:
  Ask: Identify drinking activity at each contact.
  Advise: Strongly urge to abstain.
  Assess: Determine willingness to attempt abstaining.
  Assist: Aid the patient in developing a plan to abstain.
  Arrange: Schedule a follow-up contact.

30. Is there any additional action/advice that is a standard recommendation?

ACEP also encourages for:

- *All Patients.* "We recommend that you never drive after drinking."
- *At-Risk/Harmful Drinkers.* Give recommended drinking limits and encourage follow-up with the primary care physician.
- *Positive Screen (but unsure if dependent drinker).* Abstain and refer for further assessment.
- *Dependent Drinker.* Abstain and refer to a detoxification center, Alcoholics Anonymous, and primary care.

31. What is meant by "elicit a response"?

Simply obtain some sense of the patient's reaction to this discussion. Ask, "How does this sound to you?"

32. Describe the steps to "clarify" and "confirm action" and telephone referral.

It serves a summation purpose. For instance, indicate you have completed a screening test for alcohol problems that may lead to an increase risk of illness or injury; you are giving a recommendation for what is known to be safe drinking limits, and there is a desire for the patient to follow-up, just as would be done for any patient who screened positively for other health problems (diabetes, etc.). Offer to let a patient with a positive screen speak to an alcoholic counselor (even if on the phone) or to have the ED call for a referral appointment now.

33. What aspect could triage do?

In triage, the nurse could ask the screening questions and/or give a handout.

34. Discuss the screening tool AUDIT.

This screening tool consists of ten questions, with three potential answers (and different points) for each one. It is used more frequently with inpatients as a result of its longer length and complexity. It has better detection of risky drinking levels. For more information, see the website listed in the Internet Resources Box at the end of this chapter.

35. Does screening make a difference?

Yes. For "at-risk" and "harmful" drinkers that are not dependent, goal setting within safe limits, discharge instructions, and a referral to primary care is all that may be needed. For those who are dependent or that you are unsure of their position along the spectrum of alcohol problems, the brief intervention is a negotiation process to seek further assessment and referral to a specialized treatment program.

- The interventions led to decreased drinking in 12 controlled studies. The proportion of people who decreased their drinking increased by 10% to 19%.
- D'Onofrio and Degutis (2002) review of 32 studies showed positive effects and concluded that screenings and brief interventions should be part of ED practice.

36. Do the screening recommendations apply to adolescents?

The USPSTF concluded the evidence was insufficient to recommend for or against screening and counseling of adolescents (Recommendation: I).

37. Where can I obtain resources and additional information?

Copies of the CAGE tool can be obtained from the National Highway Transportation and Safety Administration (nhtsa.dot.com) or the American College of Emergency Physicians (acep.org). In addition, ACEP will provide a sample brochure (Alcohol How Much is Too Much?) and a list of national resources. They also offer a full explanation of ED DIRECT and a quick reference card.

Key Points

- It is estimated that 7.9% of all ED visits are alcohol-related.
- Benzodiazepines are used for alcohol withdrawal. Agitation in an older adult person without alcohol abuse should *not* be treated with benzodiazepines as a result of the risk of a paradoxical reaction.
- The MCV is low in patients with chronic alcohol abuse.
- Use the SBIRT approach.
- Never assume a patient is "just a drunk."

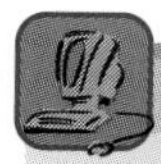

Internet Resources

Emergency Department Alcohol Education Project: Screening, Brief Intervention, Referral and Treatment (SBIRT)
www.ed.bmc.org/sbirt/index.htm

Helping Patients With Alcohol Problems: A Health Practitioner's Guide
http://www.niaaa.nih.gov/publications/Practitioner/HelpingPatients.htm

National Institute on Alcohol Abuse and Alcoholism
www.niaaa.nih.gov

Join Together Online: Take Action Against Substance Abuse and Gun Violence
www.jointogether.org/tx

Summary of the Evidence: Behavioral Counseling Interventions in Primary Care to Reduce Risky/Harmful Alcohol Use by Adults. U.S. Preventive Services Task Force
http://www.ahrq.gov/clinic/3rduspstf/alcohol/alcomissum.htm

Screening and Behavioral Counseling Interventions in Primary Care to Reduce Alcohol Misuse
http://www.ahrq.gov/clinic/3rduspstf/alcohol/alcomisrs.pdf

Alcohol Use Disorders Identification Test (AUDIT)
www.niaaa.nih.gov/publications/audit.htm

Bibliography

Baker SP, Braver ER, Chen LH, Li G, Williams AF: Drinking histories of fatally injured drivers, *Inj Prev* 8:221-226, 2002.

Cherpitel CJ: Screening for alcohol problems in the US general population: A comparison of the CAGE and TWEAK by gender, ethnicity, and services utilization, *J Stud Alcohol* 60(5):705-711, 1999.

D'Onofrio G, Degutis LC: Preventive care in the emergency department: Screening and brief intervention for alcohol problems in the emergency department: A systematic review, *Acad Emerg Med* 9(6):627-638, 2002.

D'Onofrio G, Mascia R, Razzak J, Degutis LC: Utilizing health promotion advocates for selected health risk screening and intervention in the ED, *Acad Emerg Med* 8:543(abstract), 2001.

Ellickson PL: Ten-year prospective study of public health problems associated with early drinking, *Pediatrics* 111:949-955, 2003.

Emergency Department Alcohol and Education Project: *Scope of the problem*, 2004, available: www.ed.bmc.org/shirt/scope.htm.

MacLean SL, Perhats C: Preventing death, injury and illness through a brief ED Intervention: Alcohol awareness intervention, *ENA Connections* 28(5):1, 10-13, 2004.

Marx JA: Alcohol-related disorders. In Markovchick VJ, Pons PT, editors: *Pons' emergency medicine secrets*, ed 3, Philadelphia, 2003, Hanley & Belfus, 366-370.

Masters JA: Moderate alcohol consumption and unappreciated risk for alcohol-related harm among ethnically diverse, urban-dwelling elders, *Geriatr Nurs* 24(3):155, 2003.

Naimi TS, et al: Binge drinking among US adults, *JAMA* 289:70-75, 2003.

O'Brien PG: Addictive behaviors. In Lewis SM, Heitkemper MM, Dirksen SR, editors: *Medical-surgical nursing*, ed 6, St Louis, 2004, Mosby.

St. Mars T: Routine alcohol screening for all ED patients: Ask the questions! *J Emerg Nurs* 30(3):257-258, 2004.

US Preventive Services Task Force: Screening and behavioral counseling interventions in primary care to reduce alcohol misuse: Recommendation statement, *Ann Intern Med* 140:554-556, 2004.

Whitlock EP, et al: Behavioral counseling interventions in primary care to reduce risky/harmful alcohol use by adults: A summary of the evidence for the US Preventive Services Task Force, *Ann Intern Med* 140:557-568, 2004.

Section X

Disaster and Terrorism Issues

Chapter 62

Weapons of Mass Destruction/ Mass Casualty Incident

Sharon Saunderson Cohen and Kevin Richard Brooks

1. What constitutes a mass casualty incident?

A good general definition of mass casualty incident (MCI) is when the number of patients and the severity of their medical condition or injuries exceed the capability of the facility, hospital, and staff.

2. During an MCI, do you triage the casualties the same way you would on any normal presentation?

No. Typically triage must be modified; patients sustaining major injuries who have the greatest chance of survival with the least expenditure of time, equipment, supplies, and personnel are managed first. This differs from standard triage methodology in which we evaluate the patient and treat the most critical first. This method would deplete a facility of their personnel and supplies very quickly on many patients that ultimately will not survive. In addition, it is rare to declare any person "hopeless" or black in ordinary triage.

3. Why are weapons of mass destruction a concern to the triage nurse?

The effects from terrorists' acts in weapons of mass destruction (WMD) events usually have related traumatic injuries. The common dispersal device for WMD events often is incendiary or explosive. Both methods of dispersal have the potential to cause an MCI.

4. Define terrorism.

The Department of Justice defines terrorism as a violent act or an act dangerous to human life in violation of the criminal laws of the United States to intimidate or coerce a government, civilian population, or any segment thereof in furtherance of political or social objective.

5. Define bioterrorism.

Bioterrorism is the deliberate use of microorganisms to cause disease with the intention of achieving a purpose or promoting a cause.

6. Before beginning triage and care for a patient with a potential exposure to an unknown substance or agent, what types of harm to self must the triage nurse consider?

An easy way to remember potential harm or exposure is the acronym TRACEM:
Thermal exposure
Radiologic exposure
Asphyxiation
Chemical
Etiologic exposure
Mechanical harm

7. What is the fastest and safest way for the triage nurse to avoid exposure when triaging patients during any MCI or WMD incident?

In most exposures, 80% of decontamination of the patient occurs with removal of the patient's clothing. (And leave them outside of the department.) This is the best method to reduce exposure or cross-contamination to the triage nurse. Obviously full decontamination is the best method to ensure cross-contamination cannot occur.

A way to remember basic safety strategies is SAFE
Safety comes first
Assess the situation before doing anything
Focus on the hazard—avoid contacting it
Evaluate the situation and report to proper authorities

8. What are the principles of triage during an MCI or WMD event?

An MCI or WMD event employs principles of triage, which state that triage must be:

- Ongoing all along the rescue chain
- Efficient and effective
- As objective as possible (removing subjectivity and emotion).

9. What is START?

START is a method of triage during an MCI or WMD incident. The acronym stands for:
Simple
Triage
And
Rapid
Treatment

10. Why would I use START instead of my daily triage methodology of my hospital?

- During an MCI or WMD event the situation is not like the everyday presentation of a patient to the emergency department or clinic.

- An extended history of each patient will not be feasible as a result of the large number of victims that may present in a short period of time.
- The acuity of each victim may be higher requiring quicker treatment and intervention if available.
- Decontamination of victims must occur before allowing the patients to enter any building, facility, or hospital.

11. Is using the START methodology a quicker way to triage?

Yes. Practically, victims are categorized into one of four groups: immediate care (red); delayed care (yellow); minor (green); morgue/unsalvageable (black). The triage category is based on three assessments and ambulation only:

	Normal Findings
Respirations	Present and <30 beats per minute
Pulse	Present radial pulse and capillary refill <2 seconds
Mentation	Follows simple commands

12. How do I use the START methodology?

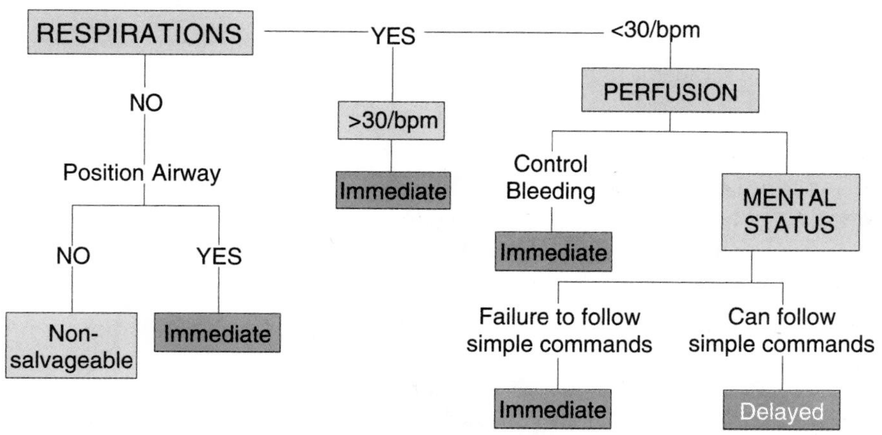

START triage.
From the Office for Domestic Preparedness, US Department of Homeland Security.

13. Do I use the START methodology the same on adults as pediatrics?

Children have unique physiologic and anatomic characteristics and differ from adults in several ways. Because of this, JumpSTART was developed for pediatric patients between the ages of 1 and 8 years.

14. How is JumpSTART different from START?

JumpSTART is also based on the assessment of RPM, with one modification for respirations. If a pediatric between the ages of 1 to 8 years is found with no spontaneous respiration the triage nurse should attempt to open the airway, reassess for spontaneous respiration, and if none exists, proceed to assess a pulse. If there is a pulse the triage nurse would then "jumpstart" the child with 15 seconds of ventilation and reassess for spontaneous respirations. If no spontaneous respirations are noted, the child is categorized as black or morgue/unsalvageable.

15. Should I triage children before adults?

Generally, the principles of triage are the same for children and adults, although the priority of children over adults within the same categories is controversial. The Save the Children Fund in 1923 and UNICEF in 1990 declared that children must receive relief first, but this recommendation is not universally accepted.

16. About how much time should the triage nurse spend on triaging each victim using START?

Each victim should be triaged and a color or category assigned in approximately 15 seconds.

17. Where do I begin to triage in an MCI?

Depending on institutional or hospital policy and procedures, a predetermined triage area may be designated if the MCI event occurred external to the medical building. If the medical building or hospital was part of the incident, then triage would begin right where the triage nurse stands.

18. What is the first step of triage utilizing START in an MCI?

The triage nurse should ask all victims that can ambulate to the green (minor) area to do so. A large number of victims will then triage themselves "green." All remaining victims will then need to be triaged also using the START method.

19. Is there any other triage method to use in an MCI/WMD incident other than START?

Several researchers introduced assessment tools to aid clinicians in the triage process during an MCI/WMD incident. One such tool utilizes the Pediatric Trauma Score with the Eichelberger modification and another is an algorithm proposed by Mackway-Jones et al. Both of these, however, have been found to have some major limitations and are not superior to START.

20. What is the Sacco Triage method?

The Sacco method is an evidence-based and outcome-driven triage and resource management system that can be utilized in an MCI incident. This methodology is not currently widely used by many prehospital medics or hospitals.

21. What amount of training is needed to perform a specialized method of triage such as START?

There is no set amount of time mandated in training to become proficient in performing START. With this said, in a stressful event such as an MCI or WMD the nurse will need a familiarity with the START methodology to be able to accurately and efficiently perform a rapid triage on a large number of victims. Like most anything, to become proficient, it has been recommended that ongoing and continual training and coordinated drills be done.

22. Where is the best place to set up a triage area during an MCI or WMD incident?

Ideally the triage site is located outside the emergency department (ED), between the area for ambulance unloading and the entrance to the ED. The most important concept is that the triage site is *outside* the hospital and away from the ED's air handling intake system!

23. Why is it so important to have the triage site outside the ED?

The most important factor in keeping the triage site outside the ED is to protect the staff and patients from contamination. Victims will have potential for exposure to a chemical, biologic, or radiologic agent(s) that in turn may contaminate anyone who is not properly suited in personal protective equipment. The recent SARS epidemic is a good example of an agent that caused contamination and the resultant closing an entire hospital to incoming patients in Toronto, Canada.

24. Talk about the purpose of triage.

Triaging patients is actually the art of "sorting" patients based on injury or illness acuity. Triage allows the medical and nursing staff to use valuable resources more efficiently and effectively to prioritize and treat the most patients. In addition, triaging allows control of the flow of patients through the ED.

25. Why are victims assigned a color or characteristic?

Assigning a color or characteristic (e.g., immediate, delayed) shows all health care personnel that the patient has been triaged, the severity of the injury or illness of the victim, and helps to maintain the flow of patients through the ED.

26. Where does a victim get "tagged" with the triaged color or characteristic?

Typically the assigned colored ribbon or tag is tied onto an upper extremity (or any intact extremity).

27. Is the triage tag very common?

A triage tag similar to the one shown on the facing page has been recognized across the United States and in some other countries.

Comment Information

Patient's Name

RESPIRATIONS R ☐ Yes ☐ No

PERFUSION P ☐ + 2 Sec ☐ - 2 Sec

MENTAL STATUS M ☐ Can Do ☐ Can't Do

Move the Walking Wounded ▶ MINOR

No Respirations After Head Tilt ▶ MORGUE

☐ Respirations - Over 30 ▶ IMMEDIATE

3

☐ Perfusion - Capillary Refill Over 2 Seconds ▶ IMMEDIATE

☐ Mental Status - Unable to Follow Simple Commands ▶ IMMEDIATE

Otherwise ▶ DELAYED

PERSONAL INFORMATION		
NAME		
ADDRESS		
CITY	4 ST	ZIP
PHONE		
COMMENTS	RELIGIOUS PREF.	

MORGUE Pulseless/Non-Breathing

IMMEDIATE Life Threatening Injury | **IMMEDIATE** Life Threatening Injury

DELAYED Serious Non Life Threatening | **DELAYED** Serious Non Life Threatening

MINOR Walking Wounded | **MINOR** Walking Wounded

CONTAMINATED CONTAMINATED

EVIDENCE EVIDENCE

Personal Property Receipt/ Evidence Tag

Destination ______

Via ______

TRIAGE TAG

☐S Solution ☐L Lacrimation ☐U Urination ☐D Defecation ☐G GI Distress ☐E Emesis ☐M Miosis

AUTO INJECTOR ☐1 ☐2 ☐3 ☐4 ☐5

Yes	No	PrimaryDecon
Yes	No	SecondaryDecon
Solution		

	Burn Trauma
	Burn
	C-Spine
	Cardiac
	Crushing
	Fracture
	Laceration
	Penetrating Injury

1

Age____

☐ Male ☐ Female

Other: ______

VITAL SIGNS

Time	B/P	Pulse	Respiration

Time	Drug Solution 2	Dose

MORGUE

IMMEDIATE | IMMEDIATE

DELAYED | DELAYED

MINOR | MINOR

Triage tag.

From the Office for Domestic Preparedness, US Department of Homeland Security.

28. Why is patient flow so important during an MCI or WMD event?

Patient flow must be in one direction only. This:

- Minimizes confusion and miscommunication.
- Aids in patient tracking.
- Eliminates cross-contamination of staff or patients.

29. Should a nurse or a physician be doing the triage during an MCI or WMD event?

Consensus is not yet out on this one. Initially, in the prehospital or incident scene initial triage is done by the field medics and patients are then sent to the most appropriate hospital to meet their needs (trauma, burn, closest, etc.). Once the patients begin to arrive at the hospital some critics say triage should be performed by a trained nurse as the physician(s) is a limiting resource. Others will say that a physician trained in emergency medicine is needed. Yet others say a nurse-physician team is the best. Either way, established hospital policy and procedures that have been tested and drilled should dictate who performs triage. Remember training is imperative for whoever is assigned the role of triage!

30. If the victims of an MCI are contaminated, do triage personnel need to don personal protective equipment?

Absolutely! The number one rule in caring for others is to protect oneself. Think safety! If the majority of the health care workers are taken out with a contaminant, who will assist them or the other victims? Depending on the agent, personal protective equipment (PPE) can range from fully encapsulated suits with self-contained breathing apparatus to a much lower, less-protected level of goggles, gowns, gloves, and booties.

31. What are the classic signs and symptoms the triage clinician will see on victims exposed to a chemical agent?

An easy way to remember the signs and symptoms is the acronym SLUDGEM:
Salivation
Lacrimation (tearing)
Urination
Defecation/diarrhea
Gastrointestinal distress (cramps)
Emesis (vomiting)
Muscle twitching (seizures)

32. Why is it important for the triage nurse to recognize SLUDGEM?

A victim presenting with exposure to a chemical agent is potentially life threatening to the triage personnel and they need to don PPE.

33. What is the rule of thumb for decontamination?

Dilution is the solution to reduce patient skin contamination.

34. If the triage personnel have donned PPE: protective suit, gloves, mask with powered air purifying respirator and boots, is there a limit on the amount of time they can spend in the suit performing triage?

- PPE is always limiting even in the simplest of terms.
- Gloves limit tactile sensation
- Any mask (powered air purifying respirator [PAPR] or other) has visual limitations and often feelings of confinement.
- PPE suits are hot, bulky (if sized correctly), and time-consuming to don.
- The most limiting factor is the time one is able to spend in the suit considering the effects of heat, health, and hydration.

35. Should more than one clinician in my hospital be trained in START or any other MCI/WMD triage methodology?

All shifts need to have trained personnel. Each shift should consider having several or all triage staff trained so rotations can be set up if the incident has large numbers of victims and lasts over a period of time. Remember PPE limitations!

36. Once the field medics have triaged the victim and they now present to my hospital/facility, do I need to retriage the victims?

Yes, each patient will need to be initially triaged on presentation to the hospital/facility as their condition may have changed during transport.

37. How do I triage patients that present to the ED during an MCI that were not part of the incident?

The answer to the question lies within the policy and procedures of your own hospital/institution. How secure is the entrance to your ED during an MCI? If patient flow is a priority (and it should be) then security personnel should be able to direct patients to the triage personnel, who then proceed to perform whatever method of triage the hospital has chosen to use in an MCI.

38. Are the START colors and terminology universal?

No. One maritime MCI system uses red, yellow, green, and blue (instead of black for the morgue/unsalvageable). The Australian Homebush Triage Standard taxonomy consists of five categories: immediate, urgent, not urgent, dying, and dead, which are given the phonetic alphabet designations of alpha, bravo, charlie, delta, and echo, respectively, to facilitate radio voice communications. Colors are assigned to each category: red (Homebush red), yellow (Homebush gold), green (Homebush green), white, and black comply with Standards Australia AS-2700 1996 Colour Standard for General Purposes, to ensure triage materials have consistent production standards. This is more proof for the case that continual training is imperative to proper use and proficiency of any MCI triage method.

39. Is it important for my local prehospital agencies and my hospital to use the same MCI triage methodology?

It would sure help to have everyone on the same page. Each agency and hospital at least should "know and understand" what the other is using. This will obviously decrease miscommunication, potential errors in triage, and improve patient tracking.

40. What is the rule of thumb in triaging victims exposed to radiation?

The people who are the farthest from the center of the site go first. The higher the dose of exposure, the earlier the onset of symptoms: Any patient with nausea/vomiting or bloody diarrhea within 3 hours has had a significant dose exposure.

41. What lessons were learned from other EDs' experience with an exposure disaster response?

- The need for total hospital participation. Decontamination is time-consuming and exhausting and the usual ED business continues as usual.
- Separate valuables (such as glasses, keys, billfolds) and decontaminate them first so they can be immediately returned.
- Maintain patient confidentiality. Hospital security needs to help control the media. However, one of the biggest problems was hospital employees who "flocked just to see what was going on."

Key Points

- Safety of triage personnel is primary:
  - Safety comes first.
  - Assess the situation before doing anything.
  - Focus on the hazard—avoid contacting it.
  - Evaluate the situation and report to proper authorities.
- Eighty percent of victim decontamination is accomplished by taking the clothes off the victim!
- Proficiency in performing a triage in an MCI or WMD incident is equaled to the time put into training!
- During an MCI or WMD incident, triage needs to be performed outside the ED.
- Patient flow is in one direction only!

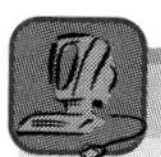

Internet Resources

Sacco Method of MCI triage
http://www.sharpthinkers.com/abc/ts_triss.htm

Australian Homebush Triage Standards
www.ncbi.nlm.nih.gov/entrez/query.fcgi?cmd=Retrieve&db=PubMed&list_uids=10472920&dopt=Abstract

Luebeck's System of MCIs at Sea (Maritime)
www.imha.net/Manila-LuDoG-s-proceedings.doc

American College of Surgeons Statement on Disaster and Mass Casualty Management
www.facs.org/fellows_info/statements/st-42.html

JumpSTART Pediatric MCI Triage
www.jumpstarttriage.com/

Emergency Medical Services Authority, California: HEICS III—Hospital Emergency Incident Command System Update Project
http://www.emsa.ca.gov/Dms2/heics3.htm

Emergency Nurses Association Position Statement on WMD
http://www.ena.org/about/position/wmd.asp

Bibliography

Brown M, Beatty J, O'Keefe S, et al: Planning for hospital emergency mass-casualty decontamination by the US Department of Veterans Affairs, *Disaster Manag Response* 2(3):75-80, 2004.

Eichelberger MR, Mangubat EA, Sacco WS, et al: Comparative outcomes of children and adults suffering blunt trauma, *J Trauma* 28:430-436, 1998.

Hudson TL, Reilly K, Dulaigh J: Considerations for chemical decontamination shelters, *Disaster Manag Response* 1(4):110-113, 2003.

Last M: Putting children first, *Disasters* 18:192-202, 1994.

Macintyre AG, Christopher GW, Eitze E Jr, et al: Weapons of mass destruction events with contaminated casualties: Effective planning for health care facilities, *JAMA* 283:242-249, 2000.

Mackway-Jones K, Carley SD, Robson J: Planning for major incidents involving children by implementing a Delphi Study, *Arch Dis Child* 80:410-413, 1999.

Proper CB, Solotkin KC: One urban hospital's experience with false anthrax exposure disaster response, *J Emerg Nurs* 25(6):501-504, 1999.

Stopford B: New report provides "benchmark" for disaster training in the ED, *ED Nurs* 12(1):166-167, 2001.

Super G, Groth S, Hook R, et al: START: Simple triage and rapid treatment plan, Newport Beach, Calif, 1994, Hoag Memorial Presbyterian Hospital.

Sweeney B, Jasper E, Gates E: Large-scale urban disaster drill involving an explosion: Lessons learned by an academic medical center, *Disaster Manag Response* 2(3):87-92, 2004.

Treat KN, Williams JM, Furbee PM, et al: Hospital preparedness for weapons of mass destruction incidents: An initial assessment, *Ann Emerg Med* 38(5):562, 2001.

US Army: *Medical management of chemical casualties handbook,* Aberdeen, Md, 1995, US Army Medical Research Institute of Chemical Defense.

US Army: *Medical management of biological casualties handbook,* Fort Detrick, Md, 1996, US Army Medical Research Institute of Infectious Diseases.

Section XI

Regulatory and System Issues

Chapter 63

Health Insurance Portability and Accountability Act (HIPAA)

Abigail R. Williams

1. What is the history of the HIPAA privacy standards?

In an effort to improve the efficiency and effectiveness of the health care system, the Health Insurance Portability and Accountability Act (HIPAA) of 1996 included "Administrative Simplification" provisions that require the department of Health and Human Services (HHS) to adopt national standards for electronic health care transactions. Congress incorporated provisions into HIPAA that mandated the adoption of federal privacy protections for individually identifiable health information.

2. What exactly does the HIPAA Privacy Rule do?

- The HIPAA Privacy Rule creates national standards to protect individual's medical records and other personal health information.
- It gives patients more control over their health information.
- It sets boundaries on the use and release of health records.
- It establishes appropriate safeguards.
- It holds violators accountable, with civil and criminal penalties.

3. Define Protected Health Information.

Protected Health Information (PHI) is individually identifiable health information related to a patient's past, present, or future health condition, health care, and/or payment for health care.

4. Describe the minimum necessary standard.

This standard requires covered entities to limit unnecessary or inappropriate access to and disclosure of protected health information. PHI should only be used for the purpose of health care services. It is based on patient confidentiality, a practice nursing has always valued.

5. Give examples of people or circumstances under which the nurse could disclose a patient's PHI.

- The patient.
- To carry out the treatment, payment, or health care operations with proper consent from the patient.

- To another clinician for continuity of care.
- Physician to physician for patient care.
- As requested with valid authorization.
- As required by law, legal requirements, and judicial proceedings (e.g., Centers for Disease Control and Prevention for infectious diseases).

6. Can clinicians engage in confidential conversations with other clinicians or with patients, even if there is a possibility that they could be overheard?

Covered entities are free to engage in communications as required for quick, effective, and high quality health care.

7. I'm worried about incidental disclosures. Will we be fined if someone overhears a conversation?

No. The HIPAA Privacy Rule does not require that all risk of incidental use or disclosure be eliminated to satisfy its standards. The Rule only requires that covered entities implement reasonable safeguards to limit incidental uses or disclosures.

As a result of necessary practices and environment, overheard communications may be unavoidable. Examples of when ordinary precautions may not be possible could include:

- An emergency situation ("Room 3 is coding!").
- A loud emergency room with competing noises.
- A hearing-impaired patient.

8. Does the Privacy Rule require hospitals to make structural changes to insure privacy?

No, structural changes are not required. This includes no private rooms, soundproofing, or encryption of communication (emergency medical radio communications or telephone systems).

9. What kind of measures could be expected as reasonable precautions to protect privacy?

In an area in which multiple patient-staff communications routinely occur, routine measures that could be used include:

- Lowering one's voice.
- Cubicles, dividers, shields, curtains. In addition, staff could talk apart from others when sharing protected health information during nonemergent situations.
- Privacy filters over computer screens so that they are not readily visibile to the public.
- Turning monitor screens so they are not easily visible from a public area.

- Sign-in sheets only listing the time and name or flow boards listing only the name or initials, as long as neither indicates the reason for the visit
- Dedicated fax to receive medical information in a secure location. It is advisable to wait by the machine if you know a sensitive patient document is currently being sent. The machine should be equipped to detect whether the number dialed matches the number on the cover sheet.

10. Give examples of activities that can occur if reasonable precautions are taken.

- Health care staff may orally coordinate services at hospital nursing stations.
- Nurses or other health care professionals may discuss a patient's condition over the phone with the patient, a clinician, or a family member.
- A health care professional may discuss lab test results with a patient or other clinician in a joint treatment area.
- A physician may discuss a patient's condition or treatment regimen in a patient's semiprivate room.
- Health care professionals may discuss a patient's condition during training rounds in an academic or training institution.

11. Can a patient be publicly addressed by name?

Yes. A person's identity is not privileged confidential health care information. Their presence in the public facility is considered public knowledge.

One hospital indicates that a patient can assume an "alias," such as John Doe, for the initial sign in. The triage nurse always asks, "What is the correct spelling of your name?" after the patient is in the private triage area to then enter the correct name.

12. How should I handle a phone call asking if someone is there as a patient?

Most departments have patients indicate if they want their presence known or not known to callers during registration. Selective choices are not permitted, as there is no way to easily confirm a person's identity over the phone. Staff respond to callers that a person is "either on the list" or "not on the list." Some will ask the patient if they want to talk to the person and who the person claims to be (if acknowledgment of the patient's presence was permitted).

13. Can clinicians leave messages for patients at their homes, either on answering machines or with a family member?

Yes. Clinicians can communicate with patients at their homes, whether through the mail, phone, or answering machine. However, information should be limited giving the hospital's phone number and asking the person to call back rather than revealing the reason for the call.

14. Are covered entities prohibited from maintaining patient medical charts at bedside or outside of examination rooms?

The Privacy Rule does not prohibit:

- Maintaining patient charts at bedside or outside of examination rooms, as long as the access to the information is relevant to the examination.
- Displaying patient's names on the outside of patient charts, or displaying patient care signs (e.g., "high fall risk" or "diabetic diet") at the patient bedside or at the doors of hospital rooms.
- Announcing patient names and other information over a facility's public announcement system.
- The Joint Commission on Accreditation of Healthcare Organizations (JCAHO) also requires that a patient's medical problem is not easily identifiable on a tracking board. Internal codes or symbols are acceptable, as is waiting for x-ray or labs (as long as the specific test is not listed). A patient-initiated concern should be honored, such as using John Doe instead of Brad Pitt.

15. Give examples of internal codes or symbols that could be used.

Ransone (2001) describes using a one-letter chief complaint diagnosis chosen based on their emergency department's (ED) most frequent presentations. It provided something to jog the mind, with the full explanatory list on the bulletin board (covered by a cover sheet). For instance "A" is abdominal pain, "B" is back pain, "C" is chest pain, "D" is dog bite, etc. They found the staff soon memorized the meaningless code from the frequent use. Another hospital ED developed a similar alphabet system, but with different meanings. For instance, they used "A" for allergic reaction, "B" for burn, "C" for cardiac, "D" for diabetes mellitus, etc.

16. My department posts the names of employees on the nurses' station bulletin board who are due for annual tuberculosis tests. Is this a violation?

No. By law, hospitals must require employees to have certain diagnostic tests, such as an annual tuberculosis-screening test. To comply, hospital must notify the employees in an organized manner and posting the time for this known standard requirement is not a violation.

17. Give examples of some common violations that can occur.

They are often routine situations that can happen without deliberate attention. Examples include:

- Talking about a patient in an identifiable way in a public arena (e.g., elevator, cafeteria).
- Taking home the daily report sheet notes with the patient name and PHI.
- Hospital staff members reading a patient's information when there is no need to know for their job performance or training (such as a transporter reading the patient's human immunodeficiency virus [HIV] result).
- In one true case, the woman's pregnancy status was revealed to her in her husband's presence. She is suing for a HIPAA violation because the baby wasn't his!

18. Explain the term "personal representative."

A person authorized (under state or other applicable law) to act on behalf of the patient in making health care-related decisions. The personal representative has the ability to act for the patient and exercise the patient's rights pertaining to the use and disclosure of the patient's protected health information.

19. Does the Privacy Rule allow parents the right to see their children's medical records?

Yes, the Privacy Rule generally allows a parent to have access to the medical records about his or her child.

20. Are there any exceptions to the parent's right to see their children's medical records?

There are three situations when the parent would not be the minor's personal representative under the Privacy Rule. These exceptions are when:

- The minor is the one who consents to care and the consent of the parent is not required under state or other applicable law.
- The minor obtains care at the direction of a court or a person appointed by the court.
- To the extent that, the parent agrees that the minor and clinician may have a confidential relationship.

In addition, a clinician may choose not to treat a parent as a personal representative when the clinician reasonably believes that the child has been or may be subjected to domestic violence, abuse, or neglect or the parent could endanger the child.

21. Does the Privacy Rule address the rights for children to be treated without parental consent?

No. The rule does not address any issues related to consent for treatment.

22. Can a family member, instead of the patient, pick up prescriptions at the pharmacy?

Yes. A pharmacist may use professional judgment and experience, with common practice, to allow a person other than the patient to pick up a prescription.

23. Elaborate on sharing protected health care information with a "business associate."

A "business associate" is a person or entity that performs certain functions or activities that involve the use or disclosure of protected health information on behalf of, or provides services to, a covered entity. An employee is not considered a "business associate"; the transporting ambulance company is.

Clinicians can disclose protected health information to "business associates" as long as the clinician obtains satisfactory written assurances that the business associate will use the information only for the purpose for which it was engaged by the covered entity, will safeguard the information from misuse, and will help the covered entity comply with some of the covered entity's duties under the Privacy Rule.

24. Is a hospital permitted to contact another hospital or health care facility, such as a nursing home to which a patient will be transferred for continued care, without the patient's authorization?

Yes. A clinician can disclose PHI about an individual, without the individual's authorization, to another clinician for that ongoing treatment of the patient. In addition, information may be released for training or quality assessment purposes.

25. Can there be communications with an ambulance company about a patient's medical information without the express permission of the patient?

Yes. This is a business associate relationship. PHI can be disclosed without the individual's authorization for the purpose of that clinician's treatment of the individual.

26. Is the U.S. Postal Service considered a "business associate" or do we need a signed contract if we mail results to the patient?

No, because the information remains inside a sealed envelope.

27. Can the hospital disclose information to a "public health authority"?

Covered entities can disclose protected health information, without authorization, to public health authorities that are legally authorized to receive such reports for the purpose of preventing or controlling disease, injury, or disability. Examples include reporting of disease or injury, reporting deaths and births, investigating the occurrence and cause of injury and disease, and monitoring adverse outcomes related to food, drugs, biologic products, and medical devices.

28. I heard that nurses couldn't discuss outside programs, such as Alcoholics Anonymous, with patients as it is construed as marketing.

Giving patients general information about the benefits of a program, such as Weight Watchers, or even directing them to a listing of such a program in the telephone directory is permitted. In addition, anyone can share anything of a personal nature if desired, such as the personal benefits of belonging to an exercise club. A violation would be active marketing of a specific program at the request of the company running the program.

29. Are hospitals or other clinicians required to provide notice of their privacy practices to patients before they are treated in an emergency?

Hospitals and other clinicians with a direct treatment relationship with individuals are not required to provide their notices to patients at the time they are providing emergency treatment. The HIPAA Privacy Rule requires only that clinicians give patients a notice when it is practical to do so after the emergency situation has ended.

30. Are hospitals able to inform the clergy about parishioners in the hospital?

Yes, as long as the patient has been informed of this use and does not object.

31. Does the Privacy Rule require providing patients with access to oral information?

No. The term "record" connotes information that has been recorded in some manner. The Rule does not require covered entities to tape or digitally record oral communications.

32. How should medical records be stored?

Records kept in the department should not be easily viewed by people passing by, such as lying open on a counter top on the nurses' station. Old medical records should be "secured," such as in a locked file cabinet. Pass codes for computer access should not be shared.

33. What should be done with our preliminary lab results or computer disks with information?

Personal health care information should not be thrown out intact (retrievable) in the trash. Shred paper (and CDs if the shredder can handle them) or ruin a disk by running a nail over it.

Key Points

- PHI can only be revealed to staff that need to know the information to do their job or for training purposes.
- A patient's identity is not PHI. Flow boards can be used if a diagnosis is not identified with the patient's name.
- Staff and hospitals are protected against accidental disclosure (e.g., an overheard phone conversation) as long as reasonable precautions for privacy were undertaken.

Internet Resources

Hypersend. Secure Internet Delivery: Health Care
www.hypersend.com

HIPAAdvisory (Phoenix Health Systems)
http://www.hipaadvisory.com/

Bibliography

Adams SJ: HIPAA patient confidentiality requirements, *J Emerg Nurs* 30(1):70, 2004.

Kobs A: Tracking boards (Managers Forum), *J Emerg Nurs* 27(1):68, 2001.

Ransone JC: Tracking boards (Managers Forum), *J Emerg Nurs* 27(1):69, 2001.

Suby C, Washburn J: HIPAA (Managers Forum), *J Emerg Nurs* 29(3):269-270, 2003.

Sullivan P: JCAHO and patient confidentiality. Re: Patient Flow Boards (Managers Forum), *J Emerg Nurs* 24(2):179, 1998.

Chapter 64

Fast Track

Polly Gerber Zimmermann

1. What are common goals of having a fast track area?

- Reduce waiting time for the less critically ill.
- Reduce the "left without being seen" (LWBS) and "against medical advice" (AMA) rate to <2%.
- Create a product line that achieves a 30% to 50% lower cost.
- Improve customer satisfaction.
- Increase revenue.

2. What are general criteria for patients who are appropriate for the fast track area?

- Noninfectious
- Medically stable
- Ambulatory (e.g., no back pain requiring a stretcher)
- No hospital admission anticipated
- No intravenous (IV) fluids or IV antibiotics anticipated
- Psychiatric patients who are calm, without any suicidal or homicidal ideation
- Children >3 months of age
- Anticipate that care will take less than 1 hour.

See Chapter 8 for an example of one emergency department's specific guidelines.

3. Can you give a guideline about when to consider opening a fast track area?

A fast track can be justified when approximately 40% or more of the ED patients are nonurgent.

4. How long should a fast track visit last?

The general model should be patients (up to 90%) for whom the evaluation and treatment visit will last 1 hour or less.

5. Is it an Emergency Medical Treatment and Active Labor Act violation to triage a patient to fast track if the patient does not request this area?

According to Emergency Medical Treatment and Active Labor Act (EMTALA) provisions, patients may be triaged to a separate, equal care area within the hospital. This would include a hospital-affiliated, on-site clinic or fast track area.

6. We do not have the volume to justify a 24-hour fast track. What hours are best?

Most emergency departments (EDs) have their largest volume between 11:00 AM and 11:00 PM, usually with the upward peak starting around 10:00 AM (e.g., initially establishing fast track hours 10:00 AM to 10:00 PM). Some stay open a few hours later to help decompress the ED before the night shift's decrease in staff. Most have at least 20% of their total patient volume that is appropriate for the area; some have up to 50%. Trend your department's patient volume, acuity, and arrival times to detect any unique patterns.

7. Give some generic policy guidelines for smooth operation of a fast track area.

- *Patient distribution.* A method to allow patient redistribution if fast track is backed up and the main ED has available capacity.
- *Designated staff.* Fast track must have designated staff. However, if the area has no patients, that staff can assist in tasks only (not patient management responsibility) or other tasks, such as call backs.
- *Adhering to patient selection criteria.* The temptation can be to put "sicker" patients in the fast track area when the main department is busy. This, however, backs up the fast track and defeats the purpose of that area by making it an ED extension.
- *Cut-off times.* Stop taking new patients about an hour before the area closes to be able to complete the care.
- *Procedure to transfer patients (as a result of their conditions) back to the main ED as needed.*

8. Provide an example of an institution's list of appropriate fast track patients.

Northwest Medical Center—Washington County (Springdale, Ark)
Source: Shawn Zimmer RN CEN BSM, ED Clinical Supervisor

- Nausea, vomiting, diarrhea without signs of dehydration.
- Low back pain without major trauma, pyelonephritis, or kidney stone signs/symptoms in patients <50 years old.
- Extremity injury without compromise of neurovascular supply or deformity.
- Children with fever excluding:
  - Less than 6 months of age with fever of more than 100°F (38°C)
  - 6 months to 2 years with 102.5°F (39.1°C)
  - Any signs and symptoms of dehydration
- Nonimmobilized motor vehicle accidents (MVAs) without chest, abdominal, or pelvic injuries.
- Minor asthma or wheezing with pulse oximetry of ≥97% and >6 years of age that will likely require only one treatment.

9. Is it advisable to staff a licensed practical nurse (LPN/LVN) as the only nurse in fast track? The patient complaints are minor and the LPN could be supervised by the ED physician and charge nurse.

Nurse Attorney Edie Brous (2004) warns against this common practice. The ED patient population is "unknown" and vulnerable, different than an established clinic setting. Fast track, in particular, is a high-risk liability as a result of:

- Fast turnover
- High need for assessing and discharge teaching
- Common practice of using physician assistants or physician residents who are inexperienced or not board certified

No state's Nurse Practice Acts allows LPNs to perform an independent "nursing assessment." The state nursing boards do not make a distinction about this based on the severity of the patient's complaint (e.g., "minor").

Although an ED charge nurse can be responsible for overseeing the fast track area, it is not realistic to expect that nurses actually "oversee" the care and nursing assessment of *each* fast track patient. The triage nursing assessment is not a factor as it was only for sorting purposes. Any patient in these circumstances can make a legitimate claim that a professional nurse never saw them. The situation is different than a physician office staffing because they are all unknown patients.

Key Points

- Fast track patients should be medically stable with a need that is anticipated to be resolved in 1 hour or less.
- Patients may be triaged to hospital's fast track (regardless if it was requested) under EMTALA provisions.

Internet Resources

Institute for Healthcare Improvement. Improvement Report: Eliminate Overcrowding in the Emergency Department
http://www.ihi.org/IHI/Topics/Flow/PatientFlow/ImprovementStories/ImprovementReport EliminateOvercrowdingintheEmergencyDepartment.htm

The University Hospital, Newark, New Jersey: Compliance Program—Policies and Procedures: Triage
http://www.umdnj.edu/uhcomweb/policy/policy02_triage.htm

California Emergency Physicians Medical Group: Immediate Bedding
http://www.cep.com/news/Perf_Imp.asp

Bibliography

Abaris Group, 700 Ygnacio Valley Road, Suite 270, Walnut Creek, CA; 888-EMS-0911, available: www.abarisgroup.com; Mike Williams, MPA/HAS.

Brous E: LPNs and fast-track staffing (Managers Forum), *J Emerg Nurs* 30(3):260-261, 2004.

Murray K: *Pediatric triage guidelines,* Philadelphia, 1997, Lippincott, Williams & Wilkins.

Chapter 65

Telephone Triage

Valerie G. A. Grossman and Polly Gerber Zimmermann

1. What is telephone triage?

Specially trained nurses do a verbal phone interview, make an assessment, and provide advice and/or treatment using standardized protocols. It has the potential to improve the quality of advice and reduce the demand for health care services. More than 100 million people in the United States are estimated to have access to a telephone triage service.

2. Is this safe to give health care advice on the phone?

Telephone triage can be performed safely if certain conditions are met, most importantly an established program in place versus "off-the-cuff" independent thoughts. The Emergency Nurses Association (ENA) Position Statement on Telephone Triage (2001) states, in part, "...sophisticated telephone triage programs provide quality health care assessment opportunities." Telephone triage has actually been in existence in some form, such as poison control centers, since the 1970s.

3. What are these conditions?

ENA indicates that essential components of a telephone triage program include:

- Experienced professional nurses with specialized education in triage, telephone assessment, communication, and documentation skills.
- Requires mandatory continuing education for all telephone advice staff.
- Clearly defined protocols.
- Policies and procedures.
- An ongoing program of continuous quality improvement.
- Documentation of each conversation and recommendation.
- Medical direction and evaluation from experienced professional emergency staff.

In addition, the position statement indicates emergency registered nurses (RNs) need training in triage, telephone assessment, and risk management. This includes the limits and capabilities of telephone triage.

The ENA's position is that when there is no established telephone triage program in place, no telephone advice is to be given. The exception is a situation with life-threatening urgency. In that case, staff should give guidance in life-saving measures (CPR) and accessing the emergency medical system (EMS).

4. We have a small community hospital. We don't have a telephone triage program but don't want to offend our callers who ask for advice. Explain how others handle this.

NorthCrest Medical Center (Springfield, Tenn)
Source: Shelley Cohen, RN BS CEN

A typed script is hung by the phone that anyone, including a clerk, can read. It states, "We understand that you are concerned about ______________ (your husband, self, etc.). However, it is not safe, nor is it in your best interest, for us to give you advice over the phone. You do have some options. If this is an emergency, hang up and dial 911. You can call your physician or whoever is on call for them. Or you can go to your closest emergency department."

Nurses indicating reasons to return during the discharge further support this policy, but indicating advice will not be given over the phone. The most important aspect is that every single staff member does the exact same thing.

University of Missouri Hospital (Columbia, Mo)
Source: Gordon Rogers, RN CEN

He listens to them describe their symptoms, sometimes even asking more questions. Then he states his standard response, "You know, it is very hard to make a diagnosis of something like you are describing over the phone. It generally takes a physician's hands-on physical examination, and possibly even some laboratory tests or x-rays, to really be sure. We would be happy to see you if you feel like this is something that shouldn't wait until you can see your regular doctor. Do you feel like you could wait until you can call your doctor, or would you like to come on in now so we can check you out?" He sometimes adds that he could not possibly recommend treatments at this point because he is not sure what he is treating.

Callers are happy because someone listened to them and did offer the best solution considering the limitations of this "telephone consultation." It is not perceived as abrupt as "Sorry we don't give advice over the phone." Most callers thank him for "helping" them. And in case the caller provides an ominous description like crushing substernal chest pain, he can say, "Hang up and dial 911 now!"

5. How is telephone triage performed safely within a program when you can't see the patient or use your stethoscope?

Telephone triage nurses (telenurses) must:

- Establish a trusting relationship with the caller to benefit from their honest interaction with the nurse.
- Be able to hear what the caller is not saying. The tone of the caller's voice and the background noise are key indicators to the telenurse regarding the environment the person is calling from (e.g., pay phone on a street corner, screaming in the background, crying baby, wheezing from the caller, etc.).

- Teach the caller to be their eyes, nose, and hands to obtain an accurate telephone assessment. Interview questions are asked in such a manner regarding teaching the caller to identify physical findings that are essential for the telenurse to make a triage decision.

6. Give some sample questions.

- What are the sizes of the bumps of the rash? The size of a pencil point? A pencil eraser? A dime? A nickel? A quarter?
- What is the size of the bruise on the leg? The size of a golf ball? Baseball?

7. How can you gather assessment data that isn't visual, like lung sounds?

When listening to a patient's breathing, ask the caller to put the part of the phone you talk into right up to the patient's mouth and watch the clock for a full 15 seconds. This enables the nurse to hear wheezing, count a respiratory rate, assess coughing, etc.

8. Is there anything to help the telephone triage nurse remember to obtain a complete history?

Rutenberg (2000) recommends these two mnemonics for telephone triage:

POSHPATE for History of the Chief Complaint
Problem
Onset
Associated **S**ymptoms
Previous **H**istory
Precipitating Factors
Alleviating/Aggravating Factors
Timing
Etiology

TICOSMO for Have I overlooked anything (e.g., considered all etiologies)?
Trauma
Infection
Chemical
Organs
Stress
Musculoskeletal
Others

9. Discuss the intuiting and emotional component in telephone triage.

There is a perceived crisis occurring in the life of the caller or he/she wouldn't be calling. Therefore, the nurse responds with compassion regardless of the complaint. The telenurse must also realize that all information leads to a working impression of the caller's situation and current state of health/illness/injury.

10. Can you give an example?

A man called about his "jock itch." Despite his ordinary term and vague, bland descriptions, the depth of his concern about such an ordinary problem raised my own level of suspicion. He finally stated, "All I can say is this is not like any rash I've ever had or seen before." I had him seek treatment that day for what turned out to be purpura caused by a drug reaction. The main thing guiding that good decision was a gut feeling regarding his emotional tone.

11. Talk about documentation.

Nursing professionals understand that "if it's not documented, it wasn't done." Documentation of each and every call must allow a future reader to understand the dialogue, decision path, education, and follow-up advice that were given by the nurse. Documentation reviews should be done regularly.

12. How does a telephone triage nurse diagnose?

Telephone triage gives treatment information or advice, not a definitive diagnosis. It is still "triage" (e.g., determining the level of care needed by the patient and assigning an acuity level). The usual conclusion of the call is seeking emergent care (911, go to the ED, etc.), office care (e.g., visit a doctor's office—some programs consider that within 12 to 24 hours; others within 72 hours), or self-care.

During the educational portion of the telephone call, the nurse will advise the caller of what changes to look for, signs or symptoms (s/s) that should cause concern, and when to call back. Depending on the program, the nurse may additionally call the patient back themselves, to perform a follow-up assessment.

13. Give an example of a protocol.

Grossman (2002) provides a sample abdominal pain protocol. It includes more than 30 items to ask about:

- History (last bowel movement, last menstrual period, possible ingestion of chemicals, plants, or medicines, etc.), assessment of the pain (PQRST)
- Behaviors (irritability, difficulty walking, etc.)
- Symptoms (nausea/vomiting, change in activity level, penile discharge, etc.)
- Risk factors (history of abdominal surgery, trauma, diabetes, etc.)

The nurse advises an ambulance when the current status is life-threatening, whether the client may deteriorate en route to the hospital, or the anxiety level is too high to drive safely. Consideration of 16 aspects are listed, including pain localized to the lower abdomen (either side) for more than 1 to 2 hours, increased pain if the patient jumps on one foot ("the hop test"), pain radiating into the scrotum or testicle, etc.

Guidelines to instruct the patient when to seek a physician visit within 12 to 24 hours include if the pain lasts longer than 24 hours or there is vaginal discharge. Home care advice includes clear liquids progressing to a bland diet. Reasons to call back are also listed to review.

14. What other factors make a telephone triage program safe?

Factors that help make telephone triage safe include appropriate staffing, equipment, resources, and documentation.

15. Discuss appropriate staffing.

While no one can predict the number of calls that will be received on a given shift, historical data can be used to predict the approximate number of calls and the approximate acuity so that enough qualified staff is available.

There should be some staffing flexibility built into the program for those unexpected periods of high call volumes. Just one news report of a communicable disease outbreak in the community can skyrocket the call volume. A common solution is having nurses on call or who can take calls from their homes in the event that the call volumes dramatically increase.

16. List some other things that should be considered, besides call volume, which can influence the need when planning the staffing.

- Weather (which impacts the activity and mobility of those in the community)
- Community health/illness outbreaks (flu season)
- Available resources (24-hour pharmacy availability)
- Time of the day or day of the week (primary care physician's office open or closed)
- Special events that may be scheduled in the community (county fair)
- Administrative support and/or back-up resources

17. Name equipment and resource essentials.

- Private, distraction-free environment
- Quality telephone equipment, with a back-up plan in place in case of power or phone outages
- Automated telephone with special features (as deemed necessary by each telephone triage program)
- Headsets and ergonomically correct workstation
- Relevant current resources within reach
- Established protocols, policies, and procedures

18. Talk about the qualifications and characteristics for personnel who work in phone triage.

- Seasoned, clinically experienced ("hands on") registered nurses (or clinicians, physician assistants, physicians, etc.) in the specialty area for which the telephone triage is being performed
- Excellent listening and communicating skills
- Precise documentation skills
- High moral and work ethics
- Precise critical thinkers, able to think "outside of the box"

- Good intuition/sensing skills
- Ability to deal with fluctuating work demands. The work flow can be just as unpredictable and chaotic as in an ED
- Comfortable working independently and autonomously

19. In my doctor's office, the secretary or the LPN takes the information and gives advice.

Many private physician practices use unqualified personnel to handle the practice's telephone triage. Some clinicians believe that a clerk can serve in this role with a good algorithm or protocol. This often works, but at substantial risk. Lawsuits around this issue are on the rise.

The danger is that objective protocols still have an element of "interpretation" about the information coming from the caller. Callers do not always volunteer complete, or the most important, information. The telephone triage nurse is always using critical thinking and experience to rule out the "zebra" when they hear the sound of hooves.

20. Tell me about studies done on this issue.

Wachter et al (1999) evaluated the application of pediatric telephone triage protocols with test scenarios. The RNs in the study averaged 14 years of work experience, 5 years of ED experience, and 1.5 years in telephone triage. They found that there was a high variability among the nurses.

In each case there was an average of three different protocols and four different dispositions determined. In the study, 58% of the RNs indicated they felt confined by the protocols and 42% made at least one deliberate deviation from the protocols according to their professional clinical judgment. The conclusion was that applying protocols doesn't necessarily result in standardized patient management. The point has been made that this is good because a seasoned nurse may need to deviate for that "zebra."

Lee et al (2003) found in their study that there was no significant difference in the advice given by physicians and that from nurse groups. However, in Baraff et al (2003), parents believed that the physician telephone advice was very good or excellent more often (76%) than the telephone advice by the clinician (56%).

21. Do people really follow the phone advice given to them?

In one study of phone advice from a pediatric physician resident there was strong agreement between the advice the physician documented as given and the parents' recollection of what was said. Even more encouraging, 90.4% of the parents followed the phone advice.

In Lee et al (2003), 20% sought unadvised care after the phone call, whether they spoke to a physician or a nurse advice group. However, only 4% of those seeking the unadvised care received "significant" care treatment, most often a prescription for antibiotics.

22. What type of previous experience is best for someone who wants to go into the specialty of telephone triage?

In my experience, emergency nurses find telephone triage a natural progression. After years of "seeing" different cases in their practice and performing face-to-face triage in their ED experience, they can make the transition to telephone triage with minimal effort.

Intensive care unit (ICU) nurses, although not proficient at triage through their ICU experience, are skilled in finding "the worst-case scenario." Office nurses, through their years of office visits, excel with minor complaints but have difficulty remembering to look for the red flag signaling a more serious cause.

23. Talk about specialized education or training courses.

Telephone triage education or special training is not yet fully available for nurses, though some colleges are now offering continuing education triage courses. The best preparation is keeping current.

Networking with other telephone triage nurses is a must and one of the best ways to stay up-to-date on the specialty's issues. Options include the ENA's and/or the American Academy of Ambulatory Care Nursing's (AAACN) Telehealth Nursing Practice Special Interest Group.

24. Should we encourage older nurses to go into telephone triage work because it is not physically demanding?

One cannot assume that age makes any nurse an automatic good fit for the telephone triage role or that this individual will be comfortable in that role.

25. How is all of this different from telephonic medicine?

Telephonic medicine usually involves specially trained clinicians who (usually in underserved areas) work in an independent setting to render direct medical care (not just advice) using only a telemedicine link with ED physicians. The most common use is supervision of trauma care. The best example is the TelEmergency System in Mississippi that enables provision of all emergency services by clinicians in rural EDs.

26. Is there a certification in telephone triage?

National Certification Corporations (NCC) offers the credentialing exam for nurses who have 2 years of experience in telephone triage (http://nccnet.org). It is designated by RN-C.

27. What does the future hold for "electronic" distance nursing?

About 69% of all American adults have Internet access. Baraff et al (2003) found that about 50% of the parents use the Internet for medical information, and about 30% used it to get information about a specific acute or chronic illness. The Pew Internet and the American Life Project found that 93 million Americans use the Web to research health topics.

Interestingly, using the Internet for health information does not necessarily lead to a health benefit. There was an increase in patients' knowledge and feelings of social support who consulted web-based programs and support groups in a review of 28 studies. However, it did not lead to behavior changes and had a striking negative effect on the patients' health outcomes of their chronic illnesses. It is speculated that this may be because the patients feel informed enough to make their own treatment decisions (and ignore proper health care advice); become unduly concerned about potential side effects; or be directed to sites that lack appropriate information. For instance, one study found that 43% of the sites identified for the term "vaccination" actually advised people to avoid them!

About 70% of survey respondents indicated they would like to be able to communicate about specific matters with their physician through email. Overall, it appears that the public is increasingly feeling comfortable with health care through other mediums than just face-to-face interactions. Futurescan (2002) predicted that many hospitals would soon (2002-2006) upgrade their electronic offerings to attract and keep satisfied patients.

Key Points

- The ENA Position Statement is that no telephone advice is given unless a telephone triage program is in place or a life-threatening emergency is occurring.
- Good telephone triage is hearing what is not said and what is said.

Internet Resources

RnCeus: Telephone Triage Continuing Education Course
www.rnceus.com/triage/triageframe.html

National Certification Corporations (NCC): 2003 NCC Task Analysis Content Validation Study
http://nccnet.org/public/files/38285_NCC.pdf

Cyberhealth Consulting—Ruth Johnson, RN, Telehealth Specialist
www.cyberhealth.bc.ca

Carol M. Stock & Assoc. E-Health Risk Management Services
www.carolstock.com

Emergency Nurses Association Position Statement: Telephone Advice
www.ena.org/about/position/telephoneadvice.asp

Bibliography

Baraff LJ, Wall SP, Lee TJ, Guzy J: Use of the internet and email for medical advice and information by parents of a university pediatric faculty practice, *Clin Pediatr* 42(6):557-560, 2003.

Briggs J: *Telephone triage protocols for nurses,* ed 2, Philadelphia, 2001, Lippincott, Williams & Wilkins.

Cohen S: Providing telephone medical advice (Managers Forum), *J Emerg Nurs* 28(5):459, 2002.

Coile RC: *Futurescan 2002: A forecast of healthcare trends, 2002-2006,* Chicago, 2002, Health Administration Press.

Grossman VGA: *Quick reference to triage,* ed 2, Philadelphia, 2003, Lippincott, Williams & Wilkins.

Lee TJ, Baraff LJ, Guzy J, Jackson D, Woo H: Does telephone triage delay significant medical treatment? Advice nurse service vs on-call pediatricians, *Arch Pediatr Adolesc Med* 157:635-641, 2003.

Rogers G: Providing telephone medical advice (Managers Forum), *J Emerg Nurs* 28(5):460, 2002.

Rutenberg CD: Telephone triage, *Am J Nurs* 100(3):77-81, 2000.

Rutenberg CD: What do we really know about telephone triage? *J Emerg Nurs* 26(1):76-78, 2000.

Schmidt B: *Pediatric telephone advice,* ed 2, Philadelphia, 1998, Lippincott, Williams & Wilkins.

Wachter DA, et al: Pediatric telephone triage protocols: Standardized decision making or a false sense of security? *Ann Emerg Med* 33(4):388-394, 1999.

Chapter 66

Prehospital/Emergency Medical Services Triage

Sharon Saunderson Cohen and Michael L. Wilkerson

1. Why do you have a chapter on emergency medical services triage?

In the United States, there are approximately 4,000 emergency dispatch centers. They assign 334,000 ambulances to transport 25 million people to emergency departments (EDs) each year. Obviously prehospital triage is a key component in the continuum of care.

2. Describe the difference between prehospital triage and hospital triage.

In the prehospital environment, emergency medical services (EMS) personnel not only triage the patient to assess severity, but to determine the appropriate hospital for the patient's destination.

3. Why do EMS personnel also triage to the most appropriate hospital?

EMS triage to the most appropriate hospital is based on the patient's needs, depending on local protocols.

4. Talk about safety for EMS clinicians.

The scene can be a hostile environment (gunman still at large), contaminated (hazardous materials), or dangerous (burning structure). Safety is always a priority! If necessary, EMS personnel may wait for a police escort or until the scene is determined to be safe.

5. List the three steps of prehospital triage.

- Someone determines that there is a need for medical attention (initial triage), and EMS is called.
- The dispatch operator sends the EMS clinicians, who triage the patient at the scene for immediate needs.
- The clinicians receive the patient when brought to the ED.

6. Differentiate between prehospital triage and medical screening.

Prehospital or field triage is a brief encounter and clinical assessment to determine the urgency of the situation. Besides determining the speed, transportation method, and hospital destination, the patient is treated using protocols. Medical screening, in comparison, is a much more detailed assessment and interview process for the purpose of determining the specifics of the patient's illness or injury and treatment.

7. Should EMS personnel triage patients to determine if patients need emergency care?

One study sent emergency medical technicians (EMTs) or firefighters as first responders to determine the need for advanced medical services. Under-triage occurred about 10.9% of the time. They had the most difficulty with patients who had multiple complaints, were poor historians, or had limited English.

Currently as many as 30% of patients are not transported after the ambulance arrives (patient refuses, etc.). Schmidt et al (2003) looked specifically at five EMS complaints: back pain, fall, bleeding or laceration, sickness, or trauma that had been triaged the lowest severity level according to dispatch criteria. They identified that 10% of these studied patients could have been safely triaged to an alternative resource, but additional work is needed before any implementation.

8. Who determines the need to call for "air rescue" to transport a patient?

Prehospital personnel, working under established protocols, make the determination.

9. What are some of the pitfalls of prehospital triage?

Failure to:

- Assess and attend to a patient complaint
- Recognize or acknowledge high-risk chief complaints
- Take a full set of vital signs
- Fully document chief complaints, assessments, and treatments
- Retriage patients
- Follow established local EMS protocols

10. Why is it important for the prehospital personnel to communicate with the ED about a patient prior to arrival at the hospital?

This communication allows the ED personnel to prepare to care for the patient. This also permits the EMS unit a quicker turn-around time to return to the field.

11. Can the prehospital personnel (after assessment) declare a patient deceased?

Typically, under established protocols, the patient can be "declared dead" in the field if the person is decapitated or has rigor mortis (with or without lividity). Some protocols require the prehospital personnel to receive a physician order for "do not resuscitate." Often the medical examiner (ME) will be notified to determine the disposition.

12. What information obtained by the EMS personnel should be communicated to the ED nurse?

All patient related information obtained by EMS personnel during triage and transportation should be communicated to the ED nurse receiving the patient. This includes information in the MIVT mnemonic.
Mechanism of injury or illness
Injuries suspected
Vital signs
Treatment given

13. Is the triage process the same for all EMS personnel?

All patients are triaged to determine the severity of injury or illness regardless of the qualifications of the prehospital clinicians. However, experience and training vary. As this book goes to press, there is increasing discussion about national standardization.

Key Points

- Prehospital triage focuses on determining the urgency to transport the patient and choice of hospital destination.
- Ongoing reassessment is necessary throughout the transport to identify any cardinal signs or symptoms of new developments.
- Basic information to communicate is MIVT (Mechanism of injury or illness, Injuries suspected, Vital signs, Treatment given).

Internet Resources

Emergency Medical Services Magazine: Prehospital Triage
http://www.emsmagazine.com/articles/emsarts/triage.html

Emergency Nurses Association and National Flight Nurses Association (NFNA) Joint Position Statement: Role of the Registered Nurse In the Prehospital Environment
http://www.ena.org/publications/statements/positionpdf/role-rn-prehospital.pdf

Bibliography

Emergency Nurses Association: *Position statement: Role of the registered nurse in the prehospital environment,* 1998, available: http//www.ena.org.

NAEMSP: EMS triage falls short, *EMS Insider* 27(2):1-2, 2000.

Schmidt T, Neely KW, Adams AL, et al: Is it possible to safely triage callers to EMS dispatch centers to alternative resources? *Prehosp Emerg Care* 7(3):368-374, 2003.

Chapter 67

Trauma Systems and Triage

Mary E. Fecht Gramley

1. How is the assessment of a trauma patient different from assessment of other types of patients?

Consideration of the mechanism of injury (MOI),which gives information related to the amount of force exerted on the body tissues and organs. This provides a high index of suspicion (HIS) for potential injury to specific body systems. Any trauma patient who has been subjected to any high level of force should be considered to have a spinal injury until proven otherwise.

2. What are the steps in the assessment of a trauma patient?

A useful format is the A-I mnemonic (from the Trauma Nursing Core Course)

- Airway
- Breathing
- Circulation
- Disability
- Expose
- Full set of vital signs/Family presence
- Give comfort measures
- Head to toe assessment
- History (use the MIVT mnemonic: Mechanism, Injury identified, Vital signs, Treatment initiated)
- Inspect the back/Identify all injuries/Initiate interventions

3. What is the goal of the primary assessment?

Identify life-threatening illness/injury and provide appropriate interventions: the ABCDs. The nurse does not move on to the next parameter of the assessment until the patient is stabilized.

4. What is the goal of secondary assessment?

Identify all illness or injuries: F through I.

5. Discuss unique characteristics about the pediatric trauma patient.

Pediatric patients are not small adults! Their special anatomy considerations include:

- Smaller body mass so there is more force per unit area. They are more prone to multiple injuries.
- High body surface area-to-volume ratio results in significant loss of body heat. They are more likely to get hypothermia early.
- Smaller airway diameter, large tongue, floppy epiglottis, and increased lymphoid tissue. They are more prone to airway obstruction. The sniffing position (slight superior and anterior positioning of the midface) is preferred.
- Mobile mediastinum. They are more likely to develop a tension pneumothorax than an adult with a similar chest injury.
- Strong vasoconstriction and compensatory mechanisms. Tachycardia is the primary response to hypovolemia. Hypotension in the pediatric patient indicates the child has lost 45% of his/her blood volume and at this point is more likely to manifest as bradycardia.
- A child's incomplete calcification of the skeleton. They can have internal organ damage without overlying fractures.

Do not be fooled by an initial apparent stable condition. Once their compensatory mechanisms are depleted, they start to deteriorate rapidly. For more discussion, see Chapter 11.

6. Elaborate on how x-ray findings might be different for a child.

Two-thirds of children with spinal cord injury had normal spine radiographs (spinal cord injury without radiographic abnormality [SCIWORA]). It results from a nondisruptive and self-reducing intersegmental deformation because of the relative elasticity of their spinal cord.

Child's compliant chest walls can result in life-threatening internal contusions without accompanying rib fractures.

7. What is a handlebar injury?

A bicycle handlebar (or elbow) striking the child in the right upper quadrant or epigastrium, causing an injury (typically a duodenal hematoma or pancreatic injury).

8. What is the seat belt complex?

Ecchymosis of the abdominal wall and a flexion-distraction injury of the lumbar spine. Consider the possibility of a fracture and intestinal or mesenteric injury.

9. Talk about concerns of trauma in the older adult.

Older adult trauma victims have six times the mortality of younger patients. They have:

- Increased propensity for long-bone fractures
- Decreased physiologic reserve of all organs
- Many take beta-blockers, which can cause "false" normal vital signs

10. What presentations in geriatric trauma are associated with an extremely high mortality?

- Automobile-pedestrian accidents
- Presenting systolic blood pressure <130 mm Hg
- Acidosis (pH <7.35)
- Multiple fractures
- Head injury (67% of unconscious older adult trauma patients die)
- Pelvic fractures

11. Tell me what is important to distinguish in an older adult patient who has a fracture related to a fall.

The cause of the fall. Was the cause external environment (e.g., tripping on a rug and awareness of falling) or was the problem related to the patient's condition (e.g., syncope, "blacking out")?

12. What is essential to remember in any trauma triage?

Always use a systematic assessment process, such as A through I. Then an omission of an important step is less likely to occur. It will help avoid the "silent trauma," an injury that is hidden.

On the other hand, beware of the "Oh my god!" distractor, for example, an obvious, horrendous finding (e.g., a severed arm) that could automatically draw your focus. No matter what other injuries are present, if the airway is not open, the patient will die.

13. Discuss "The Silent Resuscitation" technique for a trauma victim.

A lot of dramatic commotion often occurs when a trauma patient arrives. Triage First, Inc. recommends that the patient is kept on the emergency medical services (EMS) stretcher for the first 60 seconds, and everyone remains quiet. During this time, only the paramedic and lead physician talk so everyone hears the same report. If the patient is too ill to lie on the stretcher for 1 minute, then he or she probably needs to go to diagnostics or surgery immediately and bypass all emergency department (ED) interventions.

After the 60 seconds, the patient is then moved and the physician verbalizes out loud the initial primary and secondary examination while the primary nurse documents and coordinates the preparation and implementation of treatment. This step prevents duplication of effort.

14. Any other suggestions to help with the initial triage of trauma patients?

ED/Trauma Nursing Administrative Director Maryann Henry recommends:

- Hanging trauma scissors from the ceiling of the trauma bay. Nurses do not always have scissors readily available to cut off clothing
- Clip endotracheal tubes on the wall at the head of the trauma bed for quick access.

- Store computed tomography (CT) contrast dye (with weight-based dose chart) in the department to avoid diagnostic delays.

15. How are trauma patients categorized in a three-tier triage system?

Category I patients: need resuscitation. The American College of Surgeons (ACS), Committee on Trauma indicates it is preferred to treat these patients in a trauma center. Criteria for these patients include:

Glasgow Coma Scale (GCS): <14 or
Systolic blood pressure: <90
Respiratory rate: <10 or >29
Revised trauma score: <11

- Penetrating injuries to head, neck, torso, extremities proximal to elbow and knee
- Flail chest
- Combination of trauma and burns
- Two or more long bone fractures
- Pelvic fractures
- Open and depressed skull fractures
- Paralysis
- Amputation proximal to wrist and ankle
- Major burns
- Ejection from automobile
- Death in same passenger compartment
- Extrication time >30 minutes
- Falls >20 feet
- Rollover
- High speed auto crash (>40 miles per hour [mph], >20 inches vehicle deformity, >12 inches intrusion into passenger compartment)
- Pedestrian hit or run over
- Motorcycle crash >20 mph or rider separated from bike
- Patient <5 or >55, pregnant, concurrent chronic medical condition

16. What are Category II patients in a three-tier system?

These urgent (yellow) patients are stable, but have a condition that has the potential to deteriorate, or needs to be seen as soon as possible. Condition may be described as acute, but not "severe." Examples include:

- Open fractures
- Minor burns
- Surgical abdomen

17. Describe Category III in a three-tier system.

These patients are nonurgent (green), frequently called the "walking wounded." Examples would include a minor laceration (bleeding controlled) or a stable extremity fracture.

18. How are trauma patients categorized in the Emergency Severity Index five-tier triage system?

The Emergency Severity Index (ESI) uses an algorithm that considers the patient's level of responsiveness, the presence of a high-risk situation, number of resources needed to care for the patient and vital sign danger zone chart to categorize a patient at triage. Resources include lab tests, electrocardiogram, radiographs, intravenous (IV) fluids, IV or intramuscular (IM) medications, specialty consultation, etc. At any time the vital signs move into the danger zone, the patient would be moved up to the next higher category. For more information on this system, see Chapter 79.

- Category 1 (Resuscitation): The patient is apneic, pulseless, or unresponsive and may be intubated or require intubation.
- Category 2 (High risk): The patient is confused, lethargic, or disoriented, or in severe pain or distress.
- Category 3: Two or more resources are needed and vitals fall within a danger zone.
- Category 4: One resource is needed, vital signs stable.
- Category 5: No resources/simple exam (abrasion).

19. How are trauma patients categorized in the Canadian Emergency Department Triage and Acuity Scale five-tier triage system?

Level I (Resuscitation): Major Trauma

- Severe injury of any single body system or multiple system injury (Injury Severity Score [ISS] >16)
- Head injury with a GCS score <10
- Severe burns (>25% total body surface [TBS] or airway problems)
- Chest/abdominal injury with any or all of: altered mental state, hypotension, tachycardia, severe pain, respiratory signs, or symptoms

Level II (Emergency): Severe Trauma

- High-risk mechanisms and severe single system symptoms or multiple system involvement with less severe signs and symptoms in each (ISS ≥9)
- Normal or nearly normal vital signs (abnormal vs. equal to Level I)
- Moderate to severe pain
- Normal mental status

Level III (Urgent): Moderate Trauma

- Fractures, dislocations, sprains
- Severe pain (8 to 10/10)
- Stable

Level IV (Less Urgent): Minor trauma

- Minor fractures, sprains, contusions, abrasions, lacerations requiring intervention
- Moderate pain (4 to 7/10)
- Stable

Level V (Nonurgent): Minor trauma

- Contusions, abrasions, minor lacerations (not requiring closure by any means), sprains, and overuse syndromes

20. What is an important principle to remember regardless of a patient's category?

Reassess frequently and move the patient up a severity category as necessary.

21. When do you consider organ procurement?

The potential for organ procurement should be considered if an arriving patient requires resuscitation. Even patients who are pronounced dead on arrival to the ED may be candidates for tissue donation.

22. When may a trauma patient be transferred?

The Emergency Medical Treatment and Active Labor Act (EMTALA) is a federal government law that regulates the conditions when an unstable patient may be transferred. Components include:

- Request for transfer (by patient, attending physician, ED physician because of unique services available).
- Benefit of the transferred-to facility's treatment outweighs the risk of the transfer and is discussed with patient.
- Accepting physician, with whom transferring physician confers.
- Confirmed space and availability for the patient at the receiving hospital.
- Transferring hospital must provide for resuscitation and stabilization of the patient within its capabilities prior to transfer.
- Copies of all pertinent ED documentation including diagnostic results and consent for treatment accompany patient.
- Transfer uses proper equipment and personnel.

23. What is a trauma system?

A trauma system designs and carries out an organized plan within a state, region, or area to prevent, treat, and minimize the impact of trauma injury. The ACS Committee on Trauma definition of a trauma system includes administration of, access to, and designation of the system's trauma care. It includes components of prevention, acute hospital care, rehabilitation, medical audit, and research activities.

24. Who regulates the function of a trauma center?

Trauma systems are regulated by the federal government through the passage of legislation that provides funding to states to develop systems of trauma care. The state legislatures also pass laws defining how the trauma system will operate and how the monetary resources will be allocated within their state.

25. Why is trauma prevention important?

It is the fourth leading cause of death in the United States, exceeded only by heart disease, cancer, and stroke. Trauma has been described as the "disease of the young" because traumatic injury affects primarily the 1- to 40-year-old age group. It is estimated that one fatal injury occurs every 5 minutes and that a disabling injury will occur approximately every 5 seconds.

26. How are trauma centers designated?

A determination is made by the designated state agency based on the documents (application describing the institution's ability), site survey, and interviews. States use the ACS criteria for designation and accreditation of trauma centers.

27. What are the criteria for designation for each category of trauma center?

Many states have similar descriptions as the ACS Committee on Trauma. The ACS identified four levels of trauma center designation. A simplistic overview of the level components includes the following:

Level I: A regional resource that provides tertiary care and lead hospital in the region. They are expected to admit at least 1,200 trauma patients annually with an ISS of at least 15. An attending trauma surgeon must be available in house 24 hours a day.

Level II: Provides comprehensive trauma care. The attending trauma surgeon responds within a reasonable time to provide care to the trauma patient.

Level III: Must have continuous general surgical coverage and the capability to manage the care of a trauma patient until transfer. A resuscitation team must be available.

Level IV: Provides initial evaluation and assessment. A physician covers the ED 24 hours a day, but specialty coverage may not be available.

28. What is a trauma registry?

A trauma registry is one component of a trauma system. All trauma patients cared for in an individual trauma center are entered into the database of the trauma registry. The data are collected, coded, sorted, stored, and reported to appropriate agencies. Each state decides which registry software program will be used within the trauma agency in the individual state.

29. What is the continuous quality improvement process for a trauma center?

Trauma registry data parameters are monitored, such as specialty service response, complications of surgical procedures, transfusion reactions, or length of stay. A National Trauma Data Bank has been established by the ACS to review outcomes and develop strategies of care.

30. What data are collected for the trauma registry and how are they used?

The collected data are related to the injury event, severity of injury, care provided, and outcome of the injury. The various federal and state agencies compile and publish the data annually to help identify needed injury prevention initiatives.

31. Discuss videotaping trauma.

Videotaping is useful for educational and quality improvement purposes. The Joint Commission for Accreditation of Healthcare Organizations (JCAHO) has several requirements about the process, related to confidentiality and consent:

- Informed consent to be taped must be obtained. However, if the patient is unconscious or incompetent, and no family or surrogate decision maker is present, taping can still begin immediately.
- An informed consent (verbal or written and documented) is obtained before using the tape.
- The videotape remains secured by the health care organization.
- The community is informed that videotaping may take place.

32. What are the education requirements for a registered nurse (RN) in a trauma center?

Required courses include:

- Basic Life Support for Healthcare Professionals (CPR)
- Advanced Cardiac Life Support (ACLS)
- Pediatric Advanced Life Support (PALS)
- Trauma course
- Pediatric course
- Triage course
- Prehospital communication course (such as ECRN [Emergency Communications Registered Nurse])
- It is recommended nurses become certified in the specialty of emergency nursing (CEN).

33. Name some courses that would meet those requirements.

I recommend the courses from the Emergency Nurses Association (ENA):

- TNCC (Trauma Nursing Core Course)
- CATN (Course in Advanced Trauma Nursing)
- ENPC (Emergency Nursing Pediatric Course)

34. How does mass casualty triage differ from standard triage of an individual patient?

Mass casualty, military, or disaster triage is performed on the basis of the "greatest good for the greatest number." The system is based on the incident command system. It follows a four-tier triage format.

Class I: Red: Emergent: Critical, life threat: shock, airway compromise, hemorrhage.

Class II: Yellow: Urgent: Major illness or injury. Treatment necessary as soon as possible (30 minutes to 2 hours): major illness or injury, open fracture, chest injury.

Class III: Green: Nonurgent: Delayed care, may wait more than 2 hours to be treated: sprain, strain, closed fracture, "walking wounded."

Class IV: Black: either dead or anticipated to die shortly: massive head injury or full-thickness burns.

35. How does this relate to our hospital's disaster plan?

Many hospitals use this triage system in their disaster plans, as it is assumed there will be multiple trauma victims in this type of incident. The JCAHO requires every hospital to develop a mass casualty response plan (disaster plan) with annual drills. For further discussion, see Chapter 62.

36. Name some courses that will help assess injured patients in other settings besides a hospital ED.

- ENA's TNCC
- Red Cross or American Heart Association First Aid Course
- School Nurse Emergency Course
- A triage course

Key Points

- It is preferred for a Category I patient to be treated at a Level I trauma center.
- Trauma triage includes the MOI to provide a HIS of potential injury to a specific body system.
- Pediatric patients are more prone than adults to have multiple injuries, hypothermia, airway obstruction, and internal injuries without overlying fractures.
- Organ procurement potential should be considered on any trauma patient requiring resuscitation or pronounced dead.
- A trauma registry program collects, stores, and reports data related to the care of injured patients to appropriate agencies.
- The ACS has established a National Trauma Data Bank to review trauma care outcomes and develop strategies to improve care to trauma patients.

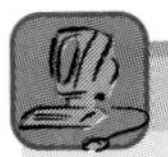

Internet Resources

National Trauma Data Bank 2003
http://www.facs.org/trauma/ntdbannualreport2003.pdf

Triagefirst.com
www.Triagefirst.com

The Abaris Group: Innovative Solutions for the Emergency Care Field
www.abarisgroup.com

Canadian Association of Emergency Physicians
www.caep.ca

Emergency Nurses Association: Trauma System Development in the United States
http://www.ena.org/publications/onlineconnection/2004/sep/traumasystemdevelopment.asp

Bibliography

American College of Surgeons, Committee on Trauma: *Resources for optimal care of the injured patient,* 1999, available: http://www.facs.org/trauma/index.html.

Barkin RM, Rosen P: *Emergency pediatrics: A guide to ambulatory care,* ed 6, St Louis, 2003, Mosby.

Biffl WL, Biffl HU: Pediatric trauma. In Markovchick VJ, Pons PT, editors: *Pons' emergency medicine secrets,* ed 3, Philadelphia, 2003, Hanley & Belfus.

Canadian Association of Emergency Physicians: *Canadian Emergency Department Triage and Acuity Scale: Implementation guidelines,* Ontario, Canada, 1993, Canadian Association of Emergency Physicians.

Emergency Nurses Association: *Course in advanced trauma nursing (CATN II), Chapter 11: Trauma care systems, defense systems,* ed 2, Dubuque, Ia, 2003, Kendall/Hunt Publishing.

Emergency Nurses Association: *Trauma Nursing Core Course (TNCC),* ed 5, Des Plaines, Ill, 2000, Emergency Nurses Association, 39-64.

Gilboy N, et al: *Emergency Severity Index (ESI),* Des Plaines, Ill, 2003, Emergency Nurses Association, 6-9, 12-33.

Henry M: Improving trauma services (Managers Forum), *J Emerg Nurs* 29(6):559-560, 2003.

Illinois Emergency Medical Services for Children (EMSC): *School nurse emergency care course,* Maywood, Ill, 2003, Loyola University Medical Center, 9-11, 93-104.

Jackimczyk KC, Tripp W: Geriatric emergency medicine. In Markovchick VJ, Pons PT, editors: *Pons' emergency medicine secrets,* ed 3, Philadelphia, 2003, Hanley & Belfus.

Jordan KS, editor: *Emergency Nurses Association Emergency Nursing Core Curriculum,* ed 5, Philadelphia, 2000, WB Saunders, 681-683.

Killian M, editor: *Standards of emergency nursing practice,* ed 4, Des Plaines, Ill, 1999, Emergency Nurses Association, 23-28.

Knaut AL, Knaut CS: EMTALA. In Markovchick VJ, Pons PT, editors: *Pons' emergency medicine secrets,* ed 3, Philadelphia, 2003, Hanley & Belfus.

McNair RS: Improving trauma services (Managers Forum), *J Emerg Nurs* 29(6):559, 2003.

Newberry L: *Sheehy's emergency nursing: Principles and practice,* St Louis, 2003, Mosby, 75-83.

Staten PA: Videotaping trauma cases (Managers Forum), *J Emerg Nurs* 26(6):601-602, 2003.

Chapter 68

Occupational Health Considerations

Jan Frustaglia

1. Does the occupational health nurse do patient care?

Yes. But the "patient" is the employee of a workplace, not from the outside community. The "care" may vary from hands-on assessment of a workplace injury to follow-up counseling.

2. Do occupational health nurses administer medications?

Some clinics work with a physician present to provide orders; others have standing medical protocols that usually include over-the-counter (OTC) drugs and appropriate vaccinations. Usually facilities located farther from hospitals have more extensive options.

3. Is triage different for the occupational health nurse?

The standards of care, protocols, and priorities of a nursing triage assessment and treatment are universal.

4. What triage levels do most nurses working independently (e.g., occupational health nurses, clinic, school nurses) routinely make?

Levels of four routine occupational health "triage" are usually protocols, for example:

Level 1 Critical, needs medical doctor (MD) now, call 911, and send to hospital
Level 2 Acute, as soon as possible (ASAP), urgent, see MD today
Level 3 Semi-urgent, in a timely fashion, see MD if no improvement
Level 4 Nonurgent, stable, not acute, when convenient/reassure/educate

To make a determination of the triage level, the nurse also considers the employee's history and concerns. An employee's self-assessment of being unable to safely do their job is always taken at face value.

5. Give examples of how this might work.

Blood pressure 230/140, complaining of dizziness	Level 1	To the emergency department (ED)
Blood pressure 180/100, dizziness, 60-year-old	Level 2	To primary care physician (PCP) today (In reality, during after-hours, the patient must often go to an ED.)
Blood pressure 150/90, no symptoms	Level 3	Call PCP
Blood pressure 140/88 today, normally 130s/70s	Level 4	Education

6. Are there "real" emergencies in the occupational setting?

Yes. No matter where you work, there is always the potential for environmental concerns and acute injuries. All workers could be exposed to slippery floors, steps, chemicals, outdoor environment, noise, fumes, radiation, electricity, or unsafe equipment. Consider these scenarios:

- Chemical splash to skin and eyes
- Inhalation of cleaning products
- Electric shock while operating construction equipment
- An allergic reaction to a new antibiotic while driving a truck on the job

7. How does the occupational health nurse handle an employee coming in with a medical need?

Initially the occupational health nurse (OHN) would:

- Assess the employee's injury or medical complaint and medical stability.
- Provide treatment per the standing medical protocols. (This would include arranging transportation to emergency room/urgent care/hospital if deemed necessary and communicating with the receiving facility.)
- Document.
- Advise the injured worker what to expect medically and advice on employer's expectations.
- Liaison with the worker's supervisor/department regarding the cause and the work status of the employee.

8. Give an example of how this all works.

- A 42-year-old woman worker who comes to the OHN on a Tuesday morning complaining that her job is causing pain in her right arm.
- The nurse documents the provided facts of the injury. Questions might be more detailed than a routine ED triage regarding the triggers or cause of the pain.
  - "Where and how does the pain occur?"
  - "What task are you doing that makes your arm hurt?"
  - "Why do you think this pain is related to the job tasks you do?"

- Appropriate teaching can be offered. You still offer appropriate care, but who pays for the health care service/product may vary depending on the cause.

9. What if the employee doesn't want to go to the hospital or do what the nurse thinks is best?

It can be alarming to have an overweight, hypertensive, diaphoretic older adult male with chest pain who refuses to go to an ED. The reality is that, just as any medical facility, a competent adult has the right to refuse care. As one ethicist summarized, "You have a legal right to be an idiot!"

Try the broken record technique to penetrate what is often fear or denial. One script that can work to encourage cooperation is, "You came here because you have a concern about this symptom. I share that concern. Let's get you the care you need."

If all else fails, the OHN can determine the person is "unsafe" to continue to work and pull the individual from the job. A medical clearance by a physician will be required to return.

10. What is the next step?

- Follow-up with the treating facility's recommendations
- Initiate appropriate workers' compensation paperwork and requirements, when appropriate

11. I don't understand. If the condition happened at work, won't workers' compensation cover it?

Not necessarily. The problem must be job-related. So although a hand caught in a drill press is covered, a heart attack would be covered under the employee's health benefits. This is why documentation is key. For instance, after a weekend an employee may claim he just sprained his ankle today at work but the nurse notes yellowish-green ecchymosis, suggesting that the injury occurred several days ago.

12. Give another illustration.

Two workers both get thermal burn to the forearm that becomes infected. Injury #1 occurred in a hospital's sterile processing department and was reported to the supervisor; Injury #2 occurred at a home. Two days later each injured worker decides to have the badly infected injury assessed by the OHN.

Injured worker #1 will report to his supervisor, then to employee health. The OHN will assess and refer employee to a medical clinician for further treatment, and initiate the workers' compensation. The workers' compensation administrator will now determine benefits. No expenses came out-of-pocket from the worker; sick days are not used. The worker will have requirements for follow-up with the OHN. If there is delayed healing, the OHN might initiate investigation for potential diabetes and encourage the employee to discuss it with his/her PCP.

Injured worker #2 will also be assessed (including ability to work), but referred to a PCP. Worker #2 will pay the expenses of doctor, treatments, and prescription using the employer health benefits and will lose pay (or take sick days) for his 2 days off work. There are no OHN follow-up requirements unless restrictions are written by the PCP.

13. After giving treatment, can the worker's case be filed away?

No. The OHN's "care plan" for "case management" has just begun.

- Full documentation of the accident. Many times the OHN and the safety officer visit the accident site performing a root-cause analysis. Prevention activities must be initiated to abate another injury of the same type.
- Follow-up of the patient's condition. This includes how the employee is physically doing, what the treating physician indicated, the regulations of workers' compensation in that state, and the determination by the work place administrator of the workers' compensation.
- Education. Many employees do not realize that tighter rules apply in a worker's compensation case. For instance, in one airline company, the follow-up requirements for "blocked" ears in flight attendants differ. If the ears blocked during a flight, then within workers' compensation, the employee must have the ears tested every other day. If the ears blocked during the employee's time off and they are using their own medical benefits, they must only have their ears tested a minimum of once every 5 days.
- Build toward a quick, successful return to work. Establish a rapport and begin ongoing communication of the progress, even if employees choose to see their primary care physician. Set up positive expectations. The goal of OHN is to return a worker as soon as safely possible to minimize a negative financial impact.

14. Isn't this a blurring of nursing's professional obligation to give nonjudgmental care?

Needed care is rendered regardless of whom the payer is. All appropriate cases are considered workers' compensation eligible. The OHN role is to complete the necessary forms and to document a detailed history immediately after a workplace event. It gives evidence to support—or not support—benefits and compensability.

However, the determination of benefits and compensability is done by the workers' compensation carrier/administrator. Traditional qualifying criteria include "in the course of" and "arising out of employment." However, because workers' compensation systems are state administered, determination may vary from state to state.

15. Can this be difficult at times for the OHN to have this distinction?

It can be. For instance, the airline employee indicates their ears had been plugged up the last few days and was hesitant to fly but didn't call in sick because he/she has no sick days left. The nurse notes cold symptoms, including frequent nose-blowing. The nurse knows that documenting this information will probably result in a denial of the worker's compensation claim for the ear "blocking" that occurred during the flight. However, the nurse maintains integrity and does complete objective charting, just as when it is not a factor.

16. Is the OHN the one who enforces the restrictions an employee is given?

No. The OHN assists the department supervisor to accommodate the worker under the restrictions written by the medical clinician. The worker "owns" how they work and the assumption is that they will adhere to the medical restrictions. The workplace supervisor or the human resource department essentially enforces the restrictions. If the employee feels the supervisor is not adhering to the restrictions, the OHN can be notified, who then requests appropriate superior or administrator involvement.

17. Do employees have trouble understanding this distinction?

Often. After all, no other source of health care provision tells someone that the medical need cannot be met because of the problem's time or onset or origin. (Some organizations do have "expanded services," which include nonoccupational health services for a fee.)

18. How do you handle that?

- Let the employees tell their whole story. Otherwise, they feel "cut off."
- Indicate, "We are not allowed (avoid 'unable,' which implies a lack of capability) to care for this health need."
- State up front the anticipated negative reaction, "I know it probably seems as if I am disregarding your problem" or "I know it is frustrating not to be able to receive this care here."
- Keep the tone empathetic and regret. Otherwise, the employee may misconstrue the nurse as "not caring."
- Provide an alternative option.

19. What are key differences in occupational health nursing?

- Employment-related. Occupational health nursing provides free care to the employees, but only for job-related concerns. This may include postoffer, preplacement health assessment, and drug screening, ongoing safety screening, preventive immunizations, job-related health teaching, and on-the-job injuries. At times, the distinction can get tricky. Is the gastroenteritis for a flight attendant from eating the airline food or just an everyday "flu"? Flight attendants traveling to undeveloped countries receive free hepatitis A immunization; airline employees traveling for vacation do not.
- Ongoing management. Similarly, occupational health provides case management for job-related concerns, but not for chronic illnesses such as high blood pressure. The nurse will screen for high blood pressure, but then

refers the employee to his or her PCP for management (using the health insurance benefit).

- Employers will be informed. Patient confidentiality is primary in an ED; an ED nurse would never call an employer and tell them the patient arrived drunk. Any statement or behaviors, although, during an occupational health visit are reportable.
- Epidemiology. The OHN might take more responsibility to note patterns, collect epidemiology data, and/or seek facility-wide changes to aid the "patient" employees as part of the job responsibilities. The role can include recognizing, evaluating, and controlling workplace conditions that may cause adverse health effects. A hospital nurse may be involved in community preventive measures ("Don't drink and drive," etc.) but usually out of a sense of public service.
- Outside regulation. There is an ever-present awareness that every case is a potential lawsuit, subject to government regulations, and/or union issues. Documentation is detailed and thorough, and the physician authority is strong.
- Reason for existence. Hospital nursing roles exist to provide health care so the value of many activities, such as routine blood pressure screening, is obvious. In occupational health, the company exists for business and financial reasons and nursing's purpose is to meet requirements and keep the workforce working. Health care is a small minor element.
- Educational needs. Employees ask about many generic health concerns and how to use the (often previously unfamiliar) company's health care or workman's compensation benefits. For many workers, the OHN is the only consistent contact with a health care professional.

20. What about malingerers?

The OHN's responsibility is to remain objective and documents what the employee states. The nurse does not have to determine the "legitimacy." For instance, one employee became too "stressed" to work "safely" every time the worker did not receive the preferred assignment. He reported to the OHN and the incident and need to go home was documented.

When a pattern is noted, the supervisor can request a medical examination confirming that the employee is healthy enough to perform the job. If the employee is, it becomes a discipline issue. If not, a medical leave is recommended until the health issues are resolved. The subjective judgment is removed for the nurse.

21. In a hospital setting, what is the difference between the infection control clinician and the OHN?

The infection control clinician (IC) monitors infection transmission and control from the patients' perspective. The OHN professional monitors infection transmission and control from the employee's perspective. Everyday scenarios involve numerous political balances (and some overlap) between health care fiscal dollars, public relations, employer expectations, public health, worker rights, and medical needs for both the IC and OHN professional. For example, both the IC and OHN would monitor an outbreak of chickenpox in a pediatric department.

Key Points

- The priorities of a nursing triage assessment are the same in occupational health as in an ED.
- OHNs' extent of care and follow-up depends on whether the problem is job-related.
- The OHN has an increased role in epidemiology and prevention.

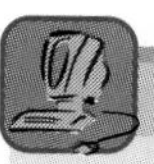

Internet Resources

American Association of Occupational Health Nurses (AAOHN)
www.aaohn.org

Association of Occupational Health Professionals in Healthcare (AOHP)
www.aoph.org

Bibliography

Gruden M: Report of AOHP 2000 Membership Survey and Needs Assessment, *J Assoc Occupational Health Professional Healthcare* Fall 1999.

Rogers B: *Occupational health nursing concepts and practice,* Philadelphia, 1994, WB Saunders.

Zimmermann PG: Airline nurse, *J Emerg Nurs* 22(6):549-551, 1996.

Zimmermann PG: Improving employee communication in the clinical setting: A nurse's perspective, *AAOHN J* 50(11):515-519, 2002.

Chapter 69

Violence and Security Issues

Bernard "Bo" Ball, Nina M. Fielden, and Rebecca S. McNair

1. What are the risk factors of community violence?

Risk factors of community violence include: adolescent or young adult males, low socioeconomic status, previous history of fighting, access to firearms, alcohol and drug use, gang involvement, exposure to domestic violence or child abuse, and media violence.

2. Who is more prone to violence?

Violence has decreased over the past decade, but there is still a culture of violence in the United States. There are two groups: the early onset, before puberty (around age 10); and the late onset, in adolescence. Most violence begins in the second decade of life (according to the Report of the Surgeon General [see Internet Resources box]) but the early onset group has more serious offenses that persist into adulthood.

3. Tell me the source of injuries in victims of violence.

For every young person who is killed by violence, approximately 20 to 40 more individuals have injuries that require hospital treatment. The nonfatal injuries usually involve the use of fists, feet, knives, and clubs although firearms are more involved in fatal assaults.

4. How do I handle those who present with injuries from violence?

According to your state law, most violent injuries involving a weapon or serious physical harm require reporting to law enforcement. However, some (frequent) patients with vague problems or who respond poorly to medical treatment can be victims of violence. Question them further about their history with violence, as they may not admit to victimization. Some of these common complaints include anxiety, depression, or a variety of somatic complaints that arise long after the traumatic event.

5. How can I assess for the risk of violence in a patient's life?

The mnemonic GUNS can be used.

G Is there a Gun in the household?

U Does the patient associate with Users of drugs or alcohol?
N Does the patient feel the Need to protect him/herself?
S Do any of these Situations exist? Having seen or been involved in violence, feeling sadness, or school-aged children in the household?

One simple question is: "Have you been struck or harmed or threatened in the past year?" If the answer is yes, question further to determine if this is ongoing or likely to recur.

Another assessment acronym is FISTS.
Fighting
Injuries
Sexual violence
Threats
Self-defense

6. If violence is admitted, what should I document?

- Circumstances surrounding the violent event
- Who (stranger, an acquaintance, or a relative)
- Is the violence recurring?
- Did either the victim or perpetrator use alcohol or drugs?
- Has the victim obtained a weapon?
- Has his/her routine changed?
- Note any other physical clues, such as gang tattoos or scars.

7. What other question must I always ask a victim of violence?

Is the danger still present (stalking, spouse carries a gun, etc.)? If yes, alert security. There is concern for the safety of the staff and the waiting room patients.

8. What should I do if I see a weapon displayed, like a knife or gun?*

Verbalize it loud and frequently, just like the police officers are trained to do, so others become aware and the appropriate actions can be initiated. "Your KNIFE in triage is scaring me. KNIFE."

9. How does the five-tier triage system Canadian Triage and Acuity Scale view victims of violence?

The Canadian ED Triage and Acuity Scale (CTAS) categorizes physical abuse/neglect/assault (sexual less than 4 hours old) or patients with aggressive/violent behavior as a Level II (emergent, 15 minutes). Even though these patients have no life-threatening problems, they do have needs related to their mental well-

---

*Contains copyright material from TRIAGE FIRST, Inc. Available at: www.triagefirst.com. Used by permission.

being. There are requirements for evidence collection or activation for assault teams and community services.

10. Tell me how the Australian Triage Scale views them.

The Australian Triage Scale (ATS) requires humane practice to relieve severe discomfort or distress and provides a time frame from 10 to 60 minutes. Violent or aggressive patients should be categorized as Level 2 (imminently life-threatening or important time-critical treatment or very severe pain or distress).

11. Indicate the ESI rating.

The Emergency Severity Index (ESI) system recommends that victims of any sexual assault be categorized as level 2 (high-risk situation, severe pain, or distress). Combative, hostile, and hysterical patients should also be categorized as level 2.

12. And the Manchester Triage Group?

Risk of harm to others (considering the state of mind, body posture, and behavior), risk for further self-harm, or unsure of risk are all considered a Level 2. Inappropriate history, regardless of the chief complaint, is a Level 3 (urgent, 60 minutes). An inappropriate history is defined, as "the alleged mechanism does not explain the apparent injury or illness." A "significant psychiatric history," e.g., history of major psychiatric illness or event is a Level 4 (standard, 120 minutes).

13. Is violence a problem in hospitals?

The Bureau of Labor Statistics indicated that cases of workplace violence rose to 16.5 per 10,000 full-time health care workers in 2001. A preliminary report on workplace violence against nurses by the New York State Nursing Association released in 2004 found that 46.9% of nurses had experienced verbal insults or threats in the workplace, 20.7% had been physically assaulted, and 4% had been physically assaulted with a weapon. Acts of violence resulting in death have occurred in 7% of major teaching hospitals.

14. Tell me some personality types that are more prone to become violent toward staff.*

Few people wake up with the personal goal of hitting a nurse. It is usually an uncontrolled response to a trigger. Personality-wise, people prone to violence have a low tolerance for frustration, a problem with authority, limited emotional resources, and poor coping skills. Some people live by a different set of rules, such as hitting is a solution, and they are not going to change their value system because they are in a hospital.

15. Any patient/family situations or conditions to be aware of?*

- Drug and alcohol abusers
- Family members who misinterpret medical treatments
- Grief-stricken relatives
- Individuals with antisocial or gang tattoos (such as "Misfit," "Death Before Dishonor," or "Satan's Army").

16. What are signs that a patient or family member may be becoming agitated or aggressive, escalating to violence?*

A previous history of violence should be regarded seriously. Typically there are behavioral cues as the patient escalates from anxiety to agitation to violence. Signals include:

- Muscle tension
- Fidgeting in the chair or restlessness/pacing
- Clenched teeth or fists
- An angry facial expression
- Loud strident rapid speech
- Withdrawal and lack of response to questions
- Disorientation
- Verbalized fear or threats
- Obscene language
- Repetitive demands
- Argumentative demeanor
- Failure to comply with rules
- Evidence of auditory or visual hallucinations

17. List verbal responses and approaches that can help keep the patient and situation in control.*

- Remain calm and respectful. Use a soothing tone of voice. Never yell back.
- Use the patient's name.
- Acknowledge the patient's emotional response. Say, "I can see that you are angry." It does not make it worse to mention the emotion. Instead, it annoys the aggressive patient to feel ignored.
- Avoid quoting authoritative rules, such as "You can't act like that! This is a hospital." They don't care. It only increases their frustration.
- Don't make an unnecessary requests or criticism. Telling an agitated person they need to fill out these forms first just causes escalation.
- Focus questions on the concrete, basic needs. "Have you eaten anything today?" Continually focusing on these (which the nurse can immediately help) can diffuse the situation.
- Permit verbal venting. This allows the individual to release energy.
- Ignore challenge questions. Redirect the individual attention to the issue at hand. Answering questions about your training, policy, etc., just fuels a power struggle.
- Share your emotional response. Say, "Now you are scaring me" if the patient's behavior starts to escalate. It won't further agitate them, but sometimes makes them realize (for the first time) that they are losing control.

- "Talk them down" by acknowledging the patient's feelings of helplessness, fear of losing control, or being frightened by the intensity of his/her own emotions.
- Place simple, realistic; and enforceable limits on the patient's behavior.
- Try to make a verbal contract (e.g., if I do this, you will do that). For instance, "If I go get you something to eat, can you stay in this room and wait? Can you do that for me? Can you stand here and wait while I get the food?"

18. Name some physical actions that can help keep the patient and situation in control and the nurse safe.*

- Maintain eye contact.
- Position yourself away from his/her personal space (1½ to 3 feet). Introduce yourself from a distance.
- Remove availability of any potential weapons, such as glasses, sharps, etc.
- Stand angled off to the side, with your arms at your side (nonthreatening postures). Standing eye-to-eye, toe-to-toe, or folding your arms sends a challenge message.
- Be aware of your body language, movement, and tone of voice. The more an individual loses control, the less that person listens to the actual words.
- Keep backing up if the person keeps coming nearer (remain out of reach in case they strike out).
- Allow yourself a clear access to an exit. Never have the patient between you and the escape route.
- Ignore the phone ringing or anything that will distract you from the full attention of the escalating individual.
- Speak loudly so other staff can overhear when the person is clearly escalating to obtain appropriate help according to the department's disruptive violent outbreak written policy.

19. Our emergency department doesn't have a disruptive violent outbreak written policy.*

Most don't. It should. Begin creating your department's policy by asking the hospital's psychiatric unit for any of their appropriate policies. The emergency department (ED) needs a clear, coordinated method to safely obtain help when there is a patient/family member who has lost control. Include a method for the triage nurse to signal for help.

20. What is an underlying theme to handling these types of situations?*

Give up control to gain control. The nurse's authority is the brain, not "rank." Avoid getting into an unnecessary battle over authority, power, or control.

21. How do I keep myself safe at triage?*

- Listen to your "gut" when in doubt. If you feel in danger, it is probably a realistic possibility. It is not unprofessional to be afraid; it is only unprofessional to not handle it properly.

- If a family member is escalating into agitation and potential violence, move them to a less stimulating environment (e.g., private family room). Limit the "public show."
- Move the potential violent, escalating patient emergently to the main ED in which clothing and possessions can be removed safely.
- If the police bring in a patient in handcuffs, bypass triage and go to the main ED. The patient may need to be placed in restraint or seclusion after the handcuffs are removed before assessment and treatment can begin.

22. Define and describe how to manage a physical "take down."*

When a patient is out-of-control and poses a physical threat, the staff must respond in an organized, coordinated way to physically restrain the patient for the safety of the patient and others and to be able to render appropriate treatment. Additional policies and training is needed, but steps of the process include:

- Alert security.
- Keep directions simple and clear.
- Inform the patient of what is being done and why. ("You are losing control and we are going to restrain you to help you get control.") Do not taunt the patient.
- Approach the patient calmly, quickly, and with authority.
- Use five staff members, one at the head and one for each limb.
- Nursing takes the lead, not security. A "key word" (from the previous training) signals everyone to act now, such as "enough is enough."
- Use leather four-point restraints.

23. Talk about documentation.*

Always include clear, precise descriptions of the exact out-of-control or threatening behaviors that lead to justifying the application of restraints (medications, etc.). Do not just write the conclusion ("irrational") but list the specific things, such as patient keeps encroaching on nurse's physical space despite nurse backing up, threw pen at nurse, screaming swear words, etc.

24. What is a concern about gang members coming to the ED for treatment?

Whenever injured individual gang members arrive, there is a risk that the rival gang may arrive to "finish them off." The patients' fellow gang members may also come, so there is a risk of setting up a major confrontation.

The primary reason a gang member comes to the ED is the same reason as other patients: they are sick or injured. They want relief. Keep focused on that. They did not come purposefully for violence or drugs: they can get those on the street.

25. Gang members seem prone to "fly off" at minimal provocation.*

Grossman (2003) recommends remembering the three "Rs" to help prevent that.

- **Reputation** is an ultimate priority. Being perceived as "brave" is important. Never give a look or say anything to refute that.

- **Respect.** Do not mishandle any of their jewelry, ornaments, or head wraps as it can be seen as a sign of disrespect. (Keep gang members wearing different colors in separate areas of the department.) Never pass judgment on a patient's use of symbolism.
- **Retaliation and revenge.** If you fail to give them respect or threaten their reputation, revenge can be sought up to weeks later.

26. Any advice in case the worse situation happens and there is a hostage situation?*

- The first 15 to 45 minutes are the most dangerous.
- Follow instructions and treat the captor like royalty.
- Remain hypervigilant.
- Think twice about trying to escape. The person fleeing is the most common target.
- Be prepared to drop to the floor when the police take control.

27. Any comments on physical plant parameters for safety?*

- All ED doors should be secured (including the back entrance); access to the hospital itself should be limited to a few controlled entrances. In addition, consider:
  - Metal detectors
  - Continuous-surveillance, closed-circuit monitoring
  - Multiple methods of summoning police/security (without going through the hospital operator). Stony Brook Hospital (New York) is buying alarms for workers to wear to quickly alert security.
  - Proper training and equipping of hospital and security staff
  - Guard dogs

28. Talk about the use of guard dogs.

A physical presence or show of unified force, control, and structure sometimes helps people to keep themselves in control. The hospital environment, in and of itself, is a "controlled location," often supplemented with highly visible security officer.

Another option is a K-9 program using trained officers and German shepherd dogs (who respond only to commands in a foreign language known only by the officer). The guard dogs, with the officer, can be placed outside (or inside) violent patients' rooms. They've also worked well to soothe anxious children.

Programs using guard dogs have been indicated to be more effective than officers carrying a gun. Displaying a gun tends to generate violence, whereas the dogs tend to have a calming effect and defuse situations. In addition, an attack command can be stopped immediately by another command; a bullet cannot.

29. What about staff name badges?

In the 1990s, ED nurses in California spearheaded California's AB508, which was one of the first to legislate changes in the ED environment to reduce the risk of violence. As this issue has subsequently developed, the California and the Federal OSHA 2004 publication, Guidelines for Preventing Workplace Violence for Health Care and Social Services Worker took a position regarding name badges. It states, "Provide staff with identification badges, preferably without last names, to readily identify employment." The entire document can be accessed at http://www.osha.gov/publications/osha3148.pdf.

30. Can a hospital be held liable for injury to waiting patients?

In one case, *Rodriguez v. 1201 Realty, LLC*, the hospital was held liable for the injuries incurred by a waiting patient in the hospital's ED despite the fact that the injuries were caused by an unsupervised 5-year-old child (whose mother was also present). The court stated that merely warning the unruly child to behave was insufficient.

31. Any advice about security related to terrorist's attacks?

Consultant Steven S. Wilder warns that hospitals will likely become secondary targets following any initial terrorist attack elsewhere in the community. He recommends the following related considerations for disaster plans:

- Develop tight access controls to prevent unauthorized vehicles from entering the hospital campus during a community disaster.
- Do not make local police, fire, or emergency medical services (EMS) part of the hospital's disaster plan. They will probably be unavailable, committed to another location.
- Enforce all staff always wearing an identification badge. Do not ever allow vendors to be in the hospital without checking in and obtaining an authorization badge.
- Emergency Medical Treatment and Active Labor Act (EMTALA) expert consultant, Steven A. Frew, JD, also urges background checks (not just criminal arrest records) for any hospital hired personnel. It is important to prevent insider attacks, such as disabling e-attacks on the hospital computer system.

Key Points

- Use GUNS or FISTS to assess for the risk of violence in a patient's life.
- Patients or family members tend to escalate from anger to agitation/aggression to violence. Recognize the signs and attempt to diffuse.
- Acknowledge the escalating patients' emotion ("I can see you are very upset."), do not quote authoritative rules ("You can't act like that!"), and attempt to make a verbal contract (e.g., if I do this, you will do that).*
- Stand an arms length away, at an angle with your arms at the side, and allow a clear access to an exit.*
- If a weapon is displayed, loudly, repeatedly verbalize it so other staff can obtain help ("I see your GUN in TRIAGE.")*

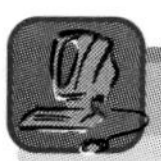

Internet Resources

Crisis Prevention Institute
http://www.crisisprevention.com/

Emergency Nurses Association (ENA) Position Statement: Violence in the Emergency Care Setting
http://www.ena.org/about/position/violence.asp

Family Violence Prevention Fund
http://endabuse.org/.

National Clearinghouse on Child Abuse and Neglect Information
http://nccanch.acf.hhs.gov/pubs/factsheets/canstats.cfm.

Nursing Network on Violence Against Women, International
http://www.nnvawi.org/assessment.htm.

World Health Organization: World report on violence and health
http://www.who.int/violence_injury_prevention/violence/world_report/en/.

Report of the Surgeon General: Youth Violence
http://www.surgeongeneral.gov/library/youthviolence/default.htm.

EMTALA Online
http://www.medlaw.com/

Bibliography

Abboud PAC: Management of the violent patient. In Markovchick VJ, Pons PT, editors: *Pons' emergency medicine secrets,* ed 3, Philadelphia, 2003, Hanley & Belfus.

Ball B (speaker): Mitigating the anger cascade. In McNair R (President): *The nature of the beast: Comprehensive triage and patient flow workshop,* Minneapolis, 2003, Triage First, Inc.

Ball B: Violence prevention (Managers Forum), *J Emerg Nurs* 31(1):99, 2005.

Campbell JC, Webster D, Koziol-McLain J, et al: Risk factors for femicide in abusive relationships: Results from a multisite case control study, *Am J Public Health* 93(7):1089-1097, 2003.

Campbell P: Guard dogs (Managers Forum), *J Emerg Nurs* 25(2):144, 1999.

Canadian Association of Emergency Physicians: Canadian Emergency Department Triage and Acuity Scale Implementation Guidelines, *J Can Assoc Emerg Physicians* 1:3, 1999.

Emergency Nurses Association: Making the right decision, Park Ridge, Ill, 1997, Author.

Grossman VAG: *Quick reference to triage,* ed 2, Philadelphia, 2003, JB Lippincott.

Mackway-Jones K: *Emergency triage,* Manchester Triage Group, London, 1997, BMJ Publishing Group.

McNair R (President): Mitigating the anger cascade. In *The nature of the beast: Comprehensive triage and patient flow workshop,* Minneapolis, 2004, Triage First, Inc.

McNair R (President): Mitigating the anger cascade. In *TRIAGE First Education: A comprehensive emergency department triage course (triaging potentially violent presentations),* Minneapolis, 2004, Triage First, Inc.

Schubert J: Violence prevention (Managers Forum), *J Emerg Nurs* 31(1):99, 2005.

Tahmincioglu E: In health and social services: A more violent workplace, *New York Times,* April 25, 2004.

Chapter 70

Waiting Room Management

Polly Gerber Zimmermann

1. Why do you have a chapter on this topic?

The waiting room is not a patient "storage area" or "floodgate control." Patients in the waiting room are the triage nurse's responsibility to assess and manage.

2. Can we ask a patient's name when they walk in or is that a violation of confidentiality under the Health Insurance Portability and Accountability Act?

HIPAA does not forbid calling people by name in public. One's identity is not protected health information (PHI).

3. So a sign-in sheet can be used?

Yes, if the reason for the visit is not listed. It can include the name, date, and time in. The temptation with a sign-in sheet, though, is to take patients in order of arrival. Triage should not become what emergency department (ED) Coordinator Barbara Weintraub calls a "deli mentality": people line up and it's first come/first served. The art and science of triage is to be able to quickly look over many persons, using observation skills and questions, to decide the order.

4. How is it possible for EDs to not have waiting rooms?

The number of treating rooms is usually increased (in one example, 35 rooms for 50,000 annual census). The triage nurse only gathers a name, date of birth, and reason for the visit before placing the patient in the room (a "streamlined" or "spot check system"). The treating nurse performs the comprehensive triage interview and examination at the bedside. Even so, there are times when all rooms are full and patients must wait. Then they used alternative spaces (e.g., internal family room or consultation room) or other hospital waiting rooms (providing the patients with beepers).

5. How do you handle multiple patients arriving at the same time?

Some form of two-tier triage or dual must take place. For instance, one nurse asks each person for the chief complaint and an "across the room" assessment (60-second rapid triage) and then prioritizes the comprehensive triage interview.

Consultant Rebecca McNair suggests a designated, observable area close to the triage station to place the patients after the rapid triage. FreemanWhite, Inc. designs a triage sub-waiting space that can accommodate 6 to 10 (or more) patients (depending on the size and projected volume of patients). The triage nurse(s) should have visual access to the patients who are waiting either to be triaged or for a treatment bed.

6. Elaborate on the concept of two-tier triage.

Larger EDs have two or more triage nurses. One does the initial sorting, including sending some to a fast track area or to the treatment room, and handles visitors. In one study, the majority of patient questions were not related to patient care ("Where is the ______ [restroom, phone], etc.?") The other nurse does the comprehensive triage interview. A variation is to schedule a second triage nurse during high census times (typically 11:00 AM to 11:00 PM).

Another growing concept is a "team" approach. It includes an ED tech to assist with the transportation, specimen collection, vital signs, or patient demographic information. TriageFirst, Inc recommends adding a second person (one can be a non-registered nurse [RN]) to triage staff once the ED census reaches around 30,000 per year.

7. How about smaller departments that cannot justify staffing two nurses?

Have an additional nurse designated to help with triage only when the need arises. EMPATH consulting emphasizes the most important thing is to have some criteria for backup assistive systems, regardless of the specifics.

TriageFirst, Inc recommends initiating a "Dual Triage" when there are five or more patients waiting or any individual patient has been waiting more than 15 minutes for a comprehensive triage. The primary triage nurse should do the rapid triage of all patients so the triage nurse will know something about all patients after the second nurse leaves.

8. Name some other measures to help manage a number of patients arriving at once.

- Write something down at least—name/complaint—or enter it into the ED computer system. It prevents "losing" someone and the patient feels "acknowledged."
- Do the rapid triage and key assessment on everyone immediately to rule out the "worst case scenario" the patient could be having with this complaint.
- Move up in priority any patients who are out of control (how can you manage them if you are already overwhelmed) or a true "mystery" patient (e.g., no idea what is wrong).
- Children before adults of the same acuity, especially if it is late at night, as a management decision. They do not have the coping skills to deal as well with the additional stress of fatigue and waiting. And, this helps the parents too!

The current trend in process improvement is to do an across the room look, rapid triage with brief information about the complaint, and quick identification registration and then placing them in an available treatment bed. This prevents triage from becoming a bottleneck. More comprehensive physical and history assessment is accomplished there. The comprehensive triage being accomplished in the triage area is then reserved only for when there is no available bed and/or staff in the treatment area and the patient is stable.

9. Can you illustrate that?

Four patients arrive at triage at the same time. They are

Patient A: A 20-year-old holding a bruised arm
Patient B: A 2-year-old whose mother states the child has a high fever
Patient C: A 50-year-old with a frequent moist cough who speaks phrases
Patient D: A 10-year-old with vomiting today

First do the across-the-room assessment/rapid triage to note obvious critical signs, such as lethargy, fainting, or hemorrhaging. The triage nurse can then assess:

- Circulation, movement, sensation (CMS), and pain in Patient A, determining stability of injury, need for analgesic, and/or give a sling/ice.
- Temperature with a thermometer or "hand method" (see Chapter 18) and last medication in Patient B, determining need for antipyretic and ruling out meningitis.
- Lung sounds or pulse oximeter in Patient C (although speaking sentences should indicate it is not emergent) and recent travel, determining stability of breathing and infectious risk.
- Capillary refill, general pulse rate and characteristics, and obtain the number of emesis for Patient D, determining dehydration.

10. Give tips (besides prioritization principles) for dealing with multiple patients.

- Look up and acknowledge the new patients when they come in (with your eyes, nod, or "I'll be with you in a minute"). The sickest patient of the day might be the next one that walks in.
- Don't assume the sickest patient will let you know. Some patients are too ill to complain.
- Do something for each patient, if possible, before beginning more comprehensive history and assessment on one patient.
- Be liberal with analgesics, food, and fluids (as appropriate).
- Give a sense of progress. Do something occasionally.
- Be sure to listen if a patient prefaces something with, "This may not be important, but . . ."

11. Discuss the concept of ongoing awareness of the waiting room.

TriageFirst, Inc. likens it to being a radar traffic controller who is always also aware of all of the planes on the radar screen, even while communicating with one specific aircraft.

I regularly look around the ED and make sure I know why everyone is there (waiting, visitor, etc.) Once I approached an "unknown" Spanish mother holding a bundled-up infant who ended up being dusky, with a heart rate of 40.

12. What is the national standard for reassessment while patients are in the waiting room?

There is no national standard, and defense attorneys recommend *not* setting a specific time limit. The Canadian Triage and Acuity Scale (CTAS) manual acknowledges its stated times to be seen (and for reassessment) are an "ideal," not an established, standard.

13. Give examples of what time ranges other EDs use as a guide.

A common example is every hour for Level 3; every 2 hours for Level 4 to Level 5. The CTAS, the same as the five-tier Australian Triage Scale (ATS), times are:

Level 1: Continuous
Level 2 Every 15 minutes
Level 3: Every 30 minutes
Level 4: Every 60 minutes
Level 5: Every 120 minutes

New Britain General Hospital
Source: Robert Flade, RN BS; Director, ED

- Vital signs at least every 4 hours (and more frequently as appropriate)
- A nursing note every 2 hours (and more frequently as appropriate)
- A complete reassessment every shift

14. What should we consider if we consistently have excessive waiting time related to triage?

- Needs-based planning for operations and design
- Team approach/use of a trained "greeter"
- Use of a reassessment nurse, (licensed practical nurse [LPN]), or ED technician

15. Who should do reassessment of the waiting room patients?

The triage nurse is ideal, as they can make comparisons to what was seen earlier. Australia introduced a new position of Clinical Initiatives Nurse (CIN) for the initiation of assessments/treatments and to reassess waiting patients. A newer concept is triage reassessment technicians to reassess according to protocols and report back to the triage nurse. In one example, this role requires a minimum of an emergency medical technician (EMT).

16. What is done on the reassessment?

Most focus the reassessment based on the presenting complaint or condition. For example:

- Temperature if an antipyretic was given
- Pain level if an analgesic was given
- CMS in extremity injuries

17. How do some hospitals guarantee a patient will be seen in a set amount of time?

Some do give specific time guarantees (15 minutes, 30 minutes, or 60 minutes); others are more vague such as "most patients are seen and treated within an hour." Some offer a token gift (e.g., rental movie certificate) if this time is not met. All have clauses that the guarantee is suspended in a regional disaster scenario with a large influx of patients.

Most have a large number of treatment beds. One ED (50,000 annual census) has 60 adult beds, 11 bed pediatric ED, and 16 observational beds, with multiple triage staff. The physician "sees" the patient to order labs, etc., even if the comprehensive ED physical and/or history are not complete. Other key factors include a streamlined triage, quick registration, and adequate physician staffing.

18. Talk about starting the work-up out in the waiting room.

A growing trend is to have triage protocols that allow some basic diagnostic work to begin in the triage area/waiting room. This includes drawing laboratory specimens, x-rays, or an electrocardiogram (EKG) (in a private area near the triage room). In their designs, FreemanWhite, Inc. usually includes a pneumatic tube station and bar-coded lab label printer in triage so any laboratory tests obtained there can be sent directly. They also have a triage restroom for patients in their designs so that urine specimens can be easily and privately obtained.

19. Give an example.

Christus Santa Rosa Hospital (San Antonio, Tx)
Source: Kevin Trainor, RN CEN, ED/Trauma Nurse Manager

Chest pain

17-35 years:	EKG, chest x-ray (CXR), partial pressure of oxygen (Po_2) if shortness of breath (SOB) or heart rate (HR) >100
Pleuritic (17-35 years):	EKG, CXR, Po_2
Nonpleuritic, resolved/brief (17-35 years):	EKG, Po_2
Atypical/anginal, >35 years:	EKG, CXR, Po_2, CBC, sequential multiple analysis (SMA-12), troponin, cardiac enzymes

Persistent upper abdominal pain (either sex) if >35 years

EKG, SMA-12, complete blood cell count (CBC), liver panel, lipase, urine dip
Add kidneys, ureter, bladder (KUB) flat plate and upright x-ray if vomiting and no bowel movement (BM) for 12-24 hours

Low back pain

Up to 55 years, atraumatic:	Dip urinalysis (U/A), wait for medical doctor (MD)
Over 55 years either sex:	Dip U/A and a liver/spleen (L/S) x-ray even without trauma

They report that, despite a 6% increase in patient volume, these protocols helped them to decrease their length of stay by 50% and reduce the number of patients who left without treatment by more than half.

20. Describe physician/nurse teams that start the work-up in the waiting area.

Manager Nancy Coombes indicates that in Kaiser Sacramento North (California) patients are assigned (on arrival for ambulance and after triage for a walk-in) to a physician and team of nurses. They begin orders and care immediately rather than waiting for an available bed. An advantage is that each team knows which patients they are responsible for managing.

21. What about physicians or nurse clinicians who actually work in triage?

EDs who use that possibility emphasize several key aspects:

- Intermittent use of the physician in triage with the physician assisting in the main treatment areas during the rest of the time.
- An "extra" physician (on call, overlapping).
- ED population that has a larger volume of patients using the ED for minor complaints.
- Some adjacent private area in which the patient can be seen.
- Limiting it to patients with "minor" problems that do not require any work-up, complete undressing, or extensive discharge instructions.

Overall, it is not a common practice because of the expense. Other hospitals will use nurse clinicians or physician assistants in a similar fashion to decompress an overflowing waiting room.

22. How do I handle someone who stops in triage to discuss a complaint but leaves without registering?

Most make the distinction that someone is not a patient until they choose to register. Just avoid giving diagnostic "advice." ED Director Robert G Flade of New Britain General Hospital indicates they create a handwritten chart for these situations. It describes the interaction and that "care was offered and refused." It provides helpful information about why someone is not in the computer system if a later call begins, "I was seen there . . ."

23. I'm concerned about the severe acute respiratory syndrome (SARS) risk in the waiting room.

Some ask all patients to wear a surgical mask and/or have triage personnel wear protective garments. A screener, or more commonly, a prominent sign (sometimes with masks), asks patients to immediately notify the nurse if they have certain symptoms with recent travel overseas.

24. What can be done about the ordinary flu spreading to a susceptible person?

Many have protocols to help prevent the spread of infectious organisms, aka "waiting room etiquette." Signs/pictures, along with masks, tissues, and hand sanitizer, are readily available in the entrances and waiting rooms. Vicki Sweet, ED Manager at St. Jude Medical Center (California), distributes "respiratory packets," containing a small Ziploc bag with a mask, antiseptic hand wipes, tissues, a disposal bag for the tissues, and bilingual instructions. Some departments create a special "respiratory" waiting room or a "flu" fast track. And, don't forget the role of handwashing.

25. Discuss "customer service" behaviors for the triage area.

The triage nurse is "on display" and sets the tone. First impressions do matter. Monitor the staff's:

- Dress code
- Phone greeting/initial greeting to arriving patients
- Responding with words to the effect that it is "not your job"
- Excessive socializing
- Eating in the triage area
- Reading nonprofessional literature in the triage area

For additional discussion, see Chapter 73.

26. No one likes to wait. Give suggestions that help make improvements to the environment.

- Make it as comfortable as possible. FreemanWhite, Inc. recommends making it more like a lobby from a hotel, with smaller groupings.
- Offer amenities, such as multiple TVs in different sections of the waiting room, magazines, fish tank/plants/nature, vending machines.
- Have a complimentary coffee cart/kiosk. Post a sign for patients to please not drink or eat until the triage nurse has talked with them.
- Eliminate clocks to reduce clock watching.
- Create a play area. Run family movies (to eliminate offensive TV content).

27. I'm concerned about contamination issues with children's toys.

The Joint Commission on Accreditation of Healthcare Organizations (JCAHO) requires washing toys after each use. Purchasing inexpensive toys that can be given to the children is one alternative option. The Oriental Trading Company, Inc. and Medibadge sell such items (small handheld toys, puzzles, coloring sheets, etc.) in bulk. One ED hands out stuffed animals donated by the members of a local church. The Starlight Foundation does donate mobile entertainment "Fun Centers" with video games to hospitals (www.starlight.org).

28. Discuss patient education about the triage process.

Brochures or videos can provide education about what can be expected in the ED, including the triage process.

- "What to Expect from Your Visit to an Emergency Care Center" can be downloaded from the members' only section on the Emergency Nurses Association (ENA) website (ena.org, 800-243-8362).
- "What You Should Know about the Emergency Department" is available from the American College of Emergency Physicians (ACEP).
- "Your Visit to the Emergency Department, by Donna Toohey RN CEN SANE CNC, posted at the Emergency Nursing World website (http://enw.org/Solutions.htm).

29. Discuss the best way to communicate the anticipated wait to patients and families when the ED is "backed up."

There is a "psychology" about waiting, the perceived time versus the actual time. Being informed about the delays is what patients value the most.

- *Overestimate, rather than underestimate, the length of the wait.* Patients bear the wait better if told a longer time and taken sooner than if told a shorter time and wait longer.
- *Announcement board indicating the wait time.* For instance, "Nonemergent patients are currently waiting 30 minutes to see a physician."
- *Frequent communication about the wait.* McNair encourages a regular "walk-through," looking at each patient, with a "statement of the department" address.

30. Don't the patients delay the nurse when walking through the waiting room?

Walk with a purposeful stance and concerned expression, not a meandering pace. Patients actually interrupt more when there is no regular communication.

31. Will these "walk-throughs" really make a difference?

Nielsen (2004) described a program of the triage nurses' waiting room "rounds" every 30 minutes (with appropriate explanations). They went from 18 complaints to just 1 complaint per month, and the patients' rating of the quality of care significantly improved.

32. Talk about the use of scripts.

It is hard to create new, satisfactory things to say throughout the day. We use "scripts" all the time, such as "Have a nice day!" Many begin by automatically apologizing for any wait. ED Clinical Manager Bob Ready's script shares the nurse's clinical judgments.

- *Communicate the physical findings.* ("Your child may have had wheezing earlier but now the lungs are clear.")
- *Give a time estimate with the reassurance of current stability.* ("Currently noncritical patients are waiting 40 minutes to see a physician. I believe your child is stable to wait.")
- *Establish ongoing availability.* ("If you feel that your child's condition worsens, please tell me and I will reassess him.")

33. Talk about the use of "pagers" similar to what restaurants use.

Sometimes it helps to give people "permission" to leave (e.g., step outside to smoke, go to the cafeteria) and a sense of freedom.

34. What are the newer trends in waiting rooms?

FreemanWhite, Inc. typically includes inner waiting rooms, within the treatment areas. These are used for stable patients who currently do not require active treatment or if a family member(s) needs to be excused during a physical examination. This type of space gives the flexibility for opening up treatment rooms more rapidly. The inner waiting rooms should be openly visible to the ED staff, with auditory privacy maintained through the use of glass-walled windows. In addition, consider separate waiting rooms for the segregated specialty treatment areas, such as pediatrics or occupational health.

Key Points

- For several people arriving at the same time, use the across-the-room look (rapid triage), chief complaint, and a key assessment(s) to rule out the worst case scenario and decide which one patient is first.
- Determine a method of "waiting room etiquette" to communicate infection control practices to waiting patients.
- It is better from a psychologic standpoint to overestimate the time of any wait. Communicate frequently during that time.

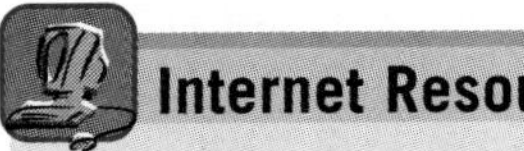

Internet Resources

Oriental Trading Company, Inc. PO
www.orientaltrading.com

Medibadge, Inc. PO
stickers@medibadge.com

Triage First
www.triagefirst.com

FreemanWhite, Inc.
www.freemanwhite.com

Bibliography

Adams SJ: HIPAA patient confidentiality requirements (Managers Forum), *J Emerg Nurs* 30(1):70, 2004.

Bruns C, Bell WA: EMTALA ED screening for non-ED patients (Managers Forum), *J Emerg Nurs* 27(1):69-70, 2001.

Canadian Association of Emergency Physicians: Canadian Emergency Department Triage and Acuity Scale (CTAS), Ottawa, Ontario, October (3 suppl), 1999, Canadian Association of Emergency Physicians.

Contino DS: Physicians in triage (Managers Forum), *J Emerg Nurs*, 28(6):565-566, 2002.

Coombes NJ: Preventing ED backup (Managers Forum), *J Emerg Nurs* 31(1):91-92, 2005.

Flade RG: Inquiring about care at triage (Managers Forum), *J Emerg Nurs* 28(6):565, 2002.

McNair R (President): The nature of the beast: Comprehensive triage course, Fairview, NC, 2004, Triage First, Inc.

McNair RS: Improving triage (Managers Forum), *J Emerg Nurs* 30(1):75, 2004.

McNair RS: Managing the waiting room, *J Emerg Nurs* 27(1):73, 2001.

Nielsen D: Improving ED patient satisfaction when triage nurses routinely communicate with patients as to reasons for waits: One rural hospital's experience, *J Emerg Nurs* 30(4): 336-338, 2004.

Trainor K: Triage protocols (Managers Forum), *J Emerg Nurs* 29(6):560, 2003.

Chapter 71

Language and Interpretation Issues

Polly Gerber Zimmermann

1. Why do you have this chapter?

There are currently more than 300 languages and dialects spoken in the United States. Nearly 47 million U.S. residents over the age of 5 speak a foreign language at home and close to a quarter of them report speaking English "not well" or "not at all."

One out of 3 children, and 29% of the U.S. population, is a member of an ethnic or racial minority group. It is predicted that by 2025, almost 40% of Americans and about half of all U.S. children will be minorities.

2. What are the requirements to deal with language issues?

Title VI of the U.S. Civil Rights Act requires health care facilities to provide a means of communication for patients with limited English proficiency (LEP). The Joint Commission on Accreditation of Healthcare Organizations (JCAHO) and the American Hospital Association (AHA) have made this accommodation a condition of accreditation. Federal guidelines recommend offering written materials for each group of non-English-speaking patients that constitutes 5% of the health care organization's patient volume.

3. How do I answer co-workers who believe people living in America should learn to speak English?

Patients with LEP have rights. Whatever a person's personal opinion is, all clinicians must obey these related federal laws.

4. What are the Emergency Medical Treatment and Active Labor Act regulations about language translation?

Emergency Medical Treatment and Active Labor Act (EMTALA) does not directly address interpreters for LEP patients. However, nothing should discourage a patient from receiving his or her medical screening examination (MSE). A lack of the nurse's ability to understand the patient's chief complaint in a timely manner could be significant.

5. Can I just automatically use a family member?

No. The patient may not want the family member to interpret, especially about issues of a more sensitive nature. The Office of Civil Rights indicates "family, minor children, and friends are not competent to act as interpreters and could compromise the effectiveness of the services, result in a breach of confidentiality, or reluctance on the part of individuals to reveal personal information critical to their situations . . ." However, in some circumstances, or if the patient desires to use a family member, it should be allowed.

6. Any other considerations with using a family member besides confidentiality and ethics?

- Family members may omit information, such as side effects, because they believe it would improve the patient's compliance.
- Using a child to ask the mother about menstrual periods and birth control is inappropriate. In some cultures, it is considered improper for a child to know more than the adults do, and the patient may not be forthright when giving information through a child.

Consultant Shelley Cohen emphasizes that you do not know that a family member has:

- The patient's best interest in mind
- Adequate fluency in both languages
- A way of representing you in a proper professional manner

7. Can we make it mandatory that other available hospital staff interpret?

No. The Office of Civil Rights indicates "covered entities must ensure that interpreters are trained and demonstrate competency as interpreters . . ."

An employee may not have adequate skills in both languages. The staff member may not want to be placed in this role. It is a common misconception that all bilingual individuals want to translate.

8. Recommend solutions.

- Hire bilingual staff (this can include financial rewards for their increased ability)
- Reimburse staff for language courses (many patients appreciate a staff member's attempt to communicate with a few basic questions, such as name, date of birth, or pain)
- Establish a translation department
- Maintain professional translators
- Use telephone translation lines
- Use MedBridge: a handheld computer that speaks, writes, and signs key sentences for both the nurse and patient (www.medbridge.net, 888-986-3003)
- Use close-circuit TV (videoconferencing) with interpreters
- Provide written materials in various languages

9. Describe how to effectively use an interpreter or translator.

A translator should literally translate all the words of the parties involved, without addition, deletions, or summations. Do not accept a lengthy response for which the interpreter than states, "He says OK."

10. Explain how to insure quality staff interpreters.

Many establish a type of "competency" testing to "credential" eligible staff, who then receive a financial incentive (such as an additional $25/week in one program; $.50 an hour in another program). This usually includes a verbal test, with sample translations.

11. Give tips for working with a translator.

- Brief the translator first on the purpose of the encounter, the subjects to be covered, and the scope of the services needed.
- Ask if the translator is aware of any cultural beliefs that could have an impact on the encounter.
- Review patient confidentiality under the Health Insurance Portability and Accountability Act (HIPAA) if a professional, outside translator is used. Maintaining patient privacy is a part of their employment when translators are part of the hospital's staff.
- Verify the patient is consenting to use an interpreter. (Document in the chart, including the name of the translator/translator service)
- If the translator is not established, verify the ability to interpret appropriately. Simply state, "I would like to see if my English is clear to you." and then give a simple direction to follow.
- Speak directly to the patient, as if the interpreter wasn't there. For instance, say "Do you have pain in your leg?" not "Ask him if he has pain in his leg." Placing the interpreter physically behind the clinician, or the patient, can help prevent directing the conversation to the interpreter.
- Speak slowly and pause frequently to give the interpreter time to complete each idea expressed. Use simple words, and avoid medical terminology. Resist the tendency to shout.
- Continue to watch the patient's body language and ask follow-up questions based on these nonverbal cues.
- Use emphasizing gestures, facial expressions, and tone of voice to help communicate the message.
- Stop if the interpreter becomes distracted. This is often a source of errors because the clinician will continue on and assume understanding.
- Always end with asking if the patient has any questions and to having the patient repeat any instructions.
- Avoid giving vague requests to interpreters that would require their own explanation, such as "tell them to follow-up."
- Avoid the temptation to make the interaction briefer just because of the extra work.

12. Talk about telephone translation lines.

Many offer 24-hour access to interpreters of over 130 different languages, some with videoconferencing options. These include:

- Language Line Services (www.languageline.com)
- OnLine Interpreters (www.onlineinterpreters.com)
- Communication Access Center (www.cacdhh.org)
- Pacific Interpreters (www.pacificinterpreters.com)
- Language Assistance (www.languageassistance.com)

Using a three-way conference call can enhance the process.

13. If I have an interpreter, then can I know for sure there is accurate communication?

Not necessarily. In one of the most comprehensive studies on this topic, there was an average of 31 interpreter errors that occurred on each of 13 doctor visits.

- Sixty-three percent were serious enough to have medical consequences because the incorrect translation altered the description of illness, misstated diagnostic or treatment options, or affected a parent's understanding of a child's condition or need for follow-up. One of the most serious errors included telling the mother to put an oral antibiotic into her child's ears!
- Fifty-two percent involved the omission of a key word or phrase.
- Sixteen percent involved the incorrect use of a word or phrase ("false fluency").

At times the interpreters would editorialize or interject their personal views. However, the study found (not surprisingly) that more errors occurred when nonprofessional translators are used.

14. Give a resource for written materials.

- Care Note Systems (English and Spanish) (www.micromedex.com/products/healthcare)

One system actually created bilingual triple-copy forms. The provider could check off appropriate areas on top in English, and the translated instructions were on the same area of the copy below.

15. Is language competency the same as cultural competency?

No. Statistics show that blacks and Latinos are hospitalized and undergo surgery at lower rates than white patients, even when their access to care, diagnosis, and illness severity are the same. Aston et al (2003) suggest disparities result from the context of patient interactions. Patients from different ethnic groups may vary their health narrative (how they view their condition and its cause), may use different terms to describe the same phenomenon, and may screen out views that they think the doctor will find unacceptable. Ethnic and cultural norms are also an influence. See Chapter 15.

16. Do they offer any suggestions to help overcome this?

They suggest that during each patient encounter, the clinician uses openings and prompts to help a patient do four things:

- Provide a health narrative
- Ask questions
- Express concerns
- Be assertive

They even suggest providing patients with pocket cards and waiting room videotapes on "how to talk with your doctor."

17. What about deaf and hearing-impaired patients?

In one study, deaf and hard-of-hearing adults were asked about their communication concerns and suggestions for improvement. Their responses included:

- Ask about their preferred method of communication instead of requiring them to use an ineffective method, such as writing notes or family members.
- Speak more slowly, repeating critical information.
- Put critical information in writing, in addition to the verbal instructions.
- Use lights as signals for required actions, such as holding one's breath.
- Have alternatives to lengthy phone message menus, such as the possibility of communicating by email or fax.
- Have a teletypewriter or telecommunications device.

18. Is it required to have a translator accompany a transfer if one was used for the MSE?

Consideration for an accompanying interpreter might be when ongoing evaluations, such as mental/neurologic status, are needed. It is not considered necessary when the patient's condition does not require ongoing verbal communication.

Key Points

- Health care facilities are legally required to provide a means of communication for patients with LEP.
- It is not acceptable to routinely or automatically use family members.
- When using interpreters, speak directly to the patient and have them literally translate your words.

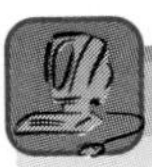

Internet Resources

United States Department of Health and Human Services: Limited English Proficiency (LEP)
www.hhs.gov/ocr/lep

MedBridge Software for LEP and Hearing-Impaired Patients
www.medbridge.net

LEP.gov: Meaningful Access for People who are Limited English Proficient
www.lep.gov

Bibliography

Ashton C, Haidet P, Patemiti DA, et al: Racial and ethnic disparities in the use of health services, *J Gen Intern Med* 18:146-152, 2003.

Cohen S: *101 triage tips,* Hohenwald, Tenn, 2002, Health Resources Unlimited.

Does your ED supply interpreter services? *ED Manag* 15(6):67-69, 2003.

Flores G, Laws MB, Mayo SJ, et al: Errors in medical interpretation and their potential clinical consequences in pediatric encounters, *Pediatrics* 111(1):6-14, 2003.

Grossman VGA: *Quick reference to triage,* ed 2, Philadelphia, 2003, Lippincott, Williams & Wilkins.

Higginbotham E: How to overcome a language barrier, *RN* 66(10):67-69, 2003.

Lezzoni LI, O'Day BL, Killeen M, Harker H. Communicating about health care: Observations from persons who are deaf or hard of hearing, *Ann Intern Med* 140(5):356-362, 2004.

Moy MM: *The EMTALA answer book, 2002,* New York, 2002, Aspen Publishers.

Office of Civil Rights of the Department of Health and Human Services: *Policy guidance on the Title VI prohibition against national original discrimination as it affects persons with limited English proficiency,* Washington, DC, 2000, Author.

U.S. Census Bureau: *Table 1: Language use, English ability, and linguistic isolation for the population 5 years and over by state: 2000,* Census 2000, Summary File 3, Washington, DC, 2002, Author.

Chapter 72

Ethics in Triage: One Ethicist Speaks

Bernard Heilicser

"Is it ever morally right to make judgments about the worthiness or unworthiness of persons who lay claim to our services?"

—Ernie W.D. Young

1. Are there ethical issues in the triage process?

Absolutely! Every patient we see has the potential to create an ethical dilemma in terms of priority of treatment and allocation of resources. Essentially, the proverbial "red flag" is raised every time we triage a patient.

2. Why has ethics become a part of triage?

The ethics of triage has been present since the concept of triage, or "selection," was first used during the Napoleonic Wars. Military triage was founded on the survival of the community. This implies that the least seriously wounded would be treated first (considering the limitation of battlefield resources and the need to return to combat). This basically rejects the principle of the independent and equal value of each human life. The common good prevails.

3. Does the common good still apply to current triage?

Although we would all like to believe all patients are treated equally, honest reflection proves not. The common good is still a major aspect of triage. We tend to treat the firefighter or policeman before the criminal. Can we truthfully say the hospital administrator will be made to sit in the waiting room although the homeless drunk gets seen quicker?

4. Have we then lost all our sense of fairness?

Fortunately, we have not. Unless we are faced with a mass casualty incident (MCI) or a disaster threatening our very social survival, triage allows us to treat those in greatest need first.

5. So, what is triage?

We can consider contemporary triage as the process of sorting patients based on their need, relative to the type of problem, the severity of the problem, and the resources available.

6. Then, what is not triage?

Triage determines the order to receive the best care available. It is not the allocation of resources to determine who gets, who doesn't get, and what quality they will get.

7. So, who goes first?

Barring a catastrophic event in which doing the greatest good for the greatest number would be appropriate; priority should go to the life-threatened patient. This would be followed by the patient who is at risk for a more deleterious outcome. The walking wounded would then be treated. This is the basic red-yellow-green triage classification. The black category includes the dead or futile.

However, a gas station robbery suspect who has been drinking crashes into a police barricade. The police officer sustains a compound femur fracture and has slightly abnormal vital signs but is fully alert. The bad guy spiders the windshield with his head and has altered mental status. His vital signs are somewhat more abnormal. Who goes by helicopter and who by ground ambulance? What would you do?

8. Does every patient have a right to be triaged into the emergency care system?

Every patient has the right to medical care. Although, some politicians and business types would not fully agree, our worth as a society demands this. Triage is there to help prioritize this medical care based on immediacy, not judgment of overall need. What may appear to be an abuse of medical resources often surprises us:

- The 29-year-old patient presenting with costochondritis who has a myocardial infarction (MI).
- The 45-year-old patient presenting with back pain who has an abdominal aortic aneurysm.
- The 6-year-old patient presenting with an ear ache at 3:00 AM who has meningitis.

9. How objective should the triage process be?

Triage should be accomplished with impartiality. Race, nationality, gender, religion, attractiveness, or unattractiveness, wealth, or social habits should be irrelevant. If one is not comfortable with this moral concept, then they should be doing something else. Remember, the drug addict may have some responsibility for his plight, but the chief executive officer who eats red meat and smokes has no less culpability.

10. Is triage confidential?

It should be, but reality tends to differ. We should be aware of governmental regulations regarding disclosure of identifying information in a public place. The patient's complaint should not be overheard or visible. An MCI would not necessarily apply. Would you want your chest pain or urethral discharge known to others?

11. Discuss triage of a minor.

A minor should not be at risk and should not be in pain. Awaiting parental or legal guardian consent is unethical if the minor is in jeopardy. Would the parents be considered negligent if they did not seek treatment for the presenting condition? If so, treat!

12. Beware of telephone triage!

So, your specific job description requires you provide telephone triage, or you occasionally are in such a position. This is not an innocuous function. When you answer the phone, ask how you can help and start to give advice, a legal duty has begun. What if your protocol for the telephone complaint indicates no emergency department (ED) referral, but basic office follow-up? Yet, you feel this patient should go to the ED. Ethically, you want to direct this patient to the ED. However, your business protocol differs. What would you do?

- Consider, your compliance with policy will reflect on your bonus at the end of the year.
- Do you want to be in this position?

13. What about my safety? Do I have an ethical obligation to put myself at risk?

The geographic location of a triage area is always of concern. Depending on your facility, this can become rather precarious. At no time should your safety be a question. There is no ethical obligation to put yourself at risk. The emergency medical services (EMS) tenet of scene safety first applies to everyone in the medical setting. Always be in a personally safe environment.

14. How far do I take the triage process?

This is facility specific. Triage should not be synonymous with a screening exam for Emergency Medical Treatment and Active Labor Act (EMTALA) purposes. It is definitely not patient stabilization. Be careful of the position you are placed in.

15. What are my triage responsibilities for the patient leaving without treatment?

Again, facility policy should be specific. Nevertheless, if a patient has entered your facility and has not formally signed in, but demonstrates erratic behavior, should they be allowed to leave (this is not an "against medical advice" situation)? I would maintain that a patient who has entered "your house" is your responsibility. Ethically, if any danger to their leaving is present, they should be evaluated before leaving. *All* patients should be made comfortable to return to your facility at any time.

16. Are triage and health maintenance organizations on the same planet?

Sometimes. Various federal and individual state enactments have certainly improved the way patients are let into the health care system. The triage nurse should still be vigilant for situations which could impede appropriate medical evaluation and stabilization. Insurance information is not part of the triage process, nor should we allow it to be. Patient concerns over potential insurance coverage are reasonable. However, as ethical individuals we must be an advocate for the patient's well-being. Financial matters are important, but the triage process should also be an opportunity to comfort the patient, both physically and emotionally.

17. Is there any relationship between triage and a gatekeeper function?

It is important to mention that there are limited medical resources in our society. Indeed, we must be careful not to abuse what is available, and not to foolishly disregard this problem. The triage process demands not only action, but also determined thought in what is carried out.

The ethics of the ED truly tests our objectivity and commitment to medicine. We are forced to prioritize treatment from basic office cuts and bruises to emergency life and death situations. This is all performed in the presence of the mean and the nice, the rich and the poor, the important and the ignored, and all in the context of very diverse cultural backgrounds. The end result reveals our humanity.

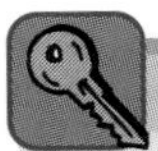

Key Points

- Accomplish triage with impartiality, including religion, unattractiveness, wealth, or social habits.
- Managed care (i.e., managed reimbursement) should be for the patient's legitimate needs and benefit, not a deterrent to care and caring.
- Triage can be rather humbling. Remember, everybody has a terminal event at some time.
- There is no ethical obligation to put yourself at risk.
- *All* patients should be made comfortable to return to your facility at any time.
- Tests and x-rays ordered from triage should have legitimate clinical basis and not be the result of a cursory evaluation or for expediency.

Internet Resources

The Center for Ethics and Human Rights
www.nursingworld.org/ethics

NursingEthics.ca—Your Resource for Nursing Ethics!
www.nursingethics.ca

Bibliography

Heilicser B: Ethics. In Zimmermann PG, editor: *Nursing management secrets,* Philadelphia, 2002, Hanley & Belfus, 201.

Iserson KV, Sanders AB, Mathieu D: *Ethics in emergency medicine,* ed 2, Tucson, 1995, Galen Press, 308-313.

Jonsen AR, Siegler M, Winslade WJ: *Clinical ethics,* ed 3, New York, 1992, McGraw-Hill, 142-143.

Malloy C: Managed care and ethical implications in telephone-based health services, *Adv Pract Nurs Q* 4:30-33, 1998.

Mezza I: Triage: Setting priorities for health care, *Nurs Forum* 27:15-19, 1992.

Pellegrino ED, Thomasma DC: *For the patient's good,* New York, 1988, Oxford University Press, 172-189.

Rodney P, Varcoe C: Towards ethical inquiry in the economic evaluation of nursing practice, *Can J Nurs Res* 33:35-51, 2001.

Young EW: Current ethical issues in emergency care, *J Emerg Nurs* 12:301-304, 1986.

Chapter 73

Customer Service/Patient Satisfaction

Polly Gerber Zimmermann

1. Why have a chapter on this subject? Isn't it just important that nurses have excellent clinical and technical skills?

Those are key aspects of competency and "quality patient care." However, patient perception of the clinicians and the care they provide also influences health. Patients are more likely to comply with the regimen if they are satisfied with and trust the clinicians. The newer concept is "patient experience" and includes all aspects such as the physical aesthetics of the building.

2. I just want to give good care.

Customer service/patient satisfaction is partly just effectively communicating the good care in a way the patient can understand. As the saying goes, people don't care how much you know until they know how much you care.

3. Aren't most people happy with their care?

There is an increase to 46% (up from 39%) in 2001 of patients who were extremely or very satisfied with their care. This means that more than half were not satisfied. Even the quality of primary care doctor-patient relationships has eroded (Safran, 2003). There is room for improvement.

4. Does customer satisfaction result in better profits in health care?

Coile (2002) indicates that a 5% increase in patient satisfaction can result in a 25% increase in business. Others have not found a clearcut relationship. Either way, it is more rewarding when the provided care is appreciated.

5. Talk about what can enhance customer satisfaction during the initial contact.

- Look up, "beam," and smile. Say "Hi."
- Face them with a physically unobstructed heart area and lean slightly forward.
- Avoid verbal triggers.

6. Explain this heart area thing.

How to Make People Like You in 90 Seconds or Less (Boothman, 2002) explains that anyone can give a first impression of being sincere, safe, and trustworthy within the first 3 to 4 seconds of contact. Keep the heart and body area uncovered and facing toward the person (e.g., no crossed arms or legs). An almost imperceptible forward tilt subtly indicates an interest. Using eye contact, "lighting up," and offering a pleasant greeting round out the presentation package of a "warm welcome."

7. What are verbal triggers?

These are phrases that tend to trigger a negative response in most adults. Key examples include:

- "You have to . . ." Adults don't like to be told they "have to" do anything. As the old saying goes, *you only have to pay taxes and die.* Instead, say "The next time that happens . . ."
- "Hang on a second." You and the patient know it is going to take more than one "second." Give a more honest statement. "I'm finishing this and I can take care of you in about 2 minutes."
- "No" at the beginning of the sentence. The "yes philosophy" is starting the sentence with a "yes" even when conveying a negative answer. "Yes, you may have something to drink after the antiemetic medication takes effect."
- In addition, universal irritation includes staff laughing, eating, or "standing around doing nothing."

8. How do I handle someone coming up to talk to me when I am on the phone?

Signal awareness by holding up the forefinger as an acknowledgment while completing the phone conversation. This helps the person to feel as if you are not ignoring them.

9. Share some physical suggestions to enhance my triage interview.

- Sit down close to the patient and look them in the eye. This is particularly important while the patient is stating the chief complaint. (The patient will perceive the time lasted two to three times longer than it did.)
- Do not write while the patient is talking to you. Efficient nurses tend to multi-task, but writing while patients are talking often leads them to feel ignored.
- Never walk out of the room while the patient is talking. If necessary, interrupt the patient and explain why you need to leave. (An alternative is to walk out of the room while you are talking.)
- Do not point or shake your finger at a patient.
- Touch the patient. This is especially true with older people.
- Wash your hands (or use an alcohol sanitizer) before touching the patient. Do it physically in front of the patient.
- Always examine the part of the body that the patient complains about. Physically touch the area.

10. Sounds like you emphasize listening.

Let the person tell you what is on his/her mind: you can learn a lot. One study found that, the majority of the time, the patient is interrupted by the clinician before 23 seconds into communicating about their problem.

11. Give tips for enhancing the triage interview.

- Use their name as often as possible. A name is the patients' most precious commodity.
- Involve the family, if possible.
- You can never go wrong with commenting how cute a child (or grandchild) is. (Now you are obviously a perceptive nurse.) You can also try "sweet" or "precious."
- You can never go wrong telling young children how "big" they are. One nurse will directly ask the middle-aged child if she/he is ___ years old, deliberately overestimating the age by 3 years. The child beams while "correcting" the nurse.
- Repeat patients' complaints in their exact words. Now the patient feels "heard." Mimicry increases rapport and interpersonal closeness. Studies found that wait staff that parrot back the order receive more tips. The tendency is to paraphrase the complaint by translating it into medical terminology for the documentation. For example, the patient states, "I hurt my arm." The nurse, noting a 5-cm by 8-cm purplish ecchymosis on the right forearm states, "You have a bad bruise."
- Never appear shocked by anything the patient tells you.
- Use repetitive, expansive speech. The familiarity of the medical complaints can make it easy to rattle off routine, rote questions and instructions. To the unfamiliar patient, it sounds like an abrupt rendition of a foreign language.
- Share what is found on assessment. Now you are involving the patient in the care. "Right now your child's fever is normal, although it probably was elevated earlier as you said."
- Praise what they have done right. Anyone can be hypersensitive to perceived criticism. Counter that with liberal praise; people usually do try to do the right thing. Even if the home treatment had some lacks, praise the proper aspect. "It was good that you gave little Jimmy some Tylenol. He's growing and now needs more, so give him 2 teaspoons the next time."
- Never indicate nothing is wrong. Even if the diagnosis turns out to be "well baby visit," the patient/person thought something was wrong (and perhaps it was earlier). Everyone receives a medical screening examination (MSE) regardless. Discounting the concerns during triage is perceived as insulting and demeaning.
- Find out what they want.
- Use reassuring phrases.

12. Explain what you mean by finding out what they want.

All patients have expectations. Determining what they are will help the nurse shape them, perhaps meet them, or explain why the expectation will not be met. For instance, explain immunization timing if the patient wants an unnecessary tetanus shot.

13. Talk about reassuring phrases.

As a result of the frequency and familiarity, it is easy to forget the experience is unique and anxiety provoking to the patient. This is not the same as "false reassurance," which indicates something unknown or untrue, such as telling a dying patient they will get better. Reassuring phrases acknowledge the patient's reality (therapeutic technique: "showing empathy") and indicate actual care (therapeutic technique: "offering self").

14. Provide some examples.

- "That looks sore."
- "I'm sorry this happened to you."
- "We'll take good care of your wife."

15. That sounds like scripting. I want to be able to be real and spontaneous.

Then you can add to the scripts. In the hectic pace, although, it is difficult to create and remember to always give a unique, satisfying individualized response. Using standard phrases that are known to work is a help in meeting a basic, known need.

16. Any suggestions regarding voice tone?

One in 10 Americans (28 million total) has some kind of hearing loss. Besides modern society's loud sounds, a factor is aging. All people lose some hearing each year after age 50; it is estimated that there is a significant degree of hearing loss (often undiagnosed) in approximately 30% of adults in ages 65 to 74. Aging also affects the ability to pick up with the tone-of-voice cues (such humor or sarcasm).

The majority of people are unaware of their hearing loss. They adapt (even subconsciously) by becoming a better listener, watching the speaker's face, or sitting closer to the sound. Simple techniques, such as speaking at normal rate, in a slightly louder voice, and facing patients, will help them to accommodate.

17. What can help patients tolerate an unavoidable wait?

- Give generous time estimates about the wait.
- Establish the nurse's ongoing availability.
- Provide frequent contact/explanations. In Carlson et al (2003) the better the communication with the staff, the greater the patient satisfaction.
- Maintain some sense of progress by doing something every now and then.
- Be literal with analgesics and fluids, as possible. Carlson et al (2003) also found patient satisfaction was influenced by the effectiveness of analgesia.
- Remember that time is distorted when waiting for a doctor, news of a loved one, the report of an important test, or a pain medicine. See Chapter 70.

18. Some people still become irate with the wait. How do I deal with the complaints?

Talk to the feelings. Acknowledge an emotion even though the patient's complaint is stated as a fact. For example,

Patient: "I've been waiting 40 minutes!"
Nurse: "I know it is frustrating to wait."

Use the broken record technique. No matter what the patient states, repeat the same answer. The patient/parent will eventually understand (and accept) the answer is the same regardless. The tendency is for the triage nurse to keep changing the response to the patient in hopes the new one will work better. Instead, it provides fuel to keep the "debate" going in hopes the nurse will eventually give the desired answer.

19. Give an example.

Parent: "We've been waiting for a doctor for my sick child and I want to see one now."

Nurse: "I understand you are concerned about your child. I expect you will be able to see the doctor in about 30 minutes."

Parent: "This is ridiculous. I thought this was an *emergency* room."

Nurse: "I understand you are concerned about your child. I expect you will be able to see the doctor in about 30 minutes."

Parent: "This is terribly inefficient. And you call yourselves professionals."

Nurse: "I understand you are concerned about your child. I expect you will be able to see the doctor in about 30 minutes."

20. If patients are upset, why not just let them go next?

The triage nurse is on "center stage" with everyone else watching. In a positive light, this is sometimes referred to as the "Disney" concept of the need to "perform" a certain way regardless of whether we "feel" like it.

In a more negative connotation, but just as true, is that the other patients are watching how you respond. If "demanding" becomes the criteria for priority, others will soon catch on and act similarly.

21. Do you make any exceptions to this?

Threats of violence cannot be tolerated. When one man threatened to kill me if I did not take his wife in, I loudly announced (so the whole waiting room could hear), "No, you are not allowed to threaten to kill a nurse. I am calling security." A security officer stood by him, the waiting room was complaint-free for the rest of my shift, and afterward the man apologized. See Chapter 69 for additional discussion.

22. What can enhance patient satisfaction/customer service during the treatment and evaluation?

- Continue to involve the patient/parent in the diagnosis to negotiate and shape the expectations. Explain what tests are being done and why. One study found that parent's rating of their child's care was most closely associated with the communication they had about their child's condition and the sense that the care of their child was coordinated.
- Illustrate the benefit of this extended diagnostic time. "You are receiving results that would normally take 1 to 2 days in about an hour here."
- Echo any survey questions' phrasing to plant that concept in the mind. For instance, reenforce the introduction (often asked on surveys), such as "I am now introducing myself. I am your nurse and my name is Sue." Nurses tend to automatically provide their name in the first seconds of the interaction, when the patient is likely to be distracted.
- Keep the patient informed on the progress. Knowledge gives people a sense of power and control. Provide frequent, dignifying updates. "We have two of the blood tests back and are waiting for one more."

23. Name a time more likely to have patient dissatisfaction.

"Service transitions." The time for breakdown in communication or care is whenever the patient/care is handed over from one to another, such as a transfer to another department (x-ray), area (inpatient unit), or person (shift changes).

24. What can help to deal with this?

- Awareness and vigilance.
- Set a positive tone through language and introduction. For instance, "We are transferring you to intensive care so you can receive the specialized care you need."
- Provide something extra. In one study, family members identified "good care" if something extra (pillow, blanket, personal remark) was done.

25. I don't know how to handle a patient's unreasonable requests.

Repeat it back in a neutral tone. For instance, "So if I understand, you are upset because you can't have a stat MRI now, at 2:00 AM, for the back pain you've had for 3 months" (Mayer, 1999). Occasionally a patient insists on being seen now or first, even when told the staff is busy caring for someone dying. One nurse stares silently at the patient with an incredulous expression. Then she calmly states, "I am sorry you feel that way" and walks away.

26. I know you can't please all of the people all of the time. What is a realistic goal?

The national average is three to five complaints per 1,000 emergency department (ED) visits. Another indicator to watch is the number of patients who "left without being seen" (≤1% to 2%).

27. How should I handle a patient complaint about the care during their visit?

This is what the service industry calls a "point of impact" intervention. When there is a problem, intervene immediately. It is easy to mentally start building the defense (and physically start writing the documentation) rather than nipping the problem in the bud.

28. Explain how to do that.

Mayer (1999) lists these steps.

- Identify the problem with the person and address it as soon as you realize it is occurring.
- Give a "blameless apology." Establish the fact that you know there has been a break down. "I'm sorry there has been a problem."
- To the extent possible, wipe the slate clean. For instance, "I am sorry we have had a negative experience. I want to make the situation right for you as much as possible."
- Listen to their complaints, including venting. Do not "correct" them.
- Establish their expectations.
- Deal with the issue causing their anger. Trying to deal with other aspects will be futile.
- Use silence as necessary to gain their attention before responding. If the person's eyes are darting around, they are not listening.
- Demonstrate a willingness to negotiate and resolve issues. You may, at this time, want to present some facts.
- Ask them what they would like you to do now.
- To the extent possible, meet their expectations.
- Offer reasonable alternatives.
- When it still fails, offer them an alternate person to talk to or care for them.

29. I don't feel that patients should pick and choose whom they get to deal with.

Sometimes, it can just help to have someone "who is in charge" talk to the patient/parent. My peer and I were "in charge" for each other for our small ED that only had two night shift nurses. Some patients are more satisfied if they have talked to "someone in authority."

In addition, dementia experts stress that one person's sex, color, age, appearance, etc., might trigger the same negative reaction impaired people had with someone similar in their past. It is unlikely there will be a "behavior modification" at this time of personal stress. Avoid power struggles; try someone else.

30. Occasionally the triage nurse discharges a simple case from triage. Any tips for enhancing customer service at discharge?

- Thank the person for their business ("We appreciate you coming here.") We are in the business of taking care of sick and injured people. We sometimes subtly communicate that they "bothered" us.
- Wish them well. End with a pleasantry. One physician routinely ends his interactions with the patients with "I hope you soon feel better."
- Help them remember the discharge instructions.

31. How do I do that?

Patients typically forget up to 80% of the medical information given to them, and almost half of what is remembered is wrong. The problem is the patients are stressed and focus more on the diagnosis than the treatment. Write the instructions down, repeat them, and be sure to answer and emphasize the three universal questions all patients have:

- What was wrong?
- What do you need to do?
- Why is it important to do that?

32. Should customer satisfaction surveys be regarded as the ultimate authoritative tool for assessing if the patients were treated appropriately?

Rosenberg (1996) indicates the concept of measuring customer satisfaction is flawed. His five myths:

- Myth #1: Customer satisfaction is objective. Objective numbers lull one into this assumption. It is actually a complex attitude related to different operations.
- Myth #2: Customer satisfaction is easily measured. It is actually the degree to which the experience matches the expectations. It is influenced by the patients' perceptions of quality and value. In one study of physician office visits, the patient satisfaction was significantly lower if the patient spent less than they expected and high for patients who spent more time than they had expected.
- Myth #3: Customer satisfaction is accurately measured. Attitudes are hard to measure, and there is high variability among people and within the same people at different times. There is a response bias, with a tendency for halo (horn) effects.
- Myth #4: Customer satisfaction is quickly and easily changed. By nature, it is difficult and slow to change. Satisfaction occurs through repeated experiences.
- Myth #5: It is obvious who the customer is. There are many different customers with different needs, including patients, family, physicians, and insurers. Who is complaining: outliers or representation of the majority?

33. What can help deal with these survey concerns?

- Real-time surveys.
- Daily collection of data from patients, staff, and physicians by a patient representative to track trends, with a department behavioral change goal per week (Cook, 2003).

- A kiosk (similar to the check-in station used at an airport) in the waiting room for patients to provide immediate feedback (Pierce, 2004).
- Simple key question surveys. Sample questions that actually abstract more information:
  - "Of all we did for you during your visit, what did you like the best?"
  - "Of all we did for you during your visit, what did you like the least?"
  - "What should we have done?" (Or "What could we do better?")

34. What should we be sure to consider if we believe that customer service or patient satisfaction is important?

Training. The majority of clinician training is clinical, but 85% of the time the patients judge the clinician by customer service types of skills. Knowing a few tricks of the service industry trade can make a difference.

Mayer (1999) cites his own emergency department as an example. After training all of the ED staff (including physicians) in customer satisfaction skills, the complaints about their department decreased by 70%, compliments increased by 100% and the survey evaluations of the staff's competency in clinical skills increased significantly even though it was the exact same staff.

35. What else can help?

Patient education. For instance, one study found that 20% of parents incorrectly believed that most colds and flu illnesses are caused by bacteria and will get better faster with antibiotics. Nurses remain the most trusted professionals in the annual Gallup survey of public perceptions of honesty and ethics (79% indicated it was "very high" or "high"). This is better than military officers, high school teachers, clergy, policemen, or physicians (who were seventh). Use this positive public perception to help patients understand.

36. Can that really work?

In one study, 50% of the parents expected antibiotics, but only 1% of them directly asked the physician for a prescription. The physician perceived that parents' expectation only 34% of the time. However, the parents were the happiest if the physician initiated the possibility of the antibiotics, discussed why or why not, and contingency plans (even if they did not get the anticipated antibiotics). Good patient education often involves an element of ongoing initiation of relevant concerns and needed information.

37. Tell me more.

Patients want information. In one survey, >75% of adult outpatients wanted to know all the side effects of all the drugs, even if they were rare and/or insignificant. This was particularly true for those of lower educational level, had a previous experience with adverse drug reactions, and older women.

38. Discuss the role of the Internet in patient information.

It appears that a substantial minority of patients uses the Internet to educate themselves regarding health. In one survey, 31% of the participants (particularly younger, higher income, and higher education levels) had sought health information on the Internet. Of the online seekers, 75% found relevant information, but then only about 25% of those (8% of the total sample) mentioned it to a clinician. *Futurescan 2002: A Forecast of Health Care Trends 2002-2006* (Coile, 2002) predicts that Internet-powered consumers will grow in numbers and significance.

39. Any last advice for enhancing customer service/patient satisfaction?

Staff needs to take care of each other. In one survey, 56% of nurses found triage stressful, particularly the interpersonal interactions. The stress was higher in medium and larger facilities. Too often, staff "blames" the triage nurse for being busy ("the shit magnet phenomena"). Nurses need to support and affirm each other. See Chapter 76 for further discussion.

Remember that nurses do what needs to be done even if it is not appreciated. Albert Schweitzer said, "No ray of sunlight is ever lost…it not always granted to the sower to see the harvest."

Nursing's goal is to strive to give patient care, not obtain satisfied customers.

40. Explain that last statement.

One ED nurse illustrated that a customer pays for services and gets what is requested. The customer wants a toaster, pays for a toaster, and gets a toaster. Patient care is often giving the patient more or something different than what was asked for, in the patient's best interest. The scared teenage new mother wants antibiotics for her baby. The baby is examined, but the mother is instead given the needed teaching, explanation, and reassurance. That is patient care and that is what nurses do.

Key Points

- Acknowledge patients when they first arrive by looking up and smiling. If on the phone, hold up the forefinger.
- Avoid writing while the patient is indicating their key problem. Repeat (mimic) the complaint back in the same words.
- Use reassuring phrases that provide comfort, such as "We can fix that."
- Deals with complaints by talking to the feelings, using a broken record technique, and providing the blameless apology.
- Make sure all patients understand what is wrong, what needs to be done, and why.

Internet Resource

Emergency Nurses Association Position Statements Customer Service and Satisfaction in the ED
http://www.ena.org/about/position/custservemergency.asp

Bibliography

Bendall-Lyon D, Powers TL: The role of complaint management in the service recovery process, *Jt Comm J Qual Improv* 27(5):278-286, 2001.

Boothman N: *How to make people like you in 90 seconds or less,* New York, 2002, Workman.

Carlson J, Youngblood R, Dalton JA, et al: Is patient satisfaction a legitimate outcome of pain management? *J Pain Symptom Manage* 25(3):264-275, 2003.

Chen-Tan L: Is patient's perception of time spent with the physician a determinant of ambulatory patient satisfaction? *Arch Intern Med* 161:1437-1442, 2001.

Co JPT, Ferris TG, Marino BL, et al: Are hospital characteristics associated with parental views of pediatric inpatient care quality? *Pediatrics* 111(2):308-314, 2003.

Coile RC: *Futurescan 2002: A forecast of healthcare trends 2002-2006,* Chicago, 2002, Health Administration Press.

Cook S: Using real time data to improve external and internal customer satisfaction (Managers Forum), *J Emerg Nurs* 29(4):360-361, 2003.

Emergency Nurses Association: *Position statement: Customer service and satisfaction in the emergency department,* 2004; available: www.ena.org; accessed Apr 19, 2005.

Employee Benefit Research Institute: *American satisfaction with health care rises, but pessimism about future remains* [press release], Washington, DC, 2001, Employee Benefit Research Institute.

Finkelstein JA: Reducing antibiotic use in children: A randomized trial in 12 practices, *Pediatrics* 108:1-7, 2001.

Friedman JF, Lee GM, Kleinman KP, et al: Acute care and antibiotic seeking for upper respiratory tract infections for children in day care, *Arch Pediatr Adolesc Med* 257:269-374, 2003.

Hammerschmidt R, Meador CK: *A little book of nurses' rules,* Philadelphia, 1993, Hanley & Belfus.

Herzlinger R: *Market-driven healthcare,* New York, 1997, The Free Press.

Mangione-Smith R: Parent expectations for antibiotics, physician-parent communication, and satisfaction, *Arch Pediatr Adolesc Med* 155:800-806, 2001.

Mayer TA, Cates RJ, Masorovich MJ, Royality D: Emergency department patient satisfaction: Customer service training improves patient satisfaction and rating in physician and nurse skill, *J Health Care Manage* 43:427-441, 1998.

Mayer TA, Zimmermann PG: ED customer satisfaction survival skills: One hospital's experience, *J Emerg Nurs* 25(3):187-191, 1999.

Pierce B: Real time customer satisfaction surveys (Managers Forum), *J Emerg Nurs* 30(4):355-356, 2004.

Rosenberg J: Five myths of customer satisfaction. *Quality Progress* 29:57-60, 1996.

Safran DG: Defining the future of primary care: What can we learn from patients? *Ann Intern Med* 4(138):248-255, 2003.

Zimmermann PG: The problems of healthcare customer satisfaction surveys. In Dochterman JM, and Grace HK, editors: *Grace's current issues in nursing,* ed 6, St Louis, 2001, Mosby, 255-260.

Zimmermann PG: Improving employee communication in the clinical setting: A nurse's perspective, *AAOHN J* 50(11):515-519, 2002.

Section XII

Triage Personnel Issues

Chapter 74

Personnel Qualifications

Polly Gerber Zimmermann

1. Who should do triage?

The Emergency Nurses Association (ENA) Comprehensive Standard VII on Triage (1999) states that the ENA "believes that safe, effective, and efficient triage can be performed only by a registered professional nurse who is educated in the principles of triage and who has a minimum of 6 months' experience in emergency nursing" (p. 23).

2. What are other typical requirements for triage that hospitals have?

The Joint Commission for Accreditation of Healthcare Organizations (JCAHO) requires documentation of clinical competence but does not specifically define how to do that. One study found that only 43% of surveyed hospitals had a special education program designated for nurses in triage.

Many individual hospitals and other countries have additional objective criteria for the triage nurses that reflect the ENA publication, *Triage, Meeting the Challenge*. They include:

- Mastery of a triage instructional program and demonstrated competency-based orientation program
- Additional registered nurse (RN) or emergency department (ED) experience: Examples from individual facilities range from 1 to 2 years of any nursing experience (in addition to the 6 months of ED experience) to 2 or more years ED experience before triaging.
- Certifications: ACLS, PALS, ENPC, TNCC, CEN

See Chapter 75 for further discussion.

3. List some other recommendations regarding the triage nurse characteristics besides work experience and formal certifications.

Grossman's (2003) list also includes more nebulous, but just as important, factors involving nursing style, nursing skills, and local resource knowledge factors. They include:

- Working knowledge of intradepartmental policies
- Understanding of local emergency services
- Possessing precision assessment skills
- Having well-developed skills in handling patients with special needs or barriers

- Demonstrating interpersonal and communication skills in the areas of interpersonal relationships, conflict resolution, supervision/delegation, telephone communication, and decision-making
- Serving as a role model
- Exhibiting flexibility, adaptability, the ability to anticipate and plan to potential occurrences, and common sense

Murphy's (1997) list of qualifications also includes:

- Rapid critical thinking skills
- Excellent prioritization skills
- Ability to adapt to stress
- Effective communication skills for all categories of people (e.g., patients, families, health care clinicians, community)

Others include tact, discretion, patience, organizational skills, and the key ability to recognize "sick" versus "not sick."

4. Why are these qualifications desired?

Triage can be one of the hardest roles in emergency nursing. Consultant Rebecca McNair identifies that it includes 16 different components.

Patient flow is unpredictable and cannot be controlled. Patients have multiple needs of varying acuity that can rapidly change. Patients' condition presentations are at different places in the continuum.

Patients vary in the ability to articulate their symptoms. The expert triage nurse not only hears what the patient says, but picks up on what is left said. In addition, there is a public relations factor in the constant interface with often distressed, demanding patients.

Because of all these factors, most departments use "seasoned" nurses in the triage role. Good triage decisions and prioritization of the patient flow is essential to a smoothly operating department.

5. Do the qualifications of the person doing triage make a difference in the time needed to perform triage?

Travers (1999) found that although there was no significant correlation between the nurse's experience and the time to complete the patient's triage, there was a positive correlation between the number of times the nurse had triaged before and the nurse's time to accomplish a patient's triage. There was a negative correlation between the number of certificates the nurse had and the triage time. This was attributed to the more educated, qualified nurse being more aware of what to ask and assess.

Paulson (2004) found that the wait time decreased by 73 minutes and the number of patients who left without being seen (LWBS) decreased by 85% when nurses, instead of unlicensed assistive personnel (UAP), performed the triage role. This was despite the nurses taking on the additional responsibilities of administering antipyretics for fever according to protocol, ordering radiographs and laboratory tests, maintaining traffic control, and transporting patients to radiology.

6. Should every experienced staff nurse rotate through triage?*

There are two schools of thought. Certain staff nurses prefer and perform well in the role and some departments tend to mainly use them. Other departments believe everyone works together better if all regularly experience the triage role.

Consultant Rebecca McNair advocates having a triage core group composed of staff who meet all the qualifications, prefer or have a special interest in the role, and are willing to champion the needs and work for on-going improvement for this role.

7. How long should the same nurse do triage in one day?

Triage, if done correctly, is physically and emotionally exhausting. Most limit the triage nurse to 8 hours, but some limit triage to 4-hour shifts. Regardless of the length, it is important to remember to relieve the triage nurse for breaks, just as any other staff nurse.

Key Point

- The ENA believes that safe, effective, and efficient triage can be performed only by a registered professional nurse who is educated in the principles of triage and who has a minimum of 6 months' experience in emergency nursing.

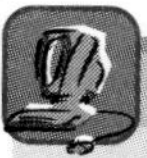

Internet Resources

Emergency Nurses Association
www.ena.org

Canadian Association of Emergency Physicians
www.caep.ca

Triage First Inc.
www.triagefirst.com

*This answer contains copyrighted material from Triage First, Inc., Fairview, NC (www.triagefirst.com)

Bibliography

Canadian Association of Emergency Physicians: Canadian Emergency Department Triage and Acuity Scale Implementation Guidelines, *J Can Assoc Emerg Physicians* 1(3 suppl), 1999.

Emergency Nurses Association: *Standards of Emergency Nursing Practice,* ed 4, Des Plaines, Ill, 1999, Author.

Emergency Nurses Association: *Triage: Meeting the challenge,* ed 2, Des Plaines, Ill, 1997, Author.

Grossman VGA: *Quick reference to triage,* ed 2, 2003, Philadelphia, JB Lippincott.

McNair R (President): *The nature of the beast: Comprehensive triage and patient flow Workshop,* Fairview, NC, 2003, Triage First, Inc.

McNair R: (President): *TRIAGE First EDucation: A comprehensive emergency department triage course,* Fairview, NC, 2004, Triage First, Inc.

Murphy KA: *Pediatric triage guidelines,* St Louis, 1997, Mosby.

Paulson DL: A comparison of wait times and patients leaving without being seen when licensed nurses versus unlicensed assistive personnel perform triage, *J Emerg Nurs* 30(4):307-311, 2004.

Travers D: Triage: How long does it take? How long should it take? *J Emerg Nurs* 25(3):238-240, 1999.

Chapter 75

Education and Training for Triage Nurses

Polly Gerber Zimmermann

1. Name some important components of an educational program that prepares emergency department nurses to triage.

- *Didactic information.* This often includes passing a written posttest.
- *Demonstration of competency.* This includes the ability to apply the attained knowledge.
- *Precepting/supervision.*
- *Audits and ongoing evaluation.*

2. Why is there an emphasis on knowledge when the Emergency Nurses Association indicates a registered nurse?

The Emergency Nurses Association's (ENA) Standards of Emergency Nursing Practice (1999) indicates, ". . . safe, effective, and efficient triage can be performed only by a registered professional nurse who is *educated in the principles of triage* . . . " Performing triage encompasses a specialized body of knowledge and skills.

3. Talk about competency in the application of knowledge.

Competency involves technical skills, interpersonal relations skills and critical thinking. Critical thinking is usually regarded as the most important because of patient safety. Consultant del Bueno emphasizes four critical thinking components of clinical judgment:

- Can the nurse recognize the patient's problem?
- Can the nurse safely/effectively manage the problem within the scope of practice?
- Does the employee have a relative sense of urgency?
- Does the nurse know why he or she is doing the action included? In other words, does the nurse do the right thing for the right reason?

4. Do most nurses really need this?

Del Bueno found that only 85% of experienced emergency department (ED) nurses had initial acceptable results of his or her simulated video testing assessments of nursing critical thinking. The result for all nonspecialized nurses was only 60% to 65%.

Only 25% to 30% of nurses with less than 1 year of experience had initial acceptable results (range: 12% to 60%). There was no difference between the educational preparation and/or previous health care experience. The acceptable results for inexperienced nurses have been declining each year from 43% in 1995/1996 to 26% in 2001. Simulated testing has limitations, but del Bueno indicates that, in her experience, only 5% to 7% (at best) who had unacceptable simulation testing actually perform well in the clinical setting.

5. Is additional education required for newly graduate nurses?

Basic level nursing education prepares the nurse for entry-level practice: a registered nurse (RN) license only assures the public that the nurse has met minimum standards for practice. Emergency nursing is a specialty that is highly complex and dynamic. The triage process requires proficient and rapid decision making, plus the ability to do skilled prioritization among changing patient problems. These are skills a newly graduated, inexperienced nurse usually does not have.

Patricia Benner's *From Novice to Expert* describes the five stages of nursing proficiency: novice, advanced beginner, competent clinician, proficient clinician, and expert clinician. An advanced beginner is marginally competent and experiences difficulty in formulating priorities. Her model (validated by Hom, 2003) indicates competent clinicians need 2 to 3 years' experience to be able to coordinate several complex demands simultaneously. The skills and knowledge needed for safe triage would be someone who has attained a more advanced stage than advanced beginner.

6. How do we improve the educational experience we provide?

Del Bueno emphasizes remediation must focus on the *applications* of knowledge and clinical practice. Internships for new registered nurses and good precepting experiences are a part of the equation.

7. List some ways to promote application in a classroom setting.

Unfolding case scenarios. This cooperative learning technique provides the information about a patient situation in staggered amounts, punctuated with questions such as, "What could be happening here?" and "What actions should be taken first?" and "What else do you need to know?"

For instance, start with a 40-year-old male, weighing 190 pounds, who has upper left abdominal pain. Triage vital signs are 100/70, 100, 20. "What do you want to consider?" Then add that he fell 8 hours ago. What are you thinking now? What is important to assess? Add that he takes propanolol (Inderal) for hypertension. How does that affect your thinking about his vital signs?

8. How can I make the use of unfolding scenarios the most effective?

Delay providing answers (or affirmation of correct given answers) until all of the learners have mentally worked through the situation, made a decision, and can then learn whether the choice was the best and why. Students remember what they think about.

The 10 seconds of silence after posing a question is when an individual's most productive thinking and learning takes place. I literally have to count off my fingers while I wait because that time period can seem like an eternity. Sharing why you are deliberately waiting with the learners usually makes them more willing to actively participate rather than just passively wait.

An alternative is to ask someone with a correct response to defend it and/or explain why another response was not the best. Examples of follow-up questions include "How does that work?" and "What does that mean?" or "Why didn't you do _____?" Playing the devil's advocate can promote a deeper understanding, different logical path, or an integration of key data.

9. What type of scenarios should be used?

Consultant Shelley Cohen recommends that triage training include a scenario for each of the following different types of patients: pediatric, geriatric, adult, trauma, mental health, and victim of abuse. She focuses on identifying what information and which questions are essential to solicit from *this* type of patient. Others also include the importance of a rapid response with any body fluid exposure.

10. What clinical areas might need more focus?

Del Bueno finds that nurses in general have the greatest limitations in recognition and management of patients with renal and neurologic problems.

11. Where can I get sample scenarios to use?

In addition to case study books, use actual cases from the department (similar to physician's morbidity and mortality conferences) or journals. I use the older Triage Decision columns (so that they are unfamiliar) from the *Journal of Emergency Nursing.*

12. Describe another version of cooperative learning techniques.

Think, pair, and share. Give the learners a generic situation, such as "What are the most important things to assess and consider in a young female with abdominal pain?"

- Participants have 1 minute to think and write something down. The writing is known to be an important aid to thinking.
- The participants are then paired (preferably someone as different as possible from themselves). Each must share their thoughts with the other, rather than just agree with the first person's comments.

- *After* this time (so they both pay attention during the sharing), the instructor announces the random, "fun" selection criteria (most siblings, longest hair, etc.) to choose a spokesperson for the pair.
- Spokespeople stand and then some are randomly selected to repeat one piece of key information from their paired sharing.

A key benefit is that everyone must participate. It accommodates those learners who need more time to think or have trouble speaking before others. They are "rehearsing" with their partner, usually to positive feedback, and can choose to "enhance" their own response with the partner's comments. Participants are conceiving, writing, teaching, hearing both themselves and others speaking about it, and considering alternative options.

The repetition and variety is penetrating. Repetition is the mother of learning. Think, pair, and share is one of the best methods of an active process (learner teaching a learner because "He who teaches learns the most") rather than a passive process (the "expert" tells all the answers).

13. List other techniques to enhance active learning.

- *Show actual clinical material.* For instance, put up lab results: "What do you think?" Show a picture of purpura: "What is your assessment?"
- *Use visual aids.* Having colorful aids increases long-term retention by 14% to 38%.
- *Peripheral learning.* Have posters on walls so information is seen (and subconsciously picked up) no matter where the eyes wander.
- *Take a break every 40 to 50 minutes.* It creates many beginnings and ends: people tend to remember the first thing and the last thing.
- *Play music before class and during breaks.* Baroque's beat particularly matches the heartbeat to stimulate natural rhythms.
- *Have passion.* "The mediocre teacher tells. The good teacher explains. The superior teacher demonstrates. The great teacher inspires."

14. Which method is best for triage classroom time?

Vary the method. Learning occurs through auditory, visual, and kinesthetic approaches. Although most have a preferred major learning style, everyone uses some of each. Accelerated learning occurs when there is a multisensory mix of all three (activating both the logical left side of the brain with the artistic right side).

15. What content should be included for triage education of staff nurses?

Many hospitals develop their own courses, which often include self-study modules. Contents include the triage system (including the process and acuity criteria), protocols and policies, red flags, regulations (Emergency Medical Treatment and Active Labor Act [EMTALA], Health Insurance Portability and Accountability Act [HIPAA], etc.), customer service (including skills for assertion, defusing, and patient relations), infection control, and supplementary resources (security, social service, etc.). The ENA sells a triage curriculum (www.ena.org).

16. Describe the Triage Game.

Terenzi (2000) developed this method to practice triage principles. A tri-fold project display board represents the emergency department. Computer graphic pictures are arranged to represent the department's layout of beds, hallway stretchers, and waiting room. "Patients" are computer graphics with a picture and chief complaint on the front, with a brief history and set of vital signs on the back. Velcro is attached to each "patient" and corresponding areas in the patient care area.

Each learner picks a "patient" from the box and reads the information, assigns an acuity score (sharing the reasoning) and places the patient in the appropriate area. Once placed, a patient can be moved to another appropriate area (including the waiting room) as needed, but no "patient" can be discharged. In addition to improving application of triage knowledge per se, it promotes respect for the charge nurse in managing patient flow as the ED "fills up" and allows "teachable" moments.

17. How do other departments track competencies for triage?

Many departments include an initial written examination to measure attainment of knowledge. They then use a check-off list that includes essential skills to help track application and competency. Besides equipment, the lists include interventions by protocol, physical assessment, and evaluation of observed interactions. Audits of charts allow evaluation of decision-making process, documentation completeness, and handwriting legibility.

18. How long should the precepting experience be?

Most use 8 to 24 hours of triage time precepting with an experienced triage nurse. *Triage: Meeting the Challenge,* indicates up to 1 to 2 weeks may be necessary for novice nurses.

19. What are ways to help promote ongoing competency of a triage nurse?

The Joint Commission for Accreditation of Healthcare Organizations (JCAHO) includes competencies. *Triage: Meeting the Challenge* suggests on a yearly basis. Many hospitals have some form of staff competency day(s)/clinical skills fair. Covered information/skills include areas that are high-risk/low-volume, mandatory regulations, new skills/procedures, change in skills/procedures, or problem-prone issues.

Ongoing random chart audits can also be an effective tool. One hospital audits 15 of each triage nurse's charts looking for

- Appropriate subjective data relevant to the patients' complaint
- Appropriate objective data that supports the designated triage priority
- Primary and secondary survey (as appropriate)
- Vital signs and parameters
- Appropriate generic triage content (e.g., allergies, means of arrival)

20. Any other recommendations related to competency?

Ann Kobs, consultant and former Associate Director for the Department of Standard Interpretation Unit at JCAHO, indicates that competency can be validated by two possible methods: observing actual behavior and documenting the absence of errors. She suggests using a formal process of a supervisor documenting actual observed behavior or the absence of error after watching the individual's day-to-day performance.

Key Points

- ENA Standard of Emergency Nursing Practice (1999) indicates that safe, effective, and efficient triage can be performed only by a registered professional nurse who is educated in the principles of triage. Triage is regarded as a specialized body of knowledge and skills that require training and validation to ensure competency.
- Critical thinking components of clinical judgment include recognizing the problem, managing the patient, perceiving the relative sense of urgency, and doing the right thing for the right reason.
- Triage courses in hospitals should include didactic information, application in clinical scenarios, competency verification, and precepting elements.

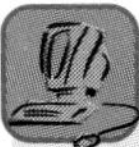

Internet Resources

Emergency Nurses Association
www.ena.org

Triage First, Inc.
www.triagefirst.com

Health Resources Unlimited
www.hru.net

Bibliography

Benner P: *From novice to expert: Excellence and power in clinical nursing practice,* Menlo Park, Calif, 1984, Addison-Wesley.

Cohen S: Verifying staff competencies (Managers Forum), *J Emerg Nurs* 30(3):266, 2004.

Del Bueno DJ: Assessing new hire competencies (Managers Forum), *J Emerg Nurs* 29(3):270-271, 2003.

Del Bueno DJ: Buyer beware: The cost of competence, *Nurse Econ* 19:250-257, 2001.

Glendon K, Ulrich D: *Unfolding cases: Experiencing the realities of clinical nursing practice,* Upper Saddle River, NJ, 2001, Prentice Hall.

Hom EM: Coaching and mentoring new graduates entering perinatal nursing practice, *J Perinat/Neonat Nurs* 17(1):35-49, 2003.

Kobs A: Verifying staff competency (Managers Forum), *J Emerg Nurs* 2795:495, 2001.

Lavin M: *Accelerated learning: Multisensory teaching and multisensory learning,* Presentation at Harry S Truman College, Chicago, Ill, Feb 2, 2002.

Miller R: Verifying staff competencies (Managers Forum), *J Emerg Nurs* 30(3):266, 2004.

Morrison S: Verifying staff competencies (Managers Forum), *J Emerg Nurs* 30(3):266, 2004.

Salter C: Sixteen ways to be a smarter teacher, *Fast Company* 5(5):114-126, 2002.

Staiger D, Auerbach D, Buerhaus P: Expanding career opportunities for women and the declining interest in nursing as a career, *Nurs Econ* 18:230-236, 2000.

Terenzi C: The triage game, *J Emerg Nurs* 26(1):66-69, 2000.

Willingham DT: How we learn: Ask the cognitive scientist: Students remember what they think about, *Am Educator* 27(2):37-41, 2003.

Zimmermann PG: Orienting ED nurses to triage: Using scenario-based test-style questions to promote critical thinking, *J Emerg Nurs* 29(3):256-258, 2003.

Zimmermann PG: Some practical tips for more effective teaching, *J Emerg Nurs* 29(3):283-286, 2003.

Zimmermann PG: The difference between teaching nursing students and registered nurses, *J Emerg Nurs* 28(6):574-578, 2002.

Zimmermann PG: Tricks for the ED trade, *J Emerg Nurs* 29(5):453-457, 2003.

Zimmermann PG: Unfolding case study instruction, *J Emerg Nurs* 28(3):246-247, 2002.

Chapter 76

Taking Care of Yourself and Your Staff

Polly Gerber Zimmermann

1. Is this going to tell me to eat well, exercise, and get plenty of rest? I know that.

Well, those known actions will enhance your health and well-being. However, self-care for a nurse also involves issues of destressing, colleague interaction, and the effects of fatigue.

2. Talk about the effects of stress.

In one survey, 56% of emergency department (ED) nurses find triage stressful. Stress results in increased distractibility, and decreased concentration. Chronic stress adversely affects health; an increase of 63% mortality in one study, from the increase in proinflammatory cytokines, interleukin-6 (IL-6). Retaining hostility was a predictor of risks for smoking, alcohol consumption, depression, high blood pressure, obesity, and low social support.

3. List individual ways to deal with stress.

- *Laugh.* Laughter reduces the levels of stress hormones (cortisol and epinephrine) and boots immunity. Even looking forward to a future event in which laughter is anticipated will reduce stress.
- *Slow breathing.* Deliberately slow the breathing to 6 deep breaths a minute (inhale for 5 seconds, exhale for 5 seconds). Tense people tend to take quick, shallow breaths. Deep breaths force the shoulders to stretch. This 10-second cycle tends to match the cardiovascular rhythm and has a calming effect.
- *Positive self-talk.* At the end of every shift, name at least one thing you did that made a difference to a patient, family member, or staff person (Cohen, 2002).
- *Think happy.* Focus on someone or something you care deeply about for 15 seconds to 5 minutes.
- *Praise a nurse.* Appreciate and affirm peers, not just assistants.
- *Eat a low-fat carbohydrate.* Carbohydrates, such as pretzels, increase the production of serotonin, which has a calming effect about 20 minutes later.
- *Be gentle with yourself.* Remember that you cannot change others, only how you respond.
- *Mentally step back ten paces to keep the incident in perspective.* One technique is to rate a stressful event on a scale of 1 to 10. Ten is a catastrophic event, like a death. It helps to realistically place the irritation in the grand scheme of life.

- *Listen to music.* Study participants report less stress when doing a task while listening to music. On the other hand, loud music with a beat tends to energize.
- *Walk.* Walking results in less stress, steadier blood pressures, and better sleep.
- *Relationships.* Giving others support may be even more beneficial than receiving it.
- *Surround yourself with happy people.* People tend to assimilate the emotional responses of the people they have a relationship with.
- *Get involved in another organized outside activity.* It will involve a commitment, real demands, and force you not to think about work all the time.
- *Take a vacation that does not involve nursing.* Plan in advance, and share your plans with your other commitments. It prevents a last-minute crisis derailing you.
- *Meditation.* Improved mindfulness over time relates to decline in mood disturbances and stress.
- *Do nothing.* At least once a day, take 5 or 10 minutes to sit quietly and do nothing. It slows the heart rate, lowers the blood pressure, and increases a sense of control.

4. Talk about a critical incident stress management debriefing.

Laposa et al (2003) survey of ED personnel found that 20% considered changing jobs as a result of a traumatic incident at work and most (67%) feel they did not get the support needed from administration. Only 18% attended critical incident stress management (CISM) debriefing and none sought outside help. The need is probably highest after a traumatic incident. Some use an informal approach of compassionate listening, reassurance, and education in a nonstructured personalized, peer-oriented environment; formal CISM is more structured.

5. Does CISM work?

In Laposa's survey, those who did attend CISM indicated feeling more support and less interpersonal conflict. Bledsoe (2003) found CISM to be ineffective in preventing posttraumatic stress disease (PTSD), but others criticize the methodology of these studies. All agree it should not be mandatory. One hospital offers sessions of free counseling sessions with an outside licensed psychologist as an alternative.

6. Talk about the effect of interpersonal conflict.

Friendly workers get more done, including being better at picking up the indirect meaning of the verbal conversations. In contrast, interpersonal conflict was closely linked with nurses' PTSD symptoms (Laposa, 2004). Conflict lessens the supportive social relationships that can reduce workplace stress. There has been a growing body of studies that identified collaboration as an important predictor of positive patient outcomes. Yet Rosenstein (2002) found that 96% of registered nurses had witnessed physician disruptive behavior.

7. How should a physician outburst be handled?

Plan for staff to gather in a semicircle behind the person being verbally attacked and look with a disapproving stare (a "code pink" or "code white"). Be quiet, still, and firm. Usually the person will walk away in a huff. If this does not work, the charge nurse or manager should say, "We need to take this away from here," turn, and walk away. The person either joins the nurse to move to the new location or, more commonly, refuses to go. Either way, this clearly sends the message the current barrage will stop now. Write up this type of incident, including witnesses and if it was within earshot of patients.

8. What can be done to prevent it in the first place?

- *Awareness.* Communication styles and goals are often different. Physicians indicate they want more factual information presented in an organized way, whereas the nurses are more likely to focus on the interpersonal relationship.
- *Collaborative Practices in Care.* The National Joint Practice Commission identified necessary system elements, such as integrated records, joint practice committees, and joint interdisciplinary orientation.
- *A Disruptive Clinician Policy.* All staff, including physicians, must sign a Code of Conduct. Inappropriate behaviors are progressively counseled, with the possible eventual loss of privileges.
- *Repercussion-Free Reporting Avenues.* Both nurses (and physicians) must be able to freely register a complaint about verbal abuse.

9. Discuss the effects of fatigue.

Anyone who has 19 hours of prolonged wakefulness will have the cognitive and psychomotor effects of a blood alcohol level of .05%; after 24 hours it is the same as if the person was legally drunk (0.1% alcohol level). Fatigue slows reaction time, saps energy, and diminishes attention to details. In addition to acts of commission, there is concern that the decreased alertness results in a "failure to rescue" a deteriorating patient.

10. Can't someone overcome this with coffee?

No, these are basic physiologic responses that cannot be altered. In fact, with aging the effects intensify. Coffee gives short-term alertness, but the subtle focus is still missing.

11. Relate this to nurses' work schedules.

There is a growing concern over the effects of nurses' workloads and work hours. The Institute of Medicine (IOM) in a 2003 report indicated that nurses' long work hours was one of the most serious threats to patient safety. The IOM recommends that nurses not be allowed to work more than 12 hours a day and 60 hours a week. Rogers found that 14% of nurses worked at least 16 straight hours at least once during the month-long study. Nurses who work shifts lasting at least 12.5 hours were three times more likely to commit an error than nurses who worked less than 8.5 hours. Working unplanned overtime at the end of a shift also increased the likelihood of making a mistake, regardless of the shift length.

12. Anything to help besides limiting an individual nurse's hours?

- *Allow power naps.* Central Health (Lynchburg, VA) encourages night shift staff to sleep 30 minutes, with 5 minutes before and 5 minutes afterwards (total 40 minutes). They also have a massage chair on the units for staff use.
- *Provide break time on all shifts.* A true "break" of only 5 minutes every 2 hours makes one more alert and refreshed. Yet 46% of nurses routinely "skip" breaks, and 43% of those taking breaks were not truly relieved of their responsibilities.
- *Exercise during work.* A short (15 to 20 minutes) exercise break during the shift enhances on-the-job alertness and morale. Examples include walking, climbing stairs, or riding a stationary bicycle.
- *Drink fluids.* Fatigue is one of the first signs of dehydration.
- *Avoid "double-back" staffing.* Working a "night" shift with a "day" shift the next morning leaves less than 8 hours off. Nurses who are sleepy on the job averaged only 6.2 hours of sleep per night (compared to others' 6.9 hours of sleep).
- *Forbid back-to-back doubles.*
- *Curtail the use of 12-hour shifts.* Rogers et al (2004) recommend that because more than three-fourths of the shifts scheduled for 12 hours exceeded that time frame, routine use of 12-hour shifts should be curtailed. They also recommend that overtime associated with 12-hour shifts should be eliminated.

13. Aren't these measures extreme?

Many of these practices are routine in other countries, such as Australia, and other safety-concerned industries, such as aviation occupations. It will involve a major culture and attitude change.

Key Points

- Use slow, deep breathing, walking, and pleasant thoughts to deal with stress during the shift.
- Disruptive colleague behavior has a negative impact on the quality of patient care.
- Avoid double-back shifts, back-to-back doubles, and missing breaks to limit effects on fatigue and safety.

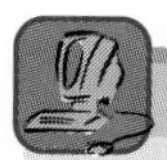

Internet Resources

Emergency Nurses Association Position Statements: Stress Management Strategies
http://www.ena.org/about/position/stressmanagement.asp

STRESS!—It's Everywhere! And It Can Be Managed!
http://www.nursingworld.org/tan/julaug99/stress.htm

Critical Incident Stress Management (CISM): Benefit or Risk for Emergency Services?
http://www.bryanbledsoe.com/CISM%20(Bledsoe).pdf

Bibliography

Answerson C, Keltner D, John OP: Emotional convergence between people over time, *J Pers Soci Psychol* 84(5):1054-1068, 2003.

Bagg JG, Schmitt MH, Mushlin AI, et al: Association between nurse-physician collaboration and patient outcomes in three intensive care units, *Crit Care Med* 27:1991-1998, 1999.

Balas MC, Scott LD, Rogers AE: The prevalence and nature of errors and near errors reported by hospital staff nurses, *Appl Nurs Res* 14(4):224-230, 2004.

Bethune G, Burnette CK: Nurse retention (Managers Forum), *J Emerg Nurs* 30(4):353-354, 2004.

Bledose BE: Critical incident stress management (CISM): Benefit or risk for emergency services? *Prehosp Emerg Care* 7(2):272-279, 2003.

Brown KW, Ryan RM: The benefits of being present: Mindfulness and its role in psychological well-being, *J Personality Soc Psychol* 84(4):822-848, 2003.

Clark K, Walsh K: Handling physician verbal abuse (Managers Forum), *J Emerg Nurs* 30(5):491-492, 2004.

Cohen S: *101 triage tips*, Hohenwald, Tenn, 2002, Health Resources Unlimited.

Davidson J: Handling a physician outburst (Managers Forum), *J Emerg Nurs* 29(6):564, 2003.

Glaser R, Robles TF, Sheridan J, et al: Mild depressive symptoms are associated with amplified and prolonged inflammatory responses after influenza virus vaccination in older adults, *Arch Gen Psychiatry* 60(10):1009-1014, 2003.

Hammonds KH: Cutting back for more balance, *J Emerg Nurs* 30(5):492, 2004.

Kiecolt-Glaser JK, et al: Chronic stress and age-relate increases in the proinflammatory cytokine IL-6, *Proc Nat Acad Sci USA* 100:9090-9095, 2003.

Kraus WA, Draper EA, Wagner DP, Zimmermann JE: An evaluation of outcome from intensive care in major medical centers, *Ann Intern Med* 104:410-418, 1986.

Laposa JM, Alden LE, Fullerton LM: Work stress and post-traumatic stress disorder in ED nurses/personnel, *J Emerg Nurs* 29:23-28, 2003.

Lee KA: Self-reported sleep disturbances in employed women, *Sleep* 15:493-498, 1992.

Mardon S: Nighwork (Managers Ask and Answer), *J Emerg Nurs* 25(2):144-145, 1999.

Mason D: Handling physician verbal abuse. In Zimmermann PG: Managers Forum, *J Emerg Nurs* 30(5):490-491, 2004.

Rogers AE, Hwang W, Scott LD, et al: The working hours of hospital staff nurses and patient safety, *Health Aff (Millwood)* 23:202-212, 2004.

Rogers AE: Sleep deprivation and the ED night shift, *J Emerg Nurs* 28(5):469-470, 2002.

Rosenstein AH: Nurse-physician relationships: Impact on nurse satisfaction and retention, *Am J Nurs* 102:26-34, 2002.

Shortell SM, Zimmerman JE, Rousseau DM, et al: The performance in intensive care units: Does good management make a difference? *Med Care* 32:508-525, 1994.

Siegler IC, Costa PT, Brummett BH, et al: Patterns of change in hostility from college to midlife in the UNC Alumni Heart Study Predict High-Risk status, *Psychosom Med* 65(5):728-745, 2003.

Chapter 77

PDA Use*

Audrey Snyder

1. What is a PDA?

PDA stands for personal digital assistant. It is a small electronic device that can hold a large amount of data. Other terminology is palmtop computing or handheld computing.

2. How can PDAs help in a health care environment?

For information to be useful in rapidly changing environments, reference materials need to be portable and easy to use. PDAs allow multiple data entry capabilities by the use of an attachable keyboard, touch screen, desktop, wireless capability, and infrared beaming.

3. Does a PDA interfere with hospital electronic equipment?

The author is unaware of any reported incidence of PDA use interfering with hospital electronic equipment. One institution has a policy that no electronic equipment can be used within 5 feet of medical equipment. Standing at the foot of most patients' beds would comply with this policy.

4. Can PDAs be incorporated with a cellular phone to be used in the health care environment?

Many hospitals currently allow digital wireless phones to be used in the hospital environment.

5. Can all PDAs share data?

All PDAs cannot share data. PDAs functioning on the same operating system can share data.

---

*Disclaimer: The author has discussed various health care applications throughout this chapter. This should NOT be construed as "promotion" of these applications. Each user should research and evaluate products and services for their benefit in his or her current health care environment.

6. What applications are available for PDA use by health care clinicians?

Applications for the PDA are available as freeware, commercial software, and demonstration versions.

- Freeware is available by CD-ROM or can be downloaded directly from the Internet at no cost to the user.
- Commercial software requires a fee for use often before the program can be downloaded.
- Demonstration versions allow you to download the software and try it out for a set period, often 30 days, prior to purchase. Many of these programs provide automatic updates to your PDA if your computer is connected to the Internet when you sync.

See the Internet Resource Box for frequently accessed programs.

7. What patient information management programs are available?

Patient charting can be accomplished with Patient Keeper and patient outcomes can be tracked with database tools like Handbase.

8. What are the minimum programs that you recommend a nurse place on a PDA when first starting to use one?

Use the basic programs (datebook, address keeper, memo pad, and expense report) that come with the PDA to organize your life as a personal information manager. The memo pad is a good way to keep small notes, often-used numbers, or passwords. A pharmacology reference, a medical consult program, and medical calculations program would be the next priority.

9. Will a PDA have enough memory to hold all those programs?

The newest PDA models come with expansion slots that can hold Compact Flash, memory sticks, or memory cards to allow for additional memory.

10. How can I keep data secure? I'm concerned about meeting Health Insurance Portability and Accountability Act regulations.

If the nurse uses the PDA primarily for reference material, the risk to confidentiality is not an issue. However, if identifiable patient data are stored on the device, the user must employ some type of security software to protect the data.

First, always password protect your device. This security feature alone, however, is not enough to comply with Health Insurance Portability and Accountability Act (HIPAA) regulations. Obtain additional information at www.hcfa.gov/hipaa/hipaahm.htm. There are encryption software programs available like File crypto, and Fsecure, Forever secure, PDA secure, and Teal Lock. See www.palmgear.com for more than 175 programs that can assist in meeting HIPAA regulations.

11. What are some examples of how a PDA can be beneficial in triage?

The following examples illustrate potential benefits of PDA usage in the triage environment.

Pharmacology: When a patient presents with a current medication list that contains medications unfamiliar to the nurse, a pharmacology program can be accessed.

Pharmaceutical and Herbal Product Interactions: A patient is taking St. John's Wort and a nurse needs to see if any of the medications ordered for the patient interact with St. John's Wort. A pharmacology program that includes herbal products with a medication check will allow the nurse to cross-reference the medications and herbal product for interactions.

Antidotes: For patients presenting with overdose or ingestion of substances, antidotes and dosages can be rapidly accessed.

Medications Containing Aspirin: Over the counter (OTC) medications containing aspirin that should not be given to children with fever can be identified.

Dosage Calculation: For ease of calculating the dose of acetaminophen at 15 mg/kg, a dose calculator such as MedCalc can be used.

Language Translation: When assessing a Hispanic patient whose primary language is Spanish, a language translator program on the PDA can be helpful in obtaining history.

Pregnancy Calculator: When a pregnant patient presents for care, a pregnancy calculator can be assessed to calculate due date.

Calendar: The calendar on the PDA can be helpful when trying to determine the date of a past injury occurrence.

Protocols: Triage protocols can be downloaded into a PDA. This can be especially helpful when orienting nurses to the triage role.

Inhaler Cap Colors: Many times patients with a history of a respiratory problem can tell the triage nurse they use an inhaler but they cannot remember the name of the medication. The nurse can use a program to look up the color of the inhaler cap to determine what inhaled medication the patient is taking.

Peak Flow: Expected peak flows can be calculated based on patient's body size.

Immunizations: When triaging pediatric patients, Shots 2004 can be helpful in determining which immunizations the patient should have received. The parent or guardian can then be consulted about the child's immunization status.

Unusual Diagnoses: When a patient presents with a past medical history of a specific disease process or problem, which is labeled by a name that is unfamiliar, the triage nurse can look in eponyms or the 5-Minute Clinical Consult to obtain information about the disease.

Temperature Conversion: When the family has taken the patient's temperature at home with a Fahrenheit thermometer and a nurse needs to convert it to Celsius for comparison, a conversion program can be helpful.

12. How can PDAs be used during mass casualty situations?

Disaster triage officers have used a PDA to keep track of the number of patients in each priority category and to document times each patient who was sent to the staging area.

13. Some PDAs have cameras incorporated. Is there any benefit in the health care arena?

Prehospital clinicians that use PDAs may take pictures of motor vehicle crash scenes. These can be beamed to the care clinician's PDA and later added to the patient's chart.

14. What are creative uses of the PDA that may become more popular in the future?

E-prescriptions is a creative use that is seen in larger cities. With e-prescriptions, the prescriber can write the prescription in the PDA and then send it to the pharmacy via wireless technology or by syncing while connected to the Internet; no paper is involved. There are several programs that will allow the user to send prescriptions in this manner: All Script, Ephysician, Iscibe, and Rx Connect.

Palmtop computers have the ability to increase the brain's capacity to recall relevant information to support triage, clinical practice, information management, quality improvement, and administrative functions. PDAs provide valuable information at the bedside and may play a role in decreasing medication errors in the future. Their role in the triage environment is just beginning to be realized.

Key Points

- Always password protect your PDA.
- Each PDA user must be familiar with the HIPAA regulations of 1996 as it relates to their work.

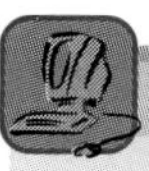

Internet Resources

HIPAA Compliance and PDAs
pdacortex.com/HIPAA_survey.htm

National Standards to Protect the Privacy of Personal Health Information
hhs.gov/ocr/hipaa/assist.html

PDA Community featuring Security Applications
palmgear.com

Free Applications: ePocrates
http://www2.epocrates.com/index.html

Medical Spanish
http://www.healthypalmpilot.com/cgi-bin/review.cgi?ID=432

MedCalc
http://medcalc.med-ia.net/download.html

Pedi-Dose
http://www.eurocool.com/review/?show=6674

Shots 2004
http://www.immunizationed.org/AnyPage.asp?Page=Palm

Handango
http://www.Handango.com

PDA Cortex: The Journal of Mobile Informatics
http://www.rnpalm.com/

MemoWare
http://memoware.com/

Palm Boulevard
http://PalmBlvd.com

SkyScape: Your Mobile Medical Library
http://skyscape.com

MedScape from WebMd
http://Medscape.com

Handheldmed
http://www.handheldmed.com

Bibliography

Eastes L: PDAs for the trauma nurse: Help or hindrance? *J Emerg Nurs* 30(4):380-383, 2004.

Gorder PF: *PDAs can help create safer shift changes, PDA Cortex*; available: www.rnpalm.com/safer_shift_changes.htm; accessed Apr 25, 2004.

Shah M: Grassroots computing: Palmtops in health care, *JAMA* 295:1768, 2001.

Stolworthy Y, Suszka-Hildebrandt S: Mobile information technology at the point of care: The grass roots origin of mobile computing in nursing, *PDA Cortex*; available: http://www.pdacortex.com/mitatpoc.htm; accessed Apr 13, 2005.

Section XIII

International Standardized Five-Level Triage Systems

Chapter 78

ENA/ACEP Five-Level Triage Work Group

Rebecca S. McNair

1. What is the Emergency Nurses Association/American College of Emergency Physicians Five-Level Triage Work Group?

The delegates present at the 2002 Emergency Nurses Association (ENA) General Assembly passed a resolution to convene a work group to review 5-level triage systems and to make a recommendation to the Board of Directors regarding the adoption of a standard five-tier system nationwide. Around the same time American College of Emergency Physicians (ACEP) moved to evaluate and make recommendations regarding five-level triage. The two organizations combined their respective work group members to form a collaborative task force in 2003 to accomplish the resolution.

2. What are the results of the work of this group?

The group published its policy statement in 2003: "ACEP and ENA believe that quality of patient care would benefit from implementing a standardized emergency department (ED) triage scale and acuity categorization process. Based on expert consensus of currently available evidence, ACEP and ENA support the adoption of a reliable, valid 5-level triage scale." In 2004, the work group indicated that either the Canadian Triage and Acuity Scale (CTAS) or the Emergency Severity Index (ESI) are good options.

3. Where can we find the results of the work group?

The article "Five-Level Triage: A Report from the ACEP/ENA Five-Level Triage Task Force" was published February 2005 in the *Journal of Emergency Nursing*.

4. Which five-level systems did the group review?

The combined ACEP/ENA work group evaluated only the literature on the four- or five-level acuity systems that have been widely published and have research available. It did not evaluate current systems in use and propose further study of these systems. The systems reviewed were CTAS, The Australian Triage Scale (ATS), Manchester Triage Scale (MTS), and ESI.

5. Are there other five-level acuity scales that were not reviewed?

Although the work group is aware of some other systems in place in facilities throughout the country, these systems have not been thoroughly researched. Some of these other systems are ascending, descending, and computerized, algorithm-driven systems.

- Sutter Triage Scale (STS), which utilizes a comprehensive five-tiered, ascending scale.
- Dot Triage Guideline, Quest care's official triage system.
- Soterion Rapid Triage System (RTS), a computerized system.

6. Why did the work group *not* recommend any particular system?

Although a uniform scale would allow a larger opportunity for evaluation, improvement, and benchmarking, the work group recommendations allow for greater exploration and research into five-level systems based on individual facility's and community's goals.

7. The ENA publishes *ESI Implementation Handbook.* Is this an implied endorsement of ESI as the recommended system?

Absolutely not. ENA's website (www.ena.org) has a clarification. ENA contracted with the ESI Triage Group, as a business decision, to publish the implementation manual. The ENA Board of Directors has not approved an association endorsement of any one particular system.

8. How should EDs proceed?

The ENA/ACEP work group paper entitled "Standardized Five Level Triage" states "We believe physicians and nurses should collaboratively evaluate the literature, come to their own conclusion and plan for implementation. At this time, the committee believes that either the CTAS or the ESI are good options."

9. What are some of the questions we should ask when evaluating the literature?

Consider the validity and reliability of the five-level triage system being examined. If using an untested system, ask, "Is the work being done to ensure reliability and validity of the system?" There are mixed opinions among the group regarding the philosophy of triage systems in general. ED nurses and physicians must answer if a triage acuity system should be based on:

- Pure-acuity OR
- Expected need for resources, OR
- Both, a blend of severity of presentation and consideration

10. Is this the final recommendation of the work group?

What has been accomplished are the first steps. The work group encourages future research and recommends an in-depth, evidence-based review of all current five-level triage systems, including those that are currently under development.

Key Points

- ACEP and ENA believe that quality of patient care would benefit from implementing a standardized ED triage scale and acuity categorization process. Based on expert consensus of currently available evidence, ACEP and ENA support the adoption of a reliable, valid 5-level triage scale.
- The committee believes that either the CTAS or the ESI are good options.

Internet Resources

A Uniform Triage Scale in Emergency Medicine
http://www.acep.org/library/pdf/triagescaleip.pdf

National Five-Level Triage System Resolution Adopted by the Emergency Nurses Association
http://www.ena.org/news/details.asp?id=19

Emergency Nurses Meet, Adopt Five-Level Triage System Resolution
http://www.nursezone.com/job/MedicalNewsAlerts.asp?articleID=9389

Bibliography

American College of Emergency Physicians: A uniform triage scale in emergency medicine [information paper], June 1999.

Fernandes CMB, Tanabe P, Gilboy N, et al: Five-level triage: A report from the ACEP/ENA Five-Level Triage Task Force, *J Emerg Nurs* 31(1):39-50, 2005.

Fernandes CMB, Wuerz RC, Clark S, et al: How reliable is emergency department triage? *Ann Emerg Med* 34(2):141-147, 1999.

Gilboy N, Travers D, Wuerz R: Emergency nursing at the millennium, *J Emerg Nurs* 25(6):468-473, 1999.

Hay E, Bekerman L, Rosenberg G, Peled R: Quality assurance of nurse triage: Consistency of results over three years, *Am J Emerg Med* 19(2):113-117, 2001.

Kosowsky JM, Shindel S, Liu T, et al: Can emergency department triage nurses predict patients' dispositions? *Am J Emerg Med* 19(1):10-14, 2001.

McCaig LF, Ly N: National hospital ambulatory medical care survey: 2000 emergency department summary, *Adv Data Vital Health Stat* 1-31, 2002.

McNair R (President): *Determining triage acuity and establishing standards of practice, lecture: The nature of the beast: Triage and patient throughput workshop,* Fairview, NC, 2003, Triage First, Inc.

Nakagawa J, Ouk S, Schwartz B, et al: Interobserver agreement in emergency department triage, *Ann Emerg Med* 41(2):191-195, 2003.

Spaite DW, Bartholomeaux F, Guisto J, et al: Rapid process redesign in a university-based emergency department: Decreasing waiting time intervals and improving patient satisfaction, *Ann Emerg Med* 39(2):168-177, 2002.

Travers DA, Waller AE, Bowling JM, et al: Comparison of 3-level and 5-level triage acuity systems [abstract], *Acad Emerg Med* 7(5):522, 2000.

Washington DL, Stevens CD, Shekelle PG, et al: Safely directing patients to appropriate levels of care: Guideline-driven triage in the emergency service, *Ann Emerg Med* 36(1):15-22, 2000.

Zimmermann PG: The case for a universal, valid, reliable 5-tier triage acuity scale for U.S. emergency departments, *J Emerg Nurs* 27(3):246-254, 2001.

Chapter 79

The Emergency Severity Index Triage Scale

Polly Gerber Zimmermann

1. What is the Emergency Severity Index triage scale?

The initial triage algorithm was conceptualized and developed by the late Dr. Richard Wuerz (at the Brigham and Women's Hospital in Boston) and Dr. David Eitel (at York Hospital in York, PA) in the late 1990s. Acuity and complexity are summarized on a 5-point scale, with level 1 representing the highest acuity and complexity and level 5 representing the lowest. It is unique in that it is based on acuity and likely resource consumption required to achieve a disposition. It expands the concept of triage from beyond *when* should the patient be seen to also *what* does the patient need.

Modifications to the original version included removing the peak flow from the algorithm, adding a vital sign criteria for children, changing the danger zone pulse oximetry to 92%, changing the danger zone heart rate criterion for those aged more than 8 years to 100 beats/minute, and asking the triage nurse to *conside*r (instead of *require*) assignment to level 2 to patients with danger zone vital signs. At the time this book went to press, Emergency Severity Index (ESI) version 4 was scheduled to be released.

2. Describe the algorithm.

After the initial decision about a life-threatening presentation (intubated, apneic, pulseless, unresponsive), the distinguishers for level 2 are acutely ill, mental status alteration (confused, lethargic, disoriented), severe pain (clinical observation and/or a rating of "7" on a 0 to 10 pain scale), or high-risk situations.

After the most acutely ill patients (ESI Level 1 and 2), the system's algorithm then incorporates the number of anticipated *different* types of resource interventions for the ultimate disposition. Examples of resources could include radiograph(s), intravenous (IV) access and medications, laboratory test(s), injections, or consults. Two items of the same type, such as two different IV antibiotics, is considered one resource.

This estimate is required only up to two resources. Resource determination is the nurse's "best guess" made according to prudent standards of practice, not a particular physician's preference. Two or more resources is ESI Level 3; one resource is ESI Level 4; and zero resources is an ESI Level 5.

After the nurse has estimated resource needs, she or he then considers if the vital signs and/or pulse oximetry are in the "danger zone." Vital signs are required to make the triage determination *only* for patients needing 2 or more resources (ESI Level 3). Patients at ESI Level 3 with abnormal vital signs *may* then be uptriaged to ESI Level 2.

3. **Our department policy requires all patients to have vital signs taken.**

   The algorithm decision and institutional policy are two different things. Many departments do vital signs for other purposes, such as health screening. Vital signs are used to make a triage level selection in this system for patients at ESI Level 3 or higher.

4. **Wouldn't all have at least one resource because they get a history and physical?**

   The emergency department (ED) history and physical, oral medications, and tetanus immunizations are not counted as resources.

5. **How is a consultation handled? Is a social worker a resource?**

   The definition of resource includes something that indicates a higher level of patient complexity. The ESI Implementation Manual indicates that a woman who "wants to talk to someone" is considered to need one resource. Departments differ regarding whether they regard a professional referral (psychiatrist, social worker, enterostomal therapist, etc.) as a resource. Consideration may reflect availability and the effect on the length-of-stay.

6. **How does the ESI regard pain in the algorithm?**

   The nurse should consider uptriaging the patient to Level 2 if the patient pain rating is >7 in a 0 to 10 scale.

7. **Tell me how the pediatric considerations are incorporated.**

   The pediatric vital sign criterion is included to help determine ESI Level 2 versus ESI Level 3. This includes fever criteria for children younger than 24 months.

8. **Discuss validity and how it related to the ESI.**

   Validity refers to the agreement between the value of a measurement and its true value. A triage scale is valid if it measures what it is supposed to measure, such as who is the sickest patient. ESI has acceptable predictive ability for predicting hospital admission, resource use, physician E & M codes, hospital charges, and 6-month mortality (Kaplan-Meier $\chi^2 = 25.9$; p <0001).

9. Define reliability related to triage scales.

Two types of reliability are relevant to triage sales: interrater and test-retest. Interrater reliability means that two raters (nurses or physicians) will rate a patient's complaint the same way based on the triage system criteria. Test-retest reliability means that the same nurse (or physician) will rate the same scenario the same way on separate occasions.

10. What is the reliability of ESI?

The validity and reliability of ESI version 3 has excellent interrater reliability, good correlation between ESI level and hospitalization rate, and accurately predicts ED resource intensity.

11. The Emergency Nurses Association publishes the ESI. Is this an implicit endorsement that the ESI is the preferred scale?

No, the publishing arrangement was a business decision, and a disclaimer indicating this is posted on the ena.org web site. ENA and the American College of Emergency Physicians (ACEP) passed a policy that supports emergency departments adapting a reliable, valid five-level triage scale. Task Force recommendation is currently that CTAS and ESI are good options.

12. What problems have people identified with the initial implementation?

Often some policy and procedure revision is necessary. Adjustments identified include:

- Requiring some type of tentative mental "diagnosis" to be made to determine the extent of resources needed, or all patients become an ESI Level 3.
- Making the distinction between what the standard practice requires in terms of diagnostic testing versus what a particular physician may uniquely do.
- Needing to standardize some treatment protocols.

13. What can assist with training for ESI?

The *ESI Implementation Handbook* can be purchased from the ENA (www.ena.org). As this book goes to press, there are plans for a training video.

Key Points

- The ESI triage scale is based on an algorithm of acuity and anticipated resource consumption. Version 3 has statistical reliability and validity.
- The ENA/ACEP Five-Level Triage Task Force recommendation adapting a five-level triage acuity system and that CTAS or ESI are good options.
- The ENA publishes the ESI, but has not officially recommended one particular 5-level triage system.

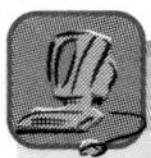

Internet Resources

NurseWeek: On the Level(s)
http://www.nurseweek.com/news/features/04-06/triage.asp

The Emergency Severity Index: ESI Recent Research: A Simulation Modeling Application
http://www.saem.org/meetings/03handouts/eitel.pdf

Pairing Emergency Severity Index 5-Level Triage Data With Computer Aided System Design To Improve Emergency Department Access and Throughput (Proceedings of the 2003 Winter Simulation Conference)
http://www.informs-cs.org/wsc03papers/249.pdf

Integration of the Emergency Severity Index System into an Existing Five-Category Triage System
http://www.ena.org/conferences/annual/2004/handouts/poster414-o.pdf

Bibliography

Eitel D, Travers D, Rosenau A, et al: The Emergency Severity Index Triage Algorithm version 2 is reliable and valid, *Acad Emerg Med* 10:1070-1080, 2003.

Gilboy N, Tanabe P, Travers D, et al: *The Emergency Severity Index implementation handbook, A five-level triage system,* Des Plaines, Ill, 2003, Emergency Nurses Association.

Tanabe P, Gilboy N, et al: Five-level triage: A report from the ACEP/ENA five-level triage task force, *J Emerg Nurs* 31(1):39-50, 2005.

Tanabe P, Gimbel R, Yarnold P, et al: Reliability and validity of scores on the Emergency Severity Index version 3, *Acad Emerg Med* 11(1):59-65, 2004.

Tanabe P, Gimbel R, Yarnold PR, Adams JG: The Emergency Severity Index (version 3) 5-level system scores predict ED resource consumption, *J Emerg Nurs* 30(1):22-29, 2004.

Travers D, Waller A, Bowling J, et al: Five-level triage system more effective than three-level system in tertiary emergency department, *J Emerg Nurs* 28:395-400, 2002.

Travers DA, Waller AE, Bowling JM, Flowers DF: Comparison of 3-level and 5-level triage acuity systems [abstract], *Acad Emerg Med* 7:233, 2000.

Wuerz R: Emergency Severity Index triage category is associated with six-month survival, *Acad Emerg Med* 8:61-64, 2001.

Wuerz RC, Milne LW, Eitel DR, et al: Reliability and validity of a new five-level triage instrument, *Acad Emerg Med* 7:236-242, 2000.

Wuerz RC, Milne L, Eitel D, et al: Outcomes are predicted by a new 5-level triage algorithm, *Acad Emerg Med* 6:398, 1998.

Wuerz R, Milne L, Eitel D, et al: Pilot phase reliability of a new five-level triage algorithm, *Acad Emerg Med* 6:398-399, 1999.

Zimmermann PG: The case for a universal, valid, reliable 5-tier triage acuity scale for U.S. emergency departments, *J Emerg Nurs* 27(3):246-255, 2001.

Chapter 80

Manchester Triage Scale

Janet Marsden and Jill Windle

1. How did "Manchester" triage get its name?

The group that developed, published, and disseminated the Manchester triage system is known as the Manchester Triage Group (MTG). It was formed in 1994 and consisted initially of a senior emergency physician and a senior nurse from each of the seven general emergency departments (EDs) around Manchester (plus a senior physician and senior nurses from the pediatric emergency service and a senior nurse from a specialist ophthalmic emergency service). We both served on this formation group.

2. What made you decide to develop a triage system?

The emergency medicine specialist audit group (EMSAG) in Manchester surveyed triage practices and found a situation aptly described as a "medieval muddle." The MTG was created with the express aim of establishing a consensus for a triage system. The group's aims became:

- Development of common nomenclature
- Development of common definitions
- Development of a robust triage methodology
- Development of a training package
- Development of an audit tool for triage

3. What conclusions did you come to about nomenclature and definitions?

The scale was developed in parallel with work done by the Royal College of Nursing Accident & Emergency Association and the British Association of Emergency Medicine and was adopted nationally in the UK:

Name	Colour	Target time (minutes)
Immediate	Red	0
Very urgent	Orange	10
Urgent	Yellow	60
Standard	Green	120
Nonurgent	Blue	240

4. How is target time defined?

Times had not been assigned in the early stages of the system development, but were added to help reflect the level of priority for each of the categories. The target time was defined as the time to first contact with a treating clinician, which could be either a physician or nurse clinician.

The nonurgent figure has been modified along with changes in government targets relating to ED waits. The goal now is that 100% of patients (exceptions only on clinical need) should be seen and have a disposition (discharged or admitted) from the ED within 240 minutes.

5. What are the key components of the system?

In general terms, a triage method can try to provide the clinician with the diagnosis, with the disposal or with a clinical category. The MTG chose a clinical priority methodology based on three major tenets:

- The aim of the triage encounter is to aid both clinical management and departmental management. This is best achieved by allocation of an accurate clinical priority.
- The length of the triage encounter is such that any attempt to diagnose a patient accurately is doomed to failure.
- The diagnosis is not accurately linked to clinical priority. Priority is determined by the clinical presentation. For instance, a patient's gastroenteritis could be minor or significant with profound dehydration.

6. Describe how clinicians use the Manchester Triage Scale.

Clinicians select from a range of presentation flow charts (organized around the patients presenting complaint rather than particular diagnoses). The triage nurse then assesses a limited number of signs and symptoms at each level of clinical priority. The signs and symptoms, which discriminate between different levels of clinical priority, are known as discriminators. The method is reductive, with the decision-making process identifying the most seriously sick and injured patients very rapidly with minimal patient data required to reach this decision.

7. What do you mean by a reductive method?

Discriminators that indicate higher levels of priority must be sought first and a patient cannot be moved from a high clinical priority until the triage nurse has eliminated the discriminators relating to that priority. The method makes no assumptions about diagnosis. So each patient presenting to the ED is assumed to be in the highest possible category until it is proved that they are not. This is in contrast to much triage work undertaken in the past that suggests that the triage nurse works on a diagnosis-based model, finding signs and symptoms to prove or disprove that diagnosis. Patients may be assumed therefore to be in a low priority unless they or the nurse can prove otherwise.

8. How many presentational flow charts are there and what are they?

At present, there are 50 presentational flow charts (named for patients' presenting complaints) with two extra charts related to dealing with major incidents.

Examples of flow charts include:

Abdominal pain	Limping child
Apparently drunk	Local infections and abscesses
Asthma	Major trauma
Back pain	Mental illness
Behaving strangely	Overdose and poisoning
Collapsed adult	Shortness of breath
Crying baby	Shortness of breath in children
Exposure to chemicals	Unwell child
Eye problems	Unwell adult
Head injury	Worried parent
Headache	Wounds

9. Why these presentations and not others?

Initially it was perceived there would be literally hundreds of presentational flow charts relating to the diverse range of patient problems seen in emergency care. However, 50 are adequate because the system is presentation rather than diagnosis based. This basic principle meant we could take out any mention of diagnosis and rely on what the patients tell us their problem is.

The list of presentations was tested during the development stage with patients. The real test has been on the millions of ED patients that have triaged using Manchester Triage Scale (MTS) since the systems adoption in more than 80% of UK EDs.

10. Have additional presentation charts been added?

The new edition of *Emergency Triage*, due for publication soon, has only two new presentational flow charts (allergy and palpitations); two existing charts, diarrhea and vomiting, were combined into a single chart. Hematologic Disease has been deleted as a result of the infrequency with which the chart is used and Truncal Injury has been renamed Torso Injury to clarify this presentation.

11. What is a discriminator?

Discriminators are factors that discriminate between patients—they allow them to be allocated to one of five clinical priorities. Discriminators are either general or specific. General discriminators apply to all patients/presentation flow charts irrespective and are the foundations of the decision-making process for MTS.

12. List and describe the six general discriminators.

- *Life threat.* Cessation of or threat to vital functions (airway, breathing, circulation) places the patient as an immediate priority. (A closed or insecure airway, stridor, absent or inadequate breathing, an absent pulse or shock always results in red/priority 1.)
- *Pain—from the patients' perspective.* Severe pain places a patient in an orange priority, moderate pain in yellow, and mild pain (any pain) in green.
- *Hemorrhage.* Exsanguinating hemorrhage results in priority 1/red, uncontrollable major hemorrhage in orange and uncontrollable minor hemorrhage in yellow.
- *Conscious level is considered separately in adults and children.* In adults, only currently fitting patients are always categorized as immediate (red), as a result of the threat to airway and breathing, although all unresponsive children are placed in this category. Adults with an altered conscious level are categorized as very urgent (orange) and those with a history of unconsciousness after trauma as urgent (yellow). An altered conscious level as a result of drugs or alcohol is as clinically important as that from any other cause.
- *Temperature—a rapid temperature measurement is available at triage as a result of the development of rapid reading tympanic measures.* A cold patient (temperature less than 89.6°F [32°C]), a hot child (over 101.3°F [38.5°C]) and a very hot adult (over 105.8°F [41°C]) are categorized as orange; a hot adult (over 101.3°F [38.5°C]) as yellow; and any mild pyrexia as green.
- Acuteness is used as it identified the time that a particular problem has been present. A recent illness or injury is defined as one, which has started or become acutely worse within the last 7 days. If the patient has had the condition for longer than this, they may safely be allocated to a nonurgent clinical priority unless they exhibit other discriminators in higher priorities.

13. Why do you feel that pain is so important?

Pain is probably the most common reason that prompts patients to attend the ED. If pain is such a defining symptom for patients, it should surely be as important to clinicians. It is for this reason that pain is a general discriminator and appears in all charts.

Pain should be assessed using a scale that encompasses the patient's perception of the pain, on a score of 0 to 10, along with behavioral indicators.

If the triage nurse asks about pain, the system must be prepared to do something about it. The triage method has acted as a catalyst in many EDs for the development of protocols for pain management at triage.

14. Describe specific discriminators.

Specific discriminators apply to individual presentations or to groups of presentations and tend to relate to key features of particular presentations. For example, in asthma the specific discriminators include no improvement with own medication or in diabetes for which the specific discriminators include capillary glucose and ketones.

15. What will happen if the triage nurse chooses the wrong presentation chart?

All discriminators that are common to more than one chart are placed in the same acuity category on each presentation flow chart. Triage acuity remains the same regardless of the chart chosen. For example, a patient presenting with signs of meningitis may state either headache or neck pain as the primary complaint. Using either of these two charts will result in the same priority.

16. How do you know that everyone is interpreting discriminators in the same way?

A discriminator dictionary is provided. It defines all discriminators and can be referred to at any time in the triage encounter. Notes page are also positioned next to presentational flow charts to allow the triage clinician to consider other charts and to define the specific discriminators.

17. You mention the use of multiple charts to triage a single patient—what do you mean?

There is no one definitive chart for each patient presentation. For example, a patient may be triaged using the "unwell adult" chart, this contains all the general discriminators and in many cases is the quickest and most appropriate route to establish a patient's priority. However, it is also important to use the system dynamically and as further information becomes available, other charts can be used such as diabetes or asthma.

18. Do vulnerable groups (e.g., children, older adults) get a higher priority?

This is one of the most common questions when training clinicians in the triage method. The answer is no because the triage category indicates a clinical priority which enables the case mix of the department to be measured and triage to be audited within and between departments. Changing triage priority because of vulnerability confuses clinical priority with department management.

However, once a particular patient has been triaged and allocated to a category based on clinical need, management decisions may include expediting certain individuals within a triage category. This is however, a management rather than a triage decision.

19. What happens if the patient's condition changes?

With the introduction of MTS, the concept of ED triage changed from an activity that occurred only as the patient arrived to a means of assessing and reassessing patient priority until the patient's ultimate discharge or admission. Any change in the patient's condition necessitates reevaluation of their clinical priority and reallocation of an acuity category. Resolution of pain as a result of effective analgesia at triage may alleviate pain to the extent that the patient's clinical priority reduces.

20. How did you convince people that it was a good idea?

The triage system was originally intended to be used only within the Manchester area so a few emergency units could evaluate their case mix and audit practice to produce consistency. Interest in the system became more widespread even before completion of the method's development. The system's goals convinced others without the MTG having to do anything!

21. How did you implement the system?

A training package was developed. Initially, regional training developed key trainers in all the units interested in implementing the system, who then trained other nurses in their units, and after a period of supervised practice, the unit moved to full implementation of the system.

22. What was the response to the system?

The response to the system was generally very positive both from nurses and emergency physicians. The main resistance seemed to come from the most experienced nurses within emergency settings who had been undertaking triage for many years and felt that this method reduced the need for their expertise. However, the system cannot replace the assessment skills and expert knowledge of emergency nurses. The right questions still need to be asked along with the expertise to interpret the answers gained. Junior nurses appreciated the benefits of a clearly articulated system with a training program.

23. What data are recorded?

The documentation of the triage decision and the allocated priority is very straightforward. All that is required is the name of which presentation chart is used, which discriminator(s) defines the category, and which category has been selected.

For example: head injury (chart), altered conscious level (discriminator), orange or very urgent (category)

Chest pain: pleuritic pain: yellow/urgent

Eye problem: red eye: green/standard

This approach to documentation not only allows for simple audit but also means that the reasons for the decision are overt.

24. What forms of delivery system are available?

A paper (charts and discriminator dictionary as a package in a folder) was developed first and was used very widely. The recognition of the need for a computer-based system to integrate with other ED systems led to the translation of the method into computer software. The computer-based system is now widely used and audits of both methods shows that departments using a computer-based system achieve significantly higher accuracy rates as the computer does not allow the clinician to make idiosyncratic decisions.

25. It sounds as although a nursing assistant could do the MTS.

MTS is designed as an expert system. All parts of the system, the choosing of an appropriate presentation chart, the reductive approach to category allocation, the recognition of discriminators (the resonation of pleuritic as opposed to cardiac pain, the assessment of consciousness, of loss of function, of a purpuric rash for example) still need experience and expertise and the decision-making capabilities that are demonstrated by an experienced emergency nurse. The system guides decision making but is not a protocol and cannot and should not replace the assessment skills required of emergency nurses.

26. Tell me more about audit and data collection.

The simplicity of the recording process (three pieces of data) allows departments to build up profiles of their case mix and allows profiles of particular presentations and diagnoses to be built up within and across EDs. Correlating the triage decision against the patient outcome may highlight system problems. EDs may be benchmarked with other EDs or regional/national benchmarks.

27. How has MTS changed practice?

MTS is accepted as the "gold standard" for triage in the UK. Its use is growing internationally and has been adopted as the national system of triage in Portugal and Holland. The system is widespread in Spain, Ireland, and Sweden and there are units in Australia, Canada, Italy, Germany, and Japan that have adopted MTS.

28. What would be your key points about the MTS?

A multidisciplinary team of expert ED clinicians developed MTS. It is based on the patient's presentation and is risk averse in that the patient is assumed to be at high, rather than low risk on presentation. It has been shown to be reproducible and accurate. System-wise, it provides for patient prioritization and allocation of resources.

Key Points

- The main distinguishing features of the Manchester Triage System are that it is a consensus model developed by a multidisciplinary expert, it is time-saving, and it is based on presentation rather than presumed diagnosis.
- General and specific discriminators within a presentation chart (not diagnosis) determine the triage acuity.
- Patients are assumed to be a high priority until proven otherwise so the system is risk averse.
- Clinical priority should not be confused with departmental management.

Internet Resource

Controversies in Emergency Care: Don't Throw Triage Out With the Bath Water
http://emj.bmjjournals.com/cgi/content/full/20/2/119

Bibliography

Cooke M, Jinks S: Does the Manchester Triage System detect the critically ill? *Accid Emerg Med* 16(3): 179-181, 1999.

Cronin J: The introduction of the Manchester Triage Scale to an emergency department in the Republic of Ireland, *Accid Emerg Nurs* 11(2):121-125, 2003.

Mackway-Jones K (ed): *Emergency triage,* London, 1997, BMJ Publishing.

Speak D, Teece S, Mackway-Jones K: Detecting the high-risk patients with chest pain, *J Emerg Nurs* 11(5):19-21, 2003.

Zimmermann PG: The case for a universal, valid, reliable 5-tier triage acuity scale for U.S. emergency departments, *J Emerg Nurs* 27(3):246-254, 2001.

Chapter 81

Australian Triage Scale: A Five-Tier Triage Emergency Scale

Toni G. McCallum Pardey

1. Give some background history.

Triage in Australia developed around the same time and along the same path as the United States (U.S.) and Canada. Casualty units, as they were then called, were developing their own triage systems guided by the literature and what they observed others to be doing. Documentation was sparse or nonexistent.

With time, the unit's name changed to Accident & Emergency (A&E) department, as designated triage nurses became routine, and documentation improved. Most had a three-tiered triage scale (emergent, urgent, and nonurgent), using either colors or 1 to 3 numbering scales.

2. What was the first version of a five-tier triage system in Australia?

Box Hill A&E Dept. a busy outer suburban Melbourne hospital in Victoria (VIC) modified a three-tier triage scale to a colored five-tier triage scale. There was an unofficial sixth code for patients who were treated as very important persons (VIPs), such as on-duty staff members, visiting officials, or those who were dead on arrival (DOA), whose care would be expedited but not take precedence over those patients requiring resuscitation. Patients were assigned a triage code based on the question, "Under optimal circumstances, this patient should be seen by a medical officer within . . ."

Seconds	Red
Minutes	Yellow
An hour	Green
Hours	Blue
Days	White
VIP	Black (usually added to one of the above colors)

By the late 1970s, the triage system was functioning smoothly and word spread.

3. Describe the role of the Ipswich Triage Scale (ITS).

Dr. Gerry Fitzgerald from Ipswich in Queensland (QLD) studied this system during the 1980s and refined it to the five-tier Ipswich Triage Scale (ITS). Dr. Fitzgerald's results, published in 1989, found the ITS was a valid and reliable measure of medical urgency. Outcome validity was demonstrated by correlation with mortality, admission rate, time spent in an intensive care unit (ICU), and time spent in a hospital. Construct validity was demonstrated by correlation with other severity indices, Trauma Score, Injury Severity Score, Asthma Score, and Cardiac Score. The ITS also related closely to numbers of investigations and operations.

Meanwhile, A&Es became busier, and there was additional interest in methods to quantify (and justify) this increased activity. Dr. George Jelinek's studies further validated the ITS. There was a growing realization that the emergency department (ED) problems would require a system-wide approach rather than "whatever works for us" individualism.

4. Discuss how this evolved into the National Triage Scale.

In the early 1990s, the Australasian College for Emergency Medicine (ACEM) developed a National Triage Scale (NTS) to be used throughout Australia in what were now known as EDs.

Category 1	Immediately	Resuscitation
Category 2	10 minutes	Emergency
Category 3	30 minutes	Urgent
Category 4	1 hour	Semiurgent
Category 5	2 hours	Nonurgent

The NTS was released in 1993 and endorsed for use in 1994 as the uniform professional standard for triage in Australia with the aim of standardizing ED triage. State, territory, and commonwealth departments of health and the Australian Council on Healthcare Standards (ACHS) quickly sanctioned it.

5. Indicate the advantages of this standardized five-tier system, NTS.

EDs quickly adapted the new NTS because it:

- Focuses on the patient
- Acknowledges the varying complexities and acuities of the patient population
- Identifies those patients in greatest need for care
- Allows for the irregularities of the ED workload

It became significant in use as a classification system and in ED management (staffing, rostering, training, and other resources).

During the mid-1990s Canada (Canadian Triage and Acuity Scale, CTAS) and the United Kingdom (Manchester Triage) adapted the NTS to local circumstances and introduced their own versions of the five-tier triage scale (see Chapters 78, 79, 80, and 82).

6. What were the problems when the NTS was implemented?

- Lack of education
- Difficulty of pediatric and mental health application
- Defining "waiting time"

- Concept of "doctor seen time"
- Irrelevance in rural settings
- Individualization (idiosyncrasies) in application

These problems should all eventually be overcome with the implementation of the Australasian Triage Scale (ATS) and the national training minimum standard for triage.

7. Talk about the problem of the lack of triage education.

There was a preexisting wide variation between hospitals in Australia in their training and experience requirements for registered nurses to triage.

- Prerequisite experience ranged from 1 month to 2 years ED experience with an average of 12 to 18 months.
- Mandatory triage educational activities ranged from none to a formal regionally based course. (The most common were self-directed learning packages.)
- Initial mentoring of beginning triage nurses ranged from 0 to 15 shifts, most common only 2 shifts.

In this environment, problems are understandable because the NTS had no accompanying training packet.

8. Explain what is meant by difficulty in defining waiting time.

There was initial confusion regarding exactly when the clock starts to measure waiting time. Was it on the patient's arrival? At the commencement of triage? At the completion of triage?

The only true indictor of waiting time was clarified as the one that measures the entire waiting period, which is from the time of the patient's arrival to the "clinician seen time" (e.g., physician or clinician). This would be equivalent to the time of the medical screening exam (MSE) in the United States.

9. I don't understand the confusion about the "doctor seen time" term.

Compliance with triage category thresholds or benchmarks was measured from time of arrival to "doctor seen time." However, not all Australian ED patients see a physician; some see other advanced clinicians. The term was changed to "clinician seen time."

10. Elaborate on the relevance in the rural setting.

The NTS was initially intended for use in EDs with 24-hour on-site medical personnel, which some rural and remote hospitals do not have. This created major compliance issues with the times. A separate rural triage scale was proposed, but it was decided that a single scale applicable to all settings was preferable.

11. Discuss the issue of individualization (idiosyncrasies) in application.

There were acceptable degrees of interrater reliability from simulated occasions of triage using the NTS system. In the "real world," however, many different individual interpretations were imposed on the application of the NTS by institutions, particularly for the pediatric and mental health patients. Some examples of the variations included:

- All children will automatically be upgraded one triage category
- All children will be triaged to category 3 or above
- All trauma team activations are automatically triage category 1
- All chest pain will be a category 2

Individual triage nurses also applied personal interpretations or "bending" of the system on top of these "cookbook" rules that contributed to:

- Changing the initial triage category when failing to meet benchmark
- Undertriaging so that waiting time by triage category statistics have greater compliance during busy periods
- Overtriaging so that the ED looks busier
- Making no patients a category 5 because they have such a significant delay in being seen

12. What is the ATS?

A comprehensive review of the NTS was undertaken and modifications resulted in the release of the ATS in 2001.

ATS Categories, Descriptions, Maximum Waiting Times, and Thresholds*†

ATS Category	Description of Category	Treatment Acuity (Maximum Waiting Time)	Performance Indicator Threshold
1	Immediately life-threatening	Immediate	100%
2	Imminently life-threatening	10 minutes	80%
3	Potentially life-threatening	30 minutes	75%
4	Potentially serious	60 minutes	70%
5	Less urgent	120 minutes	70%

*Adapted from ACEM Policy Document—The Australian Triage Scale and ACEM. Guidelines for Implementation of the Australian Triage Scale in Emergency Departments.

†Widespread improvements in the application of the five-tier triage scale have yet to be assessed and published although a study has reported improved outcomes in mental health patients.

13. How does the ATS handle waiting patient reassessment?

The ATS does not address reassessment of waiting room patients. Most EDs have a policy that the triage nurse is responsible for reassessing the waiting room patients, but they are mostly generic in nature and unworkable in reality. As the EDs became busier, the triage nurse has less time available to reassess waiting patients, yet these are the times when reassessment is needed most.

During 2003, the NSW Health Department introduced a new position of clinical initiatives nurse (CIN) into some of the busier emergency departments. The CIN is responsible for the initiation of investigations and treatment and the reassessment of waiting patients.

14. What is the national minimal standard for triage education?

During the revision of the NTS in 2000 it was acknowledged that the lack of a nationally consistent education program coinciding with the release of the NTS was the major contributing factor to the various interpretations and inconsistencies in its application. The Commonwealth Department of Health and Ageing (DoHA) funded developing a national Triage Education Resource Book (TERB), which was released in 2002. The DoHA also funded workshops in each state to assist educators in the application of the TERB. Feedback has been actively sought from the users of the TERB and a major evaluation and revision was conducted during 2004.

15. How is triage documented?

Triage documentation is widely computerized utilizing a stand-alone product known as EDIS (developed by HAS Solutions, now sold by iSOFT). This computer software was initially developed in 1993 and is used throughout Australia. EDIS is now used in some United Kingdom and Canadian EDs.

A focused triage assessment is attended on each patient on arrival and documented in free text format. The ATS code 1 through 5 is entered and any relevant vital signs and the triage form is printed. Smaller noncomputerized rural EDs document in longhand on preprinted forms.

16. How does the ATS affect the Nurses Registration Acts provisions?

There are no laws in Australia or regulations/provisions in the Nurses Registration Acts that specifically apply to triage. Australia does not have anything similar to the United States' Emergency Medical Treatment and Active Labor Act (EMTALA) or Health Insurance Portable Accountability Act (HIPAA) regulations. There is no required MSE for all patients.

17. Relate this to Joint Commission on Accreditation of Healthcare Organizations accreditation.

The Australian Council on Healthcare Standards (ACHS) is an independent, not-for-profit organization responsible for accrediting health care facilities in Australia. The ACHS provides the means for independent evaluation of health care services and encourages and assists health care organizations to continuously improve the quality of their services. It has a similar function to the Joint Commission on Accreditation of Healthcare Organizations (JCAHO) although it is not as prescriptive. The ACHS has embraced the quality benchmarks set by the ATS and look at these figures when assessing hospitals to see how individual hospitals respond to their results.

18. How does the ATS affect managed care?

There is no managed care in Australia.

19. Do you have a "triaging out" option, e.g., deferring the care to another source?

General practitioners (GPs) or EDs provide emergency health care in Australia. The exception is in remote areas in which there are no permanent GPs and "remote area nurses" provide the care there. For the majority of the population there is no alternative to EDs for after-hour care. A recent development in 2004 has seen a federal announcement of the implementation of co-located GP After-Hour Surgeries into hospitals so the practice of triaging out of the ED will become routine.

20. How does mass casualty triage (disaster triage) integrate with the ATS?

A Draft Australian Standard for Multiple Casualty Triage has been prepared under the responsibility of Standards Australia Committee HE-026, Hospital Emergency Procedures to address the lack of uniformity in the existing triage tagging systems across Australia. The draft standard is evidence based and is intended to replace all other mass casualty triage systems currently in use or being taught within Australia. How this proposed standard integrates with the ATS on the arrival of victims of mass casualties is yet to be seen.

Key Point

- Developers of the ATS emphasize the need for ED staff training in order for any triage system to succeed.

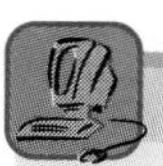

Internet Resource

New South Wales Health: Summary of Performance Data
http://www.health.nsw.gov.au/hospitalinfo/perfsumm.html

Bibliography

Australasian College for Emergency Medicine (ACEM): *Policy document—The Australasian triage scale,* 2000; available: www.acem.org.au/open/documents/triage; accessed March 4, 2004.

Australasian College for Emergency Medicine (ACEM): *Guidelines for implementation of the Australasian triage scale in emergency departments,* 2000; available: www.acem.org.au/open/documents/triageguide, accessed March 4, 2004.

Brentnall EW: A history of triage in civilian hospitals in Australia, *Emerg Med* 9:50-54, 1997.

Broadbent M, Jarman H, Berk M: Emergency department mental health triage scales improve outcomes, *J Eval Clin Pract* 10(1):57-62, 2004.

Commonwealth Department of Health and Ageing: *Triage education resource book,* Canberra, 2002, Commonwealth Department of Health and Ageing.

Fatovich DM, Jacobs IG: NTS versus waiting time: An indicator without definition, *Emerg Med* 13:47-50, 2001.

Jelinek GA, Little M: Inter-rater reliability of the Nation Triage Scale over 11,500 simulated occasions of triage, *Emerg Med* 8:226-230, 1996.

Kelly AM, Richardson D: Training for the role of triage in Australasia, *Emerg Med* 13:230-232, 2001.

Nocera A, Garner A: An Australian mass casualty incident triage system for the future based upon triage mistakes of the past: The Homebush Triage Standard, *Austr NZ J Surg* 69(8):603-608, 1999.

Standen P, Dilley SJ: A review of triage nursing practice and experience in Victorian public hospitals, *Emerg Med* 9:301-305, 1997.

Chapter 82

Canada Triage and Acuity Scale

Polly Gerber Zimmermann

1. What is the history of the Canada Triage and Acuity Scale development?

In 1995, a group of Canadian emergency department (ED) physicians at Saint John Regional Hospital (in New Brunswick) developed the Canada Triage and Acuity Scale (CTAS), based on Australia's National Triage Scale (NTS). Its use became official policy in Canada in 1997 by the Canadian Institute of Health Information (CIHI). The system is endorsed by the Canadian Association of Emergency Physicians (CAEP) and the National Emergency Nurses Affiliation of Canada (NENA).

2. What was the purpose of establishing this system?

The CTAS implementation guide indicates it is an attempt to accurately define patients' needs for timely care and allow the EDs to evaluate their acuity level, resource needs, and performance.

3. Describe the CTAS.

The CTAS is based on establishing a relationship between a group of sentinel events and the "usual" way patients with these conditions present. It includes the use of key objective data to help validate and assess the chief complaint when tiering common presentations into an appropriate triage category. The list of clinical descriptors for each level includes:

- High-risk historical factors (e.g., envenomation, toxic ingestion)
- Symptoms (e.g., abdominal pain)
- Signs (e.g., stridor, deformity, amputation, acute hemiparesis)
- Physiologic parameters (e.g., blood pressure)
- Point of-care testing (e.g., glucose, pulse oximetry)
- Nursing assessment/diagnosis (e.g., dehydration, tight cast)

Age-specific parameters and educational implementation material with tips are also included.

4. Give an example of these distinguishers applied to a common presentation.

For respiratory distress:

Level 1	Unable to speak, cyanosis, lethargic, tachycardia/bradycardia, Po_2 <90%
Level 2	Severe asthma, peek expiratory flow rate (PEFR) <40% predicted or previous best; dyspnea
Level 3	Mild/moderate asthma; frequent cough; night awakening; PEFR 40%-60% previous best and Po_2 ≤92%–94%; moderate dyspnea; shortness of breath (SOB) with exertion
Level 4	Upper respiratory illness (URI) signs/symptoms (s/s); Po_2 ≥95%
Level 5	URI; sore throat with normal vital signs

5. What is the goal time from patient presentation until nursing triage?

All patients should be at least visually assessed within 10 minutes of arrival (a primary survey or rapid assessment). It should not take more than 2 minutes and only gather enough data to assign a triage category. When there are two or more patients waiting for triage, a more detailed, thorough "primary nursing assessment" is performed later. Level 1 and Level 2 patients are sent directly to the area.

6. How are the levels of the CTAS defined?

- *Resuscitation:* Conditions that are threats to life or limb (or imminent risk of deterioration) requiring immediate aggressive interventions.
- *Emergent:* Conditions that are a potential threat to life, limb, or function, requiring rapid medical intervention or delegated acts.
- *Urgent:* Conditions that could potentially progress to a serious problem requiring emergency intervention. May be associated with significant discomfort or affecting ability to function at work or activities of daily living.
- *Less Urgent*: Conditions that related to patient age, distress, or potential for deterioration or complications would benefit from intervention or reassurance within 1 to 2 hours.
- *Nonurgent:* Conditions that may be acute but nonurgent, and conditions that may be part of a chronic problem with or without evidence of deterioration. The investigation or interventions for some of these illnesses or injuries could be delayed or even referred to other areas of the hospital or health care system.

7. What is the goal time from patient presentation until physician assessment?

Level 1	Immediate
Level 2	15 minutes
Level 3	30 minutes
Level 4	60 minutes
Level 5	120 minutes

8. Are these times absolutes?

No. The CTAS implementation guide indicates they are "ideals (objectives)" and not established care standards. In practice, the patient is usually not informed of the time associated with each triage level. In addition, the times may alter with a physician review of the chart and a verbal order for diagnostic tests or interventions to begin.

9. What are the times recommended for nursing reassessment?

Reassessments should occur until the patient is stabilized or a medical diagnosis is made. Then the frequency of nursing assessment and care depends on existing care protocols or physician orders. The recommended reassessment times are:

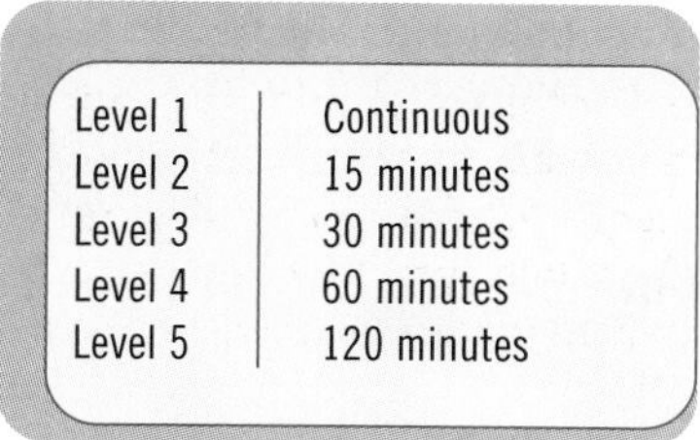

Level 1	Continuous
Level 2	15 minutes
Level 3	30 minutes
Level 4	60 minutes
Level 5	120 minutes

10. What is fractile response rate?

The CTAS defines it as "the proportion of patient visits for a given triage level in which the patients were seen within the CTAS time frame defined for that level." It does not deal with whether the absolute delay for an individual is reasonable or acceptable. They are:

Level 1	Resuscitation	98%
Level 2	Emergent	95%
Level 3	Urgent	90%
Level 4	Less Urgent	85%
Level 5	Nonurgent	80%

11. Does the system allow for a triage nurse to use his or her expertise in making the triage-level decision?

The triage assignment is based on the "usual presentation" and other objective data (vital signs, pulse oximetry, etc.). In addition there are the tiering distinguishers.

When they perceive a need, triage nurses are encouraged to use their intuition, experience, and instincts to "triage up" someone who does not fit the facts or definitions on the triage scale. The rule of thumb is "If they look sick, then they probably are." It is also suggested that it is reasonable to upgrade the triage level if the time response ideal/objective has not been met.

The triage nurse is not to use individual perception to "triage down" someone whose presentation fits a category. For instance, if the person describes visceral chest pains with vital signs changes, the nurse should not decide it is costochondritis or anxiety and give a lower triage level.

12. So triage categories can change?

Triage is a dynamic process and the category can change to reflect the patient's condition improving or deteriorating during the wait. There can also be managerial decisions to move a patient's priority. However, the initial triage level always stays, and documentation of any changes, for administrative purposes.

13. What are the CTAS admissions rates by triage level?

Level 1	Resuscitation	70% to 90%
Level 2	Emergent	40% to 70%
Level 3	Urgent	20% to 40%
Level 4	Less Urgent	10% to 20%
Level 5	Nonurgent	0% to 10%

14. What are the disadvantages of this system?

Obtaining the necessary historical details for an accurate presumptive diagnosis can be time consuming. In addition, the process (and triage decision) is hindered if the patient is a poor historian, has multiple complaints, or has a language problem.

15. Does the system have reliability?

Yes. Manos (2002) found interrater reliability in first time users (kappa 0.77) and Beveridge (1999) had interrater reliability of (0.80). Worster (2004) compared the interrater reliability of the Emergency Severity Index (ESI) and CTAS and found no difference. The CTAS and ESI have the highest reported reliability consistent from study to study.

16. What about the pediatric component?

The CTAS has recently published pediatric triage criteria based on expert consensus, i.e., it has face validity. It, as well as the other five-level scales, has not been scientifically evaluated for use in the pediatric population.

17. What is the position of the Emergency Nurses Association regarding the CTAS?

Based on expert consensus on currently available evidence, both the American College of Emergency Physicians (ACEP) and the Emergency Nurses Association (ENA) support the adoption of a reliable, valid five-level triage scale. The joint task force indicated that either the CTAS or the ESI are good options.

18. How is training handled for CTAS?

CTAS training was originally developed as a 1-day workshop, offered periodically at various sites. To improve access and to standardize CTAS training, a web-based course is now offered five times a year. Content included information (as text and graphics), course modules, interactive case studies, an online discussion area, an online tutorial, and a workplace project. To complete the course, nurses typically took 6 weeks for about 4 hours a week. Web-based pediatric CTAS course and CTAS refresher course are being developed.

19. How can I obtain a copy of the CTAS implementation guidelines?

Order from the CAEP, 1785 Alta Vista Drive, Suite 104, Ottawa, Canada ON K1G 3Y6; phone 613-523-3343 or 800-463-1158; guidelines@caep.ca.

Key Points

- The CTAS is based on sentinel events and the usual presentation, providing objective data to help validate and assess the condition when establishing a triage level.
- Clinical descriptors include high-risk historical factors, signs, symptoms, physiologic parameters, point-of-care testing, and nursing assessment/diagnosis.
- The CTAS has acceptable statistical reliability. The ACEP/ENA task force indicates that the CTAS is a good option for a valid five-level triage scale.

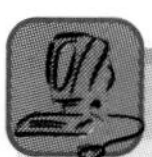

Internet Resource

Canadian Association of Emergency Physicians
www.caep.ca

Bibliography

Atack L, McLean D, LeBlanc L, Luke R: Preparing ED nurses to use the Canadian Triage and Acuity Scale with web-based learning, *J Emerg Nurs* 30(3):273-274, 2004.

Beveridge R, Ducharme J, Janes L, et al: Reliability of the Canadian ED Triage and Acuity Scale: Inter-rater agreement, *Ann Emerg Med* 34:155-159, 1999.

Beveridge R: The Canadian Triage and Acuity Scale: A new and critical element in health care reform, *J Emerg Med* 16:507-511, 1998.

Canadian Emergency Physicians: Canadian Emergency Department Triage and Acuity Scale (CTAS) implementation guidelines, *Can Emerg Med J* 1(3 suppl), 1999.

Jelinek G: Canadian Triage and Assessment Scale, *Can Emerg Med J* 8:229-230, 1996.

Manos B, Petrie D, Beveridge R, et al: Inter-observer agreement using the Canadian Emergency Department Triage Scale, *Can J Emerg Med* 4:16-22, 2002.

Tanabe P, Gilboy N: Five-level triage: A report from the ACEP/ENA Five-Level Triage Task Force, *J Emerg Nurs* 31(1):39-50, 2005.

Worster A, Gilboy N, Fernandex CM, et al: Assessment of inter-observer reliability of two five-level triage scales: A randomized controlled trial, *Can J Emerg Med* 6(4):240-245, 2004.

Zimmermann PG: The case for a universal, valid, reliable 5-tier triage acuity scale for U.S. emergency departments, *J Emerg Nurs* 27(3):246-254, 2001.

Chapter 83

Process of Changing an Emergency Department from a Three-Level to a Five-Level System

Rebecca S. McNair

1. How do we know if we should change from a three-level to a five-level triage system?

Evaluate the effectiveness of the present system you are using. Consider (McNair, 2004):

- *Mistriage.* Do chart reviews. Is there significant evidence of mistriage (inappropriate acuity assigned), which may also be evidenced by inappropriate dispositions?
- *Sentinel Events.* Does risk management have documented sentinel events that occur either during the triage process or result from the triage decisions? Joint Commission on Accreditation of Healthcare Organizations (JCAHO) reported in a Sentinel Event Alert (2002) that emergency departments (EDs) were a source of more than half of all hospital-reported sentinel event cases that resulted in disability or death because of delays in treatment. In 31% of the cases, overcrowding was identified as a key factor.
- *Continuous retriage.* Do ED staff frequently change acuity rating from the initial decision?

2. Why should our ED have a Five-Level Triage Acuity Scale?

Five-level acuity systems show stronger interrater reliability and validity (Travers, 2000). They are able to more clearly evaluate patient acuity level and resource needs and performance.

3. Will changing to a five-level acuity system solve all our problems?

The triage acuity scale is not a cure-all. Nurse-led triage is a complex system involving many aspects beyond assigning an acuity level. Ensure every triage nurse receives education regarding all of the key aspects of managing triage in a systematic approach. In my consulting work, I find *most* problems associated with a consistent triage performance as a result of a lack of education.

4. List other aspects in the triage process besides the decision regarding the acuity level.

The aspects include, but are not limited to, (McNair, 2004):

- Physical plant
- Documentation tools
- Acuity category systems
- Clinical expertise
- Systematic decision-making skills
- Hospital and federal mandates
- Collaboratively derived protocols
- Violence prevention and de-escalation training
- Customer service
- Pain management
- Interpersonal violence screening
- ED Triage concepts and process education
- Effective patient throughput (chart management, appropriate disposition, patient tracking, outcomes measurement, bed management, communication technology)

5. What is the preparation and planning needed for implementing a five-level acuity scale?

Create an implementation team composed of nurses and/or physicians who

- Are thoroughly familiar with and committed to the chosen acuity system
- Show excellent triage and leadership skills
- Have a command of the triage and patient throughput process
- Are available to educate, precept, and evaluate
- Have full administrative support

Review the policies and procedures regarding what will be impacted by the change in triage.

6. What are the steps to changing to a five-level acuity system?

There are six steps that must be accomplished if you are to expect success.

- Know the limitations of any acuity category scale and its impact on the triage process.
- Educate yourself and everyone that the move to a five-level triage acuity category scale is the correct thing to do.
- Decide which five-level scale is the most appropriate for your facility and community.
- Complete preparation and planning work needed.
- Create an implementation team and review policies and procedures.
- Educate, educate, educate.

7. Staff in our department are resistant to change. What will help them adapt this change?

- Include the staff in the implementation; keep them informed and solicit their input.

- Explore staff's reasons for their resistance to change. Common concerns include:
  - The new system will force more work on them
  - The new five levels will be too difficult to remember
  - They will make mistakes
- Identify a few (no more than three) staff registered nurses (RNs) who are respected by their peers and who support the change (or are the least resistant). Select these individuals carefully—they can make or break your change. These RNs are the "gatekeepers" because they will provide an opening or pathway from management to staff for implementation.

8. Describe how having some staff as "gatekeepers" can help.

These individuals are trusted by the staff because they are "one of us." Their message about the change have a lot of credibility. These "gatekeeper" nurses will help facilitate the change by:

- Promoting the change among peers.
- Keeping their "fingers on the pulse of change" within the ED.
- Helping plan and implement the training process.

9. Discuss what education and training should include.

Adequate learning opportunities are essential so no one feels unprepared.

- Point out the similarities between the old way and the new way. Many aspects of triage do remain the same regardless of the triage-acuity level system.
- Explain the rationale for the change. Cite "higher authorities," such as the American College of Emergency Physicians (ACEP)/Emergency Nurses Association (ENA) work group. Five-level triage *is* becoming the professional standard that a nurse will eventually answer to in court.
- Include role-playing and case studies to teach the new system.
- Consider an arrangement for your staff to shadow triage nurses in another ED in which the change has been successfully implemented.
- Consider "renting" a nurse from another ED in which the 5-level system has been successfully implemented to precept your staff during early implementation.

10. What should a training program include?

Training programs need to include:

- Pretest
- Background information on the need for change
- Method of communicating changes
- Description of system
- Clarification of discriminators
- Practice cases
- Posttest

11. What are the necessary elements of the education format?

The initial information should be standardized, quick, and easy to learn with didactic and clinical components. In my consulting, I recommend a formal education for the initial change and implementation to set a standard, help ensure quality, and establish expectations. Lack of formal education was cited as a problem during the adaptation of standardized scales in other countries.

12. After the education, how do we ensure compliance and proper use?

Necessary components to include both during the educational process and as an ongoing resource and review. These include:

- Practice cases or simulations facilitated by expert triage nurses and educators
- Related policies distributed in packets
- Posters placed in clinical areas
- Pocket guides to triage categorization
- Chart review
- Direct observation of triage practice

13. How can I motivate the staff to embrace this new system?

- Relate it to improved patient care. Provide statistical evidence of the previous three-level or four-level inadequacies, stressing the desire to be grounded in evidence-based practice.
- Provide example from your own department of the difference between how a three-level and a five-level system would handle the same patient or where undertriage occurred. (If there are no examples of mistriage in your department, maybe a change isn't needed.)
- Share other emergency departments' successes with adapting five-level triage. Invite an ED staff nurse from a hospital in which the system has been successfully implement to meet with your staff to discuss the changes, including the "growing pains."

14. What will help in the transition phase?

- Be aware that initial venting and "overreacting" can occur. Give it time, but set boundaries. For example, accept griping at a staff meeting but not in front of patients.
- Anticipate more difficulties the beginning weeks and deal with it as soon as possible.
- Assign one nurse who is knowledgeable about the five-tier system to be a support person or "troubleshooter" for the first week or so during implementation.
- Consider assigning an extra nurse to triage during the transition because the triage time might initially be longer during the phase-in.
- Take the attitude that now, after preparation and this initial implementation, the change is required. It is the "way we do things here."

15. List criteria to determine that the implementation has been completed effectively.

Some type of quality assurance tool can be developed or purchased. Methods can include:

- Perform random chart audits/direct observation on various nurses and shifts. Have a threshold of correct application (usually 90% or more).
- Track the indicators that were the impetus for the change, such as mistriages noted in chart reviews, sentinel events, or retriaging.
- Track indicators that reflect the effect on patient flow. Has the left without being seen (LWBS) and against medical advice (AMA) statistics changed?
- Anecdotally, is the terminology and application now used frequently and/or automatically within staff communication? Do you sense staff has "moved on" to other issues?

Key Points

- Most mistriage occurs as a result of lack of education, inexperience, and empathy burnout.
- Consider any five-level triage system's statistical reliability and validity before adaptation.
- Consider whether the triage process is easily understood, rapidly applied, has high rates of interobserver agreement, facilitates appropriate placement, and predicts clinic outcomes.
- Gaining staff buy-in to the proposed change in triage systems is essential to the success of the change. Address staff's concerns early in the process of change.

Internet Resources

American College of Emergency Physicians: The Dynamics of Organizational Change
http://www.acep.org/1,33908,0.html

Triage First
http://www.triagefirst.com

Soterian Rapid Triage System
www.soterionrts.com

Emergency Nurses Association
www.ena.org

On the Level in Nurseweek.com
http://www.nurseweek.com/news/features/04-06/triage.asp

Emergency Nursing World!
www.enw.org

Bibliography

Australasian College for Emergency Medicine: *Guidelines for implementation of the Australasian triage scale in emergency departments,* 2000; available: http://www.acem.org.au/open/documents/triageguide.htm, accessed April 14, 2005.

Australasian College for Emergency Medicine: *The National Triage Scale: A user manual,* Australia, 1997, Author.

Beveridge RC, Ducharme J, Janes L, Beauliu S, Walter S: Reliability of the Canadian ED Triage & Acuity Scale: Inter-rater agreement, *Ann Emerg Med* 34:155-159, 1999.

Beveridge R, Clarke B, Janes L, et al: Implementation guidelines for the Canadian Emergency Department Triage & Acuity Scale (CTAS), *Can J Emerg Med* 1(3 suppl), 1999.

Gill JM, Reese CL, Diamond JL: Disagreement among health-care professionals about the urgent needs of emergency department patients, *Ann Emerg Med* 28:474-478, 1996.

Glower MM: Managing change. In Zimmerman PG, editor: *Zimmerman's nursing management secrets,* Philadelphia, 2002, Hanley & Belfus.

MacLean S: ENA national benchmark guide: Emergency departments, Des Plaines, Ill, 2002, Emergency Nurses Association.

McNair R (President): Acuity categorization. In *The nature of the beast: Comprehensive triage and patient flow workshop,* Fairview, NC, 2003, Triage First, Inc.

McNair R (President): Use of a five-acuity scale. In *The nature of the beast: Comprehensive triage and patient flow workshop,* Fairview, NC, 2003, Triage First, Inc.

McNair R (President): Acuity lab and debate. In *The nature of the beast: Comprehensive triage and patient flow workshop,* Fairview, NC, 2003, Triage First, Inc.

McNair R (President): Implementing a five-acuity category scale (lecture). In *The nature of the beast: Comprehensive triage and patient flow workshop,* Fairview, NC, 2003, Triage First, Inc.

McNair R (President): Determining acuity and establishing standards of practice. In *TRIAGE First EDucation: A comprehensive emergency department triage course,* Fairview, NC, 2004, TRIAGE First EDucation, Inc.

McNair R (President): Acuity lab and debate. In *TRIAGE First Education: A comprehensive emergency department triage course,* Fairview, NC, 2004, TRIAGE First EDucation, Inc.

McNair R (President): Implementing a five-acuity category scale (lecture). In *TRIAGE First Education: A comprehensive emergency department triage course,* Fairview, NC, 2004, TRIAGE First EDucation, Inc.

National Triage Task Force: Canadian pediatric triage and acuity scale: Implementation guidelines for emergency departments, *Can J Emerg Med* 3(4):S1-S27, 2001.

SRPC-ER Working Group: Canadian Emergency Department Triage and Acuity Scale (CTAS): Rural implementation statement, *Can J Rural Med* 7(4):271-274, 2002.

Tanabe P, Gilboy N, et al: Five-level triage: A report from the ACEP/ENA Five-Level Triage Task Force, *J Emerg Nurs* 31(1):39-50, 2005.

Travers DA, Waller AE, Bowling JM, et al: Comparison of 3-level and 5-level triage acuity systems (abstract), *Acad Emerg Med* 7(5):522, 2000.

Wuerz RC, Fernades CMB, Alarcon J: Inconsistency of emergency department triage, *Ann Emerg Med* 32:431-435, 1998.

Zimmermann PG: The case for a universal, valid, reliable 5-tier triage acuity scale for U.S. emergency departments, *J Emerg Nurs* 27(3):246-254, 2001.

Index

Page numbers followed by t indicate tables; b, boxes.

B

C

F

G

I

M

N

O

P

Q

R

S

T

W

X

Z